FECAL
&
URINARY
DIVERSIONS

MANAGEMENT PRINCIPLES

FECAL & URINARY DIVERSIONS

MANAGEMENT PRINCIPLES

JANICE C. COLWELL, RN, MS, CWOCN
Clinical Nurse Specialist
University of Chicago Hospitals
Chicago, Illinois

MARGARET T. GOLDBERG, RN, MSN, CWOCN
Delray Wound Treatment Center
Delray Beach, Florida

JANE E. CARMEL, RN, MSN, CWOCN
Program Co-Director
Wound Ostomy Continence
Nursing Educational Program
Wicks Educational Associates, Inc.
Mechanicsburg, Pennsylvania

*With **95** illustrations*
*Including **25** color plates*

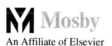

An Affiliate of Elsevier

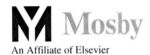
Mosby

An Affiliate of Elsevier

11830 Westline Industrial Drive
St. Louis, Missouri 63146

NOTICE

Medical Assisting is an ever-changing field. Standard safety precautions must be followed, but as new research and clinical experience broaden our knowledge, changes in treatment and drug therapy may become necessary or appropriate. Readers are advised to check the most current product information provided by the manufacturer of each drug to be administered to verify the recommended dose, the method and duration of administration, and contraindications. It is the responsibility of the treating physician, relying on experience and knowledge of the patient, to determine dosages and the best treatment for each individual patient. Neither the Publisher nor the author assume any liability for any injury and/or damage to persons or property arising from this publication.

The Publisher

International Standard Book Number 0-323-02248-0

Executive Publisher: Darlene Como
Developmental Editor: Laura M. Selkirk
Publishing Services Manager: Deborah Vogel
Senior Project Manager: Mary Drone
Book Design Manager: Gail Morey Hudson

Transferred to Digital Printing in 2009

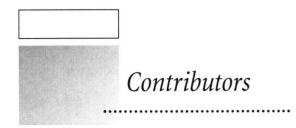

Contributors

JANICE M. BEITZ, PhD, RN, CS, CNOR, CWOCN
Associate Professor, Director of Certificate and
    Distributive Learning Programs
La Salle University, School of Nursing
Philadelphia, Pennsylvania

JANICE BESCHORNER, RN, MS, AOCN
Oncology Clinical Nurse Specialist
University of Chicago Hospitals
Chicago, Illinois

JOY BOARINI, RN, MSN, WOCN
Manager, Clinical Education and Professional Services
Hollister, Inc.
Libertyville, Illinois

RUTH A. BRYANT, RN, MS, CWOCN
Director, Web WOC Nursing Education Program
Partner, Bryant Rolstad Consultants, LLC
Minneapolis, Minnesota

VICTOR CRENTSIL, MD
Fellow, University of Chicago
Chicago, Illinois

DAVID C. CRONIN, II, MD, PhD, FACS
Assistant Professor of Surgery
University of Chicago
Chicago, Illinois

GILBERT J. CUSSON, RPh, BCNSP
Clinical Specialist Nutrition Support,
    Department of Pharmaceutical Services
University of Chicago Hospitals
Chicago, Illinois

DOROTHY DOUGHTY, MN, RN, CWOCN, FAAN
Director, Wound Ostomy Continence Nursing
    Education Center
Emory University
Atlanta, Georgia

VICTOR W. FAZIO, MD, BS, MS, FRACS, FACS, FRCS
Rupert Turnbull Chairman and Professor
Department of Colorectal Surgery
The Cleveland Clinic Foundation
Cleveland, Ohio

CRINA V. FLORUTA, RN, MSN, ANP, CWOCN
Nurse Practitioner
The Cleveland Clinic Foundation
Cleveland, Ohio

BEVERLY FOLKEDAHL, BSN, RN, COCN, CWCN
Advanced Practice Nurse
University of Iowa Hospitals and Clinics
Iowa City, Iowa

PHILIP H. GORDON, MD, FRCS(C), FACS
Professor of Surgery and Oncology—McGill University
Director of Colorectal Surgery—SMBD-JGH and
    McGill University
Montreal, Quebec

MIKEL GRAY, PhD, CUNP, CCCN, FAAN
Professor and Nurse Practitioner
Department of Urology and School of Nursing
University of Virginia
Charlottesville, Virginia

STEPHEN B. HANAUER, MD
Professor of Medical and Clinical Pharmacology
Director of Section Gastroenterology and Nutrition
University of Chicago
Chicago, Illinois

BETH HARRISON, RN, MSN, CWOCN
Nurse Consultant-ET
Children's Hospital Los Angeles
Los Angeles, California

BARBARA J. HOCEVAR, BSN, RN, ET, CWOCN
Manager, Enterostomal Therapy Nursing
The Cleveland Clinic Foundation
Cleveland, Ohio

TRACY L. HULL, MD
Staff Surgeon, Department of Colon and Rectal Surgery
The Cleveland Clinic Foundation
Cleveland, Ohio

DORTHE HJORT JAKOBSEN, RN
Research Nurse
Hvidovre University Hospital
DK-2650 Hvidovre, Denmark

ALAINE KAMM, RN, MSN, ACNP
Acute Care Nurse Practitioner, Department of Surgery
University of Chicago Hospitals
Chicago, Illinois

HENRIK KEHLET, MD
Professor, Department of Surgical Gastroenterology
Hvidovre University Hospital
DK-2650 Hvidovre, Denmark

CONNIE KELLY, RN, MS, CWOCN
Advanced Practitioner, Ostomy and Wound Care
Northwestern Memorial Hospital
Chicago, Illinois

RAVI P. KIRAN, MBBS, MS, FRCS
Research Fellow, Department of Colorectal Surgery
The Cleveland Clinic Foundation
Cleveland, Ohio

JUDITH LANDIS-ERDMAN, BSN, RN, ET, CWOCN
Enterostomal Therapy Nurse
The Cleveland Clinic Foundation
Cleveland, Ohio

ROBERT MADOFF, MD
Adjunct Professor
University of Minnesota
Minneapolis, Minnesota

PETER W. MARCELLO, MD
Staff Surgeon, Department of Colon and Rectal Surgery
Lahey Clinic
Burlington, Massachusetts

DAVID E. McGINNIS, MD
Clinical Assistant Professor of Urology
Bryn Mawr Urology Group
Thomas Jefferson University
Bryn Mawr, Pennsylvania

LAURIE LOVEJOY McNICHOL, MSN, RN, GNP, CWOCN
Clinical Manager, Clinical Quality Resource Team
Advanced Home Care
High Point, North Carolina

DEBRA NETSCH, RN, MSN, CAPN, CWOCN
Family Nurse Practitioner, WOC Nurse
Mankato Clinic, Ltd.
Mankato, Minnesota
Associate Director and Faculty
Web WOC Nurse Education Program
Minneapolis, Minnesota

LINDA D. PRUITT, RN, MS, ET
Director, Medical Education
ConvaTec, a Bristol-Myers Squibb Company
Guthrie, Oklahoma

BONNIE SUE ROLSTAD, RN, BA, CWOCN
Administrative Director, WOC Nurse Specialist
Web WOC Nursing Education Program
Minneapolis, Minnesota

JODY SCARDILLO, MS, RN, CWOCN
Clinical Nurse Specialist, ET Nursing
Albany Medical Center
Albany, New York

ANNE SCHEURICH, RN, BS, CWOCN
Wound and Ostomy Care Specialist
Northwestern Memorial Home Health Care
Chicago, Illinois

KATHLEEN SHORTRIDGE, BSN, RN
Transplant Nurse Coordinator
University of Chicago Hospitals
Chicago, Illinois

AMY J. THORSEN, MD
Adjunct Instructor in Surgery
University of Minnesota Division of Colon and
    Rectal Surgery
Minneapolis, Minnesota

**NANCY TOMASELLI, RN, MSN, CS, CRNP,
    CWOCN, CLNC**
President and CEO
Premier Health Solutions, LLC
Cherry Hill, New Jersey

PAULA ERWIN TOTH, MSN, RN, ET, CWOCN, CNS
Director, Enterostomal Therapy Nursing and Education
The Cleveland Clinic Foundation
Cleveland, Ohio

CAROL-ANN VASILEVSKY, MD
Assistant Professor of Surgery
McGill University
Montreal, Quebec

**CRAIG A. WHITE, BSc, Clin Psy D, PG Cert, C
    Psychol, AFBPsS**
Macmillan Consultant in Psychosocial Oncology
Honorary Research Fellow, Section of Psychological
    Medicine
University of Glasgow
NHS Ayrshire Arran
Irvine, Ayrshire, Scotland

Preface

························

The person undergoing a surgical procedure that will result in the creation of a fecal or urinary diversion presents with many needs. The stress of dealing with the diagnosis of a chronic or acute illness begins the process for the patient and his or her family. The news that he or she will live temporarily or permanently with a stoma can cause the patient undue stress. Before surgery the patient requires support and education. After surgery the patient begins to recognize the bodily changes, as well as the many new skills that will be required. The process of acceptance continues for many months as the patient tests his or her ability to return to normal activities. It was the recognition that the care of a person with a fecal or urinary diversion encompasses not just stoma management, but a solid understanding of the disease process necessitating the creation of a stoma as well as the adjustments that must be made that provided the foundation for *Fecal & Urinary Diversions: Management Principles.*

Changes in the management of a patient with a stoma have evolved over the last 10 years. Most fecal diversions created are generally temporary, because of the improved skills and techniques of surgeons and innovative medical treatments. Early identification and treatment of conditions such as colorectal cancer, ulcerative colitis, and Crohn's disease have provided today's patient with a number of treatment options, several of which do not demand that a patient live with a permanent stoma. Major changes in the management of a person with bladder cancer offer these patients local treatment or, in many cases, reconstructive surgery using the native sphincter and ultimately achieving continence. Equipment choices for the patient with a stoma have also evolved and include skin barriers that not only protect peristomal skin but provide a safe, reliable seal that can be custom fitted, as well as pouches that are available in a multitude of shapes, materials, films, and sizes.

This text has been written by experts who participate in the care of persons with fecal and urinary diversions. The pathophysiology of disease conditions that often result in the creation of a fecal or urinary diversion is covered from the neonate to the adult. The nuances of stoma patient management are described in chapters that include preoperative and postoperative management, ostomy adjustment, and complications. The issues surrounding the management of a person with fecal or urinary diversion, such as intestinal transplantation, medications, telemedicine, and accelerated surgical stay programs are included.

We are keenly aware of the need for additional clinical and behavioral research to provide a further understanding of the interventions and outcomes in stoma patient management. Principles for management are presented in this text, and it is hoped that they will provide a foundation to examine practice and further the science and art of ostomy management. The reader is encouraged to apply the principles in a given setting, tailoring them to the needs of the patient. It is the fervent hope of the editors of this text that it stimulates the research necessary to continue improving our practice and that it does indeed assist in the management of the person with a fecal or urinary diversion.

Acknowledgments

....

We are greatly indebted to all of the people who have contributed to the production of this text, especially the expert clinicians who generously gave of their time and expertise, as well as all of the patients who have allowed us to participate in their care and thus help us to learn daily from them.

We would also like to thank the family of Diane Singer, RN, CETN, who most generously donated to us her slide collection; we have used many of her slides in this book. We are pleased to honor the memory of this fine clinician with the inclusion of some of her work in this text.

My gratitude to my colleagues at the University of Chicago who share my passion for the delivery of care to patients with ostomies and who readily made themselves available for questions, clarification, and support. Special thanks to my husband Jim, who gave his time to allow me the time to devote myself to this project.

Janice Colwell

I thank my father Patrick Maguire, who gave me my love for books; Mike D'Orazio, who nurtured my love of all things ostomy; and Jan Colwell, whose vision and determination brought this book to fruition.

Margaret Goldberg

It has been a privilege to work with Jan and Margaret during the past 2 years to create this text. This could not have happened without the support and encouragement of my colleagues, friends, and family. Special recognition goes to my husband Chick, who was always available to be my resident computer expert in my time of need; to my father, Bondi Comalli, who gave me courage and patience to pursue my dreams. To my former and future students, may this book be a valuable resource for you to meet the needs of your patients who will require a urinary or fecal diversion.

Jane Carmel

Contents

PART

I

OVERVIEW

History of Stoma Creation and Surgical Advances

DOROTHY DOUGHTY

OBJECTIVES

1. Identify major changes in the indications for colostomy creation.
2. Describe two advances in colostomy management.
3. Relate attempts to develop a continent colostomy.
4. List advantages of the coloanal J reservoir.
5. Describe the major advances in ileostomy surgery.
6. Describe advantages of the Brooke ileostomy.
7. Describe the historical development of continent fecal internal reservoirs.
8. Compare and contrast the differences between continent urinary diversions.
9. Discuss the evolution of the neobladder.
10. Identify two advances in the area of fecal and urinary diversion.

INTRODUCTION

The history of stoma construction is an inspiring story with many heroes. They include those surgeons whose unceasing efforts to refine and improve on the existing "standard of care" have resulted in steady and sometimes landmark improvements in patient outcomes—and the patients who were willing to be the first to undergo an untested procedure! It began with crude ostomies constructed in desperate attempts to save lives, continued with improvements in surgical techniques designed to minimize complications and optimize stoma management, and most recently has been highlighted by diversions that offer the patient continence as well as well-being. Like any complex undertaking, there have been setbacks along the way, seemingly good ideas that failed to produce the desired results; however, each idea and each modification in technique, even the apparent failures, contributed to the body of knowledge that led to the next breakthrough. Surgeons throughout time have built upon their predecessors' experiences to improve outcomes for their own patients, and have kept meticulous records of both their successes and failures as their contribution to future progress.

EVOLUTION OF THE FECAL DIVERSION

The very earliest stomas were not the result of surgical intervention, but fecal fistulas that developed spontaneously following abdominal trauma or bowel obstruction. One surgeon in the mid-18th century noted that fistula formation was associated with survival, and suggested that surgeons might take hints from nature and construct intentional openings (stomas) to manage traumatic bowel injury. However, the general thinking during the 18th century was that an opening into the bowel was much too inconvenient and that it was better to leave the injured bowel alone, close the abdominal wound, and hope for the best (Cataldo, 1999). When one considers the fact that anesthesia was not introduced until 1846, it is easy to understand that all surgical procedures were considered measures of last resort and that the associated pain was identified as a major deterrent! This situation began to change in the mid-19th century, when the advent of anesthesia, the development of forceps, and the introduction of sterilization made surgery both feasible and much safer (Hardy, 1989).

The Evolution and Current Status of Colostomy Surgery

There have been many advances in the construction of large bowel stomas; key areas of development and change include indications for stoma creation, stomal construction, and guidelines for stoma location.

Indications

The earliest recorded colostomies were performed for emergency management of bowel obstruction or intestinal trauma. One source suggests that the first colostomy was done in 1750 on a "fishwife" with an incarcerated hernia; another attributes the first colostomy to the French surgeon Pillore, who is reported to have performed a cecostomy on a patient with an obstructing rectal tumor in about 1776 (Anderson, 1982; Cataldo, 1999). In 1793 Duret reported on a colostomy he performed on a 3-day-old infant with imperforate anus; he first practiced the procedure on the body of a dead infant that he obtained from the city's poor house. Despite the lack of anesthesia and asepsis, Duret's intervention was very successful; the patient lived with his "artificial anus" until the age of 45 (Anderson, 1982; Cataldo, 1999). These isolated successes notwithstanding, colostomy remained a last-resort measure until the late 19th century, when the general surgical advances noted earlier allowed surgeons to treat patients electively and the practice of surgery began to evolve at a much faster rate.

During the late 19th century, leading surgeons began to suggest the use of a proximal colostomy to provide temporary protection for a distal anastomosis; these recommendations were based on their observation that primary anastomosis resulted in unacceptably high anastomotic leak rates. In 1903 Mikulicz-Radecki reported a reduction in mortality (from 50% to 12.5%) when he protected distal anastomoses with a temporary proximal colostomy; he therefore advocated the routine use of diversion in such cases (Cataldo, 1999). During this same period, surgeons began to treat rectal cancer with narrow resection and permanent colostomy; however, this procedure was initially associated with almost 100% local recurrence of the malignancy. Sir Ernest Miles and Dr. Charles Mayo both attributed this to failure to resect the perirectal lymphatics and both described radical rectal resection as the preferred approach to management of these patients, Mayo in 1904 and Miles in 1908 (Cataldo, 1999). Their recommended technique involved a combined abdominal and perineal approach, with removal of the rectosigmoid, anal canal, and perirectal lymphatics, and construction of a permanent descending colostomy. This procedure became variably known as abdominoperineal resection of the rectum and as the *Miles' procedure* (Atkinson, 1982; Miles, 1908).

For a century the indications for colostomy remained essentially the same: management of acute colonic obstruction; temporary diversion in cases involving intestinal disruption (either from traumatic injury or spontaneous perforation); temporary "protection" of distal anastomoses; and permanent fecal diversion for patients requiring rectal excision due to rectal cancer. However, recently there have been some changes in those indications.

For example, routine diversion is no longer recommended for management of traumatic bowel injuries or perforation secondary to diverticulitis; recent studies indicate lower morbidity and mortality rates with a single-stage procedure (i.e., resection and primary reanastomosis). As a result, single-stage procedures are gradually replacing the two-stage procedures done in the past (Demetriades et al, 2001). In addition, loop ileostomy is now the recommended diversion for protection of a distal anastomosis; again, studies have shown lower morbidity rates with loop ileostomy as opposed to loop colostomy (Edwards et al, 2001). Finally, the guidelines for curative resection of rectal cancer have been revised to require only a 2-cm distal margin, as opposed to the 5-cm margin that was held as the gold standard for many years. This modification has significantly reduced the number of patients who require permanent colostomies (Fuchs et al, 1998).

Construction

Early colostomies were skin flush loop-type stomas, constructed by incising the abdominal wall and the anterior bowel wall, then suturing the opening in the bowel wall to the opening in the abdominal wall (much like a buttonhole). This construction provided decompression of an obstructed distal bowel, but did not completely divert the fecal stream and certainly did not facilitate containment of the stool (Cataldo, 1999; Hardy, 1989). In 1888 Maydl described construction of a loop colostomy with use of a "vulcanite rod" to maintain the exteriorized loop of bowel in the extra abdominal position until the stoma had granulated to the abdominal wall (Hardy, 1989). The basics of Maydl's approach remain the standard of care today. This technique produces a protruding stoma that facilitates management; in addition, exteriorization of the entire loop with support for the posterior bowel wall provides for almost complete fecal diversion by taking advantage of the naturally occurring haustrations in the colon (when the anterior bowel wall is opened, the natural protrusion of the posterior bowel wall separates the proximal and distal bowel and provides two distinct openings into the colon) (McGarity, 1992a).

Throughout most of the 20th century, loop colostomies were exteriorized and supported at the time of surgery, but they typically were not "opened" until several days later, when the anterior bowel wall was opened at the bedside. (Not painful, this procedure frequently *was* traumatic for the patient.) Surgeons noted that the exposed serosal surface of the exteriorized loop became intensely inflamed and that this caused gradual mucosal eversion (i.e., the stoma gradually turned "inside out" until the mucosal surface had attached to the peristomal skin. This process took several weeks and was labeled "maturation" of the stoma). In the early 1950s several surgeons modified the technique for surgical construction of an ileostomy to include "surgical maturation" of the stoma; i.e., the distal bowel was everted and sutured to the skin, thus exposing the mucosal surface and eliminating the "natural maturation" process. Shortly thereafter, Dr. Rupert Turnbull began to strongly advocate

opening and maturing the loop colostomy at the time of surgery, and a surgically matured loop colostomy has gradually become the standard of care (Cataldo, 1999; Hardy, 1989; McGarity, 1992a; Weakley, 1994).

The first *end* colostomies were performed and described in 1881 and 1884, but it was Henry Hartmann who popularized this procedure in the early 1900s, when he lectured in America on his technique for management of obstructing sigmoid tumors. His technique, now known as the *Hartmann procedure*, involved resection of the diseased bowel segment, closure of the distal stump (which was returned to the abdominal cavity), and construction of a proximal end stoma (Cataldo, 1999; Hardy, 1989) (Figure 1-1). End stomas were initially constructed as skin flush openings; this approach has been modified slightly to include mucosal eversion (surgical maturation) and creation of a slightly protruding stoma (McGarity, 1992a) (Figure 1-2).

The double-barrel colostomy was first described in the early 1900s by Mikulicz-Radecki, who recommended this approach to fecal diversion

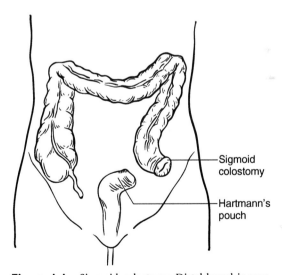

Sigmoid colostomy

Hartmann's pouch

Figure 1-1   Sigmoid colostomy. Distal bowel is oversewn and left in place to create a Hartmann's pouch. (From Hampton BG, Bryant RA, editors: *Ostomies and continent diversions: nursing management*, St Louis, 1992, Mosby.)

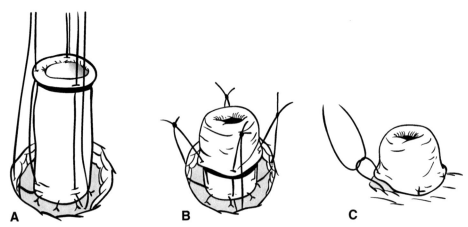

Figure 1-2   Construction of Brooke end stoma. **A**, Intestine advanced through abdominal wall; mesentery trimmed from intestine, and intestine secured to anterior rectus sheath. **B**, Sutures are placed through cut edge of intestine, seromuscular layer of intestine at skin level, and subcutaneous tissue to facilitate eversion of bowel, thus maturing stoma. **C**, Matured stoma is secured at skin level. (From Hampton BG, Bryant RA, editors: *Ostomies and continent diversions: nursing management*, St Louis, 1992, Mosby.)

following resection of diseased bowel. His technique involved resection of the involved bowel segment and anastomosis of the two limbs of the bowel to the abdominal wall as side-by-side skin flush end stomas. Once the patient had recovered from the surgery, he recommended use of a crushing clamp to create a fistula between the proximal and the distal stomas, which reestablished intestinal continuity (Figure 1-3). He reported that many of the skin flush stomas would close spontaneously once they were defunctionalized; if they failed to do so, he closed the openings surgically (Cataldo, 1999; Hardy, 1989). This procedure never became popular and is rarely, if ever, used today; double-barrel colostomies are sometimes used as a temporary diversion, but takedown involves a second surgical procedure.

Location

The earliest colostomies were abdominal stomas, created at the site of the pathology. However, in the early 1800s Amussat advocated a lumbar approach to colostomy construction; this was based on his work with cadavers, which showed that the posterior wall of the colon could be accessed and exteriorized without breaching the peritoneum (Hardy, 1989). (This of course was of major importance in the years preceding asepsis.) Unfortunately, surgeons found that lumbar colostomy was difficult to perform because the prone position that was required for the surgery caused the colon to fall forward, which made it hard to locate. As a result, this procedure was replaced by an anterior approach, once asepsis was introduced and it became safer to perform intraperitoneal procedures. The anterior approach was an improvement in that the stoma was now located on the anterior abdominal surface as opposed to the lumbar area of the back; however, placement of the stoma was usually determined by the site of the underlying problem, which meant that stomas were frequently located in the inguinal area (Cataldo, 1999; Hardy, 1989). These awkward locations of skin flush stomas, coupled with the lack of effective containment systems, made early colostomy management extremely challenging. In the late 1950s, Rupert Turnbull became increasingly aware of the impact of stoma location and patient education on long-term management of *all* patients with ostomies; this resulted in the creation of the *enterostomal therapist* role, which included

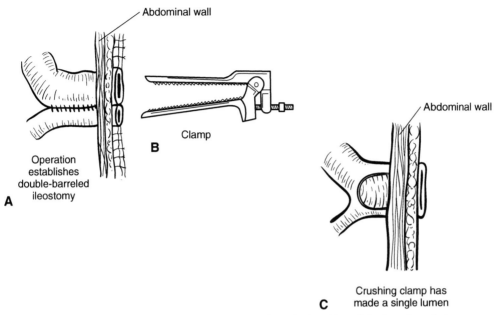

Figure 1-3   Mikulicz procedure. **A,** Anastomosis of two limbs of bowel. **B,** Insertion of clamp to create fistula between the two limbs. **C,** Crushing clamp has made a single lumen. (From Broadwell DC, Jackson BS, editors: *Principles of ostomy care,* St Louis, 1982, Mosby.)

preoperative stoma site marking (Watt, 1982; Weakley, 1994). This remains the standard of care today.

As Cataldo notes in his historical review of stoma construction, the surgical techniques used to construct large bowel stomas have changed very little in the past century (Cataldo, 1999). The major advances have been in management of the colostomy and in the development of sphincter-sparing procedures that obviate the necessity for permanent colostomy. For example, the concept and equipment for daily colostomy irrigation were developed by a California surgeon and a surgical supply company manager in 1924; this advance permitted many colostomy patients to regain continence and to manage their stomas with absorbent paper held in place by a belt (Cataldo, 1999). More recently, the development of the intestinal stapling device has contributed to surgeons' ability to manage low rectal lesions with resection and end-to-end anastomosis.

Attempts To Provide Continence for Colostomy Patients

Throughout the years, a number of attempts have been made to establish a continent colostomy. One approach involved construction of a colonic reservoir connected to an abdominal stoma by an intussuscepted colonic segment (the continence mechanism). Unfortunately, the thickness of the stool made catheter drainage almost impossible (Roberts, 1997). Another approach involved use of intestinal muscle wrapped around the segment of bowel used to construct the stoma; the goal was to create a neosphincter that would provide the patient with control. Initially the patient was taught to use small volume irrigations to stimulate evacuation; the expectation for the long term was that the patient would sense the need to defecate and apply a pouch to contain the stool. Most patients were able to achieve continence with solid and semisolid stools but were not continent for liquid stool or gas (Roberts, 1997). These poor results, along with high complication rates, caused abandonment of the procedure. Yet another approach involved placement of a magnetic ring in the subcutaneous tissue around the stoma; a magnetic "cap" was then inserted into the stoma and held in place by magnetic attraction. A charcoal filter allowed deodorized release of flatus, and patients were taught to regulate the colostomy with irrigation and to use the magnetic cap as a continence mechanism between irrigations. Unfortunately, continence rates were very disappointing (23% to 76%), and there were a number of complications; this device is no longer available (Roberts, 1997; Taylor-Mahood, 1982). However, a disposable device (the ConSeal Ostomy Plug) is used by some patients to maintain continence between irrigations; this is a soft foam plug that is inserted into the stoma to provide obstruction to leakage.

Coloanal J Reservoir

In the 1990s surgeons developed a neorectum constructed from the descending colon to provide improved outcomes for patients requiring rectosigmoid excision. These patients frequently report severe fecal urgency and possibly fecal frequency due to loss of the reservoir function of the rectum. Studies done to date on the impact of a colonic J-shaped reservoir (with anastomosis to the anal canal) have shown a significant reduction in fecal frequency and urgency (Fuchs et al, 1998).

The Evolution and Current Status of Ileostomy Surgery

The major advances in ileostomy surgery have been in the areas of stoma construction and management, issues of critical importance to a patient with a small bowel stoma, and the development of continent reservoirs as alternatives to the standard ileostomy.

Evolution of the Standard Ileostomy

The first ileostomy was reported in the late 19th century, many years after the first colostomies but only a few decades following the advent of anesthesia and sterilization. In 1879 a German surgeon reported on construction of a temporary diverting ileostomy in a patient with an obstructing malignancy of the ascending colon. Unfortunately, the patient died following reanastomosis due to an anastomotic leak (Cataldo, 1999; McGarity, 1992a).

Early ileostomy stomas were typically constructed as skin level stomas and were associated with severe and painful skin breakdown (McGarity, 1992b). The first major advance in ileostomy construction came in 1912, when a surgeon from St. Louis (Dr. John Brown) reported on a series of 10 patients in whom he had constructed a protruding ileostomy stoma. He did this by bringing the distal end of the ileum out through the incision and leaving several inches to protrude beyond skin level; the exposed serosa became inflamed and sticky, resulting in gradual eversion of the mucosal layer of the exposed bowel and eventual adherence of the mucosal layer to the peristomal skin (i.e., spontaneous maturation of the stoma) (Cataldo, 1999; McGarity, 1992b). Brown's technique was further improved during the 1930s by surgeons at the Mayo Clinic, who began bringing the ileostomy stoma out through a separate incision in the right lower quadrant; he further modified the procedure to reduce the incidence of bowel obstruction after surgery. Despite these improvements in technique, ileostomy surgery remained an option of last resort because of high mortality rates and difficulty with postoperative management (McGarity, 1992b).

The next step in making ileostomy surgery a feasible option for patients with severe ulcerative colitis was the development of an appliance that would adhere to the skin and collect the effluent. In the late 1920s, Dr. Alfred Strauss from Chicago came up with the idea of a rubber appliance that could be glued and belted in place, and he worked with one of his patients (who was also a chemistry student) to design a pouch. By the 1940s this appliance was manufactured and sold as the "Strauss Koenig Rutzen bag," and it received widespread acceptance (McGarity, 1992b).

A persistent complication of ileostomy surgery was the condition known simply as *ileostomy dysfunction*; it was characterized by cramping abdominal pain and high-volume ileostomy output (as much as 30 L/day), leading to severe fluid and electrolyte disturbances. The etiology of this condition was first explicated by Dr. Rupert Turnbull and

Dr. George Crile from the Cleveland Clinic, who attributed it to obstruction of the ileostomy stoma resulting from the intense inflammation and edema that were associated with exposure of the serosal layer and spontaneous maturation of the stoma (Crile and Turnbull, 1954). They found that they could relieve the obstruction and the associated dysfunction by passing a catheter through the stoma to provide free drainage of ileal contents. They then began to focus on strategies to prevent serosal exposure and the resulting serositis, while maintaining a protruding stoma; this focus led to development of the *mucosal grafted ileostomy stoma.* This procedure involved removal of the serosal and muscle layers of the distal half of the ileal stoma, followed by eversion of the distal mucosal and submucosal layers over the proximal half of the stoma (Crile and Turnbull, 1954; McGarity, 1992b; Turnbull, 1956; Weakley, 1994). This procedure was effective but it was technically difficult, and about the same time Dr. Bryan Brooke (an English surgeon) described a simpler procedure with the same outcomes: he left all bowel layers intact and simply everted the distal end of the stoma and sutured the mucosal layer to the skin (the Brooke ileostomy) (Brooke, 1952; McGarity, 1992b; Weakley, 1994). This procedure, first described in the mid-1950s, is still the preferred surgical approach to stomal construction; it produces a "budded" stoma and eliminates the temporary dysfunction associated with spontaneous maturation of the stoma. This advance in stoma construction significantly reduced the morbidity and mortality associated with ileostomy surgery, and quickly became the standard for stoma construction. Subsequent advances in appliance development and in programs for patient education and support had an equally significant effect on psychosocial outcomes.

Development of Continent Ileal Reservoirs

For almost a century, the primary focus in ileostomy surgery was on improved surgical techniques for stoma construction and disease management, and on improved postoperative management and rehabilitation. As a result of advances in these areas, patients experienced significantly better outcomes, both physically and psychosocially. However, the need for an external collecting device and the inability to control evacuation of stool and gas continued to be troubling for many patients, especially those who had difficulty maintaining a secure appliance seal. These concerns led surgeons to explore the possibility of an *internal* reservoir that would restore continence to these patients.

In the 1960s a Swedish surgeon named Nils Kock set out to develop a continent ileal reservoir; his idea was to create an internal reservoir connected to an abdominal stoma, and to establish some type of one-way valve between the reservoir and the stoma that would maintain continence. He tried a number of designs for both the reservoir and the continence mechanism, culminating in the development of the procedure known as the *Kock pouch.* This procedure involved construction of a reservoir and continence mechanism from 40 to 45 cm of terminal ileum; the proximal 30 cm were used to construct the reservoir, and the distal 15 cm were used to create the stoma and the continence mechanism (Kock, 1969; McGarity, 1992b). The reservoir was constructed by suturing, opening, and reconfiguring two 15-cm ileal segments to form an aperistaltic "pouch," and the continence mechanism was created by intussuscepting the segment of bowel connecting the reservoir to the abdominal stoma (Figure 1-4). Once initial healing had taken place, the patient was taught to intubate and drain the reservoir at regular intervals; the only stoma covering that was needed was a simple absorptive pad. Most patients were continent of both stool and gas; however, there was a high incidence (up to 50%) of partial or complete failure of the intussusception, which resulted in difficult intubation and compromised continence (McGarity, 1992b; Weakley, 1994). Several modifications in the design of the reservoir and continence mechanism were reported by various surgeons; the most widely adopted of these was the Barnett Continent Ileal Reservoir. Barnett incorporated several modifications to improve long-term outcomes, the most significant of which was the "living collar" (a loop of bowel fashioned as a collar around the intussuscepted segment of bowel connecting the reservoir

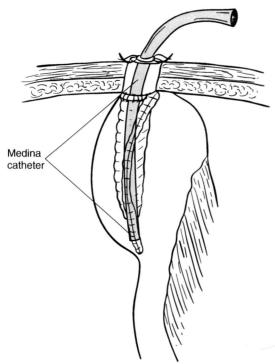

Medina
catheter

Figure 1-4 Kock continent ileostomy with Medina catheter. (From Michelassi F, Milsom JW, editors: *Operative strategies in inflammatory bowel disease,* New York, 1999, Springer.)

and the abdominal stoma). Because this ileal collar communicated with the reservoir, it filled as the reservoir filled, which provided additional resistance and support for continence. Barnett's group reported a significant reduction in complication rates, with approximately 20% of patients requiring major surgical revision or pouch removal during the first several years after surgery (Continent Ostomy Centers, 1992).

The continent ileostomy is offered at selected centers in the United States and Canada, and is a way of making a continent procedure available to patients who have previously undergone excision of the anal canal and sphincters.

Development of Pelvic Reservoirs

Despite the problems associated with continent abdominal reservoirs, these procedures represented a giant step toward continence, with most patients reporting good quality of life; in addition, the lessons learned paved the way for the construction of pelvic reservoirs controlled by native sphincters.

In the 1940s and 1950s surgeons occasionally performed straight ileoanal anastomosis for patients who required colectomy for benign disease, but the high incidence of severe diarrhea prevented any widespread acceptance (McGarity, 1992b). It was obvious that a proximal reservoir was needed to provide acceptable stool frequency and quality of life, and experience with the Kock ileostomy had made it clear that the ileum could be successfully used as a fecal reservoir. In 1976, Parks and Nicholls reported on their work with an S-shaped reservoir, and in 1980 Utsonomiya described the J reservoir (Parks, Nicholls, and Belliveau, 1980; Utsonomiya et al, 1980). Both of these approaches have been used successfully, and since that time additional reservoir designs have been developed; at this time, the J reservoir is the most widely used due to the simplicity of construction (McGarity, 1992b) (Figure 1-5). In most centers, a proximal diverting ileostomy is performed to protect the ileal pouch anal anastomosis; the ileostomy is closed following anastomotic healing. Patients are taught sphincter-strengthening exercises to optimize sphincter function, and are also taught dietary and pharmacologic measures to control stool consistency. Long-term outcomes and quality of life are good for most patients, with average stool frequency of five to six per day. The most common complications are anastomotic stricture and pouchitis; research into the causes and management of pouchitis are ongoing (Hocevar, Remzi, 2001).

EVOLUTION AND CURRENT STATUS OF THE URINARY DIVERSION

Interestingly, the evolution of urinary diversions has been parallel to that of fecal diversions, advancing from standard diversions to continent abdominal reservoirs and most recently to pelvic reservoirs anastomosed to the urethra.

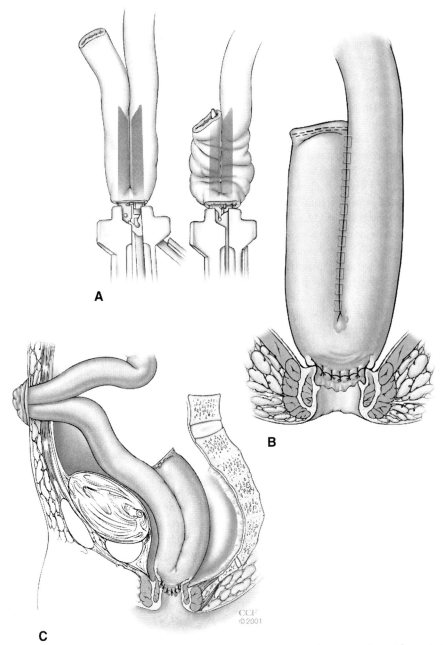

A

B

C

Figure 1-5   J-shaped configuration for ileal pouch anal anastomosis. **A**, Creation of J pouch. **B**, J pouch anal anastomosis. **C**, Temporary diverting ileostomy. (Courtesy Cleveland Clinic, Cleveland, Ohio.)

Evolution of the Standard Urinary Diversion

The earliest recorded attempts to create a urinary diversion were in the mid-1800s; however, these efforts focused on techniques for anastomosing the ureters to the rectosigmoid, as opposed to construction of an external stoma (Cohen and Novick, 1996). This approach to urinary diversion was the standard of care from the middle 1800s until almost a century later, when increasing reports of adverse effects led to alternate approaches to urinary diversion (Cohen and Novick, 1996). These adverse effects included a chronic metabolic acidosis secondary to the resorption of chloride and the excretion of bicarbonate and potassium, incontinence in individuals with compromised anal sphincter function, and, most importantly, the development of carcinoma at the anastomotic site developing 7 to 49 years following diversion in a significant percentage of patients (as high as 40%, according to some reports). This increased incidence of carcinoma was first reported in 1929 by Hammer and was supported by subsequent reports from other centers. As a result, ureterosigmoidostomy fell out of favor. At that time, the alternative approach to urinary diversion was ureterostomy. Unfortunately, this was also associated with multiple adverse outcomes, including stenosis, poor emptying, and major pouching difficulties related to the small skin flush stoma (Doughty and Lightner, 1982; Smith, 1982). This was the situation in 1950, when Bricker reported successful use of an isolated ileal segment interposed between the ureters and the abdominal wall, the ureteroileal conduit (Bricker, 1950). Bricker had begun investigating alternatives to the ureterosigmoidostomy because of his work with patients requiring pelvic exenteration procedures for advanced pelvic malignancies; ureterosigmoidostomy was of course not an option for these individuals as the rectosigmoid was included in the organs being resected. The benefits of an ureterointestinal conduit were quickly evident; the intestinal stoma was large enough to resist stenosis and to provide effective emptying, a short, straight conduit limited resorption of chloride and loss of bicarbonate, and there was no risk of incontinence or malignancy. The development of the aforementioned "Rutzen bag" provided a means for containment of the urine and facilitated postoperative management. While Bricker and others also experimented with the use of other intestinal segments, the ileal conduit has remained the ureterointestinal conduit of choice based on simplicity of construction and low complication rates. The two major disadvantages associated with the ileal conduit urinary diversion were the inability to construct a nonrefluxing anastomosis between the ureters and the ileal segment, and the necessity for an external appliance (Cohen and Novick, 1996; Doughty and Lightner, 1982).

Evolution of the Continent Urinary Diversion

The ureterosigmoidostomy did provide the patient with continence so long as the anal sphincter function remained adequate. However, as noted, the multiple complications associated with this procedure led surgeons in the mid-20th century to explore different options for urinary diversion, and the ileal conduit quickly became the urinary diversion of choice. Interestingly, at the same time that Bricker published his findings on the ileal conduit urinary diversion, Gilchrist and Merrick reported on a continent urinary diversion using the isolated ileocecal bowel; the cecum served as a reservoir, the ileum was used to construct the abdominal stoma, and the naturally occurring ileocecal valve served as the continence mechanism. This procedure failed to gain significant acceptance, possibly because management required intermittent catheterization, which was not yet viewed as a safe and effective method of management. In addition the continence outcomes were far from desirable; patients routinely experienced nocturnal leakage and many experienced daytime leakage as well, especially at higher reservoir volumes (Cohen and Novick, 1996). As a result, it was the ileal conduit that quickly became the standard of care, and it was a number of years before continent urinary diversions were again created and began to gain widespread attention and acceptance.

Camey Procedure

In 1979 Camey reported development of a neobladder fashioned from an isoperistaltic loop of ileum; the ureters were anastomosed to the ileal loop and the distal portion of the ileal segment was tubularized and sutured to the urethra. Patients voided by voluntary sphincter relaxation and use of the Valsalva maneuver. However, this procedure was associated with persistent nocturnal incontinence and failed to gain widespread acceptance (Cohen and Novick, 1996).

Kock Urostomy

The Kock urostomy was developed by Nils Kock and was patterned after the Kock pouch; the reservoir was constructed by detubularizing and reconfiguring loops of ileum, and continence was provided by intussuscepting the segment of ileum between the reservoir and the abdominal stoma. The difference in the Kock ileostomy and the Kock urostomy was the addition of an intussuscepted segment of ileum between the ureteroileal anastomoses and the reservoir, which served to provide protection against reflux. (Altogether, the Kock urostomy required 60 to 80 cm of terminal ileum; as a result, patients required lifelong supplementation with vitamin B_{12}, which was one drawback to this procedure.) The Kock urostomy provided significantly better continence than either the Camey procedure or the Gilchrist procedure; this was due in large part to the fact that the ileal segments used to construct the reservoir were detubularized, which provided a low-pressure noncontractile reservoir (DeKernian et al, 1985).

The Kock urostomy was adopted by several centers but never gained widespread acceptance, due to the complex and technically difficult operative procedure and to the relatively high complication rate (up to 30% reoperation rate) (Cohen and Novick, 1996).

Ileocecal Pouches

Ileocecal pouches were developed in the late 1980s by combining the best features of the Kock urostomy and the Gilchrist procedure, and they have proven to be an effective and straightforward approach to construction of a continent urinary diversion. Several versions have been described, including the Indiana reservoir, the Florida pouch,

and the Miami pouch; all provide a high-volume, low-pressure reservoir, an antireflux mechanism and continence mechanism, and a catheterizable channel. The reservoir is constructed by opening and reconfiguring the cecum (and possibly the right colon); detubularization successfully eliminated the problem of contractility in response to distention (as determined by Kock's work). The ureters are anastomosed to the cecal reservoir (typically in an antirefluxing fashion), and the continence mechanism is created by plicating (or folding) the cecum around a 12 Fr. catheter, which provides support for the native ileocecal valve. The distal end of the ileal segment is then sutured to the abdominal wall to create the catheterizable channel (Figure 1-6). The patient manages the reservoir by catheterizing every 3 to 4 hours and as needed; no external pouch is needed, though the stoma should be covered with an absorptive dressing (Cohen and Novick, 1996; Gowing-Farhat, 1994; Rowland and Kropp, 1994).

Surgeons around the world have used modifications of the procedures described in the previous paragraphs to construct continent urinary diversions. Various segments of detubularized bowel have been used to construct the reservoir when cystectomy is required, and augmentation of the native bladder has been used to establish an adequate reservoir in benign conditions (e.g., management of intractable incontinence in a patient with a spinal cord injury). Various structures can also be used to establish a continent, catheterizable channel; for example, the Mitrofanoff procedure uses the appendix, which is separated from the cecum, reversed, and anastomosed to the reservoir in a nonrefluxing fashion (Cohen and Novick, 1996).

Evolution of the Orthotopic Neobladder

Following the successful construction of isoperistaltic abdominal reservoirs, surgeons began to revisit Camey's concept of a urinary reservoir anastomosed to the urethra and controlled by the urethral sphincter mechanism. Alcini reported anastomosis of an ileocecal reservoir to the urethra in 1985, and Hautmann described the technique for an ileal neobladder with urethral anastomosis

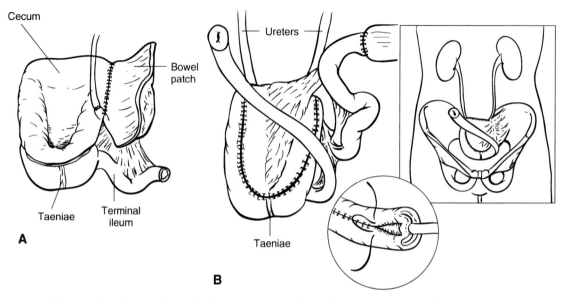

Figure 1-6   Construction of Indiana urinary pouch. **A,** Cecum and terminal ileum segment of ileum are isolated from gastrointestinal tract; another segment of bowel is resected to use as patch. Antimesenteric borders of cecum and bowel segment are opened; bowel patch is sewn to open edges of cecum. **B,** Ureters have been tunneled into taeniae coli along posterior aspect of pouch. Terminal ileum has been plicated to fit catheter and stoma created at predetermined stoma site. (From Hampton BG, Bryant RA, editors: *Ostomies and continent diversions: nursing management,* St Louis, 1992, Mosby.)

in 1988. A recent modification is the addition of a nondetubularized segment of ileum to the superior aspect of the neobladder with anastomosis of the ureters to this peristaltic segment; this modification is reported to enhance the ability to establish a tension-free anastomosis between the neobladder and the urethra (Alcini et al, 1985; Hautmann et al, 1988; Krupski and Theodorescu, 2001).

Because cystectomy involves removal of the bladder neck and proximal urethra, continence following orthotopic neobladder construction depends on a noncontractile reservoir and an intact striated urethral sphincter. Patients are taught to empty the reservoir by relaxing the sphincter and using the Valsalva maneuver to increase intraabdominal pressure. Some patients are unable to empty completely and require supplemental clean intermittent catheterization. Leakage is another potential problem, especially at night when the voluntary sphincter mechanism is relaxed; patients

are instructed in sphincter exercises to improve sphincter tone and are counseled regarding appropriate use of absorptive products. Most patients report positive outcomes, with gradual reduction in leakage and improved ability to empty spontaneously (Krupski and Theodorescu, 2001; Rolstad and Hoyman, 1992).

Recent Advances and Current Challenges

Clearly there has been tremendous progress in the area of fecal and urinary diversion; many patients now can be managed with continent procedures and those who are not candidates for continent procedures do have the benefit of improved stoma construction, which usually translates into better management. In addition to progress specifically related to fecal and urinary diversion, there has been significant progress in reducing the complications associated with radical pelvic surgery and in reducing the morbidity associated with any major surgical procedure. One significant advance is the improved ability to identify the autonomic nerves controlling sexual function, resulting in "nerve-sparing" procedures for patients undergoing radical rectal resection or radical cystoprostatectomy; these modifications have reduced the risk of long-term erectile dysfunction (Montorsi et al, 2001). Another advance is the increased use of the laparoscopic approach to abdominal and pelvic surgery, including laparoscopic stoma construction; the laparoscopic approach significantly reduces postoperative morbidity and recovery time (Price, Rubio, 1994).

CONCLUSION

Despite the tremendous progress that has been made, there are persistent challenges related to fecal and urinary diversion; one of these is the high incidence of stoma complications, particularly parastomal hernia, and another is the high incidence of pouchitis in continent reservoirs. Undoubtedly, many people are working on these challenges, and the next few decades will bring answers to these questions and continued improvements to the quality of life for those patients requiring fecal or urinary diversion.

SELF-ASSESSMENT EXERCISES

Questions

1. Surgical maturation of the stoma refers to:
   a. Allowing the stoma mucosa to age before applying a pouching system.
   b. The eversion and suturing of the distal bowel to the skin.
   c. Pulling the bowel to the skin surface at the time of the operation, and opening the stoma at the bedside 1 to 2 days after surgery.
   d. Placing a crushing clamp over the stoma to allow healing.
2. Which modification in the treatment of colorectal cancer has significantly reduced the number of patients who require a permanent colostomy?
   a. Radiation beam therapy

   b. Guidelines for curative resection of rectal cancer revised to require a 2-cm distal margin
   c. Early detection of rectal cancers
   d. The effectiveness of chemotherapeutic agents
3. Attempts to develop a continent colostomy include all *except:*
   a. Construction of a colonic reservoir connected to an abdominal stoma by an intussuscepted colonic segment.
   b. Use of intestinal muscle wrapped around the segment of bowel used to construct the stoma.
   c. Neorectum constructed from the descending colon.
   d. Abdominoperineal resection.
4. The main advantage of the coloanal J reservoir anastomosis is that it has shown a significant reduction in fecal frequency and urgency when compared to a rectosigmoid anastomosis.
   True _____   False _____
5. The major advances in ileostomy surgery include all *except:*
   a. Areas of stoma construction and management.
   b. Development of continent reservoirs as alternatives to the standard ileostomy.
   c. The development of pelvic pouches.
   d. Decreased need for follow-up in the person with an ileostomy.
6. Characteristics of ileostomy dysfunction include:
   a. Obstruction of the ileostomy stoma.
   b. Intense inflammation and edema.
   c. Exposure of the serosal layer and spontaneous maturation of the stoma.
   d. All of the above.
7. Name two advantages of the Brooke ileostomy.
8. Match the type of urinary diversion with its distinct disadvantage.
   a. Ureterosigmoidostomy
   b. Ureterostomy

   c. Ileal conduit
     i. Development of carcinoma at the anastomotic site
     ii. Stenosis, poor emptying, major pouching difficulties
     iii. No nonrefluxing anastomosis between the ureters and the ileal segment
9. Describe how an ileocecal pouch is created to be used as a continent urinary diversion.
10. Name two significant advances in the field of fecal and urinary diversions that have reduced the morbidity associated with these major surgical procedures.

Answers

1. b
2. b
3. d
4. True
5. d
6. d
7. Produces a budded stoma and eliminates the temporary dysfunction associated with spontaneous maturation of the stoma
8. a. Ureterosigmoidostomy:
     i. development of carcinoma at the anastomotic site
   b. Ureterostomy:
     ii. stenosis, poor emptying, major pouching difficulties
   c. Ileal conduit:
     iii. no nonrefluxing anastomosis between the ureters and the ileal segment.
9. The reservoir is constructed by opening and reconfiguring the cecum (and possibly the right colon); detubularization successfully eliminated the problem of contractility in response to distention. The ureters are anastomosed to the cecal reservoir (typically in an antirefluxing fashion), and the continence mechanism is created by plicating (or folding) the cecum around a 12 Fr. catheter, which provides support for the native ileocecal valve. The distal end of the ileal segment is then sutured to the abdominal wall to create the catheterizable channel.

10. One significant advance is the improved ability to identify the autonomic nerves controlling sexual function; another advance is the increased use of the laparoscopic approach, which significantly reduces postoperative morbidity and recovery time.

REFERENCES

Alcini E et al: Ileocaecourethroplasty after total cystectomy for bladder cancer, *Br J Urol* 57:160, 1985.

Anderson F: History of enterostomal therapy. In Broadwell D, Jackson B, editors: *Principles of ostomy care*, St Louis, 1982, Mosby.

Atkinson K: Abdominoperineal resection of the rectum. In Broadwell D, Jackson B, editors: *Principles of ostomy care*, St. Louis, 1982, Mosby.

Bricker E: Bladder substitute after pelvic exenteration, *Surg Clin North Am* 30:1511, 1950.

Brooke B: The management of an ileostomy including its complications, *Lancet* 2:102-104, 1952.

Cataldo P: Intestinal stomas: 200 years of digging, *Dis Colon Rectum* 42:137-142, 1999.

Cohen T, Novick A: The evolution of the urinary diversion. In Erwin-Toth P, Krasner D, editors: *Enterostomal therapy nursing: growth and evolution of a nursing specialty worldwide*, Baltimore, Md, 1996, Halgo.

Continent Ostomy Centers: Barnett Continent Intestinal Reservoir, *Clinical Summary* 1-4, 1992.

Crile G, Turnbull R: The mechanism and prevention of ileostomy dysfunction, *Ann Surg* 140:459-469, 1954.

DeKernian J et al: The Kock pouch as a urinary reservoir: pitfalls and perspectives, *Am J Surg* 150:83, 1985.

Demetriades D et al: Committee on multicenter clinical trials, American Association for Surgery of Trauma. Penetrating colon injuries requiring resection: diversion or primary anastomosis? An AAST prospective multicenter study, *J Trauma* 50(5):765-775, 2001.

Doughty D, Lightner D: Genitourinary surgical procedures. In Broadwell D, Jackson B, editors: *Principles of ostomy care*, St Louis, 1982, Mosby.

Edwards D et al: Stoma-related complications are more frequent after transverse colostomy than loop ileostomy: a randomized clinical trial, *Br J Surg* 88(3):360-363, 2001.

Fuchs K et al: Coloanal J-pouch reconstruction following low rectal resection, *Recent Results Cancer Res* 146:87-94, 1998.

Gowing-Farhat C: The Florida pouch, *Urol Nursing* 14:1-5, 1994.

Hardy K: Evolution of the stoma, *Aust N Z J Surg* 59:71-77, 1989.

Hautmann R et al: The ileal neobladder, *J Urol* 139:39-42, 1988.

Hocevar B, Remzi F: The ileal pouch anal anastomosis: past, present, and future, *JWOCN* 28(1):32-36, 2001.

Kock N: Intraabdominal reservoir in patients with permanent ileostomy, *Arch Surg* 99:223-231, 1969.

Krupski T, Theodorescu D: Orthotopic neobladder following cystectomy: indications, management, and outcomes, *JWOCN* 28(1):37-46, 2001.

McGarity W: Gastrointestinal surgical procedures. In Hampton B, Bryant R, editors: *Ostomies and continent diversions: nursing management*, St Louis, 1992a, Mosby.

McGarity W: The evolution of continence following total colectomy, *Am Surg* 58(1):1-16, 1992b.

Miles W: A method of performing abdominoperineal excision for carcinoma of the rectum and the terminal portion of the pelvic colon, *Lancet* 2:1812, 1908.

Montorsi F et al: Counseling the patient with prostate cancer about treatment-related erectile dysfunction, *Curr Opin Urol* 11(6):611-617, 2001.

Parks A, Nicholls R, Belliveau P: Proctocolectomy with ileal reservoir and anal anastomosis. *Br J Surg* 67:533-538, 1980.

Price A, Rubio P: Laparoscopic colorectal surgery: a challenge for ET nurses, *JWOCN* 21:179-182, 1994.

Roberts D: The pursuit of colostomy continence, *JWOCN* 24:92-97, 1997.

Rolstad B, Hoyman K: Continent diversions and reservoirs. In Hampton B, Bryant R, editors: *Ostomies and continent diversions: nursing management*, St Louis, 1992, Mosby.

Rowland R, Kropp B: Evolution of the Indiana continent urinary reservoir, *J Urol* 152:2247, 1994.

Smith A: Genitourinary pathophysiology. In Broadwell D, Jackson B, editors: *Principles of ostomy care*, St Louis, 1982, Mosby.

Taylor-Mahood E: Magnetic colostomy system. In Broadwell D, Jackson B, editors: *Principles of ostomy care*, St Louis, 1982, Mosby.

Turnbull R: Mucosal grafted ileostomy, *Surg Clin North Am* 36:841-847, 1956.

Utsonomiya J et al: Total colectomy, mucosal proctectomy, and ileoanal anastomosis, *Dis Colon Rectum* 23:459-466, 1980.

Watt R: Stoma placement. In Broadwell D, Jackson B, editors: *Principles of ostomy care*, St Louis, 1982, Mosby.

Weakley F: A historical perspective of stomal construction, *JWOCN* 21:59-75, 1994.

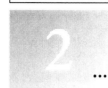

CHAPTER 2

Roles of the Ostomy Nurse Specialist: Historical Perspective, Role Potential

JOY BOARINI, JANICE C. COLWELL, LAURIE LOVEJOY MCNICHOL, JANE E. CARMEL, MARGARET GOLDBERG, and LINDA D. PRUITT

OBJECTIVES

1. Describe the early role development of the person specializing in ostomy rehabilitation services.
2. Name two developmental priorities in the history of the Wound, Ostomy and Continence Nurses Society.
3. Discuss the role of the ostomy nurse specialist in acute care, home care, long-term care, rehabilitation care, the outpatient setting, and in industry.

INTRODUCTION

In 1958 Rupert B. Turnbull, Jr., MD, enlisted Norma N. Gill to help his patients at the Cleveland Clinic overcome the shock of ostomy surgery and resume a normal, active lifestyle (Blakely, 1996). Ms. Gill, who herself had an ostomy, began a program to educate not only patients with ostomies, but also to educate nurses and surgeons in the care of a person with a stoma. Ms. Gill and Dr. Turnbull recognized the unmet needs of the person with a stoma and began the development of the profession referred to as enterostomal therapy. They became aware of the need for more people to help with this mission, and so in 1961 they established the first training program at the Cleveland Clinic. The first enterostomal therapists were required either to have an ostomy themselves or have a family member with a stoma. Over time, enterostomal therapy practice evolved into a nursing specialty, and by

1985, candidates for admission to International Association of Enterostomal Therapy-accredited education programs were required to have a baccalaureate degree with a major in nursing. The role of the enterostomal therapy nurse was developed to meet patients' unmet needs; that role is now a certified nursing specialty in the tri-specialty areas of wound, ostomy, and continence (WOC) nursing.

Included in this chapter are details of the evolution of the Wound, Ostomy and Continence Nurses (WOCN) Society and the role of the ostomy nurse specialist in acute care, the outpatient setting, home care, long-term care, rehabilitation care, and in industry.

WOUND, OSTOMY AND CONTINENCE NURSES SOCIETY

The beginnings of the WOCN Society can be traced to Norma Gill, after the need was identified for the role of the enterostomal therapist. The founding of the first organization related to ostomy came in 1962, when Ms. Gill and Archie Vinitsky founded the United Ostomy Association (UOA). As Ms. Gill and Dr. Turnbull educated students and the numbers of professionals grew, the need was recognized for a professional group that would complement the UOA. This gave rise to the American Association for Enterostomal Therapists (AAET). The group formalized their beginnings with twelve founding members in 1968 (Box 2-1). Shortly thereafter, in 1969, the organization changed its name to the North American Association for Enterostomal Therapy (NAAET). Under the second president, Henrene Honesty, the name was changed

BOX 2-1   Founding Members of the American Association for Enterostomal Therapists

Alveda Ahnafield
Jean Alvers
Charlotte Blackman-Carter
Kay Carlson
Robert Draper
Virginia Geimer

Norma Gill-Thompson
Patricia Klemens
Darlene Larson
Edith Lennenberg (President)
Bertha Okun
Jane Walker

From *History of WOCN,* Wound Ostomy Continence Nurses website: www.wocn.org.

to the International Association for Enterostomal Therapy (IAET), which was intended to reflect the widening scope of its membership.

By the early 1970s the IAET had an official publication *(The IAET Quarterly)*; it also had established standards for the education of new students, created scholarships, and developed the organization's by-laws. The organization was growing and by 1974 numbered approximately 400 active members.

In the middle and end of the 1970s the organization became structured as a professional group. Size necessitated the division of the United States into nine regions to facilitate better communication and service for members. The Canadian provinces formed a separate region, and other countries created individual organizations as well.

Because of common roots and purpose, the UOA and the IAET continued to meet for their annual meetings at the same time and location. However, as the IAET membership grew, a need for continuing professional education, along with a financial base to sustain membership (*ET Journal,* 1976) led to the separation in 1976 of the UOA and the IAET. At about the same time a nucleus of ostomy pioneers met in London at the suggestion of Norma Gill to discuss establishing the World Council of Enterostomal Therapists (WCET) (Erwin-Toth and Krasner, 1996). Two years later the WCET was formalized in Milan, Italy, when representatives of 32 different countries held the first WCET meeting.

During the seventies there were other critical initiatives that supported organizational growth and a commitment to the nursing specialty. These initiatives included the adaptation of a code of

ethics that was essential in establishing professional standards to define each individual's responsibility to this new profession (*ET Journal,* 1976), limiting admission to schools of enterostomal therapy to registered nurses, the admission of the IAET into the Federation of Specialty Nursing Organizations, and the development of the first certification examination.

During the 1980s the IAET leadership defined promotion of the specialty as a priority (Broadwell, 1981; Klein, 1985; Motta, 1988). A rapidly changing health care system forced the association to consider how the specialty would thrive and survive in the future. There were two major areas where the results of their work affected the membership during this period: a terminology change and reimbursement issues. The IAET recognized that the majority of members were nurses; thus the name change from enterostomal therapists to enterostomal therapy (ET) nurses was instituted.

The advent of diagnosis-related groups (DRGs) in the 1980s changed the face of health care in the acute-care setting, and enterostomal therapy (ET) nursing was no exception. Payment for services was related to the DRGs, groupings of disease entities; a fixed amount of money was paid for each DRG. Inpatient reimbursement was predicated on decreasing the patient's length of stay, and maintaining or improving outcomes while using fewer resources. To assist members to be proactive toward health care changes and survive in the decapitated system, in 1987 the IAET formed a task force on Health Care Financing Administration reimbursement coding. This was how the IAET began to be established as a professional organization, providing a clinical interface between the issues of government reimbursement and professional practice.

In 1982 the definitive textbook for ostomy care was published. *Principles of Ostomy Care,* edited by Debra Broadwell and Bettie Jackson and written for both the novice and the expert in ostomy care, served as the required text for students in enterostomal therapy education programs. In 1986, the ET Nursing Certification Board incorporated as a separate organization from IAET. This was undertaken to prevent the conflicts of interest that could occur if the certifying board and the professional association were the same.

In the 1990s the efforts of the IAET leadership focused on two key areas: promotion of the expanded role of the ET nurse and health care reform issues that impacted the specialty's viability. In 1993 the name of the association was changed from IAET to the WOCN Society. The professional organization supported the name change to reflect members' commitment to the expanded scope of practice. It was felt that this commitment was necessary for the overall survival of the specialty as well as members' survival in a changing health care environment. The WOCN Society launched efforts aimed at health care reforms, specifically at educating the Durable Medical Equipment Regional Carriers (DMERCs) (*WOCN News,* 1994). The DMERCs are Medicare intermediaries that determine reimbursement policies. As reimbursement drove many health care decisions, the society felt it was crucial to be involved with each of the regional carriers. It worked collaboratively with the DMERCs to correctly classify ostomy and wound products, to identify new reimbursement codes, and to review questionable claims (*WOCN News,* 1995). This helped to establish the expertise of the WOCN Society in the care of persons with wounds, ostomies and continence care issues.

Other important collaborations of the WOCN Society with governmental agencies include its work to expand coverage for surgical dressings, advise the DMERCs regarding utilization parameters for supplies, provide input on the Outcome and Assessment Information Set (OASIS) Refinement Team, and campaign to ensure Medicare coverage

of biofeedback and electrical stimulation for the treatment of incontinence (Doughty, 2001).

Also in the 1990s, the leadership of the WOCN Society identified the need to establish an evidence base that clearly documents both the cost of WOC (or ET) nursing care and the outcomes it provides (Doughty, 2000). This led to the creation of the Center for Clinical Investigation; it is charged with synthesizing and summarizing existing evidence for use by WOC nurses, assisting individual WOC nurses by completing and disseminating research based on their clinical expertise and practice, and contributing to the evidence base through research projects it coordinates (Gray et al, 2002). See Box 2-2 for a chronologic listing.

The WOCN Society continues to grow and provide various types of support for members. Report cards that summarize the evidence base in various aspects of WOC care are published in every issue of the *Journal of Wound, Ostomy and Continence Nursing,* best practice fact sheets on clinical practice issues are published and updated on a ongoing basis (see Appendix D), and guidelines for care have been developed in practice areas. While the initial mission of the organization was to provide support to clinicians in the ostomy field, its scope has widened to include increasing professional support to providers of care to persons with wounds, ostomies, and continence disorders. WOC nursing is the sole nursing specialty in the United States that focuses on nursing management of patients with an ostomy.

ACUTE-CARE SETTING

The establishment of ostomy services in the acute-care setting relies on the identification by the facility of patient needs. Depending on the model of care used in the health care setting, the ostomy nurse specialist may assume the role or roles of clinician, educator, and/or consultant. In some acute-care settings the role of the ostomy nurse specialist will consist of carrying a caseload of patients with ostomies and providing care throughout the acute-care stay and perhaps in the outpatient setting. In other organizations, the role may be that of a consultant, advising staff in areas of care. Important in

BOX 2-2   Significant Events in the History of Wound, Ostomy, and Continence Nursing

1961: RB Turnbull School of Enterostomal Therapy School at Cleveland Clinic founded

1968: American Association of Enterostomal Therapists (AAET) founded, consisting of 12 stomal therapists

1969: The AAET name changed to North American Association of Enterostomal Therapists (NAAET); membership totals 33

1971: NAAET name changed to International Association for Enterostomal Therapy (IAET)

1972: IAET by-laws established, standards for training educational programs developed, a bibliography compiled, and salary and patient census surveys conducted; first official journal published

1974: IAET membership of 304 stomal therapists
   Code of ethics, job description, and objectives of the organization developed
   Publication of ET Journal begun

1976: Membership numbers 600; only registered nurses would be admitted to Enterostomal Therapy educational programs

1978: The Enterostomal Therapy Foundation established to provide opportunities for research and development, education, and scholarship

1980: The National Board Certification Examination offered for the first time

1982: The IAET becomes accredited as a provider and approver of continuing education programs by the National Accreditation Board of the American Nurses Association

1983: A baccalaureate degree in nursing now required for admission into an Enterostomal Therapy Educational Program

1984: The House of Delegates formed

1992: The IAET name changed to Wound, Ostomy and Continence Nurses (WOCN) Society, an association of ET nurses

1993: WOC Certification Board offers specialty nursing certification exams in wound, ostomy, and continence.

1994: Journal of ET Nursing name changed to Journal of Wound, Ostomy and Continence Nursing

1998: Options for certification expanded from examination to Professional Growth Program
   Credentials change from CETN to CWOCN; the candidate must pass certification in all three specialty sections

1999: Center for Clinical Investigation (CCI) established to advance evidence-based practice

---

all roles is the education of the staff. In the acute-care setting, ostomy services are delivered 24 hours a day; thus all health care providers must have a minimal competency in ostomy care. The education of nursing staff will include basic ostomy skills: stoma assessment, pouch fitting, pouch emptying, basic problem-solving skills, and patient support strategies. Education of the surgical staff will include stoma siting, the characteristics of the "ideal" stoma, and the role of the ostomy nurse specialist.

Policy and procedure development is important in the acute-care facility. The development, implementation, and audit of ostomy-related policies and procedures are in the domain of the ostomy nurse. For example, a policy addressing the fitting of a pouching system provides the bedside caregiver with a resource. A care plan, or care path, is an example of a tool that helps the caregiver provide basic care as well as the teaching points for a person with a new urinary or fecal diversion.

The ostomy nurse specialist in the acute-care setting will be instrumental in developing the ostomy formulary. The formulary contains supplies that are used in ostomy care, as well as draining wound management, and should include the fewest number of products that will meet the majority of the patient's needs. The ostomy formulary will ensure appropriate patient care while addressing the cost effectiveness of ostomy patient management.

The nurse providing ostomy services must develop a method to collect patient data and to use this data to document productivity. Data can be collected as a manual task or via a computerized database. Minimal patient data sets should include demographic data (e.g., name, birth date, contact information, diagnosis, surgery date), procedural information (e.g., type of surgery, indication for surgery, type of stoma, surgeon), productivity information (e.g., number of visits and amount of time spent with each patient), and clinical data (e.g., type of pouching system, complications). This type of information will facilitate organized care, a means to report productivity, the examination of trends, and the ability to collect outcome data.

The acute-care ostomy nurse must develop and maintain relationships with a wide diversity of resources such as:

  Discharge planners
  Dietary staff
  Radiology
  Nursing educators
  Medical staff members
    Gastroenterologist
    Nutritional support physicians
  Surgical staff members
    General surgeons
    Colorectal surgeons
    Urologists

The relationships that are developed with the key groups clarify the role of the ostomy nurse as well as provide continuity of care. It is important for role implementation to identify the champions for ostomy care in the facility and to work closely with those champions to develop a sound ostomy service.

It is very strongly suggested that all ostomy nurse specialists practicing in acute-care settings obtain certification. Certification documents that the ostomy nurse specialist has achieved a level of competence and specialization in the ostomy field. It reinforces to the public, other clinicians, and the facility administrators that this is the most qualified nurse. Certification in ostomy care is provided by the WOCN Certification Board, an independent board accredited by the National Commission for Certifying Agencies.

The role of the ostomy nurse specialist in acute care varies according to the institutional structure. Despite these variations, ensuring the highest level of care to the person with an ostomy remains fundamental.

HOME HEALTH CARE SETTING: PROVISION OF OSTOMY SERVICES

Lengths of stay in acute care have been steadily declining since the early 1980s, when the health care environment borrowed from the business literature and introduced clinical pathways in response to the implementation of DRGs (Hood, 2001). Patients and staff nurses today would be interested in the fact that in 1980, lengths of stay in acute care for uncomplicated fecal or urinary diversion surgery averaged 14 days. Granted, these stays usually included the preoperative portion of the stay (i.e., 24 to 48 hours for bowel preparation and stoma site selection). Today's length of stay for the same diagnosis is approximately 4.5 days; all preoperative procedures take place on an outpatient basis before admission.

This is quite meaningful to the patient undergoing a surgical procedure that will entail significant alterations in bodily function and require acquisition of a specific skill set for the management of those functions at home. For many patients, it means that an ostomy nurse specialist will coordinate or provide care and support to move the patient toward independent ostomy management. However, some patients do not receive any ostomy instruction, and others are not ready or physically able to participate in ostomy education while in the acute-care setting. For others, complications from surgery may result in an open wound or a flush or retracted stoma that is difficult to manage; the patient may have compromised dexterity or learning abilities; there may even be a lack of a reliable caregiver. These are the types of patients that may require the follow-up assistance of a home health nurse following discharge from the acute-care setting. More specifically, they require follow-up by an ostomy nurse specialist who is skilled in the care of this patient population.

Qualifying Criteria

Provision of home care nursing depends on the type of health care coverage that is available to the patient. All types of third-party payers cover skilled nursing services provided in the home care setting. Typically, *home* is defined as a patient's place of residence, including his or her own house or apartment, a relative's home, a personal care home, or another type of nonskilled institution. Depending on the third-party payer, the patient may need to meet certain "homebound" criteria. In general, a patient is considered homebound if he or she has a condition caused by an illness or injury that restricts his or her ability to leave the home (except with the assistance of supportive devices such as crutches, canes, walkers, and wheelchairs, or with the assistance of another person), or if leaving the home is medically contraindicated. For home care services to be reimbursable, the services provided must be reasonable and medically necessary to the treatment of a patient's illness or injury. Through documentation and discussion with the home care provider, a case manager from the managed care company determines the necessity, frequency, and duration of ongoing home care services (Wright and McNichol, 2000).

Specifically, skilled home nursing care for a patient with a new fecal or urinary diversion is typically considered reasonable and necessary to perform:

1. Assessment and observation.
2. Complex management strategies.
3. Teaching and training of the patient and family.

For example, if on admission to home health care a patient has a flush stoma near a midline incision whose pouching system leaks frequently, he or she may require several days and perhaps weeks of daily visits to determine a pouching system that can contain the effluent while allowing the incision to begin healing. As the wound heals and an adequate pouching system is used, the wear time on the pouching system increases, and the patient is able to learn the nuances of stoma management and progress toward being able to provide self care, including making pouch changes. Gradually the frequency of the visits decreases as the patient becomes stable and independent, and capable of caring for himself or herself. The patient is discharged when he or she is able to identify resources for obtaining supplies, and can articulate signs and symptoms of exacerbation and when to notify his or her physician. If the patient is unable to accomplish self care, he or she may be discharged to the care of a capable caregiver and the oversight of his or her physician. Alternatively it may be recommended that the patient not remain at home; instead he or she may be referred to a higher level of care with increased access to skilled caregivers, such as in a long-term care setting.

Home Conditions Affecting Care Delivery

The nurse's ability to affect the patient's outcome in the home setting is influenced by the home environment. For example, the lack of an adequate water supply affects the ostomy care regimen: the tail closures of drainable pouches cannot be as easily cleaned or as well, nor can the nighttime drainage system of a patient who elects to use one following urostomy surgery be effectively rinsed. Adequate skin cleansing before pouching system application may be compromised, and hand washing may be sporadic or omitted, potentially leading to infection. However, generally the principles of infection control in home care are the same as in other settings, although adjustments can be made in specific circumstances to accommodate either the facilities or the caregiver's capabilities. The provision of privacy is often a challenge for home care patients; some require extended periods in the bathroom initially and sometimes express frustration over residual room odor or an awareness of "taking too much time" when people are waiting outside the bathroom door. For some, dependence on a mirror for the accurate placement of their pouch is established in the acute-care setting. If there is no mirror available at home in which they can comfortably visualize their stoma, and if they are unwilling or unable to attempt pouching system placement without one, one must be obtained. Finally, all home care nurses must be vigilant regarding their own and their patients' personal safety, because they visit in a variety of home environments. Conditions in the home that affect clinical care can affect the outcomes of that care (Baker, 2001).

Working With Caregivers

Inherent to the intermittent nature of home health care is the ability of patients to care for themselves between the nurse's visits, with or without the assistance of a caregiver. Although this sounds reasonable, on closer inspection it is troublesome. As the elderly population expands, an increasing number of elderly people will have health problems that prevent them from caring for themselves (Wright and McNichol, 2000).

Caregivers fall into two broad categories: (1) caregivers working for pay who are part of the formal health care sector (i.e., home care workers) and (2) unpaid "informal" caregivers (usually family members) who are motivated by a deeper commitment to the patient. The ideal situation is one of families caring for seniors or seniors caring for other seniors. In reality, demographic trends suggest that family members may not be available to provide care when needed for a variety of reasons; these might include the children's or spouse's work schedule, that children live far away from their parents, or that seniors are suffering from chronic illness when they are needed as a family caregiver.

Unfortunately for some ostomy patients, some caregivers are not willing to learn skills for bowel and bladder management. Cultural mores or lack of common knowledge regarding ostomy surgery may deter some. Although some of these people can be educated and become accepting and helpful caregivers, others cannot. A caregiver or person significant to the patient who demonstrates a disapproving or fearful attitude toward the patient, the ostomy, or the pouching system can have a deleterious effect on the patient's rehabilitation outcome. The nurse in the home has a unique opportunity to assess the integration of the ostomy into the patient's lifestyle and must be aware of the impact it has on the patient's relationships. Even when a patient is able to care for the ostomy completely on his or her own, it is often recommended that a caregiver be identified and taught the patient's ostomy routine so that care can be provided should the patient become incapacitated for any period of time due to accident, injury, or illness.

Although many patients can be taught self care after an adequate pouching system has been determined and the need for adaptive equipment assessed and addressed, there are some patients for whom a regular caregiver is necessary for the daily care and routine changing of an ostomy pouching system. If no caregiver is available and arrangements cannot be made for the regular provision of care in the home, alternate care settings (such as assisted living or long-term care) should be suggested.

Role Implications

Providing home health care for patients with urinary or fecal diversions has numerous implications for the ostomy nurse specialist role. Home care agencies are required to measure and substantiate the outcomes of the services they provide. This has created an opportunity for the ostomy nurse to be instrumental in designing outcome measurements to validate the effectiveness of ostomy care protocol. Since caring for a patient with a complex ostomy management situation can be cost prohibitive for a home health agency, it becomes essential that the care be designed, implemented, and monitored in the most cost-effective way possible. Ostomy nurse specialists are in an ideal position to offer services that accomplish just that. Initial assessments, early interventions, patient/caregiver education, staff education, policy and procedure development, case management of complex cases, quality improvement, and utilization review are a few services that the ostomy care nurse can provide the home health agency (WOCN, 1999).

Ostomy care nurses can be instrumental in establishing an effective product formulary for the management of simple and complex urinary and fecal diversions. A selection of cut-to-fit one- and two-piece pectin-based options will give many patients a reasonable range of choices. Other products may include pouches for those patients with very limited financial resources and/or deficiencies in manual dexterity or visual acuity; pouching systems for skin level or below-skin level ostomies; and barrier products with built-in convexity or separate and moldable barrier rings that provide convexity. Although some purchasing agents might attempt to discourage the addition of such products to the formulary under the guise of controlling costs, the prompt introduction of such interventions can prevent complications, enhance patient independence, decrease visit frequency, and ultimately *decrease* supply costs because of longer wear time.

Role Utilization

Many home health agencies opt to contract with a nurse specializing in the care of patients with urinary or fecal diversions instead of having one on staff, or they may have only one such employee to serve a very large geographic area. In these instances it becomes the role of the ostomy nurse consultant to educate and essentially train the generalist field nurses in the recognition of common ostomy complications and possible interventions for each. Instruction for this group should include the essentials of ostomy patient education for each type of diversion and teaching strategies for patients and caregivers. Instruction must be provided to the nurse so that she or he is able to advise the patient regarding the purchasing options for ostomy supplies after discharge from the home health agency, aspects of traveling with an ostomy, and the occasional need for the resizing of the stoma. Indications for referral to the ostomy nurse specialist should be a component of the education provided to staff nurses; some examples of these referral parameters might include a pouching system's wear time of less than 3 days, identification of symptoms indicating the patient's failure to gradually move toward acceptance of the ostomy, or any discomfort the field staff member may have regarding her or his assessment abilities. Although this system is somewhat less effective (albeit slightly more efficient) than having every patient with a urinary or fecal diversion be visited in their home by an ostomy nurse specialist, many home health agency providers have seen prompt, accurate intervention strategies implemented successfully by these trained resource nurses who follow established policies and protocols, and have realized positive patient outcomes.

The role of the ostomy nurse specialist in the home care environment continues to change and evolve, but the goal of home health care services always remains the same: to move the patient or caregiver toward independence in stoma care and toward adjustment in living with a stoma.

LONG-TERM CARE AND REHABILITATION SETTING

Long-term care, rehabilitation, and subacute-care settings offer varied opportunities and challenges for the ostomy nurse specialist. Although the actual number of patients with ostomies in these settings may be small, the patient, as well as the facility, can benefit from the services of an ostomy nurse. The employment options for the nurse specializing in ostomy care may include becoming a staff member, providing contracted services, or furnishing services on an as-needed basis. While the services of the ostomy nurse specialist depend upon the needs of the facility and patient population, the roles may include that of the clinician providing direct patient care, the consultant advising staff, and the educator assisting staff in obtaining competency in ostomy care.

The ostomy patient population in a long-term care facility is diverse and may include the person who has had a fecal or urinary diversion for 10 to 20 years who finds that he or she can no longer independently perform self ostomy care or function independently in the home setting. Other reasons for a person to require placement in a skilled nursing facility (SNF) can include dementia, a deteriorated physical condition impacting self care (i.e., Parkinson's disease), or physical and medical needs that overwhelm family members.

After surgery, ostomy patients may be transferred from the acute-care facility to the SNF setting if they are unable to become independent in their daily ostomy care or to function in the home setting. These patients present challenges for the ostomy nurse specialist as well as staff that may not be comfortable with ostomy skills. The patient with a new stoma will require both ongoing evaluation to determine whether he or she can acquire self care skills, and frequent stoma assessments as the stoma heals and changes in size and shape.

The facility's staff will need education regarding ostomy management. Other persons in the SNF may be those patients who before admission performed daily irrigations but are no longer be able to perform this skill due to other medical conditions. The ostomy nurse specialist assists the patient and the staff in developing a new ostomy care plan. The agitated resident with Alzheimer's or other dementias who pulls off the ostomy pouch can be frustrating for the staff. This resident needs the expertise of the ostomy nurse specialist, who can develop and teach the staff strategies for problem solving.

Rehabilitation Facility

In the rehabilitation setting the patient with an ostomy may be of any age, depending on the medical indication for rehabilitation. The goal in this setting is to focus on the patient becoming independent in his or her ostomy care. The person with an ostomy may have a spinal cord injury or have suffered a recent cerebral vascular accident; he or she may be participating in rehabilitation that is focused on recovering a lost function, or learning to live with the loss of function. The ostomy nurse specialist needs to be creative in developing a care plan to meet these patients' special needs. A multidisciplinary team approach is essential. Collaborating with physical and occupational therapists provides an approach that addresses the patient's needs well and results in a positive patient outcome.

The staff in rehabilitation facilities focuses on working with the patient to help him or her become independent in activities of daily living. This focus will extend to assessing the patient's ability to empty as well as to change the pouching system.

Product Formulary

The development of an ostomy product formulary is key to the provision of both the appropriate equipment for the patient as well as cost-effective ostomy care. The ostomy nurse specialist works with the SNF administration in building a formulary that meets the needs of the majority of the ostomy patients. Key contracts are evaluated for completeness as related to ostomy products, and suggestions on updated and more cost-effective supplies are made by the ostomy nurse specialist.

Payment systems in the SNF setting vary, depending on the patient's status and insurance. Medicare reimbursement uses the Prospective Payment System (PPS). The Minimum Data Set (MDS) is an assessment tool that the PPS uses to identify the patient's problems and to develop the care plan. Payment rates are based upon the data collected by the MDS. Payment is bundled; that is, the facility receives a per diem payment that covers all care provided, and there is no reimbursement for supplies. Medicaid reimbursement, too, is generally (for most states) a flat per diem rate for all care and supplies. The ostomy nurse specialist is in a position to ensure judicial use of ostomy supplies, which will be vital in controlling costs and providing a good outcome for the person with a stoma.

Educator

As an educator the ostomy nurse specialist works with a diverse patient care staff. Although the care of the SNF patient is overseen by a registered nurse, most bedside care is delivered by a licensed practical nurse or a nurse assistant. This staff may not have ostomy management skills, and tools to assist with basic assessment and interventions must be developed. Simple, step-by-step, written instructions for the patient's care are useful for the staff to follow when providing ostomy care.

Other areas of education in which the ostomy nurse specialist will be crucial include a solid ostomy orientation program, including skills checklists, and developing basic ostomy policies and procedures.

The ostomy nurse specialist in the long-term care and rehabilitation setting plays a key role in helping maintain the dignity and quality of life for the person who can no longer care for himself or herself. The demands in this area of practice will continue to increase as the aging population increases.

OUTPATIENT SETTING

The ostomy nurse specialist provides a valuable service in the outpatient setting. The role of the ostomy nurse specialist will be implemented differently depending upon the physical setting. In some clinic settings the nurse is part of the multidisciplinary team, working with a surgeon or gastroenterologist. An alternative outpatient setting might be in a private physician's office, providing ostomy services. A third setting is the nurse-managed clinic, in which the ostomy nurse specialist works with a medical director, who provides backup and assistance as indicated. Patients requiring outpatient ostomy services may include those who have been discharged from acute care without sufficient skills for self care, patients who require follow-up to ensure quality care and who need stoma and skin assessment as well as assessment of adjustment, those who have been doing well after discharge but have run into stoma management problems, or those who are referred for skilled services by the surgeon or primary care physician. Other patients seeking outpatient ostomy services may be those who have had an ostomy for some time and have developed problems or whose stoma care routines need updating.

When outpatient services or an ostomy clinic is being developed, the following issues should be addressed: space allocation including access to bathroom facilities, development of a scheduling process, creation of a record-keeping system (usually working with the Medical Records department if associated with a health care facility), and the development of documentation forms. The ostomy nurse specialist must create forms that will ensure appropriate documentation of the patient's history and stoma problem, the intervention, and the instructions given. Letters outlining the plan of care are sent to the referral source as well as to the primary care physician. In addition, policies and procedures to be followed during the visit must be formulated that are approved by the medical director and are in compliance with any local and state regulations.

Unfortunately, there is no reimbursement for outpatient ostomy services provided by the ostomy nurse specialist from most traditional insurance payers or Medicare. Advanced practice nurses in some states may qualify for reimbursement; this must be researched on an individual basis. Fee for service arrangements are usually negotiated with patients prior to consultation, although some outpatient facilities that are related to acute-care settings or even long-term care settings will provide services to the ostomy patient as a service to the community. The role of the ostomy nurse specialist in this care setting consists mainly of troubleshooting immediate problems, formulating a plan of care, and educating the patient or caregiver in the necessary interventions.

As in other care settings, the selection of a formulary of products is extremely important in order to deliver appropriate ostomy products that are cost effective. It is important to establish guidelines for the distribution of supplies to patients and to clarify whether patients will be charged for supplies used, since, if there is any reimbursement for the visit, supplies are usually included.

The adjustment to living with a fecal or urinary diversion occurs over time. With the continued decrease in length of hospital stay, as well as increasing constraints in the delivery of home care, the outpatient ostomy clinic can provide a needed resource for the person with an ostomy.

INDUSTRY

Ostomy nurses have been migrating to the wider auspices of industry for over two decades. The benefits of this shift can be seen in the businesses in which these nurses have found new careers as well as in the hospitals, long-term care facilities, and home health care agencies where many ostomy nurses first began their careers. The industry to which many ostomy nurses have moved offers career opportunities with durable medical equipment suppliers, medical device manufacturers, pharmaceutical companies, health care provider organizations, and independent medical consulting.

Of the industry positions that use an ostomy nurse's expertise, the one that comes closest to working in a hospital or clinical environment is the *medical monitor/clinical research assistant.* A medical monitor is involved in clinical trials from the proposal through protocol writing, to the monitoring of study sites, interim analyses, and the final report. A nurse in this position travels to investigator sites to observe processes and train personnel on an average of once to twice per month. While the medical monitor remains relatively close to patient care through setting up and observing trial protocols, there is very rarely any opportunity for hands-on patient care. However, this role does allow the ostomy nurse to contribute to product innovation and improving the lives of people with ostomies.

Nurses can also be very successful in *sales positions*. The ostomy nurse specialist as salesperson has the advantage of being familiar with the mindset of her or his customers as well as understanding the unique needs of a person with an ostomy. This familiarity can result in product selection that, based on the customer's needs, is a success for both the salesperson and the customer. Bringing sensitivity to the needs of the patient, clinician, and health care organization alike, the ostomy nurse specialist can assist in problem solving to meet those needs in an efficient and effective manner.

The ostomy nurse's unique perspective can also be quite valuable to a *marketing* group. Knowing the perspective of both patients and health care professionals is an asset when determining a marketing plan for that particular customer audience. The experience and knowledge an ostomy nurse brings to a marketing group can enhance and build upon information gleaned from focus groups, surveys, and other resources normally used when planning marketing strategies.

Nurses working as *independent contractors* can pursue medical writing, which permits freelancing from home and can be financially rewarding. Independent contractors can work in presentation services, developing and providing education programs. Independent ostomy nurses also contract clinical services to provide direct care services to patients. Providing clinical services to underserved markets can be rewarding for both the provider and the facility hiring the ostomy nurse independent contractor. The ostomy nurse can provide clinical services to a select group of patients, and the facility benefits from specialty nurse outcomes: patient satisfaction, a decrease in complications, and in some cases a decreased length of stay. Other job options for independent contractor ostomy nurses

exist in market research and specialty consulting, which entail patient evaluations as well as development of policy, procedures, and protocol.

The ostomy nurse specialist is a valuable asset as an *educator*. Educational sessions can be provided on an informal basis, such as a staff inservice session to introduce a new ostomy pouching system. The ostomy nurse, through the company being represented, can develop formal education programs that provide continuing education credits. The education role may also extend to informal United Ostomy Association sessions to educate the members regarding current or new ostomy products. Some ostomy companies employing an ostomy nurse provide a telephone consultation service for both the paient and other health care providers to answer questions and problems that may arise where there is no ostomy nurse specialist available. Developing teaching booklets, videos, and other educational material is an area in which the ostomy nurse can be valuable. The ostomy nurse has the expertise and skill to write clear, concise, accurate information for a new ostomy patient based on previous clinical experience in teaching ostomy patients.

The ostomy nurse specialist in industry offers many benefits to the organization. The most tangible benefits fall into two areas. First, the ostomy nurse's expertise serves to blend the clinical and business aspects of a medical equipment company to make it stronger as a whole; secondly, more credibility is given to the company in the marketplace. The nurse can act as a liaison and translator between the company and the health care worker, the patient, and the health care marketplace, and she or he can assist in marketing strategy, sales force education, customer education, and patient education about products.

The input of the ostomy nurse frequently results in better products. Strength and persistence learned through working with all levels of medical personnel have helped nurses stand their ground when advocating for products or product features that would benefit patients. Perspectives based on a caregiver's experiences with patients can enhance the development process, as can a nurse's broad understanding of the hospital environment and related issues (such as infection). Thus the ostomy nurse can guide the development of products that are designed to benefit patients and halt development of products that are not.

There are many outstanding opportunities for the ostomy nurse specialist in industry, and, although leaving the patient's side may require an adjustment for the ostomy nurse, the opportunity to effect the delivery of improved products and services to the person with an ostomy is a unique and rare challenge.

CONCLUSION

The ostomy care nurse has many opportunities for employment, working with the person who undergoes a fecal and urinary diversion or with others who perform this work. The role of the person specializing in ostomy care had humble beginnings but met an important need; it has evolved into a certified nursing specialty that is supported by the WOCN Society, a nursing specialty organization.

SELF-ASSESSMENT EXERCISES

Questions

1. Name the person who was the first enterostomal therapist.
2. List two key initiatives in the history of the WOCN Society.
3. Name two roles in the acute-care setting for the ostomy nurse specialist.
4. The main focus of the ostomy nurse specialist in providing home care services is:
   a. To monitor vital signs, looking for indications of an infectious process.
   b. To teach the patient or caregiver independence in ostomy management.
   c. To coordinate the home care and the ancillary services such as physical therapy.
   d. To be the primary deliverer of ostomy services.
5. The model for delivery of care in the skilled nursing facility:
   a. Is based on acute-care staffing standards; thus problem solving by the registered nurses should be encouraged.

b. Is based on using licensed practice nurses and nursing assistants to provide care; thus education on care should be geared toward staff who may have limited experience in managing complex ostomy patients.
   c. Does not matter when considering the provision of ostomy care services.
   d. Is not a consideration for the ostomy nurse specialist, as he or she provides direct ostomy services in all skilled nursing facilities.
6. What are two career opportunities for the ostomy nurse specialist in the ostomy industry?
7. The ostomy nurse specialist should develop outpatient ostomy services under the supervision of:
   a. The administrator of director of outpatient services.
   b. The medical director.
   c. The director of nursing.
   d. The finance department.

Answers

1. Norma Gill
2. Key initiatives include: name changes (from NAAET to IAET and then IAET to WOCN), development of a certification exam, incorporation of the ET Nursing Certification Board as a separate organization, launching of efforts aimed at health care reforms, and the establishment of the Center for Clinical Investigation (CCI) to advance evidence-based practice.
3. Roles: clinician, educator, and/or consultant
4. b
5. b
6. Working with durable medical equipment suppliers, medical device manufacturers, pharmaceutical companies, and health care provider organizations, and independent medical consulting
7. b

REFERENCES

Blakely P: Future trends in ET nursing internationally. In Erwin-Toth P, Krasner D, editors: *Enterostomal therapy nursing: growth and evolution of a nursing specialty worldwide: a festschrift for Norma N. Gill-Thompson, ET,* Baltimore, 1996, Halgo.

Broadwell D: President's Message, *JET* 8(5):5, 1981.

Doughty D: President's message: collective strength, *JWOCN* 28:119-20, 2001.

Doughty D: President's message: back to the future, *JWOCN* 27:1-2, 2000.

Erwin-Toth P, Krasner D: *Enterostomal therapy nursing, growth & evolution of a nursing specialty worldwide,* Baltimore, 1996, Halgo.

ET J Summer:9, 1976.

ET J, Summer:13, 1976.

Gray M et al: Evidence-based nursing practice: a primer for nurses, *JWOCN* 29:283-286, 2002.

Hood, FJ: Medicare's home health prospective payment system, *South Med J* 94(10):986-989, 2001.

Klein L: President's Message, *J Enterostom Ther* 12(5):155-156, 1985.

Motta J: President's Message, *J Enterostom Ther* 15(2):51-53, 1988.

Wound, Ostomy and Continence Nurses Society: Professional practice fact sheet: reimbursement/home health: reimbursement options for WOC (ET) nurses in home health, Laguna Beach, Calif, 1999, WOCN, available at website: www.wocn.org, under Publications, Fact Sheets.

WOCN News, Oct/Nov:11, 1994.

WOCN News, Spring:13-14, 1995.

Wright K, McNichol LL: Home environment: Implications for wound care practice development. In Bryant R, *Acute and chronic wounds: nursing management,* ed 2, St Louis, 2000, Mosby.

PART

II

Fecal Diversions

Anatomy and Physiology of the Gastrointestinal Tract

3

RUTH A. BRYANT

OBJECTIVES

1. Describe the structures of the gastrointestinal tract, including the accessory organs, and their corresponding functions.
2. Describe the four layers of the bowel wall, including the differences between the layers of the small bowel and colon.
3. Explain the role of the pharyngoesophageal and esophagogastric sphincters and the ileocecal valve.
4. Describe the mechanisms that normally protect the gastric and duodenal mucosa from ulceration.
5. Identify factors that modulate gastric secretion production.
6. Explain the role of intrinsic factor in the prevention of pernicious anemia and the implications for the patient who has had a gastrectomy.
7. Discriminate between the peritoneum and the mesentery.
8. Describe the physiologic processes that regulate intestinal motility.
9. Compare and contrast the volume, composition, and function of the fluid secreted daily by the salivary glands, stomach, small intestine, pancreas, and biliary system.
10. Describe vascular supply and venous drainage for the small intestine and the colon.
11. Explain the role of the enterohepatic circulation.
12. Correlate the production of gas and odor with the presence of normal bowel flora within the ileum and different locations in the colon.
13. Correlate the sensory function of the anal epithelium above and below the dentate line with bowel continence.
14. Describe the relationship between the external sphincter, the puborectal muscles, and the levator ani muscles.
15. Compare the internal and external anal sphincters in terms of function, innervation, and response to rectal distention.
16. Describe the normal defecation process.
17. Describe the exocrine functions of the pancreas.
18. Identify factors that affect the liver's rate of regeneration.
19. Explain why the liver is a common site of metastasis for gastrointestinal malignancies.
20. List key functions of the liver.
21. Explain the role of the gallbladder in digestion of fats.

INTRODUCTION

The gastrointestinal (GI) tract is a constellation of complex organs that provide numerous functions without conscious input. These organs are responsible for complex digestive, secretory, absorptive, and excretory processes that involve multiple physiologic activities: (1) GI motility (propulsion and mixing), (2) secretion of digestive juices, (3) digestion of nutrients, (4) absorption of nutrients, and (5) preparation of unabsorbed particles for excretion. GI tract function also has a significant impact on fluid-electrolyte balance, because large volumes of fluid are secreted into and resorbed from the lumen of the bowel every day during the processes of nutrient digestion and absorption (Table 3-1).

The organs within the GI tract can be divided into those of the alimentary canal and the accessory organs. The alimentary canal is a continuous tube approximately 9 m long, extending from the mouth to the anus and including the mouth, the esophagus, the stomach, the small intestine, the colon, the rectum, the anal canal, and the anus. Accessory organs are those organs located outside the alimentary canal that contribute to the ingestion and digestion of nutrients: the liver, the gallbladder, and the pancreas (Figure 3-1).

A clear understanding of normal anatomy and physiology provides the framework for understanding pathologic states and physiologic changes induced by medical disorders and surgical procedures. Thus the nurse caring for the patient with an ostomy or continent diversion must understand normal GI tract function to provide appropriate care and education. This chapter addresses GI tract anatomy and physiology with an emphasis on structure and functions that are likely to be altered in the patient requiring a fecal diversion. The first section deals with the alimentary canal; each structure along the canal is discussed in terms of key structural characteristics, major functions, vascular supply, and innervation. By means of the same organizational approach the final section of the chapter discusses accessory organs.

ALIMENTARY CANAL

General Structure

The histologic characteristics of the alimentary canal are essentially the same throughout its length, with minor variations, and comprise four tissue layers: the mucosa, the submucosa, the muscularis, and the serosa, or adventitia (Figure 3-2). Common characteristics of the tissue layers are described in this section; any variations are identified in the discussions specific to that individual organ.

Mucosa. The innermost layer of the gut wall is the mucosal layer, which itself is composed of four distinct tissue layers: the mucous epithelium, or surface layer, the lamina propria (a connective tissue layer), the muscularis mucosae layer (a thin layer of circular muscle that separates the mucosa from the submucosa), and the mucosal layer, which contains multiple mucus-secreting glands (i.e., goblet cells). The mucosal layer is particularly significant because it maintains a moist inner surface that lubricates the innermost gut layer, facilitates the forward movement of the food bolus, and prevents mucosal abrasions from coarse foods.

Submucosa. The second layer of the gut wall is the submucosal layer; key structures in this layer include connective tissue, blood and lymph vessels, nerve fibers, and a number of reticuloendothelial cells.

Muscularis. The third layer of the gut wall is the muscularis, which consists of the inner circular and outer longitudinal layers of smooth-muscle fibers. These smooth muscles are responsible for

TABLE 3-1   Characteristics of Gastrointestinal Fluid (24-hr volume)

FLUID	pH	SODIUM (mmol)	POTASSIUM (mmol)	CHLORIDE (mmol)	BICARBONATE (mmol)	WATER (ml)
Saliva	6.0-7.0	20-80	16-23	24-44	20-60	1000
Gastric Juice	1.0-3.5	20-100	4-12	52-124	0	2000
Bile	7.8	120-200	3-12	80-120	30-50	800
Pancreatic Juice	8.0-8.3	120-150	2-7	54-95	70-110	1200
Intestinal Juice	7.5-8.9	80-130	12-21	48-116	23-30	3000

Modified from Givens BA, Simmons SA: *Gastroenterology in clinical nursing*, ed 4, St Louis, 1984, Mosby; Urden LD, Stacy KM, Lough ME: *Thelan's critical care nursing: diagnosis and management*, ed 4, St Louis, 2002, Mosby.

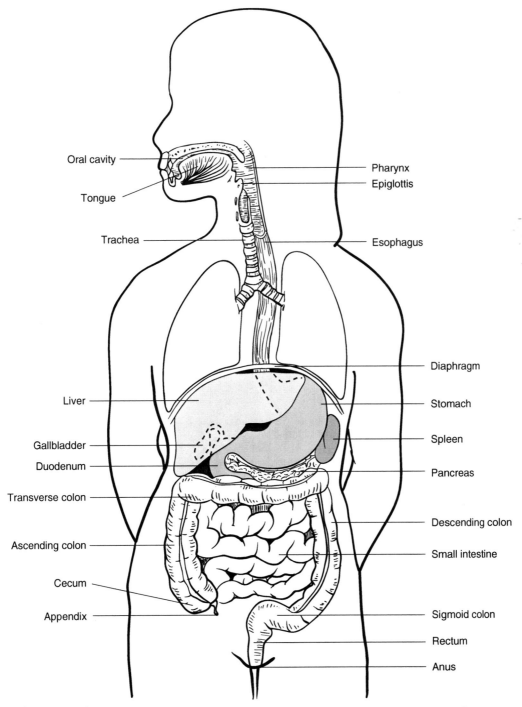

Figure 3-1   Anatomy of gastrointestinal system. (From Broadwell DC, Jackson BS: *Principles of ostomy care*, St Louis, 1982, Mosby.)

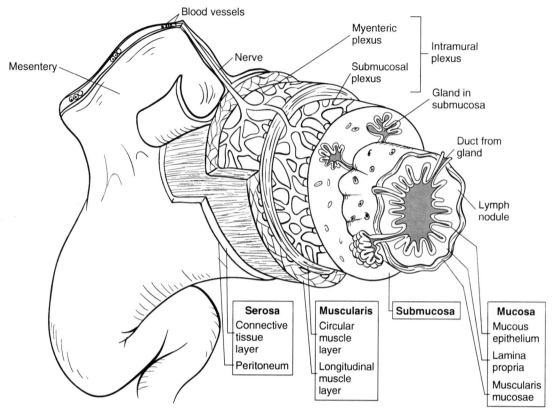

Figure 3-2   Basic structure of digestive tract in cross-section. (From Thibodeau GA, Patton KT: *Anatomy & physiology,* ed 4, St Louis, 1999, Mosby.)

the mixing of the food bolus throughout the stomach and intestine and for the forward movement of the food bolus.

Serosa. The outermost layer of the alimentary canal is a serous membrane. Structures located within the peritoneal cavity are covered by serosa, a connective tissue layer that in turn is covered by the visceral peritoneum. This continuity with the visceral peritoneum is a factor in the severe abdominal pain frequently experienced by patients with transmural inflammatory bowel disease; if the inflammation involves the serosa, it also may involve the peritoneum, resulting in a generalized peritonitis.

Because the serosa does not contain mucus-secreting glands, exposure to air results in inflammation, with eventual necrosis and sloughing of the serosal layer. This inflammatory response is significant to nurses caring for patients with an ostomy diversion, because stomas that are not matured (i.e., everted to expose the mucosal layer) are prone to develop an inflammation of the serosa (serositis), which is accompanied by edema of the stoma that can result in partial or complete obstruction. Stomas that are not matured at surgery must "self-mature," a process that occurs when the inflamed serosal surfaces adhere to each other, causing a gradual eversion of the stoma.

Structures located outside the peritoneal cavity, such as the esophagus, are covered with a connective tissue layer known as the adventitia.

Regulatory Agents of GI Function

Numerous compounds have been identified that have a regulatory effect on GI tract function, particularly in the small intestine. These can be classified as peptide and nonpeptide hormones. Peptide hormones such as gastrin, cholecystokinin (CCK), secretin, glucagon, growth hormone releasing factor, gastrin inhibitory peptide (GIP), vasoactive intestinal peptide (VIP), insulin, substance P, gastrin releasing peptide, transforming growth factor-alpha (TGF-α), and insulin-like growth factor (IGF) are produced and released throughout the GI tract, many within the enteric neurons. Some of these work solely on the GI structures, and some also trigger extraintestinal effects.

Nonpeptide hormones include vitamin D, aldosterone, hydrocortisone, nitric oxide, norepinephrine, epinephrine, histamine, serotonin, and platelet activating factor.

MOUTH

The mouth, also referred to as the oral cavity, represents the proximal end of the alimentary canal. It is bordered laterally by the cheeks, anteriorly by the lips, posteriorly by the throat, superiorly by the palate, and inferiorly by a muscular floor.

Structure

Key structures within the mouth include the teeth, the tongue, the hard and soft palates, and the salivary glands. The adult normally has 32 teeth, which play an important role in chewing and in speech. The tongue is a muscular organ that is covered by moist squamous epithelium; the anterior surface is covered by papillae, where the taste buds are located. The tongue is supplied with both intrinsic and extrinsic muscles, and jointly these muscles control the tongue's shape, position, and movements. The palates form the roof of the mouth, with the hard, or bony, palate located anteriorly and the soft, or muscular, palate located posteriorly. A large number of glands that contribute to production of saliva are present in the mouth; the three largest pairs are the parotid, the submaxillary, and the sublingual glands. Saliva actually represents a combination of mucus and thin serous secretions; saliva also contains amylase, which is an enzyme capable of beginning carbohydrate digestion. The usual volume of saliva production is about 1 to 1.5 L/day (Seeley, Stephens, and Tate, 1991).

Function

Major functions carried out by structures within the oral cavity include speech, nutrient ingestion, initiation of digestion, and swallowing.

Speech. Both the tongue and the teeth play an important role in the precise formation of words, required for clear speech.

Ingestion of Nutrients. Normally nutrients are taken into the body through the mouth; disease or injury resulting in inability to eat and drink necessitates alternate routes for nutrient ingestion. The tongue provides for the sensation of taste, which is mediated by means of the taste buds present in some of the papillae. Because taste is an important stimulus to nutrient ingestion, this is an important function.

Digestion. Mechanical digestion of nutrients begins in the mouth with the process of chewing, or mastication, which breaks large food particles into smaller particles and thereby increases the surface available for enzymatic action. Thorough chewing of food can contribute significantly to the efficiency of the digestive process. Structures that contribute to the ability to chew are the tongue, the teeth, and the muscles of mastication.

Enzymatic digestion of carbohydrates is also initiated in the mouth by the action of salivary amylase, which can reduce polysaccharides into maltose and isomaltose. Actually only a small percentage of carbohydrates are digested in the mouth, because most starches are covered with cellulose and therefore are "protected" from enzymatic action (Sanford, 1992).

Swallowing. An important function of the mouth and related structures is swallowing, which begins transport of the nutrients along the digestive pathway. Any condition that interferes with the ability to swallow places a person at risk for nutritional compromise because of inadequate intake.

Swallowing is a complex act that involves the tongue, the soft palate, the muscles of the oropharynx, the upper esophageal sphincter, the epiglottis, the muscles of the esophagus, and gravity. The normal sequence of events is as follows: the tongue forms a bolus of food and pushes the bolus of food into the oropharynx; the soft palate is elevated to close the opening to the nasopharynx, and elevation of the larynx and movement of the epiglottis close the opening to the larynx; the pharyngeal muscles contract, respiration is inhibited, and the upper esophageal sphincter relaxes, which pushes food through the pharynx and into the esophagus. Movement of the bolus through the esophagus is accomplished by peristaltic waves (i.e., the muscles distal to the food bolus relax while the muscles proximal to the food bolus contract and push the food along) (Chang, Sitrin, and Black, 1996).

Swallowing is initiated voluntarily but is completed as a reflex action; reflex activity takes over once the food bolus reaches the oropharynx. Swallowing is facilitated by the presence of saliva, which acts as a lubricant for the food particles.

Saliva also helps prevent infections of the oral cavity, because it constantly "bathes" the mouth and because it has some degree of antibacterial action.

ESOPHAGUS

Structure

The esophagus, which is approximately 25 cm in length, is the muscular tube that connects the oropharynx to the stomach. The walls of the esophagus are composed of the four layers common to the GI tract; the outer layer is adventitia as opposed to serosa. The muscular layer consists of striated (skeletal) muscle in the proximal portion of the esophagus and smooth muscle in the distal esophagus. The mucosal layer is composed of moist, stratified squamous epithelium.

The esophagus generally is divided into three sections: the upper esophagus, the midesophagus, and the lower esophagus. Proximally and distally the esophagus is bounded by sphincter mechanisms: the upper esophageal sphincter (pharyngoesophageal), and the lower esophageal sphincter (esophagogastric). These sphincters prevent reflux from the esophagus into the oropharynx and from the stomach into the esophagus (Georges, 2000).

Function

The major functions of the esophagus include transport of the food from the mouth and oropharynx into the stomach, and the production of mucus. Transport of food occurs via the aforementioned swallowing mechanism. A food bolus in the oropharynx causes reduced pressure within the upper esophageal sphincter; the sphincter opens and allows the food or fluid to enter the esophagus. The bolus is moved toward the stomach by peristalsis; as the bolus approaches the lower esophageal sphincter, the sphincter relaxes to allow the food or fluid to enter the stomach. The lower esophageal sphincter relaxes only with the approach of a food bolus; at all other times it is tonically contracted to prevent reflux of gastric contents into the esophagus (Chang, Sitrin, and Black, 1996).

Peristaltic waves within the esophagus are stimulated by the presence of food or fluid within the esophagus, which activates the intramural plexus; the presence of food or fluid also causes vagal stimulation, which stimulates contraction of the skeletal and the smooth muscles within the esophagus.

The esophageal mucosa is protected by thick mucus that is produced in the submucosal layer and delivered through ducts to the mucosal surface.

Blood Supply and Innervation

Vascular supply to the esophagus derives from the esophageal branch of the thoracic aorta and from the left gastric artery, which branches from the celiac trunk of the abdominal aorta. Venous drainage occurs as follows: the upper esophagus is drained by the superior vena cava, the midesophagus is drained by the azygos vein, and the lower esophagus is drained by gastric veins that empty into the portal system. The esophagus is innervated by the vagus nerve (Seeley, Stephens, and Tate, 1991).

ABDOMINAL CAVITY AND PERITONEUM

Most of the organs in the GI tract are contained in the abdominal cavity. The abdominal cavity is separated from the thoracic cavity by the diaphragm and actually is continuous with the pelvic cavity. The stomach, the intestines, the liver, the spleen, the pancreas, and the kidneys are located within the abdominal cavity, and the pelvic cavity contains the urinary bladder, portions of the colon, and the internal reproductive organs.

The peritoneum is a serous membrane that lines much of the abdominal cavity and covers most of the abdominal organs. Organs located outside the peritoneum are described as retroperitoneal. The part of the peritoneum that lines the abdominal cavity is referred to as the parietal peritoneum, whereas the peritoneum that covers the abdominal organs is known as the visceral peritoneum. The mesentery is a double layer of peritoneum with a central layer of loose connective tissue; it encircles most of the small intestine and anchors it to the posterior abdominal wall. The mesentery is a vital support structure for the bowel, in that it contains the blood vessels and the nerve fibers that nourish and innervate the intestine. The lesser omentum is the name given to the mesentery that attaches the lesser curvature of the stomach to the liver and the diaphragm, and the mesentery that attaches the greater curvature of the stomach to the transverse colon and posterior abdominal wall is termed the greater omentum. The greater omentum is also known as the "fatty apron," because it hangs down in front of the stomach and large amounts of fat tend to accumulate in and between its double folds (Fenoglio-Preiser et al, 1999).

Stomach

Structure

The stomach is a distensible J-shaped organ located in the left upper quadrant of the abdomen. It extends from the lower end of the esophagus at T11 to the duodenum at the right of L1. The size and shape of the stomach depends on body position and extent of fullness; at capacity (1 to 1.5 L) the stomach is approximately 25 to 27.5 cm long and about 10.25 cm wide (Fenoglio-Preiser et al, 1999). Anteriorly the stomach touches the abdominal wall and the inferior aspect of the left liver lobe; posteriorly the stomach is situated against the pancreas and splenic vessels, the left kidney, and the adrenal gland.

The stomach can be divided into several anatomic regions (Figure 3-3). The cardia is an indistinct, narrow, circular, transitional band that surrounds the opening from the esophagus into the stomach (gastroesophageal junction) and separates the esophagus from the gastric body and fundus and the lesser curvature from the greater curvature. The fundus is the most superior part of the stomach and is to the left of the cardia. The gastric body is the largest part of the stomach; it curves toward the right, extends from the cardia to the antrum, and is characterized by the presence of numerous deep folds known as rugae. The most inferior aspect of the stomach is known as the antrum; it lies just proximal to the pyloric sphincter. The antrum is structurally different from the rest of the stomach in that rugae are not present. The pylorus is the most distal structure of the stomach and is a muscular sphincter that controls the flow of gastric contents into the duodenum and prevents the reflux of bile from the duodenum into the stomach.

Histology

The wall of the stomach consists of the four layers common to GI tract histology and is most commonly no more than 0.5 cm in thickness (Fenoglio-Preiser et al, 1999). Additional histologic features of the stomach wall include:

1. The stomach has three muscle layers rather than two, with an inner oblique layer in addition to the middle circular and the outer longitudinal layers. This additional muscle layer increases the stomach's ability to "churn" the gastric contents, thus contributing to mechanical digestion of nutrients.

2. The submucosal and mucosal layers are arranged in rugae; these deep folds allow for "stretching" of the gastric lining as the stomach fills with food and fluid.

3. The mucosal layer contains a large number of openings known as "gastric pits"; the gastric pits communicate with the gastric glands and provide drainage for their secretions. The gastric mucosa is covered with simple columnar epithelium.

Cellular Composition. Simple columnar epithelial cells line the stomach and the millions of gastric glands that penetrate downward into the mucosa. Four additional types of cells are found within a gastric gland: mucous neck cells, parietal cells, endocrine cells, and chief cells. Surface

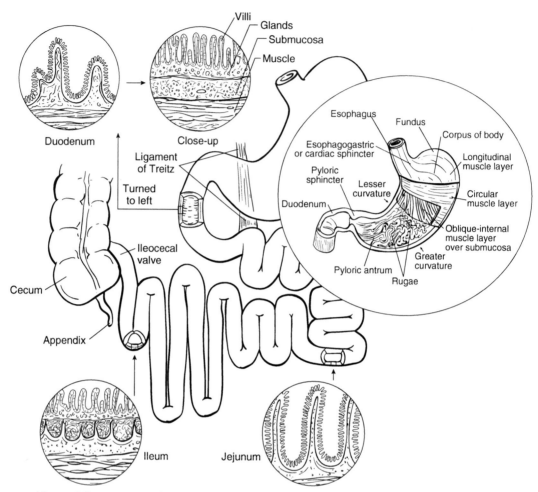

Figure 3-3 Anatomy of stomach small intestine. (Modified from Thompson JM et al: *Mosby's clinical nursing*, ed 5, St Louis, 2002, Mosby.)

mucous cells and mucous neck cells secrete a viscous and alkaline mucus that coats the superficial epithelial cells of the stomach. This mucous blanket is critical to protecting this acid-containing organ from proteolytic and acid gastric secretions. The mucus blanket these cells create is approximately 1 to 1.5 mm thick, with an adherent and consistently undisturbed innermost layer of mucus that serves to neutralize acid with mucosal bicarbonate. The pH of this innermost layer of mucus is 7.0 whereas the pH in the gastric lumen itself is typically 2.0 (Fenoglio-Preiser et al, 1999). In the

presence of gastric irritation, mucus production actually increases. An additional barrier to gastric contents is provided by the surface membranes of the mucosal cells and by the tight junctions between the mucosal cells. Gastric ulcers may result when this mucosal barrier is damaged; substances known to be "barrier breakers" include aspirin, alcohol, and bile salts, which contact the gastric mucosa when duodenal contents reflux into the stomach.

The parietal (oxyntic) cells produce hydrochloric acid (HCl), intrinsic factor, and (TGF-α).

The low pH caused by the HCL inactivates the salivary amylase and inhibits carbohydrate digestion, but it also serves to activate pepsin, which initiates protein digestion. Intrinsic factor is a substance that bonds with vitamin B_{12} and subsequently facilitates absorption of vitamin B_{12} in the ileum.

The endocrine cells produce numerous regulatory hormones that affect gastric secretion (Fenoglio-Preiser et al, 1999). For example, G cells make gastrin, a powerful stimulant to the secretion of HCl and a promoter of pepsinogen secretion and gastric motility. D cells inhibit gastric acid, gastrin, and intrinsic factor secretion by secreting somatostatin. EC cells (enterochromaffin) produce serotonin and substance P. ECL cells (enterochromaffin-like cells), the predominant histamine-containing cell of the stomach, regulate parietal cell secretion. D1 cells produce VIP and GIP.

The chief (zymogenic) cells make lipase and pepsinogen, a precursor of the proteolytic enzyme pepsin.

Function. The stomach has several important functions. It:

1. Serves as a nutrient reservoir to store ingested nutrients and controls emptying into the duodenum.
2. Continues the digestive process that began in the mouth.
3. Secretes intrinsic factor.
4. Provides a very limited amount of nutrient absorption.
5. Inhibits bacterial proliferation.

Nutrient Reservoir. The stomach serves as a reservoir for ingested nutrients and provides gradual and controlled emptying into the duodenum; this function of the stomach permits the healthy person to eat at intervals. (When the stomach is removed or bypassed, enteral feedings must be provided on a more continual basis.) A number of factors affect gastric motility and the rate of gastric emptying; these include the consistency of gastric contents, the acidity and fat content of the gastric contents, vagal stimuli, and emotional states.

Ingested foods and fluids are retained in the stomach until they have been thoroughly mixed with the gastric secretions and converted to a semifluid material known as chyme. This is accomplished by means of a combination of mixing waves and peristaltic waves. Both mixing waves and peristaltic waves proceed from the proximal end of the stomach to the distal (pyloric) end; the difference is that the mixing waves are weaker and primarily act to mix the ingested contents with the gastric secretions, whereas the peristaltic waves are stronger and actively sweep the liquid chyme toward the pylorus. The more solid material, which is toward the center of the stomach, is pushed back toward the proximal end of the stomach so that it is exposed to further mixing before it reaches the pylorus. This "mixing and moving" process continues until the gastric contents have been emptied into the duodenum (Seeley, Stephens, and Tate, 1991).

The rate of gastric emptying is primarily determined by pH, fat content, osmolality, consistency, and temperature of the chyme. Highly acidic chyme is delivered to the duodenum at a slower rate, which allows time for the chyme to be neutralized by pancreatic secretions and mucus production; meals containing significant protein content usually result in more acidic chyme because of the increased production of HCl and pepsin. Meals with high fat content also retard gastric emptying to allow for bile secretion and fat emulsification. Hyperosmolar and hypoosmolar substances empty more slowly than do isotonic substances, and solids empty more slowly than liquids. Temperature extremes can also slow gastric emptying. Other factors that affect gastric motility include vagal stimuli, medications, pathologic states, and emotions. Vagal stimulation increases gastric motility, therefore cholinergic medications such as metoclopramide enhance gastric emptying, whereas surgical vagotomy retards gastric emptying. Narcotics commonly slow gastric motility, as do a number of pathologic conditions (e.g., hypokalemia, peritonitis, and uremia), pain, anxiety, and depression.

Digestion. The stomach contributes to the digestion process through mechanical and chemical processes. The muscle layers of the stomach continue the mechanical digestion that began in the mouth by churning the gastric contents. The chemical breakdown of ingested nutrients is achieved by the production of gastrin, HCl, and pepsinogen, which mix with the food bolus to form a semifluid chyme. While the acidic pH inactivates the salivary amylase and therefore interrupts the breakdown of starches, the acidic pH provides the environment required for initiation of protein digestion. The HCl produced by the parietal cells converts pepsinogen to pepsin, which is a proteolytic enzyme that breaks intact protein down into peptide chains. Pepsin exhibits optimal activity at a pH of 3.0 or below.

The total volume of gastric secretion is normally about 2 to 3 L/day. Gastric secretion is known to occur in three phases: the cephalic phase, in which the stimulus is the thought, smell, and taste of food; the gastric phase, in which the stimulus is food in the stomach; and the intestinal phase, in which the stimulus is chyme in the intestine. Gastric secretion is regulated by neural phenomena and hormonal secretion. Neural regulation involves the autonomic and central nervous systems, in addition to local reflexes coordinated by the intramural plexus. Hormones produced by secretory cells in the stomach also affect gastric secretion. Gastrin, secreted by the stomach mucosa, is a powerful stimulant for the different specialized cells located in the gastric glands. The hormones secretin and gastric inhibitory polypeptide exert an inhibitory effect that slows stomach emptying by decreasing gastric motor activity and gastric acid secretion.

Factors known to increase gastric secretion include pleasant thoughts, the taste and smell of food, tactile stimulation resulting from chewing and swallowing, gastric distention and the presence of partially digested proteins in the stomach, and moderate amounts of alcohol and caffeine, which explains the positive effect of caffeinated and alcoholic beverages on appetite. Factors known to inhibit gastric secretion include distention or irritation of the duodenum, highly acidic duodenal contents, and hypertonic or hypotonic duodenal contents. Emotions are also thought to affect gastric secretions; anger and hostility have been noted to increase gastric secretion, whereas fear and depression are considered inhibiting factors (Seeley, Stephens, and Tate, 1991).

Intrinsic Factor Secretion. Another important function of the stomach is secretion of intrinsic factor. Intrinsic factor is necessary for effective absorption of vitamin B_{12} (cyanocobalamin) in the ileum. If the stomach is surgically removed, lifelong parenteral administration of vitamin B_{12} is required to prevent pernicious anemia.

Absorption. A much less important function of the stomach is its limited capacity for absorption; substances that can be partially absorbed in the stomach include carbohydrates that have undergone chemical digestion in the mouth, as well as alcohol and some medications (e.g., aspirin). The stomach's role in nutrient absorption is minimal.

Elimination of Ingested Bacteria. A final function of the stomach is the antibacterial effect provided by the low gastric pH; the HCl eliminates most of the ingested bacteria.

Blood Supply and Innervation

Arterial blood is supplied to the stomach through branches of the celiac trunk. Venous drainage is provided by the gastric and gastroepiploic veins, which in turn empty into the portal vein. Innervation of the stomach is autonomic, with the vagus nerve providing parasympathetic innervation and the celiac plexus providing sympathetic innervation.

Small Intestine

The small intestine in the adult is approximately 6.7 m in length and stretches from the gastric pylorus to the ileocecal valve. In the newborn infant the small intestine is only 25% of its adult length and 13% of its adult diameter. The tremendous growth of the small bowel throughout the life cycle is illustrated by the increase in small bowel length from 200 cm in the newborn to the almost 6.7 m in the adult; the infant has approximately 950 cm of absorptive surface, whereas the average adult has about 7600 cm (Keljo and Squires, Jr, 1998). The small intestine is a convoluted tube that carries out many absorptive and secretory activities, and complex movements. The small intestine is divided into three anatomic and functional sections: the duodenum, the jejunum, and the ileum. In the next sections, features common to all sections are described first, followed by a discussion of the individual sections.

Histology

The wall of the small intestine contains the four layers common to the GI tract. However, several characteristics are unique to the small intestine. The submucosal and mucosal layers are arranged in folds known as the plicae circulares, which, together with the villi, serve to significantly increase the absorptive surface.

The small intestinal mucosal layer provides a physiologic and immunologic barrier to protect the internal environment from luminal contents, which may contain pathogens and ingested noxious substances. The mucosal layer contains numerous lymphoid cells and produces more antibodies than any other body site (Fenoglio-Preiser et al, 1999). The mucosal layer also produces peptides that are essential for effective mucosal functioning and barrier function. Intestinal mucosal function and immune system mechanism (e.g., IgA concentration) is underdeveloped in the newborn (Fenoglio-Preiser et al, 1999).

The mucosal layer can be subdivided into three layers: the muscularis mucosa, the lamina propria (also known as the connective tissue layer), and the surface epithelium. The muscularis mucosa is a thin layer of circular muscle that extends into the circular folds and separates the mucosa from the submucosa. In addition to producing insulin-like growth factor (IGF), the lamina propria layer contains numerous immune-response cells: lymphocytes, eosinophils, macrophages, plasma cells, and mast cells. Aggregated lymphatic nodules are present in the lamina propria and are called Peyer's patches. The surface epithelium is composed of four types of epithelial cells: absorptive cells (enterocytes), goblet cells, endocrine cells, and Paneth cells. Both the intestinal epithelial cells and the lamina propria produce TGF-α and TGF-β, and key immunologloglobulins such as IgA (Chang, Sitrin, and Black, 1996).

The intestinal villi are significant structures of the mucosal layer and give the lumen a velvety appearance (see Figure 3-3). They are fingerlike projections, 0.5 to 1 mm in length, that cover the mucosal surface and increase the absorptive area of the small intestine. Each villus has a capillary network, a lymph vessel, and smooth-muscle fibers. Furthermore, each villus is covered with absorptive cells that have cytoplasmic extensions known as microvilli; the microvilli serve to further increase the absorptive surface. The total absorptive surface provided by the plicae circulares, the villi, and the microvilli is about 600 times greater than what may be expected from a tube with the same diameter (Georges, 2000). The microvilli form what is known as the brush border; the cells that make it up contain many enzymes and carrier substances that facilitate the digestion and absorption of nutrients. Enzymes present in the brush border include peptidases, disaccharidases, and nucleases.

The crypts of Lieberkühn, simple tubular glands, are located between the villi. Within these crypts are undifferentiated cells, mucus-secreting goblet cells, Paneth cells, and endocrine-paracrine cells.

The villi actually have the ability to elongate, or hypertrophy, which partially explains the phenomenon of bowel adaptation after partial bowel resection. The converse is also true: patients maintained on a regimen of nothing by mouth for more than a few days may have temporary atrophy of the villi, with resultant loss of absorptive capacity.

Mucosal Proliferation

Mucosal cells are reproduced on a continuing basis in Lieberkühn's crypts. These mucosal cells then migrate toward the surface of the villi, where they are sloughed into the lumen of the bowel. Mucosal cell turnover takes an average of 48 to 72 hours (Georges, 2000). The constant proliferation of mucosal cells provides rapid repair of any mucosal trauma.

Function

The small intestine is the primary organ responsible for the digestion and absorption of nutrients, vitamins, minerals, fluids, electrolytes, and miscellaneous substances such as drugs. Specific functions that contribute to the digestive process include intestinal motility, intestinal secretion (the movement from the bloodstream toward the lumen), and absorption (the movement from the lumen toward the bloodstream).

Motility. Two types of contractions occur regularly in the small bowel: segmental contractions (mixing) and peristaltic (propulsion) waves (Chang, Sitrin, and Black, 1996). Segmental contractions are multiple short (1 to 2 cm in length), ring-like contractions that produce a back-and-forth motion that mixes and churns the intestinal contents and increases the exposure of chyme to the absorptive mucosal surface. Propulsive contractions (peristalsis) act to propel the chyme distally. Luminal contents that distend the intestinal wall serve as the stimulus for peristalsis. Peristaltic waves are far less frequent than segmentation; they propel the lumen contents distally at a rate of 5 cm/min (Chang et al, 1996).

Bowel motility is controlled by both extrinsic and intrinsic innervation. The autonomic portion of the central nervous system (sympathetic and parasympathetic) provides the extrinsic innervation. Sympathetic fibers inhibit intestinal motility whereas parasympathetic fibers (vagal stimulation) increase intestinal motility. Sympathetic innervation of the GI tract originates in the spinal cord between T8 and L3 and is present in all parts of the GI tract. The hormone norepinephrine is secreted by the sympathetic nerve endings, which trigger an inhibitory effect on the smooth muscle (i.e., circular muscle) and the neurons of the GI tract's intrinsic nervous system. Therefore, simulation of the sympathetic system can be sufficient to create an ileus. Sympathetic stimulation also triggers contraction of the internal rectal sphincter.

Although parasympathetic innervation is prevalent in the esophagus and stomach (supplied by the vagus nerve), it is essentially absent in the small intestine. The vagus nerve also provides parasympathetic innervation of the first half of the colon. Parasympathetic innervation of the distal half of the colon, the rectum, and the anal canal originates in the S2-S4 segment of the spinal cord. Parasympathetic stimulation increases intestinal contraction and mucus secretion and relaxes the internal rectal sphincter.

The intrinsic nervous system of the GI tract regulates the majority of the GI functions. The intrinsic nervous system is composed of two important structures: the Auerbach (myenteric) plexus and the Meissner (submucosal) plexus. The myenteric plexus lies between the longitudinal and circular muscle layers and is primarily responsible for control of movement (peristalsis and segmentation) (see Figure 3-2). Generally, stimulation of the myenteric plexus results in an increase in the activity of the GI tract; muscular contractions increase in strength, intensity, rate, and velocity. An intact myenteric plexus can mediate both segmentation and peristalsis, even in the absence of extrinsic stimuli. Several neurotransmitters are produced by the myenteric plexus neurons: VIP, nitric oxide, peptide histidine isoleucine, and neurokinin A (Chang, Sitrin, and Black, 1996). The myenteric fibers are primarily cholinergic and secrete acetylcholine.

The submucosal (Meissner) plexus is located between the submucosa and the circular muscle and controls secretion, as well as providing a sensory function in response to stretch receptors located in the bowel wall. Motility is affected by local factors, such as distention of the bowel wall, hypertonic or hypotonic bowel contents, highly acidic chyme, and some products of digestion. Primarily the intramural plexus mediates response to these stimuli; vagal stimulation is much less important in the small bowel than in the stomach (Chang, Sitrin, and Black, 1996).

Transit time from the mouth to the colon averages 4 to 9 hours; 3 to 5 hours is spent in the small intestine, where the intestinal contents are continuously mixed.

Secretion. The small intestine contains many intestinal glands known as Lieberkühn's crypts. The secretory cells of these glands (Paneth cells) secrete as much as 3 L of extracellular fluid into the lumen of the bowel each day, with a pH of about 6.5 to 7.5. This fluid contains no enzymes; the enzymes needed to complete the digestive process are found in the cells of the brush border, as already described, and the watery intestinal fluid functions primarily to promote the absorptive process. In addition to the fluid secreted by the intestinal glands, large amounts of mucus are secreted by goblet cells located throughout the mucosal layer of the small intestine (Seeley, Stephens, and Tate, 1991).

Absorption. Nutrients undergo mechanical and chemical digestion in the mouth, stomach, and small bowel; the digestive process breaks down the complex molecules into substances that can be absorbed into the bloodstream. Absorption is then supported by the vast mucosal surface of the small intestine and by the numerous carrier systems located in the brush border of the villi. Most nutrient absorption occurs in the proximal small bowel, reflecting the tremendous absorptive capacity of this organ; however, the ileum can take over much of the absorptive function in the event of disease or surgical resection involving the proximal small bowel. The intact bowel provides significant reserve capacity for nutrient absorption; thus segmental bowel resection is usually well tolerated. The effects of any particular resection depend on the length and function of bowel removed and the length and function of the remaining bowel. For example, resection involving the ileocecal valve is more likely to result in compromised absorption than is resection of an equal length of bowel that does not involve the ileocecal valve. Similarly, removal of a jejunal segment will compromise nutrient absorption initially more than the removal of a similar length of ileum. This is a reflection of the increased nutrient-absorptive capacity of the proximal small bowel as compared to the distal bowel. Critical bowel length—that is, the length of absorptive small bowel that is essential for absorption of adequate nutrients—is difficult to determine because of differences in measurement techniques. However, removal of up to half of the small intestine appears to be tolerated from a nutrient absorption perspective (Westergaard, 1998). Notably, digestion and absorption of nutrients is more than 90% complete within the first 100 cm of the small intestine.

The small intestine also plays a vital role in maintenance of fluid and electrolyte balance through its resorption of intraluminal fluid. The proximal small bowel receives as much as 5 to 6 L of fluid per day and produces an additional amount of 3 L per day. Of this total amount, 7 to 8 L is resorbed back into the small intestine so that only 1 to 2 L of fluid passes through the ileocecal valve daily (see Table 3-1). The vast majority of this fluid is resorbed into the bloodstream; 1 to 2 L passes through the ileocecal valve daily. Any abnormal losses—for example, losses resulting from vomiting, diarrhea, or fistula drainage—may result in fluid and electrolyte imbalance. Hypokalemia, hyponatremia, and metabolic acidosis commonly occur along with fluid volume deficit, because intestinal fluid is usually neutral or alkaline and contains large volumes of sodium and potassium (Westergaard, 1998).

Digestion and absorption of specific nutrients are discussed in the section concerning the appropriate bowel segment (summarized in Table 3-2).

Blood Supply

The superior mesenteric artery supplies blood for most of the small intestine, that is, the jejunum, the ileum, and the distal duodenum (Figure 3-4). The proximal duodenum (the portion above Vater's ampulla) derives its blood supply from the celiac vessels. The superior mesenteric vein provides venous drainage for the small bowel; the superior mesenteric vein then empties into the portal vein, which drains into the liver. This vascular arrangement provides the necessary "detoxification" of the blood that passes through the intestinal tract before it reenters the systemic circulation, and this also explains the frequency of metastatic disease involving the liver in a person with a malignancy of the intestinal tract.

Bacterial Flora

The microflora of the small intestine consists of almost 400 bacteria species including streptococci, lactobacilli, *Bacteroides*, and enterobacteria (Fenoglio-Preiser et al, 1999). Bacterial counts in the small intestine are relatively low, with the distal sites having a higher bacterial population than proximal sites. The low bacterial population is probably due to the bactericidal effect of the extremely low gastric pH and the usually rapid transit of small bowel contents, which limits the potential for bacterial proliferation.

TABLE 3-2 **Nutrient Digestion and Absorption**

NUTRIENT	DIGESTIVE ENZYMES	SITE ENZYMES PRODUCED	SITE OF ACTION	SITE OF NUTRIENT ABSORPTION
Carbohydrates	Amylase	Salivary glands	Mouth	Stomach
		Pancreas	Small intestine	Small intestine
		Brush border of small intestine		
	Disaccharidase (surcase, maltase, isomaltase, lactase)	Brush border of small intestine	Small intestine	
Proteins	Pepsin	Chief cells	Stomach	Small intestine
	Trypsin, Chymotrypsin, Carboxypeptidase	Pancreas	Small Intestine	
	Peptidases	Brush border of small intestine	Small intestine	
Lipids	Bile (not an enzyme)	Liver	Duodenum	Small intestine
	Lipase	Pancreas	Small intestine	
		Brush border of small intestine		
	Esterase	Pancreas	Small intestine	

From Hampton BG, Bryant R: *Ostomies and continent diversions: nursing management*, St Louis, 1992, Mosby.

Duodenum

Structure

The duodenum is an immobile C-shaped segment of small bowel, 20 to 25 cm long, that lies just distal to the pylorus; it is secured to the pyloric region of the stomach by the ligament of Treitz, which is the dividing point between the duodenum and the jejunum (see Figure 3-3). The duodenum is located retroperitoneally and lies in close proximity to the stomach, the pancreas, the liver, the gallbladder, and the transverse colon. The cystic duct from the gallbladder and the hepatic duct from the liver merge to form the common bile duct; it and the pancreatic duct both empty into the duodenum at Vater's ampulla, approximately 9 to 10 cm from the pylorus. The sphincter of Oddi controls the flow of secretions through Vater's ampulla into the duodenum.

Function

Chyme Neutralization. The duodenum's major function is to neutralize the highly acidic gastric contents. This process is accomplished partly by secretion of alkaline mucus by the duodenal (Brunner's) glands, which are located in the submucosal layer of the duodenum. In addition, the presence of acid chyme within the duodenum causes the release of secretin, which stimulates the pancreas to secrete fluid with a high concentration of bicarbonate ions. This highly alkaline fluid drains through the pancreatic duct into the duodenum at Vater's ampulla and plays a major role in neutralizing the acidic chyme. Bile also helps neutralize the acidic gastric contents; delivery of this alkaline substance is stimulated by the presence of fats in the duodenum.

Digestion. A second function of the duodenum is to continue the digestive process begun in the proximal alimentary canal. Fatty acids and amino acids in the duodenum stimulate the release of CCK, which causes contraction of the gallbladder and secretion of enzymatic juices by the pancreas. Bile delivered to the duodenum acts to emulsify the fats, rendering them more susceptible to enzymatic breakdown. The pancreatic juice

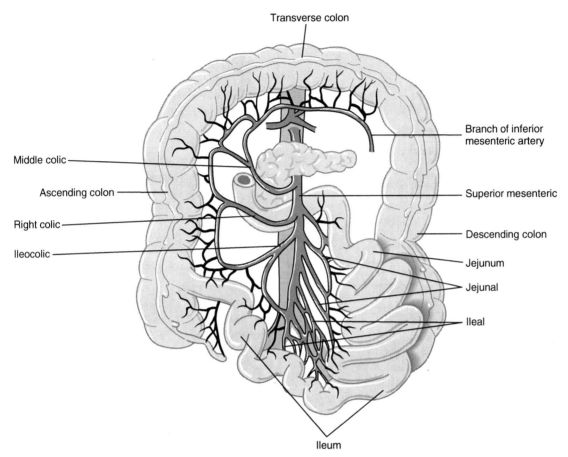

Figure 3-4 Superior mesenteric artery. (From Guyton AC, Hall JE: *Textbook of medical physiology*, ed 10, Philadelphia, 2000, WB Saunders.)

contains a number of digestive enzymes: amylase, which continues carbohydrate digestion; lipases, which continue the digestion of lipids; and the proteolytic enzymes trypsin, chymotrypsin, and carboxypeptidase. (Actually the proteolytic enzymes are secreted in precursor form; trypsin is activated in the duodenum by enterokinase, and trypsin then activates the other proteolytic enzymes.) The higher pH in the duodenum inactivates pepsin but provides an optimal environment for pancreatic enzyme activity.

Absorption. The duodenum also plays a role in absorption; substances that are absorbed in the duodenum include carbohydrates and minerals such as iron, calcium, and magnesium.

Jejunum

The jejunum is the midportion of the small intestine, considered to be the proximal 40 cm after the ligament of Treitz; it has a diameter of about 2.5 to 3.8 cm. The jejunum is the major organ for nutrient absorption; most fats, proteins, and vitamins are absorbed in this area, as well as carbohydrates not absorbed in the stomach and duodenum (Figure 3-5). The enzymes in the brush border finalize nutrient digestion, and the carrier systems

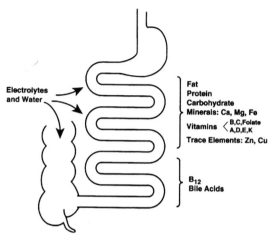

Electrolytes and Water

Fat
Protein
Carbohydrate
Minerals: Ca, Mg, Fe
Vitamins ⟨ B,C,Folate / A,D,E,K
Trace Elements: Zn, Cu

B₁₂
Bile Acids

Figure 3-5 Nutrient absorption in the gastrointestinal tract. (From Feldman M, Friedman LS, Sleisenger MH, editors: *Sleisenger & Fordtran's gastrointestinal and liver disease: pathophysiology, diagnosis, management*, ed 7, vol 2, Philadelphia, 2002, WB Saunders.)

facilitate absorption. The large volume of intestinal secretions also promotes nutrient absorption. The jejunum has prominent villi and a heavy concentration of plicae circulares, which is consistent with its role in nutrient absorption (Keljo and Squires, Jr, 1998) (see Figure 3-3). Plicae circulares are absent in the terminal ileum.

Ileum

The third segment of the small intestine, the distal 60 cm of its length, is the ileum, which is about 2.5 cm wide. Although no clear demarcation exists between the jejunum and the ileum, the ileum is narrower than the jejunum and the villi less prominent (Fenoglio-Preiser et al, 1999). The ileum provides for absorption of any nutrients not absorbed by the duodenum and jejunum. The ileum also contains the only receptor sites for absorption of the intrinsic factor-vitamin B_{12} complex and for bile salts; these sites are located in the terminal ileum (Seeley, Stephens, and Tate, 1991). Patients who have had significant lengths of the terminal ileum resected may require lifelong replacement with parenteral vitamin B_{12} to prevent pernicious anemia; fat intolerance and weight loss also may

occur in these patients. Fat intolerance results from failure to resorb bile salts in the terminal ileum, which retards production of bile in the liver. Normally the bile produced by the liver is concentrated in the gallbladder until gallbladder contraction is stimulated by CCK. The bile is then delivered to the duodenum, where it emulsifies the fats; the residual bile salts continue to pass through the lumen of the bowel until they reach the terminal ileum. At this point the bile salts are resorbed into the bloodstream and delivered back to the liver, where they are again used to produce bile. This recycling of bile salts is known as the enterohepatic circulation; it promotes bile production and therefore fat absorption (Westergaard, 1998).

Ileocecal Valve

The ileocecal valve is a one-way valve located at the junction between the ileum and the large intestine. The ileocecal valve works in conjunction with the ileocecal sphincter, a 2- to 3-cm ring of thick smooth muscle, to regulate emptying into the large intestine and to prevent reflux of contents back into the small intestine. Normally the sphincter is closed; peristaltic waves in the distal ileum cause the sphincter to relax, permitting passage of chyme into the colon. In contrast, distention of the cecum causes increased contraction of the sphincter, which protects the small bowel from reflux (Georges, 2000).

The ileocecal valve and sphincter provide some delay in the passage of chyme from the small bowel into the colon; this delay factor may be critical in the patient with short bowel syndrome or compromised absorptive capacity, because it increases the amount of time nutrients are exposed to the absorptive surface of the small bowel.

Colon

The colon is a long, hollow, distensible tube that extends from the ileocecal valve to the anus and brackets the small intestine (Figure 3-6). In the adult the colon is 5 to 6 feet in length; the diameter of the colon varies from 2.5 to 5.5 cm; largest at the cecum, the caliber decreases as it proceeds distally. The colon is subdivided into the following

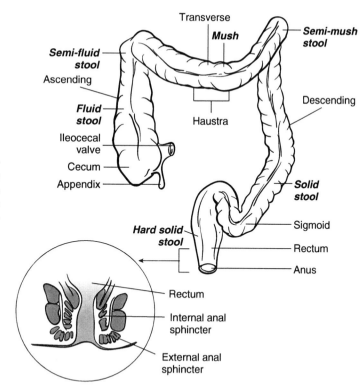

Figure 3-6　Anatomy and stool consistency of large intestine. (Modifed from Potter PA, Perry AG: *Fundamentals of nursing*, ed 5, St Louis, 2001, Mosby; and Guyton AC, Hall JE: *Text book of medical physiology*, ed 10, Philadelphia, 2000, WB Saunders.)

segments: cecum with the attached appendix, ascending colon, transverse colon, descending colon, sigmoid colon, rectum, and anal canal.

Histology

The colon wall has the same morphologic layers as the rest of the GI tract. Several features of these layers, however, are unique to the colon. The outer layer, serosa, covers most of the colon and forms peritoneal sacs that enclose fat (epiploic appendices) and hang from the bowel.

The muscular layer (tunica muscularis) has two smooth-muscle layers (longitudinal and circular), as does the small intestine. The longitudinal muscle of the colon, however, differs from the small intestine in that it is gathered into three muscular bands, or taeniae. The taeniae coli extend from the appendix to the rectosigmoid junction; at this junction the taeniae fuse into one continuous, circumferential, longitudinal muscle. Each taenia traverses one of the following surfaces of the colon: the anterior

surface, the posteroinferior surface, and the posterosuperior surface. Because the taeniae coli are shorter than the length of the colon, they are responsible for the colon's sacculated appearance, or haustra (see Figure 3-6). If a loop colostomy is opened parallel to the taenia, the natural haustrations create two separate openings, one proximal and one distal; this separation provides almost complete diversion of the fecal stream.

The submucosal layer contains small arteries, veins, and lymphatic vessels and serves to attach the muscular layer to the mucosal layer. The submucosal layer has no important distinguishing features. The inner layer of the colon, the mucosa, has several features that distinguish it from the small intestine. Tall, simple, columnar epithelial cells line the mucosa and contain numerous goblet cells and a few endocrine cells. Villi are absent, indicating that the colon provides no nutrient absorption. Lieberkühn's crypts (intestinal glands) are deeper than in the small intestine and extend into the muscularis mucosae. Paneth cells are scattered in the cecum and ascending colon but are absent in the remainder of the large intestine.

Secretions

Lieberkühn's crypts and goblet cells produce colonic secretions, which consist of water, mucus, potassium, and bicarbonate. Mucus, produced by the goblet cells, serves several functions: lubrication of the fecal bolus to aid transport of the material, protection of the mucosa from injury, and binding of the fecal material together. The parasympathetic nervous system and colonic irritants (bacterial, mechanical, or chemical) stimulate mucus production; anxiety and tension decrease mucus secretion. The secretion of bicarbonate creates an alkaline fecal matter with a pH of 7.8.

Bacterial Flora

Intestinal bacteria are vital to many colonic functions. Anaerobic bacteria present in the colon serve to putrefy remaining proteins and indigestible residue; to synthesize folic acid, vitamin K, nicotinic acid, riboflavin, and some B vitamins; and to convert urea salts to ammonium salts and ammonia for absorption into the portal circulation. Common bacteria include *Escherichia coli, Aerobacter aerogenes, Clostridium perfringens,* and *Lactobacillus bifidus.* The concentration of bacteria in the colon is higher in its more distal portions. These bacteria are partially responsible for the odor associated with feces, which explains why output from a sigmoid colostomy has more odor than does output from an ileostomy.

Bacterial action also creates intestinal gas. Swallowed air and diffusion from the blood contribute to intestinal gas production, as well. Intestinal gas is composed of oxygen, nitrogen, carbon dioxide, methane, hydrogen, and trace gases. Such gas production also creates fecal odor. Because many of these gases are flammable, an effective bowel preparation before any procedure that requires cautery (such as a surgical procedure and colonoscopy) is essential to prevent explosions.

Structure

The cecum is the first and also the widest segment of colon. Measuring 6 to 7.6 cm in length, the cecum contains the ileocecal valve. Distention of the cecum causes apposition of the two semilunar lips of the ileocecal valve, thus preventing reflux of cecal contents into the ileum; however, this antireflux mechanism is somewhat incompetent. The appendix arises from the posteromedial aspect of the cecum.

The ascending colon extends approximately 15 cm from the cecum to the right hepatic flexure and is slightly narrower than the cecum. Peritoneum covers the front and sides of the ascending colon but generally not the posterior surface.

After a sharp, 90-degree left turn, the colon continues as the transverse colon. Approximately 45 to 50 cm in length, the transverse colon is quite mobile because it is fixed only at its two end points, the hepatic flexure and the splenic flexure. In fact, the central portion of the transverse colon can gain sufficient mobility to lie in the hypogastrium near the cecum or near the sigmoid colon. The greater omentum lies in front of the transverse colon and must be elevated to expose the colon. At the splenic flexure the transverse colon makes an acute, almost 180-degree turn downward and backward to continue as the descending colon. The left splenic flexure is slightly higher than is the right hepatic flexure.

The descending colon is 25 cm long (longer than the ascending colon) and extends from the hepatic flexure to the brim of the true pelvis. Peritoneum covers the front and both sides of the descending colon; the posterior surface does not have a peritoneal covering.

The sigmoid colon begins where the descending colon passes over the psoas muscle and continues in a S-shaped curve to the upper end of the rectum. Although the length of the sigmoid varies widely, the average is 40 cm. A loop of sigmoid bowel is present when the sigmoid colon is particularly redundant. Peritoneum completely surrounds the sigmoid colon.

The rectum is a hollow, distensible, angulated structure that begins at the termination of the sigmoid colon and is marked by the third sacral vertebra; however, some experts use the sacral promontory as the landmark. The rectum measures

12 to 15 cm in length and follows the curve of the sacrum and coccyx before angulating sharply downward and backward. As the rectum passes through the levator ani muscle, it becomes the anal canal.

The diameter of the upper portion of the rectum is the same as that of the sigmoid colon; however, the lower part of the rectum, which is dilated to facilitate storage of fecal material, forms the rectal ampulla. The rectum has neither haustra nor epiploic appendices. The rectum, which normally is in a collapsed state, is surrounded by a continuous, strong, muscular coat of longitudinal fibers formed by the merging of the taeniae coli.

The rectal mucosa forms three folds in the rectum known as the valves of Houston; two valves are located on the left, and one is on the right (Figure 3-7). These folds consist of mucosa, muscularis mucosa, submucosa, and circular muscle. These structures serve as important landmarks and must be carefully negotiated during proctosigmoidoscopic examination. An additional 5 cm of length can be obtained by straightening the rectum, as is accomplished with a low anterior anastomosis. Because the distal 7 to 8 cm of rectum is below the peritoneal reflection, it is not covered by peritoneum.

The anal canal, which is 3 to 4 cm in length, is the terminal portion of the colon, extending from the anorectal junction to the anal verge. The anal verge is described as the level where the walls of the anal canal make contact in their normal resting state. The perianal skin is a 5-cm radius of skin surrounding the anal verge and is similar histologically to hair-bearing skin located elsewhere (Ajani et al, 2002). The muscles surrounding the anal canal are tonically contracted, thus completely collapsing the anal canal. An angulation of approximately 60 to 105 degrees is created by the presence of the puborectalis muscle, which loops around the anal canal at the anorectal junction.

At the midpoint of the anal canal is the dentate line (also referred to as the pectinate line) (see Figure 3-7). This is an important reference point because of the differences that exist in the tissues above and below this line. Proximal to this line, the mucosa assumes a pleated appearance known as the columns of Morgagni. The narrowing of the rectum into the anal canal creates these longitudinal folds. Above the dentate line, the anal canal is lined with columnar epithelium, whereas modified squamous epithelium lines the anal canal distal to the dentate line down to the anal verge. This transition from columnar to squamous epithelium is gradual, occurring in an area 6 to 12 mm proximal to the dentate line, known as the transition, or cloacogenic, zone (Ajana et al, 2002).

Other important differences are observed in the tissue surrounding the dentate line. The color of the epithelium changes; whereas the rectal mucosa is pink, the area proximal to the dentate line is a deep purple or plum color because of the internal hemorrhoidal plexus. Proximal to the dentate line, the epithelium is innervated with autonomic nerves; on the other hand, the submucosa distal to the dentate line contains numerous encapsulated and free sensory nerve endings. Thus, whereas the rectum is insensitive to ordinary tactile and painful stimuli, the mucosa in the distal anal canal is highly sensitive to pain, touch, and other sensations (Ajana et al, 2002). The nerve endings in the anal canal differentiate gas from liquids and solids. The area below the dentate line, referred to as the anoderm, resembles skin except for the absence of accessory skin structures (i.e., hair, sebaceous glands, and sweat glands).

Blood Supply

The superior mesenteric artery supplies the cecum, the right colon, and the transverse colon up to the splenic flexure. The inferior mesenteric artery supplies the descending colon, the sigmoid colon, and the proximal portion of the rectum. The remainder of the rectum is supplied by the middle and inferior hemorrhoidal arteries, which arise from the internal iliac arteries.

Blood is drained from the colon in a pattern similar to the arterial supply: the superior mesenteric vein drains the right colon, and the inferior mesenteric vein drains the left colon. As part of the portal system, these veins deliver the blood to the liver. The proximal portion of the rectum drains into the superior hemorrhoidal vein and

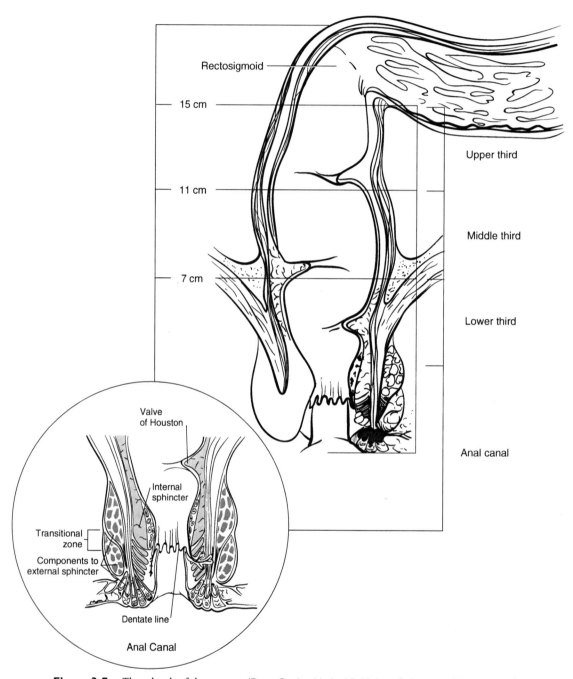

Rectosigmoid

15 cm

11 cm

7 cm

Upper third

Middle third

Lower third

Anal canal

Valve
of Houston

Internal
sphincter

Transitional
zone

Components to
external sphincter

Dentate line

Anal Canal

Figure 3-7   Three levels of the rectum. (From Quality Medical Publishing, St Louis; and Hampton BG, Bryant RA: *Ostomies and continent diversions: nursing management,* St Louis, 1992, Mosby.)

into the portal system by way of the inferior mesenteric vein. The remainder of the rectum is drained by the middle and inferior hemorrhoidal veins, which flow to the iliac veins and thus the systemic circulation.

Function

The functions of the colon include collection, concentration, transport, and elimination of intestinal waste material. Approximately 1 to 1.5 L of intestinal contents passes through the ileocecal valve to be received in the cecum daily. As the water and electrolytes (sodium and chloride), glucose, and urea are resorbed from this material, the consistency of the colonic contents changes from fluid (in the ascending colon) to semifluid (at the transverse colon) to solid in the descending colon (see Figure 3-6).

Fecal material consists primarily of bile pigments, mucus, unabsorbed minerals, undigested fats, cellulose, meat protein toxins, desquamated epithelial cells, potassium, chloride, sodium, bicarbonate, and water. Fecal composition is approximately three-fourths water (100 to 150 ml) and one-fourth solid matter. Mature absorptive cells present in the epithelium (mucus layer) are responsible for this absorption of water and electrolytes. The pH of fecal matter is 6.8 to 7.8. Elimination of intestinal waste occurs at regular intervals after a complex set of interrelated processes takes place.

Colon Motility. Motility in the colon serves to transport fecal material through the colon. In the synchronous activity of the colonic musculature, the longitudinal and the circular muscles work together to propel the fecal material through the colon (peristalsis) and to "knead" the material into a bolus (segmentation). The longitudinal muscle is primarily responsible for peristalsis, the movement of the fecal bolus through the colon. Several types of peristalsis occur. Receptive relaxation allows the cecum to fill with ileal contents; adaptive relaxation allows the fecal material to accumulate and be stored; pendulum movements (continuous back-and-forth movement of fecal material) aid absorption; and mass movement (the en masse contraction of the left colon) propels the fecal bolus into the rectum to be evacuated (Georges, 2000).

The circular muscle creates segmentation, which consists of the alternating contraction and relaxation of the haustra. Segmentation facilitates the grinding of food masses and fluid and electrolyte resorption.

Colonic motility is stimulated by hostility, anger, physical activity, colonic distention, lactose, and medications that absorb water or prevent the movement of water (e.g., bulking agents and saline cathartics). Factors that decrease colonic motility include sleep, anxiety, and fear. The average transit time from the ileocecal valve to the rectum is 18 to 24 hours (Georges, 2000).

Elimination. Feces are eliminated from the colon through the defecation process, a complex process that involves the coordination of the anal sphincters, pelvic floor muscles, and voluntary efforts.

Anal sphincter. The internal and external sphincters compose the anal sphincter (see Figure 3-7). Anatomically the internal sphincter is a continuation of the thick circular muscle and encircles the anal canal to a point approximately 1.5 cm distal to the dentate line. The internal sphincter, which is tonically contracted, is not under voluntary control because it is a smooth muscle. The external sphincter is a striated muscle that surrounds the anal canal. The superficial component is attached to the coccyx by an extension of the muscle fibers. The deep component of the external sphincter is not attached posteriorly; the proximal portion is continuous with the puborectalis muscle. The external sphincter is innervated through the pudendal nerve and is under voluntary control; the external sphincter also exhibits tonic continuous activity at rest. Rectal distention stimulates increased contraction of the external sphincter.

These two sphincters work together. In response to rectosigmoid distention, the internal sphincter relaxes at the same time the external anal sphincter contracts. This allows the sensitive epithelium of the anal canal the opportunity to "sample" the contents to determine if the contents are air, liquid, or solid. Although the internal sphincter responds only to rectal distention, the external sphincter responds with contraction to rectal distention, increased intraabdominal pressure, anal dilation, and perianal stretch, as well as to voluntary effort. Tonic contraction of the external sphincter is inhibited by voluntary effort or by the act of micturition.

Pelvic floor. The pelvic floor comprises the levator ani muscle, which forms a cone-shaped diaphragm over the perineum. Through the center of this muscle the pelvic organs exit the pelvis and enter the perineum. The levator ani muscle is divided into four components: the iliococcygeus, the pubococcygeus, the puborectalis, and the ischiococcygeus. (The puborectalis is believed to be a part of the external sphincter structure.) These striated muscles form a sling to support the anal canal and distal rectum and alter the anorectal angle to facilitate or inhibit defecation.

Elimination process. Fecal material is delivered to the rectum through mass movement. As this material is forced into the rectum and anal canal, the internal sphincter promptly relaxes while the external sphincter automatically contracts. If the individual chooses to proceed with defecation and strains to push the contents into the rectum, intrarectal pressures increase. These pressures are sufficient to overcome the external sphincter contraction. Simultaneously, the external sphincter and pelvic floor muscles relax, thus straightening the rectum and eliminating any resistance presented by Houston's valves or rectal angles. Reduced angulation is also facilitated by the squatting position. Continued relaxation of the external sphincter occurs as a result of the stimulation of the mucosa of the anal canal by the fecal material. Other textbooks (Doughty, 2000) present a more detailed discussion of the defecation process.

ACCESSORY ORGANS

The pancreas, the liver, and the biliary system are considered accessory organs to the digestive system. Each of these is discussed with emphasis on its role pertaining to digestion.

Pancreas

Structure

The pancreas is a fish-shaped, lobulated organ that weighs approximately 85 g; it is 10 to 22 cm long and 5 cm wide. The pancreas is divided into the head (which lies over the vena cava and rests in the C-shaped curve of the duodenum), the body (which extends horizontally across the abdomen and hides behind the stomach), and the tail (which contacts the spleen at the level of the first and second lumbar vertebrae (Figure 3-8).

The pancreas is described as a lobulated organ because the internal structure is composed of numerous small alveoli lined with special secretory cells called tubuloacinar cells (shaped as tiny tubes and grapes). These cells secrete digestive enzymes also known as pancreatic secretions. Clusters of the acinar cells form an acinus, which in turn forms lobules. Connective tissue joins each lobule to form the pancreas.

Each acinus contains small ducts that empty into larger lobule ducts. The ducts within the lobules receive secretions from the acinar cells and empty into Wirsung's duct, the major pancreatic duct that extends the entire length of the pancreas. Wirsung's duct empties the digestive enzymes into Vater's ampulla, located in the duodenum.

The pancreas also comprises clusters of cells that form spherical islands, known as the islets of Langerhans, embedded within the lobules of acinar tissue. These cells also are referred to as endocrine tissue, because they have no ductal system and they release their products directly into the bloodstream. Four distinct cell types are present in the islets of Langerhans: A, B, D, and F cells. A cells secrete glucagon, B cells secrete insulin, D cells secrete somatostatin, and F cells secrete pancreatic polypeptide hormone. This endocrine tissue composes less than 1% of the pancreas.

Function

The pancreas has both an endocrine and an exocrine function. The islets of Langerhans, as just described, produce the endocrine products of insulin, glucagon, somatostatin, and pancreatic polypeptide hormone; these substances are released into surrounding capillaries, empty into the portal vein, and are distributed to target cells in the liver where they enter the general circulation to reach other target tissue. (A detailed discussion of these hormones is beyond the scope of this discussion

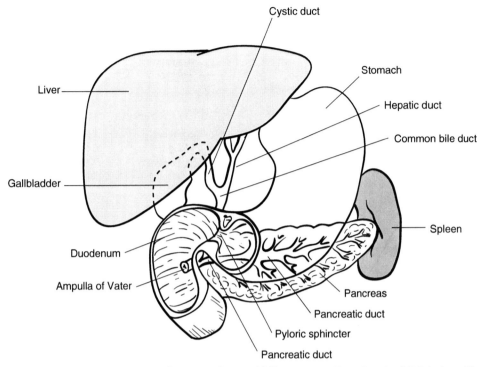

Figure 3-8   Normal anatomy of pancreas, liver, and biliary system. (From Broadwell DC, Jackson BS: *Principles of ostomy care*, St Louis, 1982, Mosby.)

and can be found in other textbooks.) Table 3-3 summarizes the stimulant, the target tissue, and the action of these hormones.

Exocrine secretions (pancreatic juices), which are produced by the acinar cells, are odorless, colorless, watery, and alkaline (with a pH of 8.3). The primary components of pancreatic juice include water (97%) and bicarbonate. Electrolytes such as sodium and potassium in high concentrations, and calcium and chloride in smaller concentrations, are also present. Enzymes in the pancreatic secretions include trypsin, chymotrypsin, carboxypeptidase, amylase, lipase, cholesterol esterase, deoxyribonuclease, and ribonuclease. Trypsin is secreted in the form of trypsinogen, a precursor, and is activated to trypsin by enterokinase, an enzyme secreted by the cells in the duodenum. This precursor mechanism inhibits autodigestion of the pancreas, which can occur with acute pancreatitis. Pancreatic juices serve to digest foodstuff (the enzymes) and to neutralize and dilute gastric hydrochloric acid (the bicarbonate, electrolytes, and water). Average daily volume for pancreatic secretions is 700 to 1000 ml.

Both hormonal and neural signals regulate pancreatic exocrine function. In response to stimulation by chyme in the intestine, the intestinal hormones secretin and CCK are released and transported to the pancreas via the portal system. In the presence of an acid chyme (pH below 4.5), secretin is released and acts on the pancreas to produce a high volume of a fluid low in enzymes but rich in water and bicarbonate. The acid chyme that is delivered to the duodenum is thereby neutralized. Other effects of secretin production include increased bile secretion from the liver, decreased gastrin-induced gastric secretion and emptying, stimulation of insulin release, increased pancreatic blood flow, and potentiation of CCK.

TABLE 3-3   **Functions of Pancreatic Endocrine Cell**

CELL	HORMONE	STIMULANT	TARGET TISSUE	ACTION (RESPONSE)
A	Glucagon	↓ Glucose	Hepatocyte	↑ Glucose in bloodstream
		Exercise	Myocyte	↑ Gluconeogenesis
		↑ Amino acids		↑ Glycogenolysis
		SNS stimulation		Mobilization fats
				Mobilization proteins
B	Insulin	Glucose	Skeletal cells	↓ Blood glucose
			Muscle cells	↓ Fat mobilization
			Cardiac cells	↑ Fat storage
				↑ Protein synthesis
				↑ Glucogenesis
D	Somatostatin	Hyperglycemia	A cells	↓ Blood glucose
			B cells	↓ Glycogen secretion
				↓ Insulin secretion
F	Pancreatic polypeptide	Acute hypoglycemia	Gallbladder	↑ Gallbladder contraction
			Smooth muscle	↓ Pancreatic enzyme

From Urden LD, Stacy KM, Lough ME: *Thelan's critical care nursing: diagnosis and management*, ed 4, St Louis, 2002, Mosby.
SNS, Sympathetic nervous system.

The release of the intestinal hormone CCK is stimulated when the chyme present in the duodenum is rich in protein and fat. CCK causes the pancreas to produce low-volume secretions that are rich in enzymes and high in bicarbonate and amylase. Additional effects of CCK include increased GI motility, increased pancreatic blood flow, slowed gastric emptying, inhibition of the lower esophageal sphincter, stimulation of sigmoid colon motility, relaxation of the hepatopancreatic ampulla, stimulation of gallbladder emptying, relaxation of the sphincter of Oddi, and release of insulin and glucagon.

Additional hormones are believed to influence the pancreas. Vasoactive intestinal peptide may mediate an increase in pancreatic fluid and bicarbonate secretion. Somatostatin, vasopressin, and calcitonin inhibit pancreatic exocrine function.

Neural influences on the pancreas are inhibitory stimulation by the sympathetic system and increased exocrine secretions and blood flow by the parasympathetic system. In addition, anticholinergic agents decrease enzyme production, whereas alcohol and histamines increase pancreatic secretions by stimulating gastric hydrochloric acid production.

Blood Supply and Innervation

Branches of the celiac, splenic, and superior mesenteric arteries form the pancreatic arteries and supply arterial blood to the pancreas. The splenic and superior mesenteric veins drain blood from the pancreas into the portal circulation.

Both sympathetic and parasympathetic fibers innervate the pancreas. The splanchnic nerves and celiac plexus (sympathetic nerves) contain preganglionic fibers for pain and postganglionic fibers for vascular control. Sympathetic fibers also innervate the acinar cells and stimulate secretion of enzymes. Parasympathetic stimulation by the vagus nerve controls both exocrine and endocrine pancreatic function and mediates the gastropancreatic reflex.

Liver

Structure

The liver, the largest organ in the body, weighs 1200 to 1600 g; it is located in the right upper abdominal quadrant below the right diaphragmatic dome (see Figure 3-8). A thick capsule of connective tissue, Glisson's capsule, surrounds the liver; it is covered by serosa and contains blood vessels and lymphatics.

The liver is held in place by intraabdominal pressure and by the falciform ligament, which is formed from the peritoneum that covers the liver. This ligament attaches the liver to the anterior portion of the abdomen between the diaphragm and the umbilicus, and also divides the liver into the right and left lobes.

Six times larger than the left lobe, the right lobe has three sections: right lobe proper, caudate lobe, and quadrate lobe. The left lobe has two sections.

The functional unit of the liver is the lobule; each lobe contains numerous lobules. Approximately 1 million lobules form the liver parenchyma. Each lobule comprises rows of hepatic cells held together with connective tissue. Between the rows of hepatic cells are capillaries, or sinusoids, that are branches of the portal vein and hepatic artery; central to each lobule is an intralobular vein that drains the lobule.

Although sinusoids are a type of capillary, they lack a definite cell wall and are lined with two types of cells: Kupffer's cells (phagocytic cells that belong to the reticuloendothelial system) and some non-phagocytic cells of modified epithelium. Kupffer's cells are significant in that they serve to phagocytose old or defective red blood cells and to detoxify harmful substances.

The liver also contains parenchymal cells, or hepatocytes. These cells secrete bile and perform metabolic (not digestive) duties.

Of interest is the liver's ability to regenerate, which is thought to result from the volume of blood supplied to the liver and the proximity of the blood flow to the individual cells. Although factors such as age, hormone levels, and diet may affect the rate, regeneration is believed to occur within 3 weeks; normal function returns within 4 months. Generally 70% of the liver can be destroyed without manifestation of symptoms (Chang, Sitrin, and Black, 1996).

Blood Supply

The liver is unusual in that it receives blood from one artery and one vein. The portal vein supplies nutrient-rich blood from the intestines, pancreas, spleen, stomach, and mesentery. The hepatic artery divides and subdivides to supply oxygenated blood to lobules and cells; it empties into the hepatic vein and the inferior vena cava. Approximately one third of the total cardiac output (i.e., 800 to 1500 ml) is carried to liver every minute through these two blood vessels (Chang, Sitrin, and Black, 1996).

The portal vein carries most of the liver's blood flow (75%) and branches into the sinusoids to supply each of the lobules. Sinusoids empty blood into the intralobular vein, which ultimately empties into the hepatic vein and the inferior vena cava.

Lymphatic vessels surround the hepatic veins and bile ducts. The lymph drains into these vessels from lymphatic spaces between parenchymal cells. Carcinoma frequently metastasizes to the liver because of the considerable lymphatic and vascular supply.

Function

The liver is a complex organ that performs many metabolic and digestive functions. (A detailed discussion of the function of the liver can be found in any physiology textbook.) Briefly, the functions of the liver include bile formation; metabolism of carbohydrates, proteins, fats, and steroids; vitamin storage; coagulation; mineral and water metabolism; and detoxification.

Bile production and secretion are continuous processes within the liver. Components of bile include water, bile salts, bilirubin, cholesterol, fatty acids, and lecithin. The predominant electrolytes present in bile are sodium chloride (145 mEq/L), chloride (100 mEq/L), bicarbonate (28 mEq/L), and potassium and calcium (each at 5 mEq/L). The liver cells form bile salts, the most abundant substance secreted into bile, with cholesterol serving as a precursor; cholesterol is either supplied by the diet or synthesized in the course of fat metabolism.

Bile salts function primarily (1) to emulsify fat globules into minute sizes to facilitate digestion and (2) to promote the absorption of lipids (cholesterol and fatty acids) across the intestinal mucosa. Fat absorption is important because when fats are not absorbed adequately, fat-soluble vitamins (A, D, E, and K) are not absorbed adequately. Bile salts also serve as a route to excrete bilirubin, cholesterol, and various hormones (sex, thyroid, and adrenal).

Resorption of approximately 94% of the bile salts occurs in the terminal ileum; the resorbed salts are returned to the liver through the portal blood. In the liver the bile salts are absorbed into the hepatic cells and then resecreted into the bile. The small amounts of bile salts lost are eliminated in the feces. This recirculation of bile salts, known as the enterohepatic circulation, is essential for maintaining normal daily flow of bile; otherwise the liver would not be able to produce enough of the salts to make the normal amount of bile. The daily volume of bile production averages 600 to 1000 ml.

Bile also serves as a mechanism for excretion of bilirubin from the body. Bilirubin, the primary pigment in bile, is derived from the heme portion of hemoglobin during the degradation of red blood cells by Kupffer's cells. When bilirubin is released into the bloodstream, it combines with albumin to form a fat-soluble, unconjugated (indirect) bilirubin. When indirect bilirubin passes through the liver, the liver cells conjugate it to a water-soluble form (direct bilirubin), which is then excreted into the intestine. Here conversion of direct bilirubin to urobilinogen compounds occurs. Some of this urobilinogen is resorbed into the portal blood and recycled, whereas other forms of the urobilinogen compounds are excreted in the feces, thus giving feces their color.

The liver serves an important role in carbohydrate metabolism and storage by synthesizing glycogen (the stored form of glucose) from glucose, protein, fat, or lactic acid. Glycogen is then broken down as necessary and released by the liver to maintain normal blood glucose levels.

The liver has a vital role in protein synthesis and amino acid metabolism. Through a complex process, amino acids can be formed from the metabolites of carbohydrates and fat. Plasma proteins important for maintaining normal serum osmotic pressure and blood clotting (such as prothrombin, factors V, VII, VIII, IX, and X, fibrogen, albumin, transferrin, and hepatoglobin) also are synthesized by the liver. Finally, the liver breaks down amino acids, thus producing ketoacids and ammonia. From these substances urea is formed, which is excreted in the urine.

Fat metabolism continues in the liver and involves conversion of triglycerides to glycerol and fatty acids, a process called ketogenesis. Synthesis of fat substances such as cholesterol, phospholipids, and lipoproteins also occurs in the liver.

Steroid metabolism is another function of the liver. Adrenocorticosteroids, glucocorticosteroids, testosterone, and aldosterone are metabolized and catabolized by the liver.

Vitamins such as B_{12}, B_1, riboflavin, B_2, nicotinic acid, pyridoxine, D, E, K, and A are stored in the liver. Bile and bile salts are required for vitamin D and K absorption to occur.

Coagulation is an extremely complex process that is influenced and regulated by the liver. The liver produces prothrombin, fibrinogen, and heparin. However, vitamin K is necessary for the synthesis of prothrombin, and absorption of vitamin K across the intestinal mucosa requires the presence of bile salts. The liver also disposes of disintegrating red blood cells.

The liver also metabolizes minerals and water. Ferritin, the storage form of iron, is stored primarily in the liver. Copper, calcium, magnesium, zinc, manganese, and cobalt also are stored in the liver.

Finally, the liver serves a unique function in the detoxification of foreign and toxic substances. For example, certain medications are detoxified and excreted in the urine, whereas other medications (such as morphine and atropine) are stored to be released at a later time into the circulation. Kupffer's cells also serve to protect the body by phagocytosis of viruses, bacteria, dyes, and foreign proteins.

BILIARY SYSTEMS

Structure

The biliary system consists of the gallbladder and the biliary ductal system, which provide a passageway for bile from the liver to the intestine (see Figure 3-8). On a daily basis the liver produces an average of 600 to 1000 ml of fluid with a pH of 7.5. This liver bile, when produced, is golden or orange-yellow. When concentrated in the gallbladder, this fluid becomes tenacious and a dark golden brown; the pH decreases to below 7.

The duct system consists of two hepatic ducts that drain the liver and the cystic duct that drains the gallbladder. These converge to form the common bile duct. The common bile duct empties into the duodenum and Vater's ampulla. The sphincter of Oddi surrounds Vater's ampulla to control the flow of bile into the duodenum.

The gallbladder is a pear-shaped organ that lies on the underside of the liver (see Figure 3-8). It is approximately 7 to 10 cm long and 2.5 to 3.5 cm wide, with a capacity of 60 ml of bile.

Blood Supply and Innervation

The hepatic and cystic arteries supply blood to the gallbladder. Venous drainage occurs via the cystic vein. Lymphatic drainage is abundant.

Innervation of the gallbladder is provided by the sympathetic (splanchnic) system and the parasympathetic (vagus) system. Sympathetic stimulation inhibits biliary smooth-muscle contraction; vagal stimulation causes contraction of the gallbladder and relaxation of Oddi's sphincter.

Function

The primary function of the gallbladder is to collect, concentrate, acidify, and store bile until it is needed for digestion. Normally the sphincter of Oddi is closed during fasting and between meals. During this time the continuous bile production by the liver increases pressure within this closed system so that as bile is passed into the hepatic ducts, it is forced into the cystic duct to be stored in the relaxed gallbladder (see Figure 3-8). Once in the gallbladder, concentration of the bile begins.

Emptying of the gallbladder and the passage of bile into the duodenum therefore depend on the tone of Oddi's sphincter. This tone is influenced by the hormone CCK, which is released in response to the presence of fats in chyme. Anticholinergic agents decrease the tone of the gallbladder and Oddi's sphincter, whereas epinephrine and cholinergic drugs produce contraction of the gallbladder and stimulate Oddi's sphincter. Sight, smell, and taste of food may stimulate the gallbladder; however, emotional states such as fear or excitement may decrease the flow of bile.

CONCLUSION

The normal anatomy and physiology of the GI tract establishes the foundation for understanding alterations in function in the presence of bowel pathology and anticipating normal function after surgical resection of any of its segments. The function of the GI tract is complex and interrelated; one part cannot be removed or altered without affecting another part. The nurse's understanding and anticipation of problems that can arise when the GI anatomy and physiology are altered are vital to providing good patient care.

SELF-ASSESSMENT EXERCISES

Questions

1. Identify the four layers of the intestinal wall, from the inside to outside.
2. Describe the structure and function of the intramural plexus.
3. Which of the following is the most important function of the structures and secretions of the mouth?
   a. Mechanical breakdown of food particles
   b. Initiation of carbohydrate digestion
   c. Initiation of protein digestion
   d. Initiation of fat digestion
4. Match the daily volume of secretions to the appropriate organ:
   a. Salivary glands _____   i. None
   b. Stomach _____   ii. 3000 ml
   c. Small intestine _____   iii. 1000 to 1500 ml
   d. Colon _____   iv. 700 to 1000 ml
   e. Pancreas _____   v. 2000 to 3000 ml
5. Swallowing is initiated voluntarily but is completed on a reflex basis.
   True _____ False _____
6. Explain the purpose of the pharyngoesophageal and the esophagogastric sphincters.
7. Explain why a transmural inflammatory process may cause a generalized inflammation of the peritoneum (peritonitis).

8. Explain the relationship between the mesentery and the peritoneum.
9. Identify two mechanisms that help to protect the gastric and duodenal mucosa from the ulcerating effects of gastric secretions.
10. Which of the following has a stimulant effect on gastric secretion?
    a. Duodenal distention
    b. Highly acidic duodenal contents
    c. Caffeine
    d. Fear
11. Briefly describe the five functions of the stomach.
12. Which of the following is known to slow the rate of gastric emptying?
    a. High-fat meal
    b. Liquid meal
    c. Carbohydrate meal
    d. Cholinergic medications (e.g., metoclopramide)
13. Which of the following structures are responsible for the highly absorptive character of the small bowel's surface?
    a. Villi
    b. Rugae
    c. Peyer's patches
    d. Taeniae coli
14. The small intestine plays an important role in maintenance of fluid-electrolyte balance.
    True _____ False _____
15. Blood flow for most of the small intestine is provided by the:
    a. Superior mesenteric artery.
    b. Inferior mesenteric artery.
    c. Celiac artery.
    d. Portal artery.
16. The major function of the duodenum is:
    a. Absorption of nutrients.
    b. Neutralization of chyme.
    c. Digestion of proteins.
    d. Secretion of intrinsic factor.
17. Most nutrients, vitamins, and minerals are absorbed in the:
    a. Ileum.
    b. Duodenum.
    c. Jejunum.
    d. Cecum.
18. Explain the impact of massive ileal resection on absorption of vitamin B_{12}.
19. Describe the structure and purpose of the ileocecal valve.
20. Explain the effects of the taeniae coli on the colon wall and implications for construction of loop colostomies.
21. The colonic mucosa contains villi and provides significant absorption of nutrients.
    True _____ False _____
22. Which of the following is not a function of the anaerobic bacteria found in the colon?
    a. Synthesis of folic acid and some vitamins
    b. Breakdown of indigestible residue
    c. Production of intestinal gas
    d. Production of colonic mucus
23. Total colonic length in the adult averages:
    a. 1.52 to 1.83 m
    b. 6.1 to 6.71 m
    c. 0.61 to 1.22 m
    d. 3.05 to 3.66 m
24. Explain the significance of valves of Houston.
25. The rectum normally is empty.
    True _____ False _____
26. Differentiation among gas, liquid, and solid is provided by sensory receptors located in the:
    a. Rectal wall.
    b. Anal canal proximal to the dentate line.
    c. Anal canal distal to the dentate line (anoderm).
    d. All of the above
27. Which of the following accurately describes the response of the anal sphincters to rectal distention?
    a. The internal sphincter contracts; the external sphincter relaxes.
    b. The internal sphincter relaxes; the external sphincter contracts.
    c. Both sphincters relax.
    d. Both sphincters contract.
28. "Mass movements" occur primarily in the left colon and are responsible for propelling the fecal bolus into the rectum.
    True _____ False _____

29. Briefly describe the endocrine and exocrine functions of the pancreas.
30. The liver is capable of regeneration.
True _____ False _____
31. List the key functions of the liver.
32. The gallbladder's primary function is the collection, acidification, concentration, and storage of bile.
True _____ False _____

Answers

1. Mucosa, submucosa, muscularis, serosa or adventitia
2. Meissner's plexus, located in the submucosal layer, and Auerbach's plexus, located in the muscularis, are jointly known as the intramural plexus. It is composed of nerve cell bodies and nerve fibers, or processes; the nerve fibers originate in receptor cells located in the bowel wall. These receptors are sensitive to local stimuli, such as stretch. The intramural plexus is the primary mediator of intestinal secretion and motility. Autonomic nerve fibers synapse on nerve cells in the intramural plexus and serve to modify its response, but autonomic stimulation is not critical to intestinal secretion or motility.
3. a
4. a; iii
   b; v
   c; ii
   d; i
   e; iv
5. True
6. The pharyngoesophageal sphincter prevents reflux of food and fluid from the esophagus into the mouth; the esophagogastric sphincter prevents reflux from the stomach into the esophagus.
7. The outer layer of the bowel wall, the serosa, is continuous with the visceral peritoneum, which covers abdominal organs. Inflammation of the serosa may spread to involve the peritoneal structures.
8. The mesentery is a double layer of peritoneum that encircles most of the small intestine and anchors it to the posterior abdominal wall. The mesentery is a vital support structure because it contains the blood vessels and nerves that nourish and innervate the bowel.
9. Two protective mechanisms are the surface membranes of the mucosal cells and the tight junctions between the mucosal cells and the blanket of viscous and alkaline mucus that coats the mucosal surface.
10. c
11. a. The stomach serves as a reservoir for ingested nutrients and provides controlled emptying into the duodenum. b. The stomach begins enzymatic digestion of proteins. The parietal cells produce HCL acid, which converts pepsinogen (secreted by the chief cells) into pepsin. Pepsin is a proteolytic enzyme. c. The parietal cells secrete intrinsic factor, which is essential for absorption of vitamin B_{12}. d. The stomach provides for limited absorption: some carbohydrates, alcohol, some medications. e. The low pH of the stomach eliminates most of the ingested bacteria.
12. a
13. a
14. True
15. a
16. b
17. c
18. Absorptive sites for vitamin B_{12} are located only in the terminal ileum. Significant ileal resection places individual at risk for pernicious anemia and may necessitate lifelong replacement of vitamin B_{12}.
19. The ileocecal valve is a one-way valve located at the junction between the ileum and the large intestine; it serves to regulate emptying into the large intestine and to prevent reflux of colonic contents back into the small intestine.
20. The taeniae coli are three muscle bands that create sacculations in the colon wall known as haustrations. If a loop colostomy is opened parallel to the taeniae, the natural

haustrations create two separate openings, one proximal and one distal; this separation provides almost complete diversion of the fecal stream.

21. False

22. d

23. a

24. The valves of Houston are three folds located in the rectum, two on the left and one on the right; they serve as landmarks and must be carefully negotiated during proctoscopic examination.

25. True

26. c

27. b

28. True

29. Endocrine: Production of insulin, glucagon, somatostatin, and pancreatic polypeptide hormone
Exocrine: Secretion of pancreatic juices containing water, bicarbonate, and digestive enzymes. Acidic chyme stimulates production of fluid rich in bicarbonate and low in digestive enzymes. Chyme that contains significant amounts of protein and fat stimulates production of fluid rich in enzymes and bicarbonate.

30. True

31. Bile formation; carbohydrate, protein, and fat metabolism; steroid metabolism; vitamin storage; coagulation; mineral and water metabolism; detoxification

32. True

REFERENCES

Ajani JA et al: Anal canal cancer. In Kelsen DP et al, editors: *Gastrointestinal oncology: principles and practice*, Philadelphia, 2002, Lippincott, Williams & Wilkins.

Chang EB, Sitrin MD, Black DD: *Gastrointestinal, hepatobiliary, and nutritional physiology*, Philadelphia, 1996, Lippincott-Raven.

Doughty D, editor: *Urinary and fecal incontinence*, St Louis, 2000, Mosby.

Fenoglio-Preiser CM et al, editors: *Gastrointestinal pathology: an atlas and text*, ed 2, Philadelphia, 1999, Lippincott-Raven.

Georges JM: Gastrointestinal function. In Copstead LEC, Banasik JL, editors: *Pathophysiology: biological and behavioral perspectives*, ed 2, Philadelphia, 2000, WB Saunders.

Keljo DJ, Squires RH Jr, Anatomy and anomalies of the small and large intestines. In Feldman M, Sleisenger MH, Scharschmidt BF, editors: *Sleisenger & Fordtran's gastrointestinal and liver disease*, ed 6, Philadelphia, 1998, WB Saunders.

Sanford PA: *Digestive system physiology*, ed 2, London, 1992, Edward Arnold.

Seeley R, Stephens T, Tate P: *Anatomy and physiology*, ed 2, St Louis, 1991, Mosby.

Westergaard H: Short bowel syndrome. In Feldman M, Sleisenger MH, Scharschmidt BF, editors: *Sleisenger & Fordtran's gastrointestinal and liver disease*, ed 6, Philadelphia, 1998, WB Saunders.

Inflammatory Bowel Disease: Medical Management

4

VICTOR CRENTSIL and STEPHEN B. HANAUER

OBJECTIVES

1. Describe the population distribution, the most common age of presentation, and the cultural distribution of inflammatory bowel disease.
2. Identify the suspected inherited predisposition, the possible environmental factor of smoking, and the role of appendectomy in the development of ulcerative colitis and/or Crohn's disease.
3. Explain why the hypothesis that inflammatory bowel disease may be an aberrant response to environmental factors in genetically susceptible hosts is supported.
4. Discuss why the genetic discovery of NOD2 is one of the most significant findings in inflammatory bowel disease pathogenesis in years.
5. Identify the clinical, radiographic, and endoscopic findings of ulcerative colitis and Crohn's disease.
6. Define the term indeterminate colitis.
7. List two principles of treating ulcerative colitis and Crohn's disease.
8. Identify two indications for the use of the following antiinflammatory drugs in the treatment of inflammatory bowel disease: aminosalicylates and corticosteroids.
9. Discuss the role of the immunomodulatory agents azathioprine, 6-mercaptopurine, methotrexate, and cyclosporine in the induction and remission of ulcerative colitis and Crohn's disease.
10. Define the biologic agent infliximab and its role in treatment of Crohn's disease.
11. Name two extraintestinal manifestations of inflammatory bowel disease.
12. Discuss the issues of supportive care, pregnancy, and nutritional therapy as they relate to the patient with ulcerative colitis or Crohn's disease.
13. List the complications of inflammatory bowel disease and their medical management.

INTRODUCTION

The inflammatory bowel diseases (IBDs) are a group of chronic intestinal disorders of unknown etiology that most commonly affect adolescents or young adults, but can first arise at any age. Although they are uncommon and usually nonfatal, their importance is highlighted by their typical presentation around the high school or college years and the ensuing economically productive years. Though the term IBDs may connote a broad spectrum of gastrointestinal (GI) disorders, it has been most commonly reserved for Crohn's disease (CD) and ulcerative colitis (UC).

The medical management of IBD has undergone significant advances over the past several decades, in part due to increased understanding of the pathogenesis of the diseases, and in part to the unraveling of the immune and inflammatory events leading to acute and chronic intestinal inflammation. Medical management of patients with IBD is complex. Its challenge is related to the spectrum of medications available and the special requirements of different subpopulations of IBD patients with different disease activity and distribution. In addition, the potential adverse effects of therapy demand a sound understanding of the clinical behavior of the diseases and the clinical pharmacology of the available therapeutic agents.

The impact of IBD often goes beyond what meets the eye of the less experienced clinician. Frequent sources of untold psychologic distress to the patients include the unpredictable extraintestinal manifestations; disfiguring complications such as fistulas and potential ostomies; the lack of cure by surgery in CD and the common need for multiple operations throughout the lifetime of a patient; and the socially disrupting symptoms of diarrhea, chronic abdominal pain, and bleeding. The goal of the medical management of UC and CD is to induce and maintain clinical remissions while minimizing side effects and maintaining patients' quality of life through the course of the chronic illness. The health care team needs to take a holistic view toward not only medical therapy, but also to nutritional and psychosocial support, comprehensive health of the patient and support for the family, and indications for and timing of surgery.

EPIDEMIOLOGY

The insidious onset and heterogeneous manifestations of IBD create a challenge to epidemiologic studies of CD and UC. Geographic differences in incidence rates due to factors such as environment and genetics can be significantly blurred by the diagnostic awareness of CD and UC of medical practitioners in that region (Loftus and Sandborn, 2002). The highest incidence and prevalence rates of IBD have been reported from the United Kingdom, Scandinavia, and the United States.

In North America the incidence of CD ranges from 3.1 to 14.6 per 100,000 person-years, and that of UC from 2.2 to 14.3 per 100,000 person-years; this translates into 9,000 to 44,000 new diagnoses of CD and 7,000 to 43,000 new UC patients each year. In Europe a north-south gradient of IBD incidence and prevalence, with the highest rates in the north, has been repeatedly observed.

Although in general there are no substantial differences in the gender distribution of IBD, there may be a slight female predominance in the prevalence of CD. A bimodal distribution of age at diagnosis has been described for both UC and CD, with a first peak in the second or third decade of life and a second, less prominent, peak at the sixth or seventh decade. IBD has always been more predominant in the Caucasian population, and in particular, in Jews of Ashkenazic descent. Nevertheless, ethnoracial differences in IBD incidence and prevalence are beginning to change as persons of Hispanic and Asian descent who are at lower risk of IBD in their native countries migrate to more Westernized locations. Such studies of epidemiologic changes after migration indicate the significant influence of environmental factors on the risk of IBD.

ETIOLOGY

The infectious origin of IBD has been pursued for decades; however, no specific agent has been significantly associated with UC or CD. Atypical mycobacteria—a chronic, measles-like infection—and *Listeria monocytogenes* have been hypothetically linked to CD without adequate confirmation (Sartor, 1997).

The theory of inherited predisposition is gaining more support as clues for genetic associations of IBD increase. Foremost, multiple studies have proposed a four- to twentyfold increase in the risk of IBD (compared to the general population) in first-degree relatives of affected patients, and a 7% absolute risk of first-degree relations of patients has been suggested (Tysk et al, 1988; Orholm et al, 1991). Second, identical twins have a 60% concordance for CD and a 20% concordance for UC, leading to the inference that the genetic contribution to CD may be more significant than to UC. An identification of a proband (the person in whom a disease originally manifests itself) suggests a 20% risk of IBD occurring in a second family member, and the risk doubles if the proband is a child (Hanauer, 2001). The risk of IBD occurring in offspring is almost 50% if both parents have IBD; although it may present as CD or UC, there seems to be a family concordance for the disease type.

Cigarette smoking is an important "environmental factor" that impacts the pathogenesis and course of IBD (Rubin and Hanauer, 2000). Although cigarette smoking is strongly associated with CD in adults, smoking has a protective effect that acts against the development of UC. Smokers with CD are more refractory to medical treatment, as are ex-smokers who develop UC. Nicotine has not been confirmed to be a prime factor in these intriguing relationships; however, delivered transdermally it has a modest ameliorating effect on UC, albeit less potent than resumption of cigarette smoking.

Appendectomy, through a mechanism that has yet to be clarified, may be protective against UC and is associated with the development of CD (Andersson et al, 2001; Duggan et al, 1998). Investigations into other suspected etiologic factors, such as oral contraceptives, sugar intake, and breast-feeding, are conflicting, and no specific agent has been confirmed to have a role in the development of IBD.

PATHOGENESIS

The hypothesis that IBD may be an aberrant response to environmental factors in genetically susceptible hosts is supported by two key observations. The first is the lack of development of intestinal inflammation in animals maintained in a germ-free environment (Fiocchi, 1998; Sartor, 1997). Second, many IBD cases seem to have been triggered by acute GI infections, such as gastroenteritis and traveler's diarrhea, and even by antibiotic use. The importance of susceptibility is suggested by the paradoxic observation that exposure to microorganisms during childhood may reduce the future risk of development of IBD; therefore the potential of acute infections to trigger IBD is not universal. Despite these observations the exact role of genes, germs, and an inappropriate mucosal immune response to luminal, gut-associated flora—or the combination of all three—in the pathogenesis of CD and UC remains an enigma and an area of ongoing research. Whatever the initiating event, IBD patients, as opposed to unaffected individuals, have an impaired ability to down-regulate a gut inflammation once it has begun.

Chronic inflammation is normal in the gut mucosa, due to the relatively hostile environment of the intestinal mucosal immune system, and is described as chronic physiologic, or controlled, inflammation. To maintain the necessary equilibrium, a general adaptive state of suppression (tolerance) has been developed by the mucosal immune system; defects in this suppressive system, be they genetic or otherwise, initiate a cascade of events culminating in chronic gut inflammation and manifesting collectively as IBD.

In CD and UC an inappropriate and exaggerated response to an antigen by most of the mucosal immune elements, including mucosal T cells and tissue macrophages, is observed. These activated macrophage and T cells contribute to the recruitment of nonspecific mediators of inflammation, such as neutrophils, that are final arbiters of tissue damage. The inflammatory responses also include cytokines, chemokines, growth factors, and metabolites of arachidonic acid (e.g., leukotrienes and prostaglandins), as well as reactive oxygen metabolites and nitric oxide (Swidsinski et al, 2002; Fiocchi, 1998).

The cytokine response and the balance of cytokines seem to differ between CD and UC, and may be responsible for some of the dissimilarities between the disease phenotypes. Several studies have shown increased mucosal interleukin (IL), specifically IL-1 and IL-6, and tumor necrosis factor (TNF)-α in CD and UC; however, CD features a more prominent Th1 cytokine response (IL-2, IL-12, interferon-γ, and TNF-α), whereas UC demonstrates a relative Th2 predominance, manifested by elevated levels of mucosal antibodies, plasma cells, and B cells. In addition, increased elaboration of antineutrophil cytoplasmic antibodies (ANCAs) and IgG antibodies reacting with a 40 kD tropomyosin protein has been described in UC (Targan, 1999; MacDermott, 1999). CD, on the other hand, has been associated with an increased likelihood of developing antibodies to *Saccharomyces cerevisiae* (common brewer's yeast) (Targan, 1999).

GENETICS

The complex genetics of IBD and potential genetic-environmental interactions are increasingly borne out by the identification of specific candidate genes. The genetic roots of IBD were previously supported by epidemiologic data based on familial aggregations of IBD and the significantly higher monozygotic twin concordance for IBD compared to dizygotic twins. Because of the ethnic-based difference in the risk of IBD among family members of affected patients, the complex polygenic nature of IBD genetics is favored over a simple mendelian model of inheritance (Yang and Rotter, 1995).

Histocompatibility locus antigen (HLA)-B5 and HLA-Bw35 have been linked to UC in Japanese and Israeli Jewish populations respectively (Hiwatashi et al, 1980; Delpre et al, 1980). Three polymorphisms in the TNF-α–promoter sequence have been associated with CD in Japanese patients; one of the three polymorphisms in TNF-α has similarly been linked to CD in the United Kingdom (Kinouchi et al, 2001; Negoro et al, 1999). Genetic linkage studies have confirmed the linkage between CD and a locus on chromosomes 16 and 14q, namely, the IBD1 and IBD4 loci, respectively. A locus on chromosome 12q (IBD2 locus) has been associated with IBD (especially UC), and a link between IBD (especially CD)

and chromosome 6p (IBD3 locus) has been confirmed (Hampe et al, 1999).

Further work on the IBD1 led to the identification of the NOD2 genetic variants that seem to change the response of the innate immune system to bacterial agents (Ogura et al, 2001). The discovery of NOD2 (also called CARD 15, or caspase activation and recruitment domain) is one of the most significant findings in IBD pathogenesis in years. Individuals homozygous for NOD2 variants may have a relative risk for CD of 14.3 to 44, especially for ileal disease (Cuthbert et al, 2002; Hugot et al, 2001; Ogura et al, 2001). There is no significant association between NOD2 and UC.

DIAGNOSIS OF INFLAMMATORY BOWEL DISEASE

The clinical distinction between CD and UC is paramount, since the type of IBD may dictate the therapeutic approach. Smoking status and clinical and endoscopic manifestations may form the cornerstones for differentiation of CD from UC (Table 4-1).

TABLE 4-1   **Clinical Distinction between Ulcerative Colitis and Crohn's Disease**

FEATURE	ULCERATIVE COLITIS	CROHN'S DISEASE
Inflammation	Superficial	Transmural
Mucosal appearance	Continuous involvement with granularity, friability, and pinpoint ulcerations	Focal, discontinuous involvement with aphthous ulcerations progressing to linear/irregular shaped ulcer; granulomas can be present
Location	Limited to colon	Any part of gastrointestinal tract (mouth to anus)
	Rectum always involved	Rectal involvement variable
	Small intestine not involved	Terminal ileum and cecum most commonly involved
	Perianal area normal	Perirectal abscess/disease can be present
Clinical symptoms	Pain not typical	Pain more likely due to transmural inflammation
	Rectal bleeding	Bleeding present with colonic disease
	Diarrhea present as more colonic involvement presents	Diarrhea depends on location of disease (colonic involvement = diarrhea)
		> percent obstructive symptoms (due to fibrosis and narrowing of intestinal lumen)
		Weight loss more common (because of small bowel involvement)

Ulcerative Colitis

Chronic persistent or intermittent diarrhea and/or rectal bleeding in the absence of infection should increase the index of suspicion for UC. Since the rectum is always affected, UC can easily be identified or ruled out by flexible sigmoidoscopy. The contiguous superficial inflammation is generally limited to the colonic mucosa. It may comprise any extent of the colon; approximately one third of patients are seen with proctitis, one third with left-sided colitis, and one third with disease proximal to the splenic flexure. This inflammation usually spares the small bowel, except in extensive disease when the terminal ileum may manifest a similar superficial inflammation termed "backwash ileitis." The extent of colitis is usually maintained from the onset through the course of the disease; although it sometimes may increase or diminish, it does not determine the disease's severity. However, the mucosal extent is of prognostic significance (e.g., risk of neoplasia) and is relevant to therapeutic approaches.

UC has an insidious onset in general; the most consistent manifestation is rectal bleeding. Reduced compliance of the rectum may cause urgency and tenesmus. Although crampy abdominal pain before bowel movements may frequently occur, the signal of fulminant disease is often the occurrence of fever, night sweat, diarrhea, and weight loss.

Physical examination, including perianal examination, is normal; abdominal tenderness is typically limited to severe disease, and, in contrast to CD, significant perianal changes (e.g., fistulas, fissures) are always absent. Endoscopically, the normally glistening smooth bowel mucosa becomes edematous, granular, and erythematous (Color Plate 1). Microscopic or "pinpoint" ulcerations are manifestations of mild to moderate disease, whereas gross ulceration and spontaneous hemorrhage represent severe disease. Protuberances of granulation tissue, in severely affected areas, reepithelializes to form "pseudopolyps," which may mimic adenomatous polyps.

Flat plate abdominal x-rays are valuable for the exclusion of complications such as free air and toxic megacolon. Although air contrast barium enemas can demonstrate the mucosal granularity and ulcerations and the extent of the disease, in most instances the diagnosis and follow-up are based on colonoscopic determinations of the mucosal extent and severity; there is also the possibility of performing biopsies to exclude other colitides and to survey for dysplasia. Occasionally an indium- or technetium-labeled leukocyte scan is performed for severely ill patients to noninvasively and rapidly determine the extent, severity, and continuity of gut inflammation and to exclude small bowel involvement.

Crohn's Disease

The diagnosis of CD is also based on clinical manifestations and the radiologic, endoscopic, and histologic findings. The inflammation of CD may involve any part of the GI tract from mouth to anus. In contrast to the contiguous, superficial (mucosal) inflammation of UC, the inflammation of CD is transmural, predisposing to intestinal strictures (stenosis) and fistulas, and focal. The terminal ileum and cecum are the most commonly involved parts of the GI tract, and, similarly to UC, the pattern and location of the inflammation usually remains unchanged in any particular patient.

The clinical picture may include abdominal cramping, postprandial pain with nocturnal bowel movements, watery stools, and rectal hemorrhage. Other features such as weight loss, fever, and night sweat are not uncommon. Nausea and vomiting usually reflect stricturing of the small intestine; diarrhea in CD can be due to malabsorption or active inflammation in the small or large bowel. The presence of perirectal abscesses or fistulas and skin tags distinguish CD that is confined to the colon from UC. Toxic megacolon is an uncommon but severe complication of either CD or UC. CD is typically present with chronic symptoms; however, an acute presentation may mimic appendicitis, manifested by severe abdominal pain with or without bleeding, or an acute bowel obstruction.

Physical examination reveals stigmata of chronic illness, such as weight loss and pallor, and many patients are seen with oral aphthae, a right lower quadrant inflammatory mass, perianal skin tags, fistulas, or finger clubbing. Endoscopically CD presents as focal inflammation (aphthous, linear, or irregularly-shaped ulcerations) in any portion of the GI tract (Color Plate 2). Stricture formation may limit or preclude complete colonoscopic examinations. Contrast radiographic examination with barium is useful and convenient for evaluating the upper GI tract (including small bowel) and colon, especially in the presence of complications such as fistulas and strictures. Mucosal cobble-stoning and asymmetric focal findings (e.g., ulcers located at the antimesenteric border) support a diagnosis of CD. Imaging studies such as computed tomography scans, ultrasonography, magnetic resonance imaging, and leukocyte scanning are generally used when a complication is suspected. Although the serum anti-*Saccaromyces cerevisiae* antibody (ASCA) test is only about 30% sensitive, its specificity for CD is high (Targan, 1999). Nonspecific tests such as C-reactive protein or an erythrocyte sedimentation rate may be helpful to follow disease activity.

Despite current knowledge of the features that distinguish CD from UC, symptoms in as many as 10% of patients with IBD are limited to the large intestine and may not meet the criteria of classification of either UC or CD; thus, the term "indeterminate colitis" is used to describe this group of IBDs.

THERAPEUTICS OF INFLAMMATORY BOWEL DISEASE

The therapeutic approach to IBD is determined by its type (UC or CD), location, and severity. Therefore an accurate diagnosis is paramount. Although a multifaceted plan increases the rate of therapeutic success, medical management forms the backbone of therapy most of the time. However, certain complications are amenable only to surgery; thus, an interdisciplinary collaboration should be established in a timely fashion to minimize morbidity and mortality in the event these complications occur. The ever-increasing variety of drugs available for IBD increases the challenge for the health care provider; an organized, stepwise approach to medical treatment, with less active drugs initiated at the beginning and a response-driven escalation in drug

potency, seems to be the general treatment protocol of most physicians.

The principles in treating UC and CD are to first induce, and then maintain, remissions. Remission implies resolution of inflammatory signs and symptoms with evidence of mucosal healing. The choice of agents depends on severity and location of disease. At all times, therapies are selected to improve and maintain the patient's quality of life with minimization of side effects (Box 4-1).

Antiinflammatory Agents
Aminosalicylates

Mild to moderate UC and CD are primarily treated with aminosalicylates, derivatives of 5-aminosalicylic acid (5-ASA). These agents act by inhibiting the synthesis of leukotrienes and prostaglandins and blocking oxygen radical production; they are free-radical scavengers. Additionally, they interfere with monocyte and lymphocyte function, immunoglobulin production, and nuclear factor-kB activation.

The prototype of the aminosalicylates is sulfasalazine. Sulfasalazine has an antibacterial moiety (sulfapyridine) linked by an azo-bond to 5-ASA (mesalamine). Sulfasalazine is minimally absorbed in the stomach and small bowel. In the colon the azo-bond is "split" by azoreductase activity of colonic bacteria. The sulfapyridine is then absorbed, metabolized by the liver, and excreted by the kidneys. The 5-ASA moiety remains in the colon and is eliminated in the feces. In effect, sulfasalazine functions as a "prodrug" to make 5-ASA available to the colon, its primary site of action. 5-ASA has been demonstrated to provide the primary therapeutic properties of sulfasalazine, whereas the sulfapyridine moiety is attributed to the majority of the adverse effects. These findings formed the basis of development of sulfa-free aminosalicylates (i.e., mesalamine, olsalazine, and balsalazide).

All of the aminosalicylates share the active component mesalamine that, if delivered in an unprotected form, is absorbed from the small intestine. Therefore, to protect mesalamine from proximal absorption, alternative delivery systems are required. Oral formulations include pH-dependent

BOX 4-1   Medical Therapy

Antiinflammatory Agents
Aminosalicylates (used to treat mild/moderate ulcerative colitis and Crohn's disease)
Sulfasalazine (Azulfidine)
Olsalazine (Dipentum)
Mesalamine (Asacol)
Mesalamine (Pentasa)
Mesalamine enema (Rowasa)
Mesalamine suppository (Canasa)
Corticosteroids (used to treat moderate-to-severe ulcerative colitis and Crohn's disease)
Prednisone
Budesonide (Entocort)

Immunomodulatory Agents
Azathioprine (AZA) (used in the induction and maintenance of remission in ulcerative colitis and Crohn's disease)
6-mercaptopurine (6-MP) (used in the induction and maintenance of remission in ulcerative colitis and Crohn's disease)
Methotrexate (used in steroid-dependent active CD and CD remission maintenance)
Cyclosporine (used in hospitalized UC patients who have failed to respond to enteral or parenteral steroids)

Antibiotics
Metronidazole (used to treat Crohn's disease of the colon and perineal fistulas)

Biologic Agents
Infliximab (Remicaide) (used to treat patients with Crohn's disease unresponsive to aminosalicylates, AZA, 6-MP, corticosteroids, and antibiotics, or patients with cutaneous and perianal fistulas)

coatings that deliver mesalamine into the distal ileum and colon (Asacol), encapsulation of mesalamine into ethylcellulose beads that deliver into both the small bowel and the colon (Pentasa), or the alternative azo-bond formulations olsalazine (Dipentum) and balsalazide (Colazal). These formulations are equally effective, at equal doses of mesalamine, as long as the active moiety is delivered to the intestinal or colonic site of inflammation. In addition, mesalamine can also be administered as an enema (Rowasa) or suppository (Canasa) to the left colon or rectum, respectively.

Dose-dependent adverse effects are anorexia, nausea, vomiting, malaise, and headaches. Hypersensitivity reactions such as fever, hepatitis, rash, agranulocytosis, pneumonitis, hemolytic anemia,

pancreatitis, and worsening colitis may occur in a dose-independent fashion. Side effects unique to sulfasalazine are folate malabsorption and sperm abnormalities (reversible). Olsalazine may cause dose-dependent diarrhea.

Aminosalicylates are effective at inducing remission in mild to moderate UC, as well as at preventing relapse and maintaining remissions. In CD, these agents are somewhat less effective, but can be used to treat mild-to-moderate disease and, for responders, to maintain clinical remissions.

Corticosteroids

Corticosteroids are the mainstay of treatment of moderate to severe UC and CD. However, they are not efficacious for remission maintenance in UC and CD. Corticosteroids are usually used when aminosalicylates fail to control disease activity, or for patients with moderate to severe disease. In IBD, corticosteroids are used for their antiinflammatory and immunomodulatory properties; they can be given in preparations that exhibit enhanced efficacy at specific locations in the gut and reduce systemic exposure. Oral corticosteroids are the main therapeutic agents used to treat moderately severe UC in the outpatient setting. The average dosage in the majority of cases is 40 mg/day of prednisone. Topical corticosteroids (e.g., rectal hydrocortisone enemas or foam) are useful for patients with distal UC or ulcerative proctitis. Patients hospitalized with severe or fulminant UC are generally treated with parenteral corticosteroids. Topical corticosteroids are at times used as adjuncts to parenteral corticosteroids in patients with severe disease. For quiescent UC, corticosteroids do not prevent relapse (Kornbluth and Sachar, 1997).

Corticosteroids are also the main treatment for moderate-to-severe CD. In addition to prednisone, budesonide is a corticosteroid that combines a high topical activity with a low bioavailability. In an enteric formulation designed to deliver into the distal ileum and proximal colon (Entocort), budesonide is mainly useful for patients with mild-to-moderate ileal and right-sided colonic CD. However, budesonide, like other steroids, is not effective for the prevention of relapse in CD. It is important to circumvent preventable side effects of corticosteroids such as osteoporosis with adequate calcium and vitamin D supplementation and, in the presence of osteoporosis, with a bisphosphonate.

Immunomodulatory Agents

The role of immunomodulatory agents in the induction and maintenance of remission in UC and CD continues to expand (Sandborn, 1996). Agents that have been effective are azathioprine (AZA), 6-mercaptopurine (6-MP), methotrexate, and cyclosporine.

Azathioprine and 6-Mercaptopurine

AZA and 6-MP have been used to treat IBD for more than a quarter of a century. In spite of early concerns regarding the potentially increased risk of neoplasia (e.g., lymphoma) neither agent has been demonstrated to increase the risk of malignancies other than basal cell and squamous skin cancers (Podolsky, 2002; Lewis et al, 2001; Farrell et al, 2000). Although the exact mechanism of action of AZA and 6-MP in IBD remains unknown, inhibition of a subgroup of long-lived T cells is credited for their therapeutic effects, and that may account for the 3 to 6 months needed for an observable response to either drug.

AZA and 6-MP are most often used as steroid-sparing agents and to prolong remission in both UC and CD (Present et al, 1980; Bouhnik et al, 1996). Clinicians generally consider the use of AZA and 6-MP when they are faced with difficulty in tapering patients off corticosteroids for more than 6 weeks. Both agents are generally well tolerated; however, adverse effects such as bone marrow suppression, pancreatitis, hepatitis, nausea, rash, and fever may limit their use. Continuous monitoring of the complete blood count is necessary, at a minimum of on a quarterly basis, to watch out for delayed bone marrow suppression.

Methotrexate

Methotrexate inhibits DNA synthesis by blocking dihydrofolate reductase. Although the actual mechanism of its antiinflammatory action is not fully known, inhibition of the elaboration of inflammatory mediators, antibody production, and cell division are potential components of activity (Egan and Sandborn, 1996). Methotrexate has been effectively used in steroid-dependent, active CD and CD remission maintenance. Available evidence favors intramuscular or subcutaneous dosing at 25 mg/week over oral administration. There is no positive evidence to support a role for methotrexate in the treatment of UC.

Side effects such as myelosuppression and hepatic fibrosis are uncommon, but serious, and can be minimized by regular follow-up of blood counts and liver function tests. Folic acid supplementation can decrease side effects such as nausea, vomiting, and diarrhea. Pregnancy is a contraindication for methotrexate use.

Cyclosporine

Cyclosporine derives its potent inhibitory effects on T cells from inhibiting IL-2, TNF-α, and interferon-γ, among other cytokines. It has a dramatic effect on severe acute IBD, and its onset of action is more rapid than AZA and 6-MP. The main role for cyclosporine in IBD is in treating hospitalized, severe UC patients who have failed to respond to enteral or parenteral steroids. In these refractory UC patients, 50% to 80% will respond to cyclosporine (Kornbluth and Sachar, 1997) in the short term; about 80% of those who respond avoid colectomy if AZA or 6-MP is used to maintain remissions. Intravenous cyclosporine has shown efficacy in fistulizing and steroid-resistant CD, but the efficacy of the oral form has not been demonstrated. With the advent of infliximab, the role of cyclosporine in CD management has been greatly diminished.

There is a poor correlation between serum cyclosporine levels and therapeutic response and toxicity. Its narrow therapeutic margin has limited its widespread use. The adverse effects are nephrotoxicity and opportunistic infections (notably *Pneumocystis carinii* pneumonia). Another calcineuron inhibitor, tacrolimus, has been reported to be efficacious in IBD; however, it has not reached significant clinical utility in either UC or CD.

Antibiotics and Probiotics

Antibiotics have shown efficacy in the treatment of subpopulations of patients with CD, primarily those with mild to moderate colonic involvement or perianal fistulas or abscesses. There is no defined role for antibiotics in UC outside of the perioperative setting in fulminant colitis. This variance may suggest a differential contribution of gut microflora in these two types of IBD.

Metronidazole has been effectively used to treat CD of the colon and perianal fistulas. High dosages may be required; therefore neurotoxicity (peripheral neuropathy) may limit its use. Reports of small studies advocate ciprofloxacin as an alternative to metronidazole. Antibiotics have been efficacious for the treatment of pouchitis after ileoanal anastomosis in UC.

The apparent importance of luminal microflora in the pathogenesis of IBD in the susceptible host has been the driving force behind the proposition and administration of probiotics, or "healthy

bacterial food agents," to change the intestinal microflora. Nonpathogenic organisms that have been used include *Lactobacillus*, noninvasive coliforms, and *Saccharomyces boulardii*, among others. Probiotic lactobacilli may be capable of blocking inflammation and reducing the development of colonic malignancy as suggested by its demonstrated effects in IL-10 knockout in a mice model of enterocolitis (Shanahan, 2001). To date the most convincing evidence for the effectiveness of probiotics is the therapeutic response obtained in patients with pouchitis (Gionchetti et al, 2000). Their general lack of systemic adverse effects is a definite plus, but it remains to be determined whether any other roles for probiotics will be defined in controlled clinical trials.

Biologic Agents

Infliximab

As the first agent in its class to be approved by the Food and Drug Administration for the therapy of CD, infliximab represents an entry into a new therapeutic era of IBD. Though infliximab is a chimeric monoclonal antibody to TNF-α, the mechanism of its action is not fully understood. It is composed of a human IgG constant region (the complement-fixing part) and a murine-derived variable region (the antigen-binding part).

In one study, a single infliximab infusion (5 mg/kg) resulted in a clinical response in 80% of patients with CD unresponsive to aminosalicylates, AZA, 6-MP, corticosteroids, and antibiotics (Targan et al, 1997). Almost one half of these CD patients attained remission, and this was maintained for 8 to 12 weeks. Other studies have demonstrated that reinfusion of infliximab at 8-week intervals maintained the remission (Rutgeerts et al, 1999). The positive therapeutic response in CD patients with cutaneous and perianal fistulas is noteworthy. However, the efficacy of infliximab in UC remains to be demonstrated.

Infliximab is generally well tolerated; unique side effects such as development of anti-DNA antibodies and human antichimeric antibodies occur in about 1 in 10 treated patients. Reactions resembling serum sickness have been reported in patients who resume infliximab treatment after a prolonged period of discontinuation. The minimal risk of lymphoma suspected from earlier trials remains unconfirmed.

Other anti-TNF therapies, such as CDP571, are in their developmental stages. Etanercept, a fusion protein of the ligand-binding domain of TNF and an IgG common region, has limited effectiveness in CD. Another emerging anti-TNF therapeutic agent is thalidomide; however, its teratogenic potential has led to strict precautions, such as requiring proof of contraception in women of childbearing potential.

MEDICAL MANAGEMENT OF EXTRAINTESTINAL COMPLICATIONS

Not all of the extraintestinal complications of IBD exhibit an intestinal disease-dependent activity. However, pyoderma gangrenosum, peripheral arthritis, episcleritis, and erythema nodosum have an occurrence that parallels the activity of intestinal disease. Therefore their presence requires intensification of antiinflammatory therapy for bowel disease when appropriate. Nonsteroidal antiinflammatory drugs (NSAIDs) must be avoided because of their potential to exacerbate IBD; acetaminophen may be used for mild articular symptoms.

Ankylosing spondylitis and sacroiliitis may require treatment with prednisone, methotrexate, or hydroxychloroquine, as well as physical therapy. These arthritides, primary sclerosing cholangitis, uveitis, and iritis show a colitis-independent activity. Ocular complications should be managed in conjunction with an ophthalmologist. (See Box 4-2 for further extraintestinal complications.)

NUTRITIONAL THERAPY

The perceived relationship between antigens in the diet and immune activation in IBD supports the importance of nutritional therapy in IBD. Although nutritional manipulations have been effective in active CD, UC patients do not respond to dietary approaches. Peptide-based and elemental diets are as efficacious as steroids or total parenteral nutrition (TPN) in certain patients. Similarly, TPN and total bowel rest in combination is an equally effective alternative to steroids for the short-term induction of remission. However, neither TPN nor enteral diets can maintain remission.

A fish oil formulation (enteric-coated) has been observed to be efficacious in maintaining CD remission; this form of treatment may provide an alternative therapeutic modality if validated. Omega-3 fatty acids at higher dosages have been effective to some extent in refractory UC.

Poorly absorbed nutritional agents such as sucrose, Olestra, and fats may cause bloating, diarrhea, and increased flatulence. Patients with lactase deficiency may benefit symptomatically from a lactose-free diet.

SUPPORTIVE CARE

Symptoms unrelated to active inflammation are commonly encountered in IBD, and they are a significant cause of morbidity and reduced quality of life. The prevalence of irritable bowel syndrome (IBS) mirrors what is seen in the general population; therefore the identification of the correct cause(s) of symptoms is essential to the expeditious resolution of patient complaints. A complete dietary history may reveal that nutritional agents may trigger certain symptoms and that the patient may be better served by avoiding them.

Antispasmodics and antidiarrheal agents may be helpful for the control of certain IBS symptoms. Malabsorption of bile salts causing diarrhea after resection of the bowel usually responds to bile-salt sequestrants such as cholestyramine. Steatorrhea generally improves after reducing dietary fat. Antimotility agents should be avoided in severe disease due to their ability to precipitate toxic megacolon.

NSAIDs may precipitate disease exacerbation or refractory disease; therefore, analgesics such as acetaminophen are favored for pain control. The need for narcotics is rare. Persistent pain may be inflammatory in origin; thus, the primary cause should then be removed with antiinflammatory IBD treatment. In addition, because of the chronicity of painful complaints, habit-forming drugs should be avoided as much as possible.

BOX 4-2   Extraintestinal Manifestation of Inflammatory Bowel Disease

Musculoskeletal
Sacroilitis, peripheral arthropathy, ankylosing spondylitis, osteopenia, hypertrophic osteoarthropathy, osteoporosis, osteonecrosis, osteomalacia, relapsing polychondritis

Ophthalmologic
Episcleritis, scleritis, uveitis, iritis, conjunctivitis, retinal vascular disease

Dermatologic
Angular stomatitis, psoriasis, erythema nodosum, pyoderma gangrenosum, pyostomatitis vegetans, Sweet's syndrome, erythema multiforme, epidermolysis bullosa acquisita, metastatic CD

Genitourinary
Glomerulonephritis, nephrolithiasis, membranonephritis, fistulas, obstructive uropathy, amyloidosis

Hematologic
Anemia of chronic disease, iron-deficiency anemia, B_{12} deficiency, folate deficiency, hypercoagulable state, autoimmune hemolytic anemia, leukopenia, leukocytosis, thrombocytosis, thrombocytopenia, coagulation abnormalities

Cardiovascular
Endocarditis, myocarditis, cardiomyopathy, pericarditis

Neurologic
Seizures, meningitis, neuropathy, myopathy, vasculopathy

Pulmonary
Bronchitis, bronchiolitis, fibrosing alveolitis, bronchiectasis, pulmonary vasulitis, apical fibrosis, tracheal stenosis, granulomatous pulmonary disease

Hepatobiliary
Primary sclerosing cholangitis, cholelithiasis, pericholangitis, cirrhosis, steatosis, liver abscess, autoimmune hepatitis, portal vein thrombosis, granulomatous hepatitis, cholangiocarcinoma

Pancreatic
Granulomatous pancreatitis, CD of the ampulla

From Su CG et al: Extraintestinal manifestations of inflammatory bowel disease, *Gastroenterol Clin North Am* 31:308-309, 2002.
CD, Crohn's disease.

INFLAMMATORY BOWEL DISEASE AND PREGNANCY

Uncontrolled disease affects menstrual regularity and libido and increases the risk of early fetal loss; however, fertility is intact in both women and men; similarly, the course of pregnancy is unaffected when the disease is quiescent.

Sulfasalazine-related sperm abnormalities (which are reversible) and folate malabsorption may occur. Immunomodulators and aminosalicylates are safe in pregnancy and with lactation; thus treatment should not be withheld. Ensuring disease control before and throughout pregnancy is the best approach to obtaining the best fetal outcome.

COMPLICATIONS OF INFLAMMATORY BOWEL DISEASE AND THEIR MEDICAL MANAGEMENT

Intestinal complications of IBD are bleeding, toxic megacolon, fistulas, strictures, and malignancy.

Bleeding

The severity of bleeding that usually occurs depends on the depth of inflammation, which is in turn characteristic of the type of IBD under consideration. Profuse hemorrhage, therefore, is rare in UC, barring complications such as toxic megacolon; on the other hand, CD patients may experience significant bleeding because of the depth of their ulcers and the transmural nature of bowel inflammation. Coagulation abnormalities may complicate the picture. Thus iron deficiency anemia is common in both UC and CD; iron replacement therapy and other methods of maintaining an adequate hematocrit are often necessary.

Toxic Megacolon

This is a potentially life-threatening complication of UC (less common in CD), in which the colonic wall decompensates from severe inflammation (fulminant colitis). It may be precipitated by the use of narcotics, antidiarrheals, anticholinergics, and barium enema. The patient usually becomes febrile and may have leukocytosis and generalized abdominal tenderness with signs of systemic toxicity. The characteristic radiologic picture of an edematous and dilated colon with a thin wall emphasizes the friability of the colon; thus initial medical management is aggressive and includes volume resuscitation, broad-spectrum antibiotics, intravenous steroids (high dose), and bowel decompression. Almost half of patients respond to medical therapy; the lack of improvement in 48 to 72 hours or the presence of perforation or peritonitis is an indication for surgery.

Fistulas

CD patients are predisposed to fistulas because of the transmural nature of their bowel inflammation. Though perianal fistulas are the most common, enterocolic, enterovesical and rectovaginal fistulas may form. Metronidazole, ciprofloxacin, AZA, 6-MP, cyclosporine, and infliximab are some of the therapeutic agents that have shown efficacy for the management of fistulas. The dramatic effect infliximab has had on fistulas in CD is worth mentioning. The amount of discharge from high-output fistulas may decrease after treatment with octreotide and a proton-pump inhibitor. Associated abscesses need to be drained.

Strictures

The transmural inflammation with fibrosis and the cicatrization occurring in CD make stricture formation more characteristic of CD than UC. Sometimes inflammation, edema, and spasm of the terminal ileum may masquerade as a stricture; this condition usually reverts to normal after the inflammation is controlled.

In UC, reduction in luminal caliber may be due to the smooth muscle thickening seen during the active phase of disease, explaining the reversibility of this narrowing with the control of active inflammation. The presence of strictures that are fixed in patients with UC suggests malignancy or dysplasia.

Multiple strictures, particularly in the small intestine, cause recurrent obstruction (partial or complete), which may eventually necessitate surgical resection. Because of the short-gut syndrome that occurs after the resection of multiple strictures, a functional side-to-side enteroenterostomy or strictureplasty is performed whenever possible as an alternative to resection.

Adenocarcinoma

Colonic neoplasias in the setting of IBD have features that distinguish them from sporadic adenomas and carcinomas. In contrast to the general population, in whom adenomatous polyps and adenocarcinomas are related to age and family history, colonic cancers in IBD are most commonly preceded by flat or nodular areas of dysplasia that are related to the duration and extent of IBD, and the neoplasia risk is accelerated by the presence of primary sclerosing cholangitis. In contrast, the risk for neoplasm has no relationship to disease activity or the type of IBD.

For management of UC, colonoscopic surveillance starts 8 to 10 years following diagnosis. Thereafter, an individualized program is advised. A common recommendation is a surveillance colonoscopy every 2 to 3 years for patients who have had UC for 10 to 20 years, and every 1 to 2 years for patients with a history of UC greater than 20 years.

Indefinite dysplasia is a reason to aggressively control inflammation and repeat colonoscopies every 3 to 6 months; confirmation of low-grade dysplasia is adequate evidence to recommend a colectomy.

In the case of CD, additional risk factors are chronicity and the location of bowel inflammation. Unlike UC, there are no standard surveillance guidelines for bowel neoplasia, because CD is segmental in nature and heterogeneous in location. Although stricture formation may preclude a full colonoscopic evaluation at times, the surveillance program for UC may be applied.

INDICATIONS FOR SURGERY AND POSTSURGICAL MAINTENANCE THERAPY

Proctocolectomy with an ileostomy cures and improves quality of life in refractory UC; in CD it is only curative in those patients with disease limited to the colon. However, most young persons (of a physiologic age below 65) with UC are candidates for sphincter-saving ileoanal anastomoses and pelvic pouches. Occasionally patients with colonic CD without any stigmata of small bowel or perianal disease may also undergo successful sphincter-saving procedures, although the outcomes are not quite as good as with UC.

Indications for emergency surgery are complications such as severe hemorrhage, persistent fulminant colitis, toxic megacolon, and perforation. In CD, obstruction may require urgent surgery, just as chronic refractory colitis and medical complications such as steroid psychosis may precipitate urgent surgery in a UC patient.

Elective surgery may be needed for a variety of reasons, in particular because of medically intractable disease and a significantly poor quality of life; other indications include intolerance or significant adverse reactions to drugs (e.g., aseptic necrosis after steroids) and chronic steroid dependence.

After intestinal resections for CD, recurrence at the anastomotic site is nearly inevitable. Mesalamine has been demonstrated to reduce recurrence after surgery, although the statistical number needed to treat to prevent one recurrence is nearly 20 patients (i.e., 20 patients would have to be treated after surgery with mesalamine to prevent one patient from developing a postoperative recurrence).

Metronidazole given for 3 months after surgery at a high dose (20 mg/kg) has been effective in reducing recurrence, and most recently 6-MP has also been shown to reduce postoperative recurrence for at least 24 months after surgery.

Pouchitis is the most prevalent long-term complication of proctocolectomy (with an ileoanal anastomosis) in UC. The pathogenesis is not known; however, recurrence of UC in a colonlike mucosal lining has been proposed. Many agents have been tried to treat pouchitis, but antibiotics such as metronidazole or ciprofloxacin are those most commonly used. Recent experience shows that high amounts of the probiotic VSL#3 may also help to prevent pouchitis or treat refractory symptoms after a course of broad-spectrum antibiotics. Early trials also suggest a potential role for topical budesonide (Sambuelli et al, 2002).

FUTURE DIRECTIONS

Due to expanding knowledge regarding the pathogenesis of IBD, the focus of drug design and clinical trials has begun to target specific sites along the immunoinflammatory cascades. The inability of conventional IBD treatment to significantly modify the natural history of the disease has made the need for superior therapeutic agents imperative.

Biologic therapy targeting specific pathways of inflammation is an option that has shown significant promise. The preliminary success with infliximab, natalizumab, and CDP571 supports the impression that antiinflammatory cytokines and biologic immunomodulators may change the therapeutic approach in the near and distant future, particularly if they prove to modify the long-term disease activity. Other biologic agents in development include onercept (p55 TNF-binding protein), anti–IL-12 antibody, interferon-β and anti-interferon-γ, p65 anti-sense oligonucleotide, anti-CD4 antibody, colony-stimulating factors, human growth hormone, epithelial growth factor, and anti–IL-2 receptor antibody (Sandborn and Targan, 2002). Pilot studies have demonstrated the efficacy of α-4 β-7 integrin chimeric antibody for UC, and the beneficial effects of α-4 integrin subunit monoclonal antibody in CD has been observed in a large study (Gordon et al, 2001). In addition, therapeutic agents against nuclear factor-kB and p38 antagonists are targets of interruption of signal pathways of leukocytes and macrophages in IBD.

Adhesion molecules are involved in antigen presentation, and they also control the migration of leukocytes to both inflamed and normal intestines. These molecules have been observed to be up-regulated in IBD; therefore designing therapies directed against them is a mechanistically sound hypothesis. Clinical trials with ICAM-1 and ISIS-2302 in patients with corticosteroid-resistant CD yielded conflicting results; however, natalizumab, LDP-02, and anti–α-4 integrin are agents still in clinical trials that may prove valuable (van Assche and Rutgeerts, 2002).

Extracorporeal therapy that removes activated circulating T lymphocytes is touted as a quick and safe immunomodulatory method of treating IBD. Methods such as photopheresis and leukocytapheresis have been shown to be effective in IBD. The lack of significant side effects compared to drug therapy makes it an option with a promising future (Takazoe et al, 2002).

In preclinical experiments, transforming growth factor-α cured experimentally induced colitis, and gene transfer of IL-10 prevented the spontaneous development of colitis in interleukin-10–deficient rodents (Seegers, Bouma, and Pena, 2002); however, the vector-related hurdles to overcome make gene therapy a distant possibility in IBD. Early studies of IL-11 are promising. Its benefits are mediated through blockade of inflammatory cytokines and strengthening the epithelial barrier. Clinical trials in CD and UC on a larger scale are ongoing (Sands et al, 1999).

Other agents found to be of variable effect in IBD are transdermal nicotine, rosiglutazone, fish oil, and growth hormone. Allogenic bone marrow transplantation for reasons unrelated to IBD has put many CD patients in remission for prolonged periods, probably because of the reassembly of T cells that are not pathogenic. Nonimmunologic therapies under investigation are different forms of heparin, acemannan (an aloe vera derivative) and a variety of nontransdermal nicotine formulations (including intrarectal forms) (Robinson, 1998). Most of these agents have shown varying degrees of effectiveness.

CONCLUSION

The medical management of IBD continues to be challenging for all health care professionals involved. With the further elucidation of the pathogenesis of IBD, new agents targeting specific pathogenetic mechanisms may be designed. Our understanding of the immune and inflammatory pathways associated with the acute and chronic inflammation of IBD continues to expand and allows numerous potential targets for therapeutic intervention. The recent example of infliximab, a monoclonal antibody that specifically binds to TNF, is a prime example, although numerous other cytokines or intracellular pathways also afford potential for inhibition of proinflammatory compounds, or stimulation of antiinflammatory signals. Therefore it may come as no surprise if most of our current conventional therapies become obsolete in the foreseeable future.

The limitations that IBD imposes on the lives of patients and their families can be easily overlooked as the health practitioner gets entangled in the traditional therapeutic issues that the patients bring up. The lack of complete knowledge of the origins of the disease, with its malignant potential in a population mostly at the prime of their lives, can be psychologically unsettling. Therefore it is imperative that the psychologic issues facing the patients and their families be addressed, especially if one desires to adequately control noninflammatory aspects of the disease such as irritable bowel syndrome symptoms.

The importance of a multifaceted, if not multidisciplinary, approach to the therapeutic success of the medical management of IBD cannot be overemphasized. As a disease that challenges the skills and patience of the clinician, a compassionate but optimistic strategy that routinely involves patients in decision making can often tame a disease as morbid and lifestyle-threatening as IBD.

SELF-ASSESSMENT EXERCISES

Questions

1. What is the goal of the medical management of UC and CD?
   a. To induce and maintain clinical remission while minimizing side effects and maintaining the quality of life
   b. To prevent the side effects of the medications by reducing the need for corticosteroids
   c. To cure the disease and allow the patient to lead a productive and full life
   d. To prevent surgical consult and/or surgical intervention
2. The highest incidence and prevalence rates of IBD have been reported from:
   a. The United Kingdom, Spain, and France.
   b. Japan and the United States.
   c. Third-world countries where bacterial food infestation is known to be high.
   d. The United Kingdom, Scandinavia, and the United States.
3. Which of the following would be most likely to see an inherited predisposition for IBD?
   a. Sister to sister
   b. Cousin to cousin
   c. Mother to grandmother
   d. Maternal nieces
4. What is the most important "environmental factor" impacting the pathogenesis and course of IBD?
5. Is the hypothesis that IBD *may be* an aberrant response to environmental factors in genetically susceptible hosts true or false?
6. Why is the discovery of NOD2 one of the most significant findings in IBD pathogenesis in years?
   a. NOD2 is found in the small and large intestinal ulcers of the person with IBD.
   b. NOD2 is a genetic variant that when found in individuals who are homozygous for NOD2 may have a relative risk of Crohn's disease of 14.3% to 44%.
   c. Specific medications can alter the NOD2 gene, decreasing the risk of developing CD.
   d. NOD2 indicates that a person has a high risk of developing UC.
7. The rectum is always involved in UC. True _____ False _____
8. Name three clinical distinctions that differentiate UC from CD.
9. The reason that CD patients are more likely to symptoms of abdominal pain is:
   a. The medication that is used to treat CD causes vascular friability.
   b. Related to the transmural inflammation.
   c. It is a chronic recurring disease.
   d. Related to the location of the disease.
10. Fistula formation is only seen in which of the IBDs?
11. What are the principles in treating ulcerative colitis and Crohn's disease?
12. Name two aminosalicylate drugs used to treat mild to moderate ulcerative colitis or Crohn's disease.
13. What is the average dose of corticosteroids used in the treatment of moderately severe UC in the outpatient setting?
14. Name one immunomodulatory agent used in the induction and maintenance of remission in UC and CD.
15. Which of the following antibiotics has been shown to be effective in the treatment of patients with CD and perianal fistulas?
    a. Keflix
    b. Metronidazole
    c. Ciprofloxin
    d. Clindamycin
16. The biologic agent infliximab is:
    a. A transforming growth factor.
    b. Adhesion molecules that are involved in antigen presentation.
    c. A chimeric monoclonal antibody to TNF-α.
    d. A type of interleukin substance that mediates inflammatory cytokines.

17. Colonoscopic surveillance for adenocarcinoma is recommended for a person with UC:
    a. 5 years after diagnosis
    b. 8-10 years after diagnosis
    c. Annually following the initial diagnosis
    d. 15 years after diagnosis
18. Which of the following over-the-counter drugs may precipitate disease exacerbation?
    a. Antihistamines
    b. NSAIDs
    c. Laxatives
    d. Acetaminophen

Answers

1. a
2. d
3. a
4. Cigarette smoking
5. True
6. b
7. True
8. UC: superficial inflammation; mucosal appearance denotes continuous involvement; the mucosa appearance is edematous, granular, and erythematous; the location is limited to the colon; the rectum is always involved and the small intestine is not involved; the perianal area is normal; pain is not typical; rectal bleeding may be present; diarrhea may be present as more colonic involvement presents
CD: inflammation is transmural; the mucosal appearance is discontinuous with cobblestoning; granulomas can be present; the location can be in any part of the GI tract; rectal involvement is variable; terminal ileum and cecum are most commonly involved; perirectal abscess/disease can be present; pain is more likely due to transmural inflammation; bleeding depends upon disease location; greater percent of obstructive symptoms and weight loss more common
9. b
10. CD
11. First induce remission, and then maintain remissions.
12. Asacol, Pentasa, Dipentum, Colazal, Rowasa, Canasa
13. 40 mg/day
14. Azathioprine and 6-mercaptopurine, methotrexate, cyclosporine.
15. b
16. c
17. b
18. b

REFERENCES

Andersson RE et al: Appendectomy and protection against ulcerative colitis, *N Engl J Med* 344:808-814, 2001.

Bouhnik Y et al: Long-term follow-up of patients with Crohn's disease treated with azathioprine or 6-mercaptopurine, *Lancet* 347:215-219, 1996.

Cuthbert AP et al: The contribution of NOD2 gene mutations to the risk and site of disease in inflammatory bowel disease, *Gastroenterology* 122:867-874, 2002.

Delpre G et al: HLA antigens in ulcerative colitis and Crohn's disease in Israel, *Gastroenterology* 78:1452-1457, 1980.

Duggan AE et al: Appendectomy, childhood hygiene, *Helicobacter pylori* status, and risk of inflammatory bowel disease: a case control study, *Gut* 43:494-498, 1998.

Egan LJ, Sandborn WJ: Methotrexate for inflammatory bowel disease: pharmacology and preliminary results, *Mayo Clin Proc* 71:69-80, 1996.

Farrell RJ et al: Increased incidence of non-Hodgkin's lymphoma in inflammatory bowel disease patients on immunosuppressive therapy but overall risk is low, *Gut* 47:514-519, 2000.

Fiocchi C: Inflammatory bowel disease: etiology and pathogenesis, *Gastroenterology* 115:182-205, 1998.

Gionchetti P et al: Oral bacteriotherapy as maintenance treatment in patients with chronic pouchitis: a double-blind, placebo-controlled trial, *Gastroenterology* 119:305-309, 2000.

Gordon FH et al: A randomized placebo-controlled trial of a humanized monoclonal antibody to alpha-4 integrin in active Crohn's disease, *Gastroenterology* 121:268-274, 2001.

Hampe J et al: A genome wide analysis provides evidence for novel linkages in inflammatory bowel disease in a large European cohort, *Am J Hum Genet* 64:808-816, 1999.

Hanauer SB: Inflammatory bowel diseases. *WebMD Scientific American Medicine, Gastroenterology* IV(June):1-18, 2001.

Hiwatashi N et al: HLA antigens in inflammatory bowel disease, *Tohoku J Exp Med* 131:381-385, 1980.

Hugot JP et al: Association of NOD2 leucine-rich repeat variants with susceptibility to Crohn's disease, *Nature* 411:599-603, 2001.

Kinouchi Y et al: Transmission disequilibrium testing confirms the association of the TNF-alpha 1031C allele with Crohn's disease, *Gastroenterology* 120:A456, 2001.

Kombluth A, Sachar DB: Ulcerative colitis practice guidelines in adults: American College of Gastroenterology, Practice Parameters Committee, *Am J Gastroenterol* 92:204, 1997.

Lewis JD et al: Inflammatory bowel disease is not associated with an increased risk of lymphoma, *Gastroenterology* 121:1080-1087, 2001.

Loftus E, Sandborn WJ: Epidemiology of inflammatory bowel disease, *Gastroenterol Clin North Am* 31:1-20, 2002.

MacDermott RP: Lack of current clinical value of serological testing in the evaluation of patients with IBD, *Inflamm Bowel Dis* 5:64, 1999.

Negoro K et al: Crohn's disease is associated with novel polymorphisms in the 5'-flanking region of the tumor necrosis factor gene, *Gastroenterology* 117:1062-1068, 1999.

Ogura Y et al: A frameshift mutation in NOD2 associated with susceptibility to Crohn's disease, *Nature* 411:603-606, 2001.

Orholm M et al: Familial occurrence of inflammatory bowel disease, *N Engl J Med* 324:84-88, 1991.

Podolsky DK: Inflammatory bowel disease, *N Engl J Med* 347:417-428, 2002.

Present DH et al: Treatment of Crohn's disease with 6-mercaptopurine: a long-term randomized, double blind study, *N Engl J Med* 302:981-987, 1980.

Robinson M: Medical therapy of inflammatory bowel disease for the 21st century, *Eur J Surg* Suppl 582:90-98, 1998.

Rubin DT, Hanauer S: Smoking and inflammatory bowel disease, *Eur J Gastroenterol Hepatol* 12:855, 2000.

Rutgeerts P et al: Efficacy and safety of retreatment with anti-tumor necrosis factor antibody (infliximab) to maintain remission in Crohn's disease, *Gastroenterology* 117:761-769, 1999.

Sambuelli A et al: Budesonide enema in pouchitis—a double-blind, double-dummy, controlled trial, *Aliment Pharmacol Ther* 16:27-34, 2002.

Sandborn WJ: A review of immune modifier therapy for inflammatory bowel disease: azathioprine, 6-mercaptopurine, cyclosporine, and methotrexate, *Am J Gastroenterol* 91:423, 1996

Sandborn WJ, Targan SR: Biologic therapy of inflammatory bowel disease, *Gastroenterology* 122:1592-1608, 2002.

Sands BE et al: Preliminary evaluation of safety and activity of recombinant human interleukin 11 in patients with active Crohn's disease, *Gastroenterology* 117:58-64, 1999.

Sartor RB: Review article: role of enteric microflora in the pathogenesis of intestinal inflammation and arthritis, *Aliment Pharmacol Ther* 11(Suppl 3):17, 1997.

Seegers D, Bouma G, Pena AS: Review article: a critical approach to new forms of treatment of Crohn's disease and ulcerative colitis, *Aliment Pharmacol Ther* 16(Suppl 4):53-58, 2002.

Shanahan F: Probiotics in inflammatory bowel disease, *Gut* 48:609, 2001.

Swidsinski A et al: Mucosal flora in inflammatory bowel disease, *Gastroenterology* 122:44-54, 2002.

Takazoe M et al: The present status and the recent development of the treatment for inflammatory bowel diseases: desirable effects of extracorporeal immunomodulation, *Therapeutic Apheresis* 6:305-311, 2002.

Targan SR et al: A short-term study of chimeric monoclonal antibody cA2 to tumor factor alpha for Crohn's disease, Crohn's Disease cA2 Study Group, *N Engl J Med* 337:1029, 1997.

Targan SR: The utility of ANCA and ASCA in inflammatory bowel disease, *Inflamm Bowel Dis* 5:61, 1999.

Tysk C et al: Ulcerative colitis and Crohn's disease in an unselected population of monozygotic and dizygotic twins: a study of heritability and the influence of smoking, *Gut* 29:990-996, 1988.

van Assche G, Rutgeerts P: Antiadhesion molecule therapy in inflammatory bowel disease, *Inflamm Bowel Dis* 8:291-300, 2002.

Yang H, Rotter JI: Genetic aspects of idiopathic inflammatory bowel disease. In Kirschner JB, Shorter RG, editors: *Inflammatory bowel diseases,* ed 4, Baltimore, 1995, Williams & Wilkins.

Inflammatory Bowel Disease: Surgical Management

RAVI P. KIRAN and VICTOR W. FAZIO

OBJECTIVES

1. Discuss the basic principles and indications that guide surgical decision making for the patient with Crohn's disease.
2. Identify two of the surgical procedures that are considered when treating a patient with Crohn's disease of the small bowel.
3. List three procedures that can be used to surgically manage Crohn's disease of the large bowel.
4. Discuss the rate and areas of recurrence of Crohn's disease following either a small or large bowel resection.
5. Describe the indications for surgery in patients with ulcerative colitis.
6. Compare and contrast the four surgical options for treatment of the patient with ulcerative colitis.
7. Describe the surgical procedure for construction of the ileal pouch anal anastomosis.
8. Differentiate between the one-, two-, and three-staged procedures in the creation of an ileal pouch anal anastomosis.
9. Explain the differences and the pros and cons in the stapled and handsewn anastomosis when creating an ileal pouch anal anastomosis.
10. Discuss the functional results of patients undergoing an ileal pouch anal anastomosis.
11. Describe the surgical procedure and management of the continent ileostomy.

INTRODUCTION

Crohn's disease (CD) and ulcerative colitis have a remitting and relapsing course. Patients of any age group may be affected and are first seen either in an acute phase or with chronic signs and symptoms. Since any part of the gastrointestinal tract may be involved, the focus of treatment in CD revolves around the prevention of recurrence and maintenance of adequate absorptive surface. Because the small bowel is spared, restoration of continence after resection of disease is a major concern in ulcerative colitis. Initial treatment is medical in both disorders, but a significant proportion of patients are likely to need surgery, the probability of which increases with increasing duration of disease. Timing of surgery and type of procedure performed depend on a variety of factors such as patient preference, site of involvement, response to medical treatment, age and physiologic status of the patient, comorbidity, concomitant medication, severity and duration of disease, and the risk of complications including malignancy. For example, in toxic megacolon the procedure of choice in patients with less severe colitis is subtotal colectomy with the formation of an end ileostomy. However, in the frail patient with more fulminant disease, extensive dissection may be avoided by performing a rapid decompressive procedure such as a loop ileostomy with a blowout colostomy (Turnbull procedure; see following paragraphs). Similarly, management of the distal rectosigmoid stump after an emergency subtotal colectomy depends on the condition of the colon and its consequent risk for further perforation. Surgeon factors such as previous experience and preference of procedure also determine the timing of surgery and the choice of procedure performed. Although the management of CD and ulcerative colitis is discussed separately in this chapter, there is considerable overlap in the diagnosis and management of the two disorders.

CROHN'S DISEASE

Introduction

CD is a transmural granulomatous disorder that may affect any portion of the gastrointestinal tract from the mouth to the anus. Lesions may be multifocal, with patches of diseased bowel separated by grossly normal segments. Most patients have involvement of the small bowel, 41% of CD patients have involvement of the ileocolic area, and an additional 30% have isolated involvement of the small bowel. Peak onset occurs at about 35 years of age, although it may also start later in life. The cause of the disease is unknown, and neither medical nor surgical treatment is curative. Treatment is aimed at the relief of symptoms and the prevention or management of complications. Initial therapy is always medical; surgery is only indicated when medical therapy fails, or complications occur, or the patient is unable to tolerate medication because of unacceptable side effects. The primary goals of surgical therapy include dealing with the immediate adverse effects of the disease, restoration of health and function, and permitting withdrawal of steroids and other immunosuppressive agents.

Historical Aspects

Crohn, Ginzburg, and Oppenheimer (1932) first described the clinicopathologic features of the disease in 1932. Wells described segmental colitis in CD in 1952, Brooke described granulomatous disease of the large and small intestine in 1959, and Lokhart-Mummery and Morson subsequently showed in 1960 that CD can affect the colon. The surgical procedure that was initially advocated for CD of the small bowel by both Dalziel and Berg was small bowel resection. The latter subsequently popularized bypass, and the Berg or Mount Sinai operation consisted of transection of the small bowel proximal to the involved disease site, oversewing of the distal transected end of the ileum, and anastomosis of the end of the proximal small bowel to the mid transverse colon. It was later recognized that

this procedure could be complicated by stump blowout or disease reactivation in the bypassed segment; thus resection once again became the treatment of choice for involvement of the terminal ileum and ileocolon. More recently the principle of strictureplasty, which was initially described in India for tubercular strictures of the intestine, has been adopted for CD; this reduces the risk of short bowel syndrome in these patients, who often need multiple operations. Laparoscopic-assisted resection with extracorporeal anastomosis has more recently been shown to be an effective approach in the management of these patients. A recent randomized control trial found that patients undergoing surgery by laparoscopic approach have a shorter length of stay, fewer complications, and faster recovery of function (Milsom et al, 2001). However, the potential problems of laparoscopic resection include difficulty with transection of thickened mesentery and lymph nodes, identification of proximal skip lesions, and adhesions from prior surgery.

Clinical Features

Although it may not always be possible, ulcerative colitis and CD need to be differentiated, since the procedure performed and the prognosis depend on the specific diagnosis. Clinical features that distinguish Crohn's colitis from ulcerative colitis include a normal-appearing rectum with proximal colonic disease, perianal fistula or abscess, velvety or indurated anal skin tags, aphthoid ulcers, serpiginous longitudinal ulcers with normal-appearing intervening mucosa, anal fissures which are broad and indolent, ileal disease, skip lesions or patchy inflammation, and internal fistulas to small bowel, bladder or vagina.

Farmer, Hawk, and Turnbull (1975) found that the primary site of involvement of CD was ileocolic in 41% of patients, small intestine in 28.6%, colon in 27%, and anorectal in 3.4%. After 10 years of follow-up (Whelan et al, 1985), 90% of patients with ileocolitis and 70% of those with ileal or colonic disease required operation. Patients with ileocolic disease had the highest rate of recurrence requiring another operation, compared to those with colonic and small intestinal disease. When CD is confined to the colon at initial presentation, the rate and site of recurrence are influenced by the type of procedure performed (de Dombal, Burton, and Goligher, 1971; Greenstein et al, 1975; Lee and Papaioannou, 1980; Williams et al, 1991). Recurrence is lowest after total proctocolectomy and end ileostomy, and highest after segmental colectomy.

Basic Principles of Operative Management and Preoperative Care

Since CD is a chronic disease with multiple remissions and relapses, as well as an unclear etiology, the goal of treatment is control of disease and prevention of relapse. The decision is difficult as to when to operate in the patient who has chronic symptoms that are controlled partially with medication or fully with high doses of medication. The risk of side effects of medication and the effect on quality of life must be considered when persisting with medical therapy; quality of life is of paramount importance in these patients, who are often young. However, though surgery has been shown to cause an immediate improvement in quality of life (Delaney et al, 2003), the associated risk of complications must be considered when reaching a decision about subjecting the patient to surgery. The benefit to the patient from reduction of macroscopic disease, or from treatment of obstruction from stricture formation, needs to be balanced against the potential loss of absorptive surface from resection during each operation. Radical surgery does not affect cure, and medical and operative modalities need to be used in combination to manage complications and improve quality of life.

The extent of CD is determined by contrast radiography and endoscopy. Surgery is performed after restoration of physiologic deficits. Anemia and fluid electrolyte imbalance is corrected if possible, and significant nutritional depletion is corrected with total parenteral nutrition. However, the role of preoperative nutrition is controversial, since the postoperative complication rate is not reduced despite an improvement in nutritional parameters. If there is no evidence of obstruction, mechanical

bowel preparation is administered the evening before surgery. Temporary ostomies help to make surgery safer and may help anastomotic healing in the presence of intraabdominal sepsis, excessive bleeding during surgery, multiple anastomosis, and severe hypoalbuminemia. Thus stoma siting is done before surgery. Perioperative steroid cover is given for patients on steroids, and intravenous antibiotics are used prophylactically but may need to be continued in the event of contamination. If reoperative surgery is indicated, it is best performed 3 to 6 months after the previous laparotomy in the elective setting.

Conservation is the cornerstone of therapy in CD; hence strictureplasty is preferred for small bowel disease. Resection is performed only when unavoidable, and the extent of resection is guided by the gross appearance of the intestinal segments, bowel wall thickening, thickening or induration of the mesenteric margin, and enlarged paraileal lymph nodes. Only the primary problem is dealt with surgically, and resection margins are conservative, because radical resection has not been shown to be beneficial to the patient (Fazio et al, 1996). Although some studies have published conflicting results (Berman and Krause, 1977; Martin, Heyen, and Dube, 1994; Wolff et al, 1983), most series agree that there is no significant relationship between microscopic inflammation at resection margins and the recurrence rate (Adolff, Armaud, and Ollier, 1987; Chardavoyne et al, 1986; Fazio and Marchetti, 1999; Papaioannau et al, 1979; Speranza et al, 1986).

Indications for Surgery

Failure of medical therapy and the development of complications are the primary indications for surgery in the patient with CD. Patients with failure to thrive, bowel obstruction, abscess, free perforation, fistula, obstructive uropathy (Siminovitch and Fazio, 1980), intestinal hemorrhage, perianal disease, carcinoma of the bowel, or disabling extraintestinal manifestations may require surgery. Acute obstruction and perforation are absolute indications, but when subacute symptoms occur, the pros and cons of an operative procedure need to be carefully weighed before subjecting the patient to surgery. The potential risks of surgery include metabolic and nutritional loss, possibility of a stoma, recurrence or relapse of disease, and short bowel syndrome if multiple bowel resections are undertaken. Hence patients need to be a central part of the decision-making process; patient preference, compliance, and quality of life desired have a major bearing on the procedure performed. Box 5-1 outlines indications for surgical intervention.

Malignancy that develops in the affected portion of the bowel is a rare indication for surgery (Ekbom et al, 1990; Greenstein et al, 1981; Hawker et al, 1982; Savoca, Ballantyne, and Cahow, 1990). Carcinoma complicating CD of the colon is more common than the one that is a complication of the small bowel. The risk of malignant transformation of strictured segments creates special problems in management, since biopsy and cytology of the lesion does not always result in a diagnosis. Furthermore, resection of all stricture-bearing segments cannot be performed, because this could lead to loss of large absorptive lengths. The guidelines that have hence been proposed in these patients include resection of any excluded segment of bowel that is not amenable to future restorative surgery, annual colonoscopic surveillance for non-resected segments of the colon, consideration of resection for patients who have had CD for more than 10 years with colonic strictures, and multiple biopsies of strictures with resection if dysplasia or adenoma is identified. Patients with long-standing chronic fistula in-ano require curettage of tracts and tru-cut biopsy of indurated skin and subcutaneous tissue.

Crohn's Disease of the Small Bowel

Within 5 years of the diagnosis of CD of the small bowel, 50% of patients undergo surgery, and within 10 years this rises to 66%. With concomitant colonic involvement the rate of operation rises to 75% and 90%, respectively. The probability of surgery after 20 and 30 years of CD was 78% and 90% in the National Cooperative Crohn's Disease Study (NCCDS) (Mekhjian et al, 1979). Obstruction is the most common indication for surgery. Patients who develop an inflamed ileocecal mass will benefit from conservative ileocecal resection.

Resection. This is the procedure of choice for CD of the small bowel, especially for the patient without previous surgery. In addition to reduction of macroscopic volume of disease, the other advantage of resection is the opportunity to get enough tissue for a histologic diagnosis. During resection, only mesenteric nodes that hamper resection and anastomosis are excised, because reducing nodal disease does not reduce recurrence. Only grossly involved segments of the disease are resected, and the presence of aphthoid ulcers in soft, supple, otherwise healthy bowel does not indicate a need for further proximal or distal resection. Ileocecal CD is managed by an ileocecal resection preserving as much of the right colon as possible. Equivalent results can be achieved with either a handsewn or stapled anastomosis.

Bypass. This is of historical interest, as previously mentioned in this chapter, but is more useful as a temporizing procedure for planned reexploration in instances where there is a large, fixed, inflammatory mass. Bypass is also useful for duodenal CD.

BOX 5-1 **Indications for Surgery in Patients with Inflammatory Bowel Disease**

Crohn's Disease
Failure of medical treatment
Intolerance of medical treatment
Development of complications:
    Acute obstruction
    Perforation
    Malignancy

Ulcerative Colitis
Failure of medical treatment
Intolerance of medical treatment
Dysplasia
Toxic megacolon

Strictureplasty. The safety and efficacy of strictureplasty has been corroborated by a number of studies (Ozuner et al, 1996a; Ozuner et al, 1996b; Stebbing et al, 1995). Improvement of obstructive symptoms is reported by 90% of patients. The operative mortality for resection in CD ranges from 0.3% to 3.2% (Alexander-Williams and Haynes, 1985; Michelassi et al, 1991) but in strictureplasty is perhaps lower. Strictureplasty is particularly useful in patients with multiple strictures, because it helps conserve bowel by avoiding resection. The main disadvantage is the absence of adequate tissue for diagnosis in order to rule out carcinoma or lymphoma, which may occur at stricture sites. Strictureplasty is contraindicated if there is free or contained perforation of the small bowel, inflammatory mass with internal or external fistulas, multiple strictures within a short segment of the bowel, and for colonic strictures. After strictureplasty, symptomatic recurrence is seen in the majority of patients; however, there is no definite evidence favoring frozen sections of resection margins in CD patients, since several studies have shown that recurrence of CD is independent of the presence of disease at the intestinal margin (Heuman et al, 1983; Pennington et al, 1980).

Surgical Technique. The whole length of the intestine is examined at laparotomy before definitive resection or strictureplasty is performed. Strictures are identified either by careful visual and tactile examination or by the use of a Foley catheter for calibration of the small bowel. Strictures less than 10 cm in length are treated by a Heinecke-Mikulicz strictureplasty (Figure 5-1) and longer strictures by a Finney strictureplasty (Figure 5-2). For short strictures a linear antimesenteric incision is made that extends a couple of centimeters on either side of the edge of the stricture, stay sutures are placed at the midpoints of the cut edges of the incision on either side, and using these, the incision is sutured transversely in a single layer after securing hemostasis. The site is marked with a surgiclip for future reference and identification. Biopsy of the mucosa is done to confirm the diagnosis and to exclude carcinoma. Longer strictures are treated by

an enterotomy, and the posterior layer is approximated with a continuous suture taking all layers of the bowel wall. The anterior layer is also similarly closed, thus resulting in a Finney strictureplasty. Other modifications have been described, including combination strictureplasty and isoperistaltic side-to-side anastomosis.

Crohn's Disease of the Large Bowel

Most patients with extensive Crohn's colitis do not have long-term remission with medical treatment and require surgery; therefore, the commonest indication is the failure of medical therapy. Chronic disability, bleeding, long-term or high dose steroids, extraintestinal manifestations, and troublesome perianal disease may require elective surgery. Urgent indications include toxic dilation, perforation, or massive hemorrhage; sepsis and obstruction are other occasional indications. The majority of patients with Crohn's colitis require excision of the disease, and the probability of surgery for Crohn's colitis is estimated as 35 ± 7% at 5 years and 39 ± 7% at 10 years for recent onset disease (Elliott, Ritchie, and Lennard-Jones, 1985), rising to 72 ± 6% at 6 years from the first hospital admission (Lennard-Jones, Ritchie, and Zohrab, 1976).

The specific procedure depends on the extent and site of disease, distensibility of the rectum, sphincter function, presence or absence of perianal disease, age, and attitude of the patient toward stoma and surveillance. Total proctocolectomy and ileostomy gives the best long-term results because it eliminates the risk of recurrence. Abdominal colectomy with ileorectal anastomosis is an alternative in younger patients who have good sphincter tone, since it avoids a stoma and reduces the risk of inadvertent autonomic nerve damage, but the disadvantage is the possibility of recurrent disease. Segmental resection of the colon is an alternative for isolated short-segment involvement of the colon.

Elective Procedures
Total Proctocolectomy and Ileostomy. This is the most appropriate procedure for the treatment of extensive Crohn's colitis when associated with serious anorectal disease or poor sphincter tone. It can be performed in one stage or as a staged

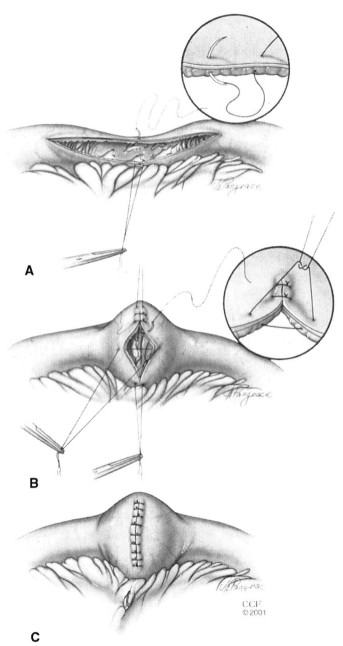

Figure 5-1   Heinecke-Mikulicz strictureplasty. **A,** Stricture and adjacent "normal" bowel incised longitudinally. **B,** Defect closed transversely. **C,** Completed Heinecke-Mikulicz strictureplasty. (Courtesy Cleveland Clinic, Cleveland, Ohio.)

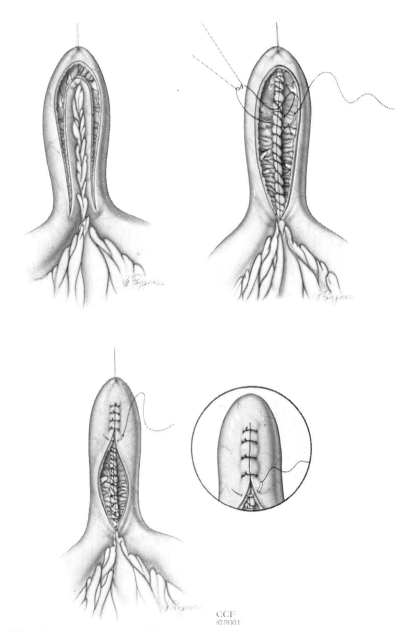

Figure 5-2 Finney strictureplasty. The two loops are opposed and antimesenteric enterotomy is made. (Courtesy Cleveland Clinic, Cleveland, Ohio.)

procedure after previous abdominal colectomy with or without anastomosis. Initial diverting ileostomy can be performed in the presence of severe perianal and rectal sepsis and in some patients who require time to get used to the idea of a stoma before a more permanent procedure. A single-stage procedure is avoided in patients with fulminant disease, toxic megacolon, severe malnutrition, or perianal sepsis. Although subtotal colectomy is the procedure usually performed for severe colonic hemorrhage, total proctocolectomy may occasionally be indicated for patients with proctoscopic evidence of significant rectal hemorrhage.

Surgical technique. During surgery, care is taken to ensure that resection of the rectum is conservative, unless there is evidence of cancer. The rectum may be dissected within the mesorectum in order to avoid damage to autonomic nerves, but this is associated with greater operative blood loss. A modified conservative dissection may instead be performed in the avascular plane between the investing layer of fascia of the rectum and Waldeyer's fascia up to the lower border of the third sacral vertebra, followed by dissection close to the rectal wall. This facilitates the proctectomy considerably, with minimal blood loss, and does not injure the nervi erigentes and the sacral sympathetic nerves. The lateral rectal dissection is kept close to the rectal wall at the level of the lateral ligament. Anteriorly the rectal dissection is carried out on the rectal side of the fascia of Denonvilliers, exposing the vertical muscle fibers of the rectum but not the seminal vesicles, and perineal proctectomy is completed by the endoanal technique. An intersphincteric dissection is performed, preserving the anal skin, external sphincter, and levator muscles, since this has been reported to be associated with a lower incidence of impotence (Leicester et al, 1984). Primary closure of the perianal wound is then performed. Alternatively, the external sphincter may be resected, or the rectum can be transected at the level of the levators and the rectal stump closed by sutures or staples, thus avoiding a perianal wound. The skin is left open if anal fistulas require simultaneous excision or deroofing. Mucosal proctectomy with or without closure of the anorectal stump has also been proposed.

Ileostomy creation. An incision is made at the marked ostomy site and the end of the ileum is delivered through the incision so that it extends above the skin surface. A full thickness bite of the open end of the ileum is first taken, followed by a seromuscular bite of the ileum at the skin level, and finally a subcutaneous bite of the skin is taken. The resultant stoma should protrude 2 to 3 cm above the abdominal wall to create a spout. Finally, sutures are placed between the cut edge of the ileum and the dermis (Figure 5-3; see also Figure 1-2).

Complications include perianal fistulas, which may persist despite these procedures, proximal small bowel recurrence (3% to 46%) (Steinberg et al, 1974), and nonhealing of the perineal wound. Up to 34% of patients may have an unhealed perineal wound compared to 11% in ulcerative colitis (Corman et al, 1978). Wounds may be managed by serial wound curettage and cautery, resurfacing with skin grafting, filling of cavities with vascularized pedicle muscle grafts such as gracilis, semimembranosus, rectus abdominis, or omentum. The

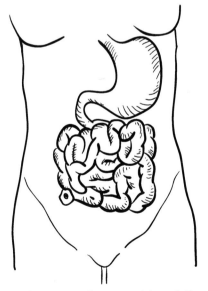

Figure 5-3 Proctocolectomy with end ileostomy. (From Hampton BG, Bryant RA: *Ostomies and continent diversions: nursing management*, St Louis, 1992, Mosby.)

inferior gluteal myocutaneous graft has also been used. Failure rates continue to remain high despite these procedures. When proctocolectomy is performed in the acute setting, it is associated with high mortality and morbidity rates. Pelvic dissection may lead to pelvic abscess, enteric fistula, or autonomic nerve damage.

Abdominal (Subtotal) Colectomy. This is indicated when a compliant rectum is spared of disease, sphincter tone is adequate, there is lack of perianal sepsis, and extensive ileal disease is absent. The disadvantage of subtotal colectomy is that it is associated with a higher incidence of recurrence than total proctocolectomy.

One-stage surgery is usually performed unless the patient has toxic colitis, intraabdominal sepsis, or significant malnutrition, or if doubt exists as to the normality of the rectal mucosa and/or moderate perineal disease. After resection of diseased colon, the rectal remnant may, with diversion and the passage of time, recover compliance and function and thus become suitable for ileorectal anastomosis. Some studies have reported favorable results with ileorectal anastomosis (primary or secondary) when mild proctitis is present (Buchmann et al, 1981; Lock et al, 1981; Longo et al, 1992), and anastomotic complications are similar irrespective of whether the ileum is anastomosed to diseased or macroscopically normal rectum; routine proximal covering ileostomy is not indicated. Equivalent results have been reported with sutured and stapled anastomoses. When in doubt, initial abdominal colectomy and ileostomy is a better procedure, with reanastomosis of the ileum to the rectal remnant at a later date once all sepsis has resolved (usually 1 year). When ileorectal anastomosis is performed, the level of rectal transection should be at the sacral promontory to preserve as much of the rectum as possible to ensure adequate capacity. Alternatively an ileosigmoid anastomosis may be performed when the distal sigmoid is free of active disease. When the rectum is preserved, it is prudent to monitor the stump by regular surveillance, since cancer has been reported to occur in both the defunctioned and anastomosed patient (Cunsolo et al, 1988; Jones, Munro, and Ewen, 1977).

Subtotal colectomy is the procedure of choice in critically ill patients. In this situation, damage to the autonomic nerves is minimized by preserving the main trunk of the inferior mesenteric artery and instead dividing the mesenteric branches. This also makes it easier for the distal stump to reach the anterior abdominal wall, which is made to lie in the subcutaneous plane in the lower end of the abdominal incision after it has been stapled across and oversewn. If it is too friable, a mucus fistula is formed (Figure 5-4); alternatively, it may be exteriorized and matured into a mucus fistula at a later date. If reanastomosis is not performed, proctectomy of the stump is best performed later because the development of a stricture in the rectal stump due to recurrent inflammation may preclude adequate surveillance after a couple of years.

Segmental Resection. Segmental ileocolic resection is the preferred treatment for ileocolitis, but the role of segmental resection in segmental colitis is less defined. This may take the form of a segmental resection and colocolic or colorectal anastomosis, or abdominoperineal resection of the

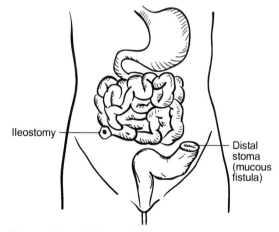

Figure 5-4 Abdominal view of descending colostomy with distal bowel in place and exiting to skin as mucous fistula. (From Hampton BG, Bryant RA: *Ostomies and continent diversions: nursing management*, St Louis, 1992, Mosby.)

rectum with a terminal colostomy. Recurrence rates after segmental resection are high (Longo, Ballantyne, and Cahow, 1988), but it may be performed when disease is limited, as a greater length of colon that is able to absorb water can be preserved.

Restorative Proctocolectomy and Continent Ileostomy for Crohn's Colitis. The role of these procedures is controversial, and they have a relatively high failure rate in CD. Recurrence rate in the small bowel is high, and the presence of perianal disease in the preoperative period is considered to be an indicator of poor subsequent pouch function (Hyman et al, 1991). Another report found that only 54% of patients had a functional pouch 10 years after surgery (Sagar, Dozois, and Wolff, 1996). However, in one study patients who had an inadvertent creation of ileal pouch anal anastomosis (IPAA) because of inconclusive initial histology reports were, surprisingly, noted to have a good functional outcome at 3 years after surgery (Hyman et al, 1991). Similar controversy exists regarding the role of continent ileostomy in CD patients. Some authors have suggested the creation of a continent ileostomy in select patients who are no longer taking steroids and those who are free of symptoms for 5 years (Bloom et al, 1986). Some patients request a continent pouch despite fully comprehending the risks, since they may be completely averse to a stoma and an external pouching system. IPAA and continent ileostomy are discussed later in this chapter. See Box 5-2 for surgical interventions in CD.

Laparoscopic Procedures. Laparoscopic ileocecal and small bowel resections are feasible. Laparoscopic techniques offered a faster recovery of pulmonary function, fewer complications, and shorter length of stay compared with conventional surgery for selected patients undergoing ileocolic resection for CD in a randomized controlled trial (Milsom et al, 2001). Resection is the most common laparoscopic procedure performed in CD, but the safety and usefulness of stricturoplasty continues to be corroborated, and new techniques are increasingly described. Other procedures that are performed laparoscopically include sigmoid colectomy and stricturoplasty (see Chapter 22).

Ileostomy. Ileostomy formation is a major advance in the management of inflammatory bowel disease. It may be temporary, used to defunctionalize the large or small bowel in patients with perianal disease or for anastomotic protection. A permanent end ileostomy is fashioned after total proctocolectomy (see Figure 5-3); the cumulative risk of receiving a temporary or permanent stoma in CD patients has been estimated as 41% (Post et al, 1995).

Operative Management of Specific Manifestations of Crohn's Disease

Fistula

The presence of an internal fistula is not an absolute indication for surgery but fistulas rarely heal with conservative treatment. Resection of the primarily involved bowel segment with closure of the secondary segment is usually performed. En bloc resection may be indicated when extensive inflammation is encountered. Colonic fistulas occur in 25% to 40% of patients, and the preferred procedure for the management of ileosigmoid fistulas is resection of the involved segment, with

---

BOX 5-2   Surgical Interventions/Crohn's Disease

Small Intestine	Large Intestine
Resection	Proctocolectomy with ileostomy
Strictureplasty	Subtotal colectomy
	Segmental resection (for ileocolitis)
	Ileal pouch anal anastomosis[*]
	Continent ileostomy[*]

*Controversial.

ileocolic anastomosis and segmental resection of the sigmoid colon. For enterovesical fistulas, the bowel segment involved with the fistula is treated by standard resection and anastomosis, whereas the bladder defect is closed primarily, with or without the interposition of a pedicled omental graft.

Perforation

Free perforation of the colon is a rare indication for surgery in CD patients; in such cases the procedure of choice is subtotal colectomy with end ileostomy.

Abscess

This usually develops as a result of sealed perforations. Computed tomography-guided drainage and antibiotics may help initial management of the abscess, following which resection may be indicated for persistent disease, complication, or absence of response to medical therapy.

Stricture of the Large Bowel

The incidence of stricture formation in the colon is 5% to 17%, and strictures usually develop as a result of fibrosis of segments of intestine that follows inflammation. Though these are usually benign, carcinoma can develop secondary to chronic inflammation in longstanding strictures. Strictures may also develop at the site of anastomosis, which can either be resected or dilated endoscopically.

Growth Retardation

Cessation of linear growth, lack of weight gain, retarded bone development, and delayed onset of sexual maturation are seen in up to 30% of children with CD. Surgery in such children is best performed in the prepubertal phase to allow catch-up growth to occur in those patients.

Extraintestinal Manifestations

With the exception of primary sclerosing cholangitis, cirrhosis, and ankylosing spondylitis, many extraintestinal manifestations improve after resection of disease. Failure of medical therapy is the usual indication for surgical resection in these cases.

Cancer Prophylaxis and Dysplasia

Unlike ulcerative colitis, patients with CD have no established dysplasia-carcinoma sequence.

Anorectal Crohn's Disease

The incidence of anorectal CD varies from 30% to 80% (Fielding, 1972; Keighley and Allan, 1986; Rankin et al, 1979), and patients with large bowel involvement are more likely to have perianal involvement. It may present as skin tags, cyanotic discoloration, fissures, canal ulceration, abscesses, fistulas, or anorectal stricture. As with disease elsewhere, the main aim of therapy for perianal CD is conservation, and most manifestations are initially managed by medical therapy. Some studies suggest that resection of active disease in the proximal bowel causes regression of perianal disease (Homan, Tang, and Thorgjarnarson, 1976; Wolff, 1986) but other studies refute the claim (Buchmann et al, 1981; Marks, Ritchie, and Lockhart-Mummery, 1981). Conservative treatment is preferred for skin tags and hemorrhoids, since surgical excision may lead to chronic, nonhealing ulcers. Fissures in CD patients are usually painless, and perianal pain usually indicates the presence of sepsis. Management is initially conservative, because they usually have a self-limiting course. If there is no improvement, lateral internal anal sphincterotomy is performed, since some studies have shown this to be effective (Fleshner et al, 1995; Wolkomir and Luchtefeld, 1993), as opposed to traditional concerns that sphincterotomy leads to nonhealing open wounds. Short segment anorectal strictures respond to dilation, whereas longer strictures with proctitis may require proctectomy. Proctectomy may eventually be required in patients with persistent anorectal CD.

Anal Fistulas

Surgery for fistulas involves the use of setons (drains that can be placed long-term into a fistula site) with or without additional conservative surgery. Treatment depends on the location and complexity and the presence or absence of proctitis. A low simple fistula can be managed by fistulotomy, but if there is concern about potential damage to the anal sphincter, seton insertion (Figure 5-5) or use of a mucosal advancement flap is preferred. High complex fistulas are managed by mucosal advancement flap or fecal diversion, and these patients may sometimes need an endoanal

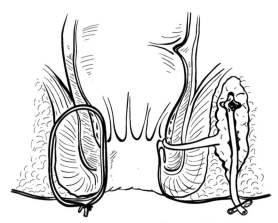

Figure 5-5   Seton drain in place on the left. (From Corman ML: *Colon and rectal surgery*, Philadelphia, 1993, Lippincott, Williams & Wilkins.)

proctectomy. Rectovaginal fistulas are a particular problem, and the traditional treatment has been ileostomy with or without a proctectomy. Rectal advancement flaps and transanal repair have been shown to produce good results in the absence of active rectal CD. In persistent cases of perianal disease, ostomy may be indicated to divert the fecal stream to help achieve quiescence of perianal disease. It is also important to consider that fistulas introduce the potential for malignant degeneration of the tract.

Duodenal Crohn's Disease

Management of CD in this location is usually medical unless persistent duodenal obstruction develops. In the past, gastrojejunostomy with or without a vagotomy was the preferred treatment. More recently, strictureplasty has been performed in duodenal CD (Worsey et al, 1999). However, bypass may still be preferable when the duodenum is brittle or enormously thick. A pedicled patch graft of the jejunum can also be employed for the strictured duodenum (Eisenberger et al, 1998).

Emergency Procedures

Indications for emergency surgery of the large bowel include toxic megacolon, perforation, or massive hemorrhage. When toxicity is less extreme, medical therapy is the initial treatment. Abdominal colectomy with an end ileostomy is the best procedure in this setting, and the sigmoid and rectal stump is exteriorized, formed into a mucus fistula (see Figure 5-4), or closed by staples or sutures. Reconstruction and treatment of the rectal stump is performed at a later date.

In fulminant Crohn's colitis, if the colon is found to be paper-thin and sealed perforations coexist, the colon is first decompressed with a large-bore needle passed through a taenia coli. Prior to mobilization of the splenic flexure, the rest of the peritoneal cavity and the wound edges are packed off, to minimize contamination in the event of spillage of fecal matter due to dehiscence of the colon wall. The lower sigmoid fistula is exteriorized and wrapped in gauze to prevent retraction. A mucus fistula can be formed at a later date (7 to 10 days).

Ileostomy and Blowhole Colostomy

The Turnbull blowhole colostomy and loop ileostomy are occasionally indicated when severe toxic megacolon is encountered in a patient in extremis. These surgical procedures were described in the 1960s and helped reduce mortality (Turnbull, Hawk, and Weakley, 1971). They are useful in extremely ill patients and in those for whom colectomy is hazardous, in instances such as a contained perforation, pregnancy, or a high-lying splenic flexure. The main advantages of the procedures are that they are simple and rapid to perform and help to reduce sepsis rapidly. The main disadvantages are that the diseased colon that is the source of the complication is left behind, which leads to persistent toxicity. These procedures are contraindicated in patients with free perforation or bleeding. After the patient has recovered, a definitive procedure is performed (6 months later).

Factors Influencing Recurrence of Crohn's Disease

The cumulative 5-year risk of reoperative recurrence has been calculated by the Kaplan-Meir method as 28%. Restricture, new stricture, or perforative disease was seen in 5% and 17% of patients during a 42-month median follow-up period in one study (Ozuner et al, 1996a). Recurrence occurs most commonly in the terminal ileum just proximal to the ileostomy after total proctocolectomy, in the ileum or rectum after ileorectal anastomosis, and in the residual large bowel after segmental colectomy. The NCCDS did not show any value in chemoprophylaxis for the prevention of recurrence and surgery (Mekhjian et al, 1979). Other studies (McLeod et al, 1995) have shown some value of chemoprophylaxis with different agents. Studies have shown that a wide-lumen stapled anastomosis leads to reduced recurrence rates compared to patients undergoing end-to-end sutured anastomosis.

Complications of Surgery for Crohn's Disease

Septic complications occur in 3% to 49% of patients, whereas perioperative septic complications occur after conventional resection for CD and in 5% to 14% of patients after strictureplasty. Bleeding is a complication that may occur after strictureplasty. Short bowel syndrome during long-term follow-up after resection is seen in 1.5% to 12.6% of cases. In total proctocolectomy, complications related to the ileostomy include recurrence, recession, fistula, stricture, prolapse, parastomal hernia, ischemic necrosis, paraileostomy ulcers, internal hernia or volvulus, and peristomal dermatitis. Malabsorption of vitamins, including B_{12} and folate, and bile acids and fluid and electrolyte disturbances may also occur. Sexual and bladder dysfunction and problems with healing of the perineal wound are other complications. Perianal complications may range from small sinuses to more extensive cavities that can be managed by debridement and skin grafting or with gracilis or rectus abdominis myocutaneous flaps. Abdominal colectomy with ileorectal anastomosis is associated with a low leak rate, but the incidence increases in the presence of sepsis. The cumulative probability of reoperation in CD is more than 50%. Thus all these factors must be carefully weighed before reaching a decision to operate, especially in patients whose symptoms are under control with medication. Intraabdominal abscesses, bowel obstruction, venous thrombosis, and wound complications are

other complications that may occur in these patients.

ULCERATIVE COLITIS
Introduction

Ulcerative colitis has been known since the nineteenth century, when it was reported in the United Kingdom. The features that help distinguish ulcerative colitis from CD have been dealt with in a previous section in this chapter, as well in Chapter 4. The risk of colectomy in ulcerative colitis is directly related to the degree of disease activity and the extent of inflammation at the time of diagnosis. Ileoanal anastomosis was performed in the 1940s (Wangensteen, 1943), but results were poor, with high rates of urgency and frequency. The creation of an ileal reservoir proximal to the anal anastomosis helps reduce frequency and urgency and has been used since the 1970s. Restorative proctocolectomy with IPAA is now considered the gold standard for the management of ulcerative colitis. Results following the procedure are good, with an acceptable complication rate and functional outcomes (Becker, 1993; Kohler et al, 1992). See Box 5-3 for surgical options for the patient with ulcerative colitis.

Indications for Surgery

Indications for surgery in ulcerative colitis include bleeding, risk of cancer, and active disease that is unresponsive to medical therapy. Colonic strictures are also reported to develop in 5% of patients with longstanding ulcerative colitis, and a fourth of these are malignant (Gumaste, Sachar, and

---

BOX 5-3   Surgical Interventions/ Ulcerative Colitis

• •

Restorative proctocolectomy with IPAA
Subtotal colectomy with end ileostomy (option for IPAA)
Proctocolectomy with end ileostomy
Continent ileostomy

IPAA, Ileal pouch anal anastomosis.

Greenstein, 1992). See Box 5-1 for indications for surgery for the patient with ulcerative colitis.

Restorative Proctocolectomy

The components of this procedure are total colectomy, rectal excision, and construction of an ileal reservoir with an ileoanal anastomosis. A compliant sac made up of loops of small bowel constitutes the reservoir. The pouch anal anastomosis is either stapled or handsewn. In the stapled technique, the anal transitional zone is preserved, and anastomosis is done one centimeter above the dentate line. This procedure leaves the anal transitional zone (ATZ), which retains some colonic epithelium. The ATZ is potentially vulnerable to neoplastic and/or acute symptomatic inflammatory change; thus an annual biopsy surveillance of the ATZ is performed. Patients who are poorly compliant at follow-up, or who have rectal dysplasia or primary sclerosing cholangitis, are best managed by additional mucosectomy of the anorectum and the handsewn anastomosis. Ileoanal pouch anastomotic options are outlined in Box 5-4.

The procedure is best performed when colitis is inactive and when patients who were on steroids have either discontinued steroid therapy or are on a low dose. In patients with mild colitis, restorative proctocolectomy with a covering ileostomy can be performed. However, in acute or fulminant colitis, subtotal colectomy with preservation of rectum and end ileostomy is a safer option. IPAA can then be considered at a later date. Restorative proctocolectomy has been shown to be effective in patients of all age groups, in both ulcerative colitis and indeterminate colitis and in the presence of malignancy. Satisfactory function has been reported in children younger than 10 years, and it can also be performed in the elderly who have reasonable sphincter function. According to one study, when restorative proctocolectomy is performed in patients with indeterminate colitis the short- and long-term results were similar to those in patients with ulcerative colitis (Wells et al, 1991; Yu, Pemberton, and Larson, 2000); however, such patients who went on to develop CD had worse outcome (Yu, Pemberton, and Larson, 2000). Although results are similar in the short term to ulcerative colitis, patients with indeterminate colitis need to be counseled regarding the possibility of long-term pouch dysfunction because of their risk of subsequent development of CD. IPAA has also been performed for patients with carcinoma complicating inflammatory bowel disease. No difference has been noted in these patients compared to patients with inflammatory bowel disease in operative complications, stool frequency, incontinence, pad use, or pouchitis. However, there is a deterioration in function of the pouch when such patients undergo radiotherapy. When fulminant colitis develops in the setting of ulcerative colitis, management is similar to fulminant colitis in CD patients as discussed earlier in the chapter. A cautious approach is taken in recommending IPAA surgery to obese patients, especially if they are male and/or have a narrow pelvis. Adequate mesenteric length may be technically difficult to achieve, preventing the pouch from reaching the pelvic floor. Thus patients need to be counseled that creation of an IPAA may not be feasible at the first procedure, and a subtotal colectomy and end ileostomy may be the initial procedure. The pouch may need to be created at a subsequent operation after the patient loses weight.

The IPAA may be performed as a single-stage procedure, proctocolectomy with straight ileoanal

---

BOX 5-4   Ileal Pouch Anal Anastomosis: Anastomotic Options

Stapled
Simpler, faster operation
Improved functional outcome
Less nocturnal incontinence
Risk of cancer, need for surveillance

Hand Sewn
Increased risk of complications
No need for surveillance

BOX 5-5   Staged Procedures: Ileal Pouch Anal Anastomosis
••
One Stage
Proctocolectomy, ileoanal pouch anastomosis

Two Stages
Stage One: Proctocolectomy, ileoanal pouch anastomosis, loop ileostomy
Stage Two: Ileostomy closure

Three Stages
Stage One: Subtotal colectomy, ileostomy
Stage Two: Ileoanal pouch anastomosis, loop ileostomy
Stage Three: Ileostomy closure

anastomosis. Another possibility is a two-stage procedure, stage one being total proctocolectomy and IPAA, with temporary loop ileostomy, and stage two the stoma closure. Lastly, a multi-stage procedure can be used: stage one is subtotal colectomy and oversew of rectal stump and end ileostomy, stage two is IPAA creation with loop ileostomy, and stage three is closure of the loop ileostomy. Box 5-5 outlines the stages of the IPAA. The choice of surgical procedure depends on the indications for surgery.

Technique of Creation of the Ileal Pouch Anal Anastomosis: J Pouch. Standard oral and mechanical bowel preparation are given before surgery. Stoma siting and preoperative preparation are provided to the patient and family. The operation is commenced by means of a midline incision, after which the colon is mobilized. High ligation of the inferior mesenteric vessels is then carried out. Dissection is continued into the pelvis using electrocautery in the plane between Waldeyer's fascia and the investing fascia propria of the rectum. Dissection in this plane is then carried down to the pelvic floor, after which the distal rectum is divided 1 cm above the dentate line. A variety of pouch techniques have been described, including the J, S, W, and lateral isoperistaltic H types. The J pouch, 20 cm in length, preferred by these authors, is fashioned from the distal ileum by the use of staples

and is anastomosed to the anal canal proximal to the dentate line (see Figure 1-5, *A* and *B*). This anastomosis is completed by the use of a circular stapling device for a stapled anastomosis or by sutures for a handsewn anastomosis. A loop ileostomy is then created in the right abdominal wall (see Figure 1-5, *C*).

IPAA Postoperative Management. Following IPAA with loop ileostomy, patients generally have high ileostomy output, from 1000 to 2000+ ml/24 hours. The ileostomy bypasses 20% or more of the distal bowel, and this can lead to dehydration. Patients are advised about the signs and symptoms of dehydration, to maintain a high level of hydration, to modify their diet to include foods that will thicken the stoma output, and to take antidiarrheal medications to slow the output and encourage absorption. The loop ileostomy, which is generally almost flush to the skin, should be managed with a skin barrier seal that can tolerate high volume output (extended-wear barrier), and convex pouching systems are frequently used to follow abdominal contours to provide an adequate seal. Teaching points related to the management of the patient with a loop ileostomy following the IPAA are outlined in Box 5-6.

At approximately 3 months, when complete healing of the pouch and the anastomosis is confirmed radiographically, the patient returns to surgery for closure of the loop ileostomy.

Other Procedures

Subtotal colectomy and ileostomy is the procedure of choice in patients who need emergency treatment in the presence of active inflammation such as toxic colitis or megacolon. Such patients can have a subsequent creation of IPAA to establish continence. This group of patients would have a three-staged procedure, subtotal colectomy/ileostomy, IPAA/loop ileostomy, and closure of ileostomy. Some studies show that there is no difference in functional results between the immediate and delayed IPAA construction. In the setting of indeterminate colitis, subtotal colectomy rather than a one-stage restorative proctocolectomy is a safer option when diagnosis of CD cannot be excluded. Thus pathology of the resected colon specimen would determine any subsequent procedure.

BOX 5-6   **Management of Patient with Loop Ileostomy following Ileal Pouch Anal Anastomosis**

....

Monitor stoma output for volume and consistency.

Use antidiarrheals to maintain output between 1000 and 1200 ml/24 hr (space over waking hours).

Plan for removal of support rod from under stoma 4 to 6 days after surgery, longer if patient on high-dose steroids or if there is excessive tension on the rod.

Use extended-wear skin barrier to prevent erosion from high-volume liquid output.

Consider use of a convex pouching system if stoma is at skin level or if there are retraction/folds/creases in the peristomal area.

Educate patient about foods that can increase the consistency of the fecal output (e.g., bananas, cheeses, applesauce, pasta, rice, pretzels).

Alert patient that rectal fullness or pressure may be present and that sitting on the toilet and expelling rectal/pouch contents is reasonable. The patient should initially expect some bloody drainage, followed by mucous. The need to evacuate the rectal/pouch area may occur up to 3 times per week.

Proctocolectomy and ileostomy is an alternative to IPAA in patients with poor anal sphincter function (see Figure 5-3). It can also be performed in cases where the patient prefers to have a one-stage procedure and wishes to minimize the chance of further procedures. See earlier sections for surgical technique.

Complications after Surgery for Ulcerative Colitis

Complications that may develop after restorative proctocolectomy include pelvic sepsis, pouch failure, pouchitis, and fistulas. Fistulas may be pouch-vaginal, pouch-cutaneous, or pouch-perineal in type. Sexual disturbances secondary to damage to the autonomic nerves during rectal dissection may also occur. Most instances of pouch failure are related to pouch sepsis. Revision of the pouch can be performed with good results for septic complications (Fazio, Wu, and Lavery, 1998) but patients undergoing planned IPAA should be informed of the possibility of a permanent stoma.

Pouchitis is a common complication after IPAA. It is a poorly defined syndrome with vague symptoms including tenesmus, diarrhea, pelvic discomfort, and sometimes hematochezia. Malaise, low-grade fever, anorexia, and extraintestinal manifestations of colitis can occur. There may or may not be endoscopic evidence of pouchitis. Pouchitis occurs more frequently in patients with primary sclerosing cholangitis, extracolonic manifestations, or early onset of disease. Smokers have a lower incidence of pouchitis than nonsmokers. Patients who have pouch formation for inflammatory bowel disease rather than for other indications (familial adenomatous polyposis), as well as those with extraintestinal manifestations and with a longer duration of follow-up, have a greater incidence of pouchitis. Anastomotic strictures and excessively large pouches that empty poorly are also thought to predispose. Frequent attacks and attacks refractory to treatment may be due to indeterminate colitis or unrecognized CD. Treatment with metronidazole usually results in prompt resolution of symptoms, but there may be recurrences. Alternatives to metronidazole include sulfasalazine, steroids, other antibiotics, and antiinflammatory agents. The cause of pouchitis is not definitely known; it may be due to stasis-bacterial overgrowth, altered levels of luminal fatty acid, and mucosal ischemia with reduction of oxygen-free radicals.

When ileorectal anastomosis is performed for ulcerative colitis, rectal cancer develops in 3.5% of patients on long-term follow-up (Fazio and Tjandra, 1992; Oakley et al, 1985). Since a 0.5- to 2-cm length of anal canal mucosa from the dentate line is retained after stapled IPAA, neoplastic transformation of the pelvic pouch mucosa in the form of dysplasia or cancer may develop in the preserved anal mucosa. Thus mucosectomy should be performed in patients who are at a high risk of developing dysplasia or cancer in the anal canal. Patients who have synchronous colorectal cancer and ulcerative colitis, rectal dysplasia, and any dysplasia in the colon identified preoperatively are at a high risk for the development of cancer. However, patients who undergo mucosectomy have also been reported to develop cancer due to incomplete stripping of the mucosa. As many as 21% of patients retain mucosal epithelial cells in the ATZ even after mucosectomy (O'Connell et al, 1987), suggesting that surveillance may be required even for these patients. When persistent dysplasia develops in the preserved canal, it can be managed by removal of the diseased mucosa with preservation of function by a transanal pouch anal reanastomosis.

Functional Results and Quality of Life

Quality of life after IPAA is rated as excellent by patients, with minimal deterioration in pouch function with time (Fazio et al, 1999). After surgery for ulcerative colitis, 90% of patients are satisfied. The mean daily stool frequency varies from 7.5 at 1 month to 5.4 at 1 year. The median stool frequency after stabilization is five during the day (Wexner et al, 1990), and function improves with time. Functioning pouch rates at 5 years are 50% to 70% for CD and 95% to 98% for ulcerative colitis. The former group consists mainly of the 5% to 10% of all patients undergoing surgery for ulcerative colitis, who are later reclassified as CD patients. Patients who undergo restorative proctocolectomy for severe distal colitis have results similar to those who have the procedure for symptomatic pancolitis.

Controversies in Configuration, Type of Anastomosis, and Defunctioning Ileostomy for IPAA

There is a general view that functional results are the same after IPAA regardless of the configuration of the pouch (J, S, or W). However, evacuation disorders are more common with the S pouch. This is minimized if the exit conduit of the S pouch is 2 cm or less, since longer conduits may lead to obstructive defecation. A randomized controlled trial comparing J and W pouches noted that the J pouch was preferable because of the simplicity of its construction (Johnston et al, 1996).

Advantages of stapled anastomosis are that it is technically simpler and quicker and causes less

trauma to the anal sphincter, because mucosectomy is avoided. A randomized controlled trial found that handsewn IPAA resulted in a greater reduction in anal resting tone from preoperative levels compared to that in patients undergoing anastomosis (Hallgren et al, 1995). Daytime continence was similar in the two groups, but the stapled group had less nocturnal incontinence. Similar results were reported by others (Reilly et al, 1997). Thus manometric and functional results are better for stapled than handsewn anastomosis (Tuckson et al, 1991a; Tuckson et al, 1991b), since the ATZ above the dentate line is preserved. A further potential advantage of the stapled IPAA is the avoidance of a muscle cuff around the anastomosis, which may harbor sepsis. Studies comparing stapled and handsewn anastomoses for the creation of IPAA found that the former leads to better function, fewer complications (including early sepsis), and a lower pouch excision rate than the latter (Gemlo et al, 1995; Ziv et al, 1996).

The role of proximal diversion with an ileoanal pouch is also a controversial issue. Randomized controlled trials suggest that there is no deleterious effect suffered by patients who undergo a one-stage IPAA compared to those who are decompressed. Unfortunately, these studies suffer from the disadvantage that the numbers of patients studied were small (Grobler, Hosie, and Keighley, 1992; Sagar et al, 1992). The current general consensus is that proximal defunctioning of an IPAA is indicated if there is technical difficulty during the procedure, evidence of air leak on testing of the anastomosis, and if the patient has features of toxicity or malignancy.

Salvage of the Failed Pelvic Pouch

The most important concern for patients who undergo IPAA is the maintenance of continence. Despite good control, symptoms such as frequency and urgency also affect quality of life. Dehiscence of IPAA, poor function, pouchitis, and perianal disease are the major causes of pouch failure in the first 2 years. Ischemia of the pouch, development of CD, chronic pouch sepsis, and refractory pouchitis may contribute to pouch failure. Complications may require pouch excision and ileostomy, but redo pouch-salvage procedures can be performed in such patients provided the anal sphincter function continues to be good. Indications for salvage surgery or major revision of the pouch include a long efferent limb, pouch- or anastomosis-associated fistula, sepsis or defect, anastomotic stricture, and previous pouch excision. Obstructive problems and evacuation disorders may be due to long exit conduit, anismus (anorectal dysfunction or failure of the pelvic floor to relax), and anal anastomotic stricture. Permanent pouch failure after restorative proctocolectomy is reported to be between 6% and 20% (Dozois et al, 1989; Galandiuk et al, 1990; Nicholls, Moskowitz, and Shepherd, 1985; Wexner et al, 1990).

Continent Ileostomy

The continent ileostomy was developed in the 1960s by Nils Kock based on the principle that detubularized bowel would not develop high intraluminal pressures and would hence serve as a reservoir. A nipple valve was subsequently designed by adding an intussuscepted length of ileum as an efferent limb. The indications for the procedure are patients with ulcerative colitis who are not candidates for the IPAA because of poor sphincter tone, and those who have a failed IPAA and who desire continence. In the latter case, the IPAA can be modified for use as a continent ileostomy pouch. The pouch consists of an S-shaped reservoir made of three 15-cm limbs of small bowel and a nipple segment that is created by intussuscepting the penultimate 12 cm into itself, followed by the last 8 cm forming the exit conduit and ileostomy segment (see Figure 1-4). The pouch is emptied by intermittent self-catheterization. Though most patients have an improved quality of life after the procedure, the long-term pouch revision and excision rates are high, predominantly attributable to slippage of the nipple valve. Various modifications have been described to help anchor the nipple valve and prevent slippage. More recently, the T pouch continent reservoir has been described; it is still under evaluation but creates a new type of valve that is unlikely to slip.

Continent Pouch Postoperative Management

When the pouch is created, a curved Medina tube is placed through the stoma into the pouch and is connected to a drainage bag (see Figure 1-4). This prevents distention of the pouch by keeping it empty of stool, so as to promote healing. The catheter is connected to straight drainage for fourteen days and is irrigated three times daily, starting on the first day after surgery. During irrigation, it is important to assess if irrigation fluid is returning around the catheter. When this occurs it may indicate that the Medina catheter is blocked or has slipped out of place. After two weeks, the patient is instructed to clamp the catheter for increasing periods of time so as to allow for expansion of the pouch. The catheter is removed on the twenty-fourth day after surgery, and the patient is taught to intubate and irrigate the tube per protocol (Cohen, 1999). A dry dressing is worn over the stoma.

CONCLUSION

Inflammatory bowel disease presents in a variety of guises. As there is considerable overlap in the presentation for CD and ulcerative colitis, distinction between the two may be blurred despite a most thorough preoperative workup. Prognosis for the two disorders is different, and patients must hence be warned about the potential for histologic surprise and the risk of a permanent stoma regardless of the initial diagnosis. Patients with CD are at risk of recurrence, and surgical procedures are aimed at improving quality of life and treating complications. In ulcerative colitis, efforts are directed towards maintenance of fecal continence after resection of all mucosal disease, which is at risk for neoplasia. Decisions regarding when to operate and which surgical procedure to use should be made judiciously to ensure maximum benefit to the patient.

SELF-ASSESSMENT EXERCISES

Questions

1. What is the primary site of involvement of CD?
   a. Small intestine

b. Ileocolic

c. Colon

d. Anorectal

2. What is the procedure of choice in the surgical management of CD of the small intestine?
   a. Proctocolectomy with end ileostomy
   b. Strictureplasty
   c. Small bowel resection
   d. Bypass

3. What operation for the treatment of CD of the colon demonstrates the lowest recurrence rates?
   a. Segmental colectomy
   b. Ileocolic resection
   c. Proctocolectomy and end ileostomy
   d. Proctectomy and sigmoid colostomy

4. Why is strictureplasty particularly useful in patients with multiple strictures?
   a. It avoids a permanent stoma, resting the bowel with a temporary diversion.
   b. The operation can be performed via a colonoscope, thus avoiding an open abdominal approach.
   c. It helps conserve bowel by avoiding resection.
   d. It calls for only a small resection of the diseased bowel, thus preserving the small bowel length.

5. Name two surgical procedures that are controversial in the treatment of Crohn's colitis because of the rate of recurrence.

6. Recurrence occurs most commonly at what site after total proctocolectomy with ileostomy?
   a. Terminal ileum
   b. Transverse colon
   c. Mid ileum
   d. Duodenal

7. What is the gold standard operative approach to surgical management of the person with ulcerative colitis?
   a. Proctocolectomy with permanent end ileostomy
   b. Restorative proctocolectomy with IPAA
   c. Temporary diversion above the point of disease

d. Loop transverse colostomy allowing the bowel to rest

8. Why is a cautious surgical approach taken in obese patients with ulcerative colitis?
   a. Because of poor wound healing complicating the pouch-anus anastomosis
   b. Because of the higher risk of diabetes in this population
   c. It may be technically difficult to achieve adequate mesenteric length, preventing the pouch from reaching the pelvic floor.
   d. The development of pouchitis in this population is over 75%.

9. List the three stages of the IPAA that can be performed in the patient with ulcerative colitis.

10. Why is the assessment and management of the high output from the loop ileostomy following the creation of an IPAA critical?

11. What is the most common complication following the IPAA?
    a. Sepsis
    b. Fistula formation
    c. Pouchitis
    d. Bleeding

12. What is the drug of choice in the treatment of pouchitis in the ileoanal anastomosis patient?
    a. Cipro
    b. Metronidazole
    c. Keflex
    d. Prednisone

13. Which type of IPAA leaves the ATZ intact?
    a. Handsewn
    b. Stapled

14. List two advantages of the stapled IPAA.

15. What is a continent ileostomy?

Answers

1. b
2. b
3. c
4. c
5. Restorative proctocolectomy with IPAA and continent ileostomy
6. a
7. b

8. c
9. Single stage: (1) Proctocolectomy with ileoanal anastomosis
Two stages: (1) Proctocolectomy with ileoanal anastomosis, loop ileostomy
(2) Takedown of loop ileostomy
Three stages: (1) Colectomy with end ileostomy
(2) Proctocolectomy, ileoanal anastomosis, loop ileostomy
(3) Takedown of loop ileostomy
10. Because 20% of the small intestine is generally located below the loop ileostomy, the resultant small bowel has less absorptive surface, and the patient is at risk for dehydration and potential pouch failure if the appropriate skin barrier is not used.
11. c
12. b
13. b
14. Advantages: less operative time, easier to construct, less nocturnal incontinence
15. A continent ileostomy is a pouch created from small intestine. The pouch provides continence by creating a nipple valve that prevents the involuntary escape of stool. The internal pouch is emptied via the stoma with a large single lumen catheter at periodic intervals.

REFERENCES

Adolff M, Armaud JP, Ollier JC: Does the histological appearance at the margin of resection affect the postoperative recurrence rate in Crohn's disease? *Am Surg* 53:543-546, 1987.

Alexander-Williams J, Haynes IG: Conservative operations for Crohn's disease of the small bowel, *World J Surg* 9(6):945-951, 1985.

Becker JM: Surgical management of inflammatory bowel disease, *Curr Opin Gastroenterol* 9:600-615, 1993.

Berman L, Krause U: Crohn's disease: a long-term study of the clinical course, *Scand J Gastroenterol* 12:5-7, 1977.

Bloom RJ et al: A reappraisal of the Kock continent ileostomy in patients with Crohn's disease, *Surg Gynecol Obstet* 162(2):105-108, 1986.

Buchmann P et al: Natural history of perianal Crohn's disease: ten-year follow-up: a plea for conservatism, *Am J Surg* 140(5):642-644, 1980.

Buchmann P et al: The prognosis of ileorectal anastomosis in Crohn's disease, *Br J Surg* 68(1):7-10, 1981.

Chardavoyne R et al: Factors affecting recurrence following resection for Crohn's disease, *Dis Colon Rectum* 29(8):495-502, 1986.

Cohen Z: Proctocolectomy with the Kock Pouch. In Michelassi F, Milsom J: *Operative strategies in inflammatory bowel disease*, New York, 1999, Springer.

Corman ML et al: Perineal wound healing after proctectomy for inflammatory bowel disease, *Dis Colon Rectum* 21(3):155-159, 1978.

Crohn BB, Ginzburg L, Oppenheimer GD: Regional Ileitis, *JAMA* 99:214-220, 1932.

Cunsolo A et al: Ileorectal anastomosis after colectomy for benign colon disease, *Int Surg* 73(1):6-9, 1988.

De Dombal FT, Burton I, Goligher JC: Recurrence of Crohn's disease after primary excisional surgery, *Gut* 12(7):519-527, 1971.

Delaney CP et al: Quality of life improves within 30 days of surgery for Crohn's disease *J Am Coll Surg* 5:714-721, 2003.

Dozois RR et al: Ileal pouch-anal anastomosis: comparison of results in familial adenomatous polyposis and chronic ulcerative colitis, *Ann Surg* 210(3):268-271; discussion 272-3, 1989.

Eisenberger CF et al: Strictureplasty with a pedunculated jejunal patch in Crohn's disease of the duodenum, *Am J Gastroenterol* 93(2):267-269, 1998.

Ekbom A et al: Increased risk of large-bowel cancer in Crohn's disease with colonic involvement, *Lancet* 336(8711):357-359, 1990.

Elliott PR, Ritchie JK, Lennard-Jones JE: Prognosis of colonic Crohn's disease, *Br Med J (Clin Res Ed)* 291(6489):178, 1985.

Farmer RG, Hawk WA, Turnbull RB Jr: Clinical patterns in Crohn's disease: a statistical study of 615 cases, *Gastroenterology* 68(4 Pt 1):627-633, 1975.

Fazio VW, Marchetti F: Recurrent Crohn's disease and resection margins: bigger is not better, *Adv Surg* 32:135-168, 1999.

Fazio VW, Tjandra JJ: Pouch advancement and neoileoanal anastomosis for anastomotic stricture and anovaginal fistula complicating restorative proctocolectomy, *Br J Surg* 79(7):694-696, 1992.

Fazio VW, Wu JS, Lavery IC: Repeat ileal pouch-anal anastomosis to salvage septic complications of pelvic pouches: clinical outcome and quality of life assessment, *Ann Surg* 228(4):588-597, 1998.

Fazio VW et al: Effect of resection margins on the recurrence of Crohn's disease in the small bowel. A randomized controlled trial, *Ann Surg* 224(4):563-571; discussion 571-573, 1996.

Fazio VW et al: Long-term functional outcome and quality of life after stapled restorative proctocolectomy, *Ann Surg* 230(4):575-584; discussion 584-586, 1999.

Fielding JF: Perianal lesions in Crohn's disease, *J R Coll Surg Edinburg* 17(1):32-37, 1972.

Fleshner PR et al: Anal fissure in Crohn's disease: a plea for aggressive management. *Dis Colon Rectum* 38(11):1137-1143, 1995.

Galandiuk S et al: Ileal pouch-anal anastomosis. Reoperation for pouch-related complications, *Ann Surg* 212(4):446-452; discussion 452-454, 1990.

Gemlo BT et al: Functional assessment of ileal pouch-anal anastomotic techniques, *Am J Surg* 169(1):137-141; discussion 141-142, 1995.

Greenstein AJ et al: Reoperation and recurrence in Crohn's colitis and ileocolitis. Crude and cumulative rates, *N Engl J Med* 293(14):685-690, 1975.

Greenstein AJ et al: A comparison of cancer risk in Crohn's disease and ulcerative colitis, *Cancer* 48(12):2742-2745, 1981.

Grobler SP, Hosie KB, Keighley MR: Randomized trial of loop ileostomy in restorative proctocolectomy, *Br J Surg* 79(9):903-906, 1992.

Gumaste V, Sachar DB, Greenstein AJ: Benign and malignant colorectal strictures in ulcerative colitis, *Gut* 33(7):938-941, 1992.

Hallgren TA et al: Ileal pouch anal function after endoanal mucosectomy and handsewn ileoanal anastomosis compared with stapled anastomosis without mucosectomy, *Eur J Surg* 161(12):915-921, 1995.

Hawker PC et al: Adenocarcinoma of the small intestine complicating Crohn's disease, *Gut* 23(3):188-193, 1982.

Heuman R et al: The influence of disease at the margin of resection on the outcome of Crohn's disease, *Br J Surg* 70(9):519-521, 1983.

Homan WP, Tang C, Thorgjarnarson B: Anal lesions complicating Crohn's disease, *Arch Surg* 111(12):1333-1335, 1976.

Hyman NH et al: Consequences of ileal pouch-anal anastomosis for Crohn's colitis, *Dis Colon Rectum* 34(8):653-657, 1991.

Johnston D et al: Prospective controlled trial of duplicated (J) versus quadruplicated (W) pelvic ileal reservoirs in restorative proctocolectomy for ulcerative colitis, *Gut* 39(2):242-247, 1996.

Jones F, Munro A, Ewen SW: Colectomy and ileorectal anastomosis for colitis: report on a personal series, with a critical review, *Br J Surg* 64(9):615-623, 1977.

Keighley MR, Allan RN: Current status and influence of operation on perianal Crohn's disease, *Int J Colorectal Dis* 1(2):104-107, 1986.

Kohler LW et al: Long-term functional results and quality of life after ileal pouch-anal anastomosis and cholecystectomy, *World J Surg* 16(6):1126-31; discussion 1131-1132, 1992.

Lee EC, Papaioannou N: Recurrences following surgery for Crohn's disease, *Clin Gastroenterol* 9(2):419-438, 1980.

Leicester RJ et al: Sexual function and perineal wound healing after intersphincteric excision of the rectum for inflammatory bowel disease, *Dis Colon Rectum* 27(4):244-248, 1984.

Lennard-Jones JE, Ritchie JK, Zohrab WJ: Proctocolitis and Crohn's disease of the colon: a comparison of the clinical course, *Gut* 17(6):477-482, 1976.

Lock MR et al: Proximal recurrence and the fate of the rectum following excisional surgery for Crohn's disease of the large bowel, *Ann Surg* 194(6):754-760, 1981.

Lokhart-Mummery HE, Morson BC: Crohn's disease (regional enteritis) of the large intestine and its distinction from ulcerative colitis, *Gut* 1:87-105, 1960.

Longo WE, Ballantyne GH, Cahow CE: Treatment of Crohn's colitis. Segmental or total colectomy? *Arch Surg* 123(5):588-590, 1988.

Longo WE et al: Outcome of ileorectal anastomosis for Crohn's colitis, *Dis Colon Rectum* 35(11):1066-1067, 1992.

Marks CG, Ritchie JK, Lockhart-Mummery HE: Anal fistulas in Crohn's disease, *Br J Surg* 68(8):525-527, 1981.

Martin G, Heyen F, Dube S: Factors of recurrence in Crohn's disease, *Ann Chir* 48(8):685-690, 1994.

McLeod RS et al: Prophylactic mesalamine treatment decreases postoperative recurrence of Crohn's disease, *Gastroenterology* 109(2):404-413, 1995.

Mekhjian HS et al: National Cooperative Crohn's Disease Study: factors determining recurrence of Crohn's disease after surgery, *Gastroenterology* 77(4 Pt 2):907-911, 1979.

Michelassi F et al: Primary and recurrent Crohn's disease. Experience with 1379 patients, *Ann Surg* 214(3):230-238; discussion 238-240, 1991.

Milsom JW et al: Prospective, randomized trial comparing laparoscopic vs. conventional surgery or refractory ileocolic Crohn's disease, *Dis Colon Rectum* 44(1):1-8; discussion 8-9, 2001.

Nicholls RJ, Moskowitz RL, Shepherd NA: Restorative proctocolectomy with ileal reservoir, *Br J Surg* 72(suppl):S76-79, 1985.

Oakley JR et al: Complications and quality of life after ileorectal anastomosis for ulcerative colitis, *Am J Surg* 149(1):23-30, 1985.

O'Connell PR et al: Does rectal mucosa regenerate after ileoanal anastomosis? *Dis Colon Rectum* 30(1):1-5, 1987.

Ozuner G et al: How safe is strictureplasty in the management of Crohn's disease? *Am J Surg* 171(1):57-60; discussion 60-61, 1996a.

Ozuner G et al: Reoperative rates for Crohn's disease following strictureplasty. Long-term analysis, *Dis Colon Rectum* 39(11):1199-1203, 1996b.

Papaioannou N et al: The relationship between histological inflammation in the cut ends after resection of Crohn's disease and recurrence, *Gut* 20:A916, 1979.

Pennington L et al: Surgical management of Crohn's disease. Influence of disease at margin of resection, *Ann Surg* 192(3):311-318, 1980.

Post S et al: Experience with ileostomy and colostomy in Crohn's disease, *Br J Surg* 82(12):1629-1633, 1995.

Rankin GB et al: National Cooperative Crohn's Disease Study: extraintestinal manifestations and perianal complications, *Gastroenterology* 77(4 Pt 2):914-920, 1979.

Reilly WT et al: Randomized prospective trial comparing ileal pouch-anal anastomosis performed by excising the anal mucosa to ileal pouch-anal anastomosis performed by preserving the anal mucosa, *Ann Surg* 225(6):666-676; discussion 676-677, 1997.

Sagar PM, Dozois RR, Wolff BG: Long-term results of ileal pouch-anal anastomosis in patients with Crohn's disease, *Dis Colon Rectum* 39(8):893-898, 1996.

Sagar PM et al: One-stage restorative proctocolectomy without temporary defunctioning ileostomy, *Dis Colon Rectum* 35(6):582-588, 1992.

Savoca PE, Ballantyne GH, Cahow CE: Gastrointestinal malignancies in Crohn's disease. A 20-year experience, *Dis Colon Rectum* 33(1):7-11, 1990.

Siminovitch JM, Fazio VW: Ureteral obstruction secondary to Crohn's disease: a need for ureterolysis? *Am J Surg* 139(1):95-98, 1980.

Speranza V et al: Recurrence of Crohn's disease after resection. Are there any risk factors? *J Clin Gastroenterol* 8(6):640-646, 1986.

Stebbing JF et al: Recurrence and reoperation after stricture-plasty for obstructive Crohn's disease: long-term results, *Br J Surg* 82(11):1471-1474, 1995.

Steinberg DM et al: Excisional surgery with ileostomy for Crohn's colitis with particular reference to factors affecting recurrence, *Gut* 15(11):845-851, 1974.

Tuckson W et al: Manometric and functional comparison of ileal pouch-anal anastomosis with and without anal manipulation, *Am J Surg* 161(1):90-95; discussion 95-96, 1991a.

Tuckson WB et al: Impact of anal manipulation and pouch design on ileal pouch function, *J Natl Med Assoc* 83(12):1089-1092, 1991b.

Turnbull RB Jr, Hawk WA, Weakley FL: Surgical treatment of toxic megacolon. Ileostomy and colostomy to prepare patients for colectomy, *Am J Surg* 122(3):325-331, 1971.

Wangensteen OH: Primary resection (closed anastomosis) of the colon and rectosigmoid, *Surgery* 14:403-432, 1943.

Wells AD et al: Natural history of indeterminate colitis, *Br J Surg* 78(2):179-181, 1991.

Wexner SD et al: The ileoanal reservoir, *Am J Surg* 159(1):178-183; discussion 183-185, 1990.

Whelan G et al: Recurrence after surgery in Crohn's disease. Relationship to location of disease (clinical pattern) and surgical indication, *Gastroenterology* 88(6):1826-1833, 1985.

Williams JG et al: Recurrence of Crohn's disease after resection, *Br J Surg* 78(1):10-19, 1991.

Wolff BG et al: The importance of disease-free margins in resections for Crohn's disease, *Dis Colon Rectum* 26(4):239-243, 1983.

Wolff BG: Crohn's disease: the role of surgical treatment, *Mayo Clin Proc* 61(4):292-295, 1986.

Wolkomir AF, Luchtefeld MA: Surgery for symptomatic hemorrhoids and anal fissures in Crohn's disease, *Dis Colon Rectum* 36(6):545-547, 1993.

Worsey MJ et al: Strictureplasty is an effective option in the operative management of duodenal Crohn's disease, *Dis Colon Rectum* 42(5):596-600, 1999.

Yu CS, Pemberton JH, Larson D: Ileal pouch-anal anastomosis in patients with indeterminate colitis: long-term results, *Dis Colon Rectum* 43(11):1487-1496, 2000.

Ziv Y et al: Stapled ileal pouch anal anastomoses are safer than handsewn anastomoses in patients with ulcerative colitis, *Am J Surg* 171(3):320-323, 1996.

Gastrointestinal Cancers: Medical Management

CRINA V. FLORUTA, JANICE BESCHORNER, and TRACY L. HULL

OBJECTIVES

1. Discuss the presentation of small bowel cancer.
2. Describe the etiology of colorectal cancer.
3. Discuss the differences between colon and rectal cancers.
4. List the risk factors for colorectal cancer.
5. Discuss the possible etiologic factors in the development of colorectal cancer.
6. Describe the preoperative workup for the patient with colorectal cancer.
7. Discuss the pros and cons of preoperative and postoperative radiation therapy in the management of colorectal cancer.
8. Describe the benefits of adjuvant chemotherapy for the patient with colorectal cancer.
9. List the two different types of anal cancer.
10. Discuss the nursing considerations for patients receiving radiation and chemotherapy.

INTRODUCTION

Colorectal cancer is a leading cause of cancer mortality in the United States. Early detection and screening is important in diagnosing early stage disease. Mortality rises when this disease is diagnosed in advanced stages. Much research is being conducted to provide information that will guide treatment decisions for people diagnosed with colorectal cancer. Although the two sites of disease are frequently spoken of as a unit, colon cancer and rectal cancer do not arise from the same malignancy. Routes of spread are different in colon cancer than in rectal cancer. Relapses of colon cancer are seen in the pelvis and also occur as disseminated disease. This differs from rectal cancer, in which relapses occur locally. The treatment approaches of each of these gastrointestinal malignancies are different. When the cancer is diagnosed, clinical and pathologic staging is done before decision making. The tumor type, differentiation, and extent of disease are used to plan the appropriate therapy. Although surgery is the curative approach, chemotherapy and radiation therapy can assist in prolonged survival and in the reduction of recurrence.

The medical management of intestinal cancers described in this chapter includes the most common colonic and rectal neoplasms. A brief discussion of small bowel and anal cancers is included. There are other tumors and tumorlike conditions affecting the gastrointestinal (GI) tract, including lesions that are very rare or difficult to manage; a discussion of these is beyond the scope of this chapter.

SMALL BOWEL CANCER

Small bowel cancer is rare. The American Cancer Society predicted 5300 new cases and 1100 deaths from small bowel cancer in 2002 (American Cancer Society, 2002; Jemal et al, 2002). The symptoms of small bowel cancer are vague and include crampy abdominal pain, intermittent episodes of intestinal obstruction in the absence of inflammatory bowel disease or prior abdominal surgery, and anemia due to chronic intestinal bleeding, which is not identified by radiography. The most common primary cancer of the small bowel is adenocarcinoma.

This tumor usually occurs in the upper jejunum and is generally treated by surgical resection (Rustgi, 2002).

COLORECTAL CANCER

Colorectal cancer is one of the most common malignancies in North America, Europe, and other regions where lifestyles and dietary habits are similar. The American Cancer Society predicted 148,300 new cases and 56,600 deaths from colorectal cancer in the United States in 2002 (American Cancer Society, 2002; Jemal et al, 2002).

Epidemiology

Colorectal cancer is the third most common cause of cancer death in the United States. It constitutes 10% of cancer death in men, behind cancers of lung and prostate. Colorectal cancer leads to 11% of cancer death in women, behind cancers of lung and breast (Hearn et al, 2000). The incidence rates are similar in men and women in the United States, although worldwide there appears to be a slight male predominance (Greenlee et al, 2001; Wakefield et al, 1998). Colorectal cancer occurs less frequently before age 40; the incidence rises progressively thereafter; the lifetime incidence is about 5%; 90% of cases occur after age 50 (American Cancer Society, 2002; Landis et al, 1999; Wakefield et al, 1998).

In the United States mortality from colorectal cancer is considerably higher in African-Americans and native Alaskans than in Caucasians, but lower among American Indians (Kroser, Bachwich, and Lichtenstein, 1997; Mayberry et al, 1995). The incidence of colorectal cancer rises in populations that migrate to the United States from areas of low risk. This was demonstrated by Japanese immigrants to Hawaii and to the continental United States during the 1950s. The cancer rate rose sharply in this population and exceeded the rate of native Japanese living in Japan, and the incidence rate of their offspring born in the United States rose to approximately that of the native white population (Corman, 1998; Ries et al, 2000).

There are marked geographic variations with regard to the incidence of colorectal cancer in the world. The Western industrialized countries have the highest incidence of colorectal cancer. The incidence is highest in Australia, New Zealand, North America, and northern and western Europe, in that order. Moderate incidence is seen in southern and eastern Europe and South America. Incidence is low in Africa and Asia. However, Japan, once a low-risk region for colorectal cancer, now has an incidence equivalent to that of Europe (Baquet and Hunter, 1995; Corman, 1998; Kroser, Bachwich, and Lichtenstein, 1997).

Epidemiologic data reveals interesting patterns in the occurrence of colorectal cancer. A regional difference in the incidence of cancer has been observed from country to country, as well as in the United States, when urban population has been compared to rural population. A moderately higher incidence of colorectal cancer was noted for urban residents, although socioeconomic status is not considered a risk factor for colorectal cancer. It is likely that environmental rather than genetic factors are largely responsible for these differences. Although some of these regional differences have persisted for a long time, they are gradually fading as lifestyles and, more particularly, dietary patterns are becoming more homogenous among the industrialized regions of the world (Coia, Ellenborn, and Ayoub, 2000; Landis et al, 1999; Wakefield et al, 1998).

Etiology

The etiology of colorectal cancer, like that of other cancers, is most likely multifactorial. It probably arises from a series of events instead of a single cause. No definite external etiologic factors have been identified as the direct cause of colorectal cancer. The etiology of colorectal cancer continues to be investigated. Most colorectal neoplasms are caused by sporadic mutations occurring in the colonocytes as a result of environmental influences. These mutations lead to genetic changes in the cells, which produce proteins that control the death, growth, and differentiation of cells. Cell growth and cell differentiation become uncontrolled, and cells escape normal maturation and death. Mutations accumulate in succeeding generations of cells in the colorectal epithelium, until ultimately cells can grow of independently. These cells may differentiate partially, defectively, or not at all. Also, they may be sensitive to various carcinogenic agents and may be transformed to malignant growth (Bond, 2001; Corman, 1998; Kronborg, 2002).

Small proportions of colorectal cancer patients suffer from syndromes in which a key mutation is inherited in the germline as opposed to mutations at the cellular level as just described. The mutation is present in the germ cell at conception and is therefore transmitted to every cell in the body of the new offspring. Some colorectal cancers are related to inherited genetic defects, such as the familial adenomatous polyposis (FAP) syndrome and hereditary nonpolyposis colorectal cancer (HNPCC), also known as Lynch syndrome.

FAP is an autosomal-dominant condition. It comprises about 0.5% of all reported colorectal cancer (Kroser, Bachwich, and Lichtenstein, 1997). The hallmark of FAP is the presence of over 100 adenomatous polyps in the large bowel. If the colorectal polyposis is untreated, colorectal cancer will certainly develop at a mean age of 39 years. Close to 100% of those inheriting the mutation develop the disease. About 20% of patients with FAP have no known family history and represent new mutations. Approximately two thirds of people with sporadic mutations have colorectal cancer at diagnosis (Corman, 1998; Kroser, Bachwich, and Lichtenstein, 1997).

The HNPCC syndrome is an autosomal-dominant condition in which colon cancer develops at an early age (mean 40 years) from preexisting adenomas. The HNPCC syndrome has two clinical variants. They are defined based on the presence or absence of extracolonic manifestations. Lynch syndrome I is an autosomal-dominant condition and is characterized by early onset of the disease, predominantly in the proximal bowel. Multiple colonic tumors are common. Lynch syndrome II is a hereditary, site-specific, nonpolyposis colon cancer associated with cancer of the endometrium, ovary, small bowel, and urinary tract.

HNPCC syndrome requires the presence of three relatives affected by the disease over two generations, two of whom must be first-degree relatives and one younger than 50 at the time of diagnosis. Patients with FAP are excluded (Corman, 1998; Kroser, Bachwich, and Lichtenstein, 1997).

Most colorectal cancer (90%) is adenocarcinoma. The tumor arises from the glandular epithelium and can spread to the surrounding microscopic blood vessels by way of lymphatics and to the distant organs, most commonly the liver and the lungs. Some rectal tumors may extend locally into the adjacent organs such as the prostate, bladder, posterior vaginal wall, and other retroperitoneal organs.

Colorectal cancer can occur throughout the large bowel. More than half of the lesions occur in the colon, with higher incidence in the sigmoid and the right colon; about 43% of the neoplasms occur in the rectum (Corman, 1998).

Risk Factors

Several studies have tried to demonstrate a correlation between diet and lifestyle and the increased risk of colorectal cancer. Dietary habits, excessive alcohol intake, obesity, sedentary life, and cigarette smoking are considered factors that predispose to colorectal cancer. The mechanism by which increased dietary fiber protects against colorectal cancer, while high fat content and overall caloric intake increase the risk of colorectal cancer, remains speculative. Due to the complex composition of many foods, it is difficult to identify the specific nutrients associated with the development of colorectal cancer (Mulcahy and Benson, 2003; Corman, 1998; Kroser, Bachwich, and Lichtenstein, 1997; Story and Savaiano, 2001). The most consistent dietary observation is that vegetable consumption is inversely related to the risk of developing colorectal cancer, whereas meat, animal fat, and protein intake are positively correlated with the risk of colorectal cancer (Kroser, Bachwich, and Lichtenstein, 1997).

Present evidence strongly indicates that the majority of sporadic colorectal cancers arise within previously benign adenomatous polyps. A polyp is a protrusion from the mucosal surface. There are a few different types of polyps that develop from the mucosal lining of the bowel lumen; however, only adenoma types of polyps will convert into cancer. Adenomatous polyps can become dysplastic as they grow larger and then become malignant. They can extend from the mucosa on a stalk (pedunculated) or have a flat appearance (sessile). The adenomatous polyps are grouped, according to their architectural appearance, into three types, the tubular, the tubulovillous and the villous adenomas. The tubular adenoma is the most frequent of all the neoplastic polyps and has a lobulated, berry-like appearance. The villous adenoma, although less frequently encountered, has a greater predisposition to changing into a malignancy than the tubular adenoma. The villous adenoma has a shaggy appearance and is found in the rectum and the cecum. The tubulovillous adenoma has characteristics of both the tubular and villous types of polyps and can turn into a very aggressive malignancy (Bond, 2001; Goodman, 1998; O'Brien, 1995).

It has become increasingly clear that genetic predisposition plays a role in colorectal cancer risk. Inherited autosomal-dominant conditions such as FAP and HNPCC syndromes, mentioned earlier in this chapter, may lead to the development of colorectal cancer.

Other colorectal cancer risk factors include family history and personal prior colorectal cancer diagnosis or a history of polyps before age 60. A prior history of colorectal cancer increases the risk of another primary metachronous lesion apart from recurrence of the original lesion (Winawer et al, 1997).

Patients with inflammatory bowel disease (e.g., ulcerative colitis or Crohn's disease) have an increased risk for developing colorectal cancer. The extent and duration of disease increase the risk for developing precancerous changes (i.e., dysplasia) and/or cancer in the bowel. The risk increases in patients with a history of the disease that spans more than 10 years (Corman, 1998; Kroser, Bachwich, and Lichtenstein, 1997). The risk for bowel cancer in patients with ulcerative colitis is 10 to 25 times higher than that in the regular population. The risk increases even more in the younger population and in persons with a history of extensive colitis (pancolitis) of more than 10 years' duration. Precancerous changes and/or cancer develop in inflamed segments of the bowel, particularly in

strictured and long-standing fistula segments. Excluded and bypassed loops of bowel are also vulnerable for developing cancer (Corman, 1998). Colorectal risk factors are summarized in Box 6-1.

Screening and Surveillance

In the context of colorectal cancer, screening is used to identify persons who are more likely to have colorectal cancer or adenomatous polyps compared to persons without symptoms of disease. Diagnosis is intended to classify persons who are suspected of having colorectal cancer or adenomatous polyps, (because of positive screening) in the categories of those who have the disease and those who do not. Surveillance monitors persons who have a history of colorectal cancer or inflammatory bowel disease (Winawer et al, 1997).

Colorectal cancer is a preventable and highly curable disease when detected early. If colorectal cancer is diagnosed at an early stage, the 5-year survival rates are estimated at 90% (Coia, Ellenborn, and Ayoub, 2000). Unfortunately only 37% of patients are diagnosed with localized disease, and 50% of the patients diagnosed with potentially curable disease will develop local recurrence or advanced metastases of the cancer (Coia, Ellenborn, and Ayoub, 2000; O'Brien, 2002; Ries et al, 2000). The key to colorectal cancer cure is early detection.

BOX 6-1   Colorectal Cancer Risk Factors

. . . .

Diet[*]
 Low fiber
 High animal fat
 Alcohol and tobacco[*]
Hereditary syndromes
FAP
HNPCC
Inflammatory bowel disease
Family history of colorectal cancer
Personal history of colorectal cancer
Polyps (adenoma)

---

[*]Remains questionable.
FAP, Familial adenomatous polyposis; *HNPCC,* hereditary nonpolyposis colorectal cancer.

Despite the fact that colorectal cancer is highly curable when detected early, the national trend shows that almost half of all Americans over age 50 have never been screened for the disease (Donegan, 1998; Winawer et al, 1997). Discussion about diseases of the colon and rectum is often considered embarrassing. That embarrassment, coupled with the perception that screening involves uncomfortable procedures, may explain some of the reluctance people have regarding these examinations. With the baby-boomer generation now either at or past the half-century mark, the American Cancer Society, the Centers for Disease Control and Prevention, and several multidisciplinary panels have produced recommendations to guide clinicians and the public in making decisions regarding colorectal screening and surveillance (American Cancer Society, 2002; Cohen, 1996; Jemal et al, 2002; Winawer et al, 1997).

In 1997 a multidisciplinary panel of experts produced guidelines and recommendations for colorectal cancer screening. These guidelines were published in the *Journal of Gastroenterology* and were endorsed by many American groups of practitioners, including the American Society of Colon and Rectal Surgeons (Winawer et al, 1997). The panel of experts provided guidelines related to screening, diagnosis, and surveillance for colorectal cancer. Screening tests recommended by the expert panel are listed in Table 6-1.

The multidisciplinary expert panel recommended that all persons without risk factors should be offered screening for colorectal cancer and the presence of adenomatous polyps, starting at age 50. The panel of experts provided specific recommendations for screening and surveillance for persons at average and high risk for colorectal cancer.

Those who are at average risk for the development of colorectal cancer include asymptomatic persons of age 50 or older, without other risk factors for colorectal cancer. Persons at increased risk for colorectal cancer include those with close relatives who had colorectal cancer or an adenomatous polyp, those with a family history of FAP and HNPCC, and those with a history of adenomatous polyps, cancer, or inflammatory bowel disease.

TABLE 6-1   Recommendations for Colorectal Cancer Screening

POPULATION	SCREENING TESTS
People at Average Risk	**Options**
>50 years of age	Annual FOBT
Asymptomatic	Flexible sigmoidoscopy every 5 years
Without other risk factors	FOBT + flexible sigmoidoscopy
	DCBE every 5-10 years
	Colonoscopy every 10 years
People at Increased Risk	
Family history	Same screening options as for average risk
Genetic syndrome (FAP, HNPCC)	(see above), starting at age 40
Colorectal cancer in 1-2 first-degree relatives	Genetic counseling and testing for genetic syndrome
Adenomatous polyps in first-degree relative <60 yr	
Personal history of adenomatous polyps, colorectal cancer	
Inflammatory bowel disease	Surveillance colonoscopy

From Winawer SJ, et al: Colorectal cancer screening: clinical guidelines and rationale, *Gastroenterology* 112(2):594-642, 1997. For specifics regarding frequency of recommended surveillance when the screening tests are positive, refer to the above journal.
DCBE, Double contrast barium enema; *FAP,* familial adenomatous polyposis; *FOBT,* fecal occult blood test; *HNPCC,* hereditary nonpolyposis colorectal cancer.

Persons at increased risk should be offered screening beginning at age 40 (Church et al, 2001; Winawer et al, 1997). The specific recommendations for each risk group are described in Table 6-1.

Clinical Presentation

Most colorectal cancers are diagnosed in symptomatic patients. The adenomatous polyps of the colon grow slowly and may be present for a number of years before any symptoms are manifested. The symptoms of colorectal cancer vary with the anatomical location of the tumor.

Since stool is relatively liquid as it passes through the ileocecal valve into the right colon, neoplasms arising in the cecum and ascending colon may become quite large, significantly narrowing the bowel lumen without resulting in obstructing symptoms or noticeable alterations in bowel habits. Lesions in the right colon commonly ulcerate, leading to chronic, insidious blood loss without a change in the appearance of the stool. Patients with tumors of the right colon may first be seen with symptoms attributable to anemia, such as fatigue and palpitations. The anemia is hypochromic and microcytic, indicating iron deficiency.

Tumors arising in the transverse and descending colon tend to impede the passage of the more solid stool, resulting in the development of abdominal cramping, occasional obstruction, and even perforation. Contrast radiographs of the abdomen may reveal characteristic annular, constricting lesions (i.e., apple-core lesion).

Neoplasms arising in the sigmoid colon and rectum often are associated with hematochezia, or passing bright red blood per rectum, tenesmus, which is defined as persistent spasm of the anus accompanied by a desire to empty the bowel, and narrowing in the caliber of the stool (Jemal et al, 2002; Kalenberg, 2002; O'Brien, 2002). Table 6-2 summarizes the symptoms of colorectal cancer.

Preoperative Testing

When cancer is suspected because of clinical signs and symptoms, or screening suggests the possibility of tumor, a multitude of diagnostic tests are performed to evaluate the status of the colon and rectum. The diagnostic workup for both colon and rectal cancer begins with a full history and physical examination, a digital rectal examination, and a rigid proctosigmoidoscopy. Further evaluation includes a colonoscopy. A full colonoscopy is preferred over a flexible sigmoidoscopy for suspected colon and rectal cancers to confirm the location of the tumor, obtain tissue for diagnosis,

TABLE 6-2   Colorectal Cancer Symptoms

RIGHT-SIDED COLON CANCER	TRANSVERSE COLON AND DESCENDING COLON CANCER	SIGMOID COLON AND RECTAL CANCER
Fatigue, palpitation due to occult blood loss	Abdominal cramps	Rectal bleeding with or without clots
Hypochromic, microcytic anemia	Abdominal bloat	Constipation
Iron deficiency anemia	New onset of constipation or diarrhea	Change in stool caliber ("pencil-thin stool")
New congestive heart failure due to anemia	Obstruction	Abdominal cramps
	Perforation	Urgency
		Tenesmus
		Passage of mucus and blood
		Sense of incomplete evacuation
		Perianal pain
		Urinary symptoms
		Vaginal fistula

remove the polyps that are discovered during the procedure, and assess the entire colon for synchronous lesions or any other abnormalities. Synchronous lesions have a reported incidence of up to 7% (Bertagnolli and Mahmound, 1997; Kalenberg, 2002; Stotland et al, 1997).

Compared to barium enema, the colonoscopy is more sensitive in detecting polyps less than 1 cm in size. The double contrast barium enema is still useful as an additional diagnostic test. It is particularly useful for right-sided lesions that may be missed by an incomplete colonoscopy or because of poor bowel preparation that did not allow for full visualization of the colon (Bertagnolli and Mahmound, 1997; Stotland et al, 1997).

In addition to the endoscopic and radiologic evaluations mentioned in previous paragraphs, other preoperative tests include blood analysis. The blood testing includes a complete blood count to identify anemia from local blood loss or chronic disease. Liver chemistries and tumor markers are also measured and may be indicators of advanced disease. Elevation in liver enzymes, specifically the alkaline phosphotase enzyme, can indicate hepatic involvement; however, abnormal liver function tests are present in only 15% of patients with liver metastasis, and false-positive elevations approach 40% (Bertagnolli and Mahmound, 1997; Kalenberg, 2002; Minsky, 1998 CRINA).

Carcinoembryonic antigen (CEA), a protein produced only in fetal tissue and tumors of the GI tract, may be elevated in patients with colorectal cancer, but colorectal cancers of all stages can be present even in the face of a normal serum CEA. Other conditions such as hepatitis, cholelithiasis, primary biliary cirrhosis, pancreatitis, and diverticulitis may cause elevation in this tumor marker. CEA levels are not used for routine screening, but instead are drawn to compare with postoperative levels (Bertagnolli and Mahmound, 1997; Duffy, 2001). A patient whose serum CEA level is elevated before surgery should respond to a curative resection with a return to normal levels within 1 month. Persistent elevation of the CEA level seems to be indicative of residual or recurrent disease (Kalenberg, 2002; Minsky, 1998 CRINA; Saddler and Ellis, 1999).

A chest x-ray is performed to establish the presence of pulmonary metastases and, if abnormal, should be followed by a computed tomography (CT) scan of the chest (Kalenberg, 2002).

Preoperative Evaluation for Colon Cancer

Although colon and rectal cancers are often grouped together, they are distinctly different, and the preoperative evaluation is very specific (Table 6-3). The preoperative evaluation for colon cancer must be specific because the treatment approach is unique. Colon cancer is treated by surgical resection, which can be done either by conventional or laparoscopic approach. Details about the operations performed for the treatment of colon cancer are presented in Chapter 7.

TABLE 6-3   Preoperative Evaluation for Colorectal Cancer

COLON CANCER	RECTAL CANCER
Colonoscopy	Colonoscopy
Chest x-ray: if positive, follow with chest CT	Chest x-ray: if positive, follow with chest CT
CBC	CBC
Chemistry	Chemistry
Hepatic panel (liver function test)	Hepatic panel (liver function test)
CEA	CEA
CT scan of abdomen and pelvis (controversial)	CT scan of abdomen and pelvis
Double-contrast barium enema	ELUS for preoperative tumor staging

CBC, Complete blood count; *CEA,* carcinoembryonic antigen; *CT,* computed tomography; *ELUS,* endoluminal ultrasound.

Preoperative CT scanning of the abdomen and pelvis is controversial in the presence of colon cancer. Staging of colon lesion by CT scan is unacceptable because the accuracy compared with final surgical pathologic staging is only 60% to 70% (Bertagnolli and Mahmound, 1997). The CT scan is intended to screen for hepatic metastases; however, most liver metastasis cannot be detected if less than 1 cm in size. Lesions in the lateral segment of the liver usually must be larger to be detected. Furthermore, despite preoperative imaging, one third of patients at time of surgery have unsuspected liver metastasis (O'Brien, 2002; Stotland et al, 1997; Yanagi et al, 1996). Therefore preoperative CT scanning in the presence of colon cancer remains controversial.

Liver metastasis can be detected by the use of magnetic resonance imaging (MRI). The MRI and CT scan have comparable accuracy, 85%, in diagnosing liver metastasis (Stotland et al, 1997). However, the most sensitive test to determine the presence of liver tumor and its resectability is the intraoperative hepatic ultrasonography (Bertagnolli and Mahmound, 1997).

Preoperative Preparation

Once the diagnosis of cancer has been made, the remainder of the preoperative evaluation focuses upon minimizing the patient's operative risk. One of the most difficult periods for cancer patients is the interval between the time they learn that they need surgery and the time they undergo the planned operation. This period is emotionally laden for patients and their families; it is a time full of fears, uncertainties, and questions.

For the patient to be effectively rehabilitated, this preoperative preparatory period must be maximized. The ideal preoperative preparation requires the combined efforts of a team working closely together. Substantial effort is invested in the preoperative planning for a patient with a problem amenable to surgery. This includes scheduling tests to establish the presence and location of the tumor (see Table 6-3), discussing the findings with the patient and family, proposing consultation with the surgeon, and consulting on the care of the patient's medical problems.

There is no consensus on the components of a general preoperative evaluation. However, in addition to a comprehensive preoperative history, every patient should have a physical examination, preoperative testing as mentioned above, and a thorough evaluation for comorbidities (e.g., cardiac, renal, and hepatic) that may increase the risk of surgery.

Mechanical Bowel Preparation

The mechanical bowel cleansing is controversial, and some institutions have stopped requiring patients to undergo bowel preparation before colorectal surgery. Zmora, Pikarsky, and Wexner (2001) state that, although several recent studies have suggested that elective colorectal surgery can be safely performed without any mechanical bowel preparation, mechanical bowel preparation remains the standard of care at least in North America at present. Even though there has been some literature opposing the use of mechanical bowel preparation, most surgeons continue to request that their patients clean their bowels before the surgery (van Geldere et al, 2002).

The preoperative bowel preparation consists of dietary restriction and mechanical cleansing. The patient is placed on a clear liquid diet for 1 to 2 days before surgery. The mechanical cleansing of the bowel for elective colorectal surgery is intended to decrease the amount of bacteria present as part of the normal colonic flora, in theory decreasing the chance of postoperative infection (Corman, 1998; van Geldere et al, 2002). It also facilitates the palpation of the entire colon during surgery and allows for the performance of intraoperative colonoscopy if indicated. During laparoscopic surgery, the chance of injury to the bowel during the manipulation of the instruments is decreased if the colon is free of stool.

The two most commonly used solutions for bowel cleaning are the polyethylene glycol (PEG) solution (e.g., GoLYTELY) and the sodium phosphate (NaP) solution (e.g., Fleet Phospho-soda) (Oliveira et al, 1997; Zmora, Pikarsky, and Wexner, 2001). The PEG solution is an osmotic balanced solution associated with low occurrence of resulting electrolyte imbalances. The most common complaints from patients taking this solution to clean their bowel for surgery include its salty taste, nausea, vomiting, abdominal fullness, and discomfort because of the large volume they are expected to consume over a short period of time (Zmora, Pikarsky, and Wexner, 2001).

The NaP solution, which is administered in a much smaller quantity, may cause electrolyte imbalances and significant dehydration. This solution is not recommended for patients with a history of chronic renal failure, hepatic disorders, or significant heart failure. Theoretically these side effects may have a more significant effect on patients undergoing surgery under general anesthesia and may lead to hypotension (Zmora, Pikarsky, and Wexner, 2001).

The choice of bowel preparation solution is usually made by the clinician. Caution should be exercised for patients with known comorbidities to prevent untoward reactions. Home bowel preparation is safe, with no demonstrable increase in morbidity or mortality; other advantages of home bowel preparation include cost reduction, decreased length of hospital stay, and increased patient satisfaction (Frazee et al, 1992; Hearn et al, 2000).

In addition to the use of one of the previously mentioned oral solutions to cleanse the bowel, antibiotics are recommended for bowel preparation. During the first half of the twentieth century, mortality from colon and rectal surgery often exceeded 20% and was mainly attributed to sepsis. With current common practices including mechanical bowel cleansing, perioperative intravenous antibiotics, and modern surgical and perioperative techniques, the infection rate has been reduced to 6% to 25% (Cohen, 1996, Corman, 1998; Zmora, Pikarsky, and Wexner, 2001).

Antibiotics are aimed at reducing the bacterial load in the colon and providing tissue levels of antibacterials, should contamination occur during surgery. The antibiotics can be administered orally the day before surgery as part of the bowel preparation and/or intravenously just before surgery. Intravenous prophylactic antibiotics that effectively cover gram-negative bacilli and anaerobes are given just before the start of the operation. The timing of antibiotic administration is the most important

aspect of their use, because none of their benefit accrues if they are given during or after surgery. Antibiotic prophylaxis is not harmless. In addition to their cost, antibiotics can be associated with side effects. Thus, one should select effective, well-tolerated, cost-effective antibiotics with a low rate of side effects (Corman, 1998; Zmora, Pikarsky, and Wexner, 2001).

Preoperative Stoma Siting

A number of the surgical procedures considered for the resection of tumors of colon and rectum will result in a temporary or permanent ostomy. Stoma siting is an extremely important component of the preoperative preparation of patients undergoing surgery for colorectal cancer. A poorly located stoma may result in leakage, stoma complications, and increased physical and emotional stress on the patient. Preoperative stoma site marking and education may reduce some of these adverse outcomes. All patients who are anticipating colorectal surgery that may result in a stoma should be given basic stoma care instructions before surgery and have their stoma site marked by a trained clinician. See Chapter 11 for additional information on stoma site selection.

Adjuvant Therapy

Patients with locally advanced large bowel cancer have a significantly increased risk of relapse after surgical resection alone. Adjuvant chemotherapy for colorectal cancer has been used since the 1960s. Early adjuvant studies often used 5-fluorouracil (5-FU) as a single agent. Many trials have been conducted since that time that incorporate 5-FU with other chemotherapeutic agents in the adjuvant and advanced disease treatment of colon cancer. In the adjuvant setting, as well as in metastatic colon cancer, 5-FU is the gold standard. Two cooperative clinical trials were done in the 1980s that suggest the use of adjuvant chemotherapy has an improved overall survival and disease-free survival rate compared to surgery alone (Wolmark et al, 2000; Laurie et al, 1989). In 1990, Moertel and colleagues reported the results from the Intergroup Trial-0035, in which stage B colorectal cancer patients were randomized to surgery alone versus adjuvant treatment with levamisole or 5-FU/levamisole.

Levamisole is an antihelminthic agent with immunomodulatory properties. The initial results were impressive. There was a 33% reduction in death rates, and a 41% reduction in disease recurrence in the adjuvant 5-FU/levamisole arm compared to surgery alone. Levamisole alone did not demonstrate any benefit.

As a result of these trials, the U.S. National Institutes of Health (NIH) issued a Consensus Statement in 1990 stating that stage III patients should receive 5-FU/levamisole if unable to be placed on a clinical trial. In the United States, this was then considered standard treatment. Future clinical trials compared investigational treatments against 5-FU/levamisole.

Since then, several studies have examined the role of 5-FU plus leucovorin (folinic acid) in the adjuvant treatment of colon cancer. 5-FU is a thymidylate synthase (TS) inhibitor that prevents formation of thymidine, and therefore impairs deoxyribonucleic acid (DNA) synthesis. When leucovorin is added to 5-FU, there is a stabilization of the 5-FU/TS complex, which prolongs the inhibition of DNA synthesis. Thus the antitumor effect of 5-FU is enhanced. 5-FU plus leucovorin (5-FU/leucovorin) has been evaluated in a variety of doses and schedules and has been used as a standard treatment regimen in advanced colon cancer. A North Central Cancer Treatment Group (NCCTG) and the Mayo Clinic study evaluated 208 patients with advanced colorectal cancer. These patients were randomized to receive 5-FU alone, or 5-FU/leucovorin in either a high dose or a low dose (Laurie et al, 1989). Improved disease-free survival was seen in the 5-5-FU/leucovorin group.

Another trial was conducted by the Intergroup Colon Cancer Surgical Adjuvant Study (INT-0089, Part II) (Haller et al, 1998). In it, 3759 patients were randomized to treatment with 5-FU/levamisole for 12 months, or either 5-FU plus low-dose leucovorin for 6 months, 5-FU plus low-dose leucovorin and levamisole for 6 months, or weekly 5-FU plus high-dose leucovorin in four 6-week cycles. The results were similar between the arms. Based on these results, 5-FU/leucovorin given for 6 months is preferred to 5-FU/levamisole given for 12 months in consideration of side effects and patient convenience.

The value of adjuvant therapy in stage III colon cancer is unequivocal, but its role in stage II disease is controversial. Clinical trials have been conducted examining the role of adjuvant therapy in stage II disease. There was a combined analysis of four National Surgical Adjuvant Breast and Bowel Project (NSABP) trials (Mamounas et al, 1999) evaluating the efficacy of adjuvant therapy in stage II colon cancer. It was concluded that adjuvant therapy in this population is beneficial (see further discussion later in this chapter). In another analysis the results of five clinical trial results were pooled and analyzed (International Multicentre Pooled Analysis of B2 Colon Cancer, or IMPACT B2, Investigators, 1999). There was no statistically significant difference in event-free or in overall survival in patients who received treatment compared to those who did not. They concluded that the biology of B2 colon cancer has a greater impact on the patient's outcome than the treatment regimen does. Of the studies published for B2 colon cancer patients, the efficacy remains to be determined.

Advanced Colon Cancer

A new chemotherapeutic agent, irinotecan, received U.S. Food and Drug Administration (FDA) approval in 1996 for metastatic colon cancer that fails to respond to 5-FU treatments. Irinotecan was the first new FDA-approved chemotherapy drug for metastatic colorectal cancer in several years. Used in this setting, it showed an improvement in survival and quality of life. A new set of clinical trials evaluated the addition of this drug to what had been considered the standard therapy of 5-FU/leucovorin. Saltz and colleagues (2000) conducted a randomized study to evaluate whether the addition of irinotecan to 5-FU/leucovorin was better than 5-FU/leucovorin or irinotecan alone in patients with metastatic colorectal cancer. These regimens were administered as the first-line therapy. The results of this trial demonstrated that the irinotecan, 5-FU/leucovorin arm had a significantly longer survival. Douillard and colleagues (2000) studied the addition of irinotecan to 5-FU/leucovorin and compared it to 5-FU/leucovorin alone. The response rate was 49% in the irinotecan arm and 31% in the arm that did not contain irinotecan. The investigators also saw that time to progression was longer in the irinotecan arm, and that the overall survival was higher.

Capecitabine is an oral fluoropyrimidine that is converted to 5-FU in tumor tissue. It is used in treating advanced colon cancer. One study (Hoff et al, 2001) compared capecitabine alone to 5-FU plus leucovorin. Capecitabine had a better anti-tumor response (24.8%) than 5-FU/leucovorin (15.5%). However, the time to disease progression was almost the same. Capecitabine was better tolerated except for the more severe toxicities of hand-foot syndrome and hyperbilirubinemia. The oral route of administration can increase the compliance of patients toward palliative chemotherapy, decrease the cost, and improve quality of life.

Oxaliplatin is the first platinum compound to show activity against metastatic colorectal cancer. It received FDA approval in August 2002 as a second-line treatment in patients with metastatic colorectal cancer who failed to respond to 5-FU/LV and irinotecan treatment. Two randomized phase III trials demonstrated a benefit in combining 5-FU/LV with oxaliplatin as first-line therapy in advanced colorectal cancer (de Gramont et al, 2000; Giacchetti et al, 2000). Response rates were improved and progression-free survival was prolonged.

Treatment of Liver Metastasis

Colorectal cancer metastasizes to the liver, a principal site of involvement. In selected patients, therapies directed toward the liver may be used. Therapies such as surgical resection, hepatic intraarterial infusion of chemotherapy agents, hepatic artery ligation, portal vein chemotherapy, chemoembolization, and cryoablation are some of the approaches used to treat liver metastasis.

The rationale for chemoembolization is to impede blood supply to the sites of liver metastasis. Tumors need nutrients to survive and they obtain those nutrients from the blood. If blood flow to the tumor is impaired, theoretically the tumor should die. Chemoembolization is a procedure that uses a foreign material, such as a gelatin sponge, that is impregnated with chemotherapy agents. Cisplatin is a commonly used chemotherapy agent, although

other chemotherapy drugs have been used. The procedure is usually performed in the interventional radiology department and involves insertion of a catheter through the femoral artery up to the hepatic artery. The chemotherapy agent-impregnated sponge is injected into the arterial catheter; it will treat the hepatic metastases with the chemotherapy and embolize the hepatic artery (Berg and Lilienfeld, 2000). In some clinical trials this therapy has shown an overall response rate of 30%, with survival times ranging between 7 to 16 months (Cascinu and Wadler, 1996). Some potential complications include pain, nausea and vomiting, and infection.

When liver metastasis is not amenable to surgical removal, regional chemotherapy via the hepatic artery may be an option. The liver has a dual blood supply. Hepatic metastases derive their blood supply from the hepatic artery, whereas the normal liver draws its blood supply from the portal vein. It might be rationalized that the administration of chemotherapy drugs directly into the hepatic artery may be more efficacious than systemic chemotherapy. An important principle for this treatment modality is that regional administration of drugs that are rapidly metabolized in the liver by a first pass effect leads to higher-level drug exposure. Another advantage to this route of administration is that systemic side effects are limited (Davidson et al, 1996). Administration of chemotherapy can occur through a percutaneous catheter or through a subcutaneously implanted pump. The more common of the two is the implantable pump. The pump is placed subcutaneously in the abdomen, and the catheter that is attached to the pump is placed into the hepatic artery. Chemotherapy agents are injected into the pump for continuous release for approximately two weeks. The pump is then emptied and sterile, heparinized normal saline is instilled into the pump. This allows for a rest period, while the heparin solution maintains catheter patency.

Floxuridine (FUDR) is the most commonly used chemotherapy drug, and it can be given alone or in combination with leucovorin. Other drugs have also been used. Toxicities of this therapy include hepatobiliary toxicity, gastritis, gastric or duodenal ulcer, and hepatic arterial thrombosis (Kemeny et al, 1999; Nordlinger and Rougier, 2002b). Dexamethasone is frequently added to FUDR to try to ameliorate the inflammatory problem of the hepatobiliary toxicity.

Pump placement complications include incomplete perfusion of the liver, pump pocket seromas, infection, and thrombosis of the hepatic artery. One of the downsides to hepatic intraarterial chemotherapy is that relapses are seen in extranodal sites where the chemotherapy is not distributed. Systemic chemotherapy would then have to be given to treat these other disease sites.

Chemotherapy infusion via the portal vein has been used as an adjuvant treatment for colorectal cancer for several years. Metastatic disease to the liver from colon cancer can occur via the portal vein. At this point, small tumors may receive their blood supply from the hepatic artery. In theory, if adjuvant chemotherapy is delivered through the portal vein, tumor cell kill may be maximized. A meta-analysis of ten studies was performed by the Liver Infusion Meta-analysis Group and published in 1997 (Liver Infusion Meta-analysis Group, 1997). Based on the results of these studies, researchers concluded that an adjuvant administration of 1 week of continuous 5-FU infusion via the portal vein may have a small survival benefit. They added that further studies with this mode of treatment are needed.

Cryosurgery is a treatment approach that attempts to establish local control of liver metastasis. A probe is inserted into the tumor and liquid nitrogen is instilled into the probe to cool it. The tumor freezes and becomes an ice ball. The tumor then becomes necrotic. There are complications associated with cryotherapy such as intraoperative bleeding, cracking of the surface of the liver, cold injury to adjacent organs, transient elevations in liver function tests, fevers, acute renal failure, pleural effusion, and others that occur less frequently (Sotsky and Ravikumar, 2002).

In some settings, radiofrequency ablation is used. A radiofrequency needle electrode is attached to a radiofrequency generator and inserted into the liver tumor. The tumor is then heated, causing cell death (Nuyttens et al, 2001). Complications related to this therapy are not common, but bleeding, infection, pain, and nausea and vomiting have been seen.

Intraperitoneal Chemotherapy

Intraperitoneal chemotherapy has been used for several years (Markham, 1999). But it is not widely used as a treatment approach because it is often viewed as palliative in nature. Intraperitoneal chemotherapy is a local or regional treatment. The rationale for using it is that peritoneal involvement from colon cancer is one of the routes of spread, and intraperitoneal chemotherapy may permit better exposure to the tumor than the systemic route of administration. But an important concern is that it is not known how much of the tumor is actually exposed to the chemotherapy (De Bree et al, 2002). Intraperitoneal chemotherapy can be used before surgery, intraoperatively, or after surgery.

The procedure requires a Tenckhoff catheter or a subcutaneous implantable Port-a-cath implanted into the peritoneal cavity. Chemotherapy agents are infused through the catheter and allowed to dwell. The patient must frequently change positions in the bed during the dwell time. Years ago this was called the "belly bath" because the intent is to bathe the peritoneal space with the chemotherapy solution to get maximum exposure to the tumor. After the prescribed dwell time, excess fluid may be drained out by opening the intraperitoneal catheter clamp. The drug most commonly used is 5-FU, but other chemotherapeutic drugs have also been used. Major toxic reactions are abdominal pain and bone marrow suppression.

RECTAL CANCER

Rectal cancer is a common malignancy in the United States. Surgery is the primary treatment modality for this disease (see Chapter 7). Local regional recurrences are common and have been noted to occur in up to 50% of these patients; they can cause significant morbidity (O'Dwyer, 1992; Barrett, 1998; Gamelin et al, 2002). Tumor stage is the main determinant of recurrence. Other factors that can play a role in recurrence include depth of tumor invasion into the rectal wall, the extent of tumor spread into lymph nodes or adjacent tissues, and tumor location in the lower rectum.

Rectal cancers offer specific therapeutic challenges; thus preoperative evaluation is very specific to aid in the selection of the best option for oncologic resection of the tumor, and to minimize the risk of tumor recurrence. The management of rectal cancers includes preoperative radiation and chemotherapy along with surgical options. For select early lesions, the treatment options include local excision and endocavitary radiation and fulguration. Fulguration involves the use of electrocoagulation to destroy distal rectal cancers.

Local excision of rectal cancer can be done with a curative or a palliative intent. Most local excisional techniques are performed transanally. Only the tumor itself is removed during this procedure. This is reserved for a select group of patients who do not have an aggressive tumor and do not show evidence of lymph node involvement. Local excision is also used for patients who have high comorbidity risk or are opposed to a more involved abdominal approach. If the tumor recurs, more extensive surgery can be performed. Rectal cancers can be surgically removed through an abdominal approach; specific procedures are outlined in the following chapter.

Preoperative Evaluation

In the presence of rectal cancer, CT scans of abdomen and pelvis are performed to identify the mass effect of the rectal tumor in the surrounding tissue. The CT scan cannot detect malignant disease in normal-size lymph nodes and has a low sensitivity and specificity in detecting local tissue invasion. For rectal cancers the CT scan specificity may be as high as 96%, but the sensitivity is 55% for local invasion (Stotland et al, 1997).

Most clinicians would agree that abdominal and pelvic CT scans should be done preoperatively if local excision of the rectal cancer will be done with curative intent. This is to verify the absence of other obvious abdominal spread, since only the tumor itself will be removed with this treatment approach.

The CT scan and MRI are also indicated in laparoscopic-assisted surgery to excise the rectal cancer, or in a situation where the patient will be entered into a preoperative protocol for radiation therapy and/or chemotherapy. Some surgeons feel these preoperative tests provide a more accurate patient prognosis before surgery. In addition they allow the surgeon to anticipate if the tumor has invaded other structures and if the surgery will be technically more difficult. If the tumor is anticipated to be small, expensive tests rarely change the type of operation and add little that will not be discovered at surgery (Bertagnolli and Mahmound, 1997; Coia, Ellenborn, and Ayoub, 2000).

The endoluminal ultrasound (ELUS) adds valuable information about rectal tumors that could not otherwise be obtained. The ELUS is ideally suited for tumor staging because it delivers detailed images of the bowel wall layers and can accurately assess the depth of tumor invasion. ELUS also evaluates, with less accuracy, lymph node invasion (N stage as described in next paragraph). ELUS gives detailed information on the relation of the tumor to the anatomic layers of the rectal wall and the surrounding structures. It also identifies the enlarged lymph nodes in the vicinity of the tumor (Corman, 1998; Hidebrant and Feifel, 1985; Yanagi et al, 1996).

Staging of rectal cancer is important because it aids in prognosis and decision making about preoperative treatment options (Hidebrant and Feifel, 1985). Preoperative staging of the rectal tumor gives the clinician more information for selecting the best approach to treat and resect the tumor. Staging refers to the assessment of the local extent of disease and determines the presence of metastases. Previous classification systems of staging were a modified Astler-Coller system and the Dukes' staging system. The TNM (tumor, nodes, and metastases) system of the American Joint Committee on Cancer is currently the accepted staging system. This model includes the extent of tumor invasion of the bowel wall (T), the presence or absence of lymph node spread and the degree of spread (N), and the presence or absence of metastases (M), all of which have prognostic value (Table 6-4) (Kalenberg, 2002; Vaughn and Haller, 1997).

TABLE 6-4 TNM Staging

The TNM staging system classifies malignant tumors according to the characteristics of the primary tumor (T), involvement of lymph nodes (N), and presence or absence of metastases (M). Stages are denoted as 0, I, II, III, or IV.

TNM STAGING SYSTEM	PRIMARY TUMOR	LYMPH NODE METASTAS IS	DISTANT METASTAS IS
0	T_{is}	N_0	M_0
I	T_1	N_0	M_0
	T_2	N_0	M_0
II	T_3	N_0	M_0
	T_4	N_0	M_0
IIIA	Any T	N_1	M_0
IIIB	Any T	N_2	M_0
IV	Any T	Any N	M_1

Adapted from Vaughn D, Haller D: The role of adjuvant chemotherapy in the treatment of colorectal cancer, *Hematol Oncol Clin of North Am* 11(4):699-719, 1997.

T_{is}, Carcinoma in situ; T_1, tumor invades submucosa; T_2, tumor invades muscularis; T_3, tumor invades through muscularis into adjacent tissue; T_4, tumor invades neighboring organs.

N_0, No regional lymph node metastasis; N_1, metastases in one to three lymph nodes; N_2, metastases in four or more lymph nodes.

M_0, No distant metastasis; M_1, distant metastasis.

Preoperative Radiation and Chemotherapeutic Treatment

Studies are ongoing to determine the efficacy of preoperative radiation therapy in patients with rectal cancer. There have been published reports demonstrating that local control is improved with preoperative radiation therapy (Nordlinger and Rougier, 2002a). Furthermore, neoadjuvant chemotherapy plus radiation therapy is receiving recognition by physicians as an acceptable treatment approach to this disease. The chemotherapeutic drug used is 5-FU. The Swedish Rectal Cancer Trial (1997) has reported that the use of preoperative short-course radiation therapy in rectal cancer results in a decrease in local recurrence, a decrease in the development of metastasis, and an overall improvement in survival (Tepper et al, 2002). In another trial, Grann and colleagues reported that preoperative administration of 5-FU and radiation therapy demonstrated the same results in 68 patients, 68% of whom had a sphincter-sparing procedure. At the time of surgery there was a 13% pathologic complete response and a 9% clinical complete response. In addition, they reported a 3-year survival of 95% (Grann et al, 2001).

There are some advantages to preoperative therapy. Of considerable importance is the potential for sphincter preservation because of reduction in the size of the tumor. Other possible benefits are decreased tumor seeding at time of operation, no postoperative small bowel fixation in the pelvis, better oxygenation within the tumor area (which increases radiosensitivity), and decreased toxicities (Moertel et al, 1990; Saltz et al, 2000). In fact, preoperative radiation might be desired over postoperative radiation because after surgery some residual tumor cells may be in fibrous scar tissue, with little vascularity, leading to a decrease in the effect of the radiation. A disadvantage to this approach is an increase in perineal wound infections.

Currently, combined modality therapy for stages II and III rectal cancer is the standard of care. Standard administration of 5-FU is 225 mg/m^2/day, given as a continuous intravenous administration. This chemotherapy can be administered before as well as after radiation therapy.

Physicians are still seeking (1) to design an effective drug combination with radiation therapy; (2) whether the timing should be preoperative, postoperative, or a combination of both; and (3) which mode of delivery is most beneficial (Wilkes, 2002).

The main disadvantage of the therapies is that there may be overtreatment in some patients because preoperative staging is not truly accurate. Neoadjuvant chemotherapy plus radiation therapy can increase the risk of postoperative complications. An example of this is seen in a study by Onaitis et al (2001), in which patients received neoadjuvant 5-FU and cisplatin plus radiation therapy. Surgery was performed 4 to 8 weeks after the combined modality treatment. They reported the following postoperative complications:

- Wound infection
- Wound dehiscence
- Bowel obstruction
- Ureterocutaneous fistula
- Ischemic ileostomy
- Peristomal hernia

On the positive side, there was significant downstaging and an increase in the number of sphincter-sparing procedures (O'Dwyer, 1992).

Intraoperative Radiation Therapy

Intraoperative radiation therapy (IORT) is radiation delivered to the operative site during the surgical procedure. Using this approach, high doses of radiation can be delivered to the area where the tumor is excised, with the goal of improving local control of the malignancy. Patients must not have advanced disease at time of resection in order to be eligible for this treatment.

There are certain requirements from the standpoint of feasibility, namely a designated operating room that has a radiation therapy unit, or a radiation therapy department that is capable of caring for an intraoperative patient. Transporting a patient from the operating room to the radiation therapy department can be cumbersome, especially if the two departments are not in close proximity to one another. Some facilities have portable IORT machines that can be moved into the operating suite. Potential complications of IORT are hemorrhage, ureteral stricture, and peripheral neuropathy.

Adjuvant Radiation Therapy and Chemotherapy

The main advantage of adjuvant radiation therapy is that the exact stage of the disease is known (Barrett, 1998). This eliminates stage I patients from being inappropriately treated with adjuvant therapy. Another advantage is that the tumor bed can be marked with surgical clips, which can aid the radiation oncologist in visualizing and planning the treatment field (Minsky, 2002). A major disadvantage to adjuvant therapy is that more small bowel is involved in the radiation port (Hu and Harrison, 2000). One group of researchers studied the amount of small bowel that was irradiated in patients treated before surgery compared to patients treated after surgery. They concluded that there is objective evidence that the amount of small bowel that is irradiated is greater in the postoperative setting (Onaitis et al, 2001). Another disadvantage is that the area to be irradiated may be hypoxic secondary to surgical scarring. Radiation needs oxygenated cells to be effective, and so additional doses of radiation may be needed to achieve the desired outcome (Minsky, 2002; Wolmark et al, 1988; Bleiberg, 1998).

Radiation therapy is a *local* treatment that has an important role in decreasing the local recurrence rates in patients with rectal cancer. It is used for patients at high risk for local recurrence. Local recurrences may be attributable to residual disease within the lymph nodes or soft tissue. Chemotherapy is a *systemic* treatment and as adjuvant therapy is used to eradicate any micrometastatic disease. Several trials have established that combination radiation therapy and chemotherapy (a 5-FU–based regimen) for stage II and stage III rectal cancer shows an increase in disease-free and overall survival (Bleiberg, 1998; Fisher et al, 1998; Gastrointestinal Tumor Study Group, 1985). When given in conjunction with radiation therapy, 5-FU is also a radiosensitizer (i.e., it enhances the effects of radiation treatment).

With radiation therapy, attempts are made to minimize the dose to the small bowel. Several approaches may be used, such as treating the patient with a full bladder, which helps to push some of the small intestine out of the radiation field, placing the patient in a prone position on a "belly board," treating with multiple fields, visualizing the small bowel through oral contrast, and placement of an absorbable mesh during surgery to move the small bowel up out of the pelvis (Onaitis et al, 2001).

Several early trials have established that postoperative radiation and a 5-FU–based chemotherapy regimen for stage II and stage III rectal cancer are effective in achieving local and regional control (Douglass et al, 1986; Fisher et al, 1998; Krook et al, 1991). (See the following section for descriptions of GITSG 7175, NCCTG 79-47-51, and NSABP R-01.) The Gastrointestinal Tumor Study Group (GITSG) protocol 7175 was a randomized study that compared observation after surgery, postoperative radiation, chemotherapy with 5-FU and semustine, and radiation therapy plus 5-FU followed by maintenance therapy with 5-FU and semustine. This study showed that chemotherapy plus radiation therapy had a significantly lower tumor recurrence rate than surgery alone. Survival also was improved. There were several toxicities seen in this trial, including three late deaths—two from enteritis in the radiation plus chemotherapy arm, and leukemia from the chemotherapy-alone group (Douglass et al, 1986). The NSABP trial R-01 was a large, randomized trial that took almost 10 years to accrue 555 patients. Patients were randomized to observation alone; to chemotherapy with methotrexate, vincristine, and 5-FU; or to postoperative radiation therapy alone. Survival was improved in the chemotherapy-alone arm versus observation, and there was a decrease in local tumor recurrence with radiation, but there was no improvement in the surgery-alone arm (Fisher et al, 1998).

In 1990 the NIH Consensus Conference recommended postoperative combination chemotherapy and radiotherapy as standard treatment for stages II and III rectal cancer (Nordlinger and Rougier, 2002a). Other trials have subsequently tried to improve both the recurrence rates and survival, with emphasis on the delivery of radiation concomitantly with radiosensitizers (Kachnic and Willett, 2001).

The Gastrointestinal Intergroup 0114 published its final results in 2002. Patients in this study had a potentially curative resection followed by two cycles of chemotherapy, then pelvic radiation therapy plus chemotherapy, and finally two additional cycles of chemotherapy. Patients were randomized to receive 5-FU alone, 5-FU plus leucovorin, 5-FU plus levamisole, or 5-FU plus leucovorin plus levamisole. The results indicated that none of the combination chemotherapy regimens were superior to 5-FU alone when combined with radiation (Bleiberg, 1998).

The NSABP Project Protocol R-02, a large study with almost 700 patients, showed that the addition of radiation therapy to chemotherapy decreased the local and regional recurrences but did not differ in disease-free or overall survival versus chemotherapy alone (Wolmark et al, 2000). This differs from the GITSG 7175 study results.

Pelvic Radiation: Side Effects

Skin reactions are common with radiation therapy and include tissue erythema, dry skin, and dry to moist desquamation. The patient may experience symptoms of itching, burning, and pain. Potential interventions are perianal hygiene procedures, sitz baths, Burrow's compresses, moisturizing ointment such as Aquaphor, and use of analgesics. The intensity of radiation skin reactions increases over time, because radiation therapy has a cumulative effect. Severe reactions of ulcerations and necrosis are rare. When the radiation therapy is completed, the skin will start to heal. This healing usually takes several weeks. The new skin has a hyperpigmentation that lasts for several months. A chronic radiodermatitis can cause a sensation of dryness, and in some cases there is hyperesthesia and significant pain. Assessment findings may include hyperpigmentation or depigmentation, telangiectasis, edema, ulceration, or necrosis. There is a risk of a secondary (meaning that it occurs as a result of therapy) squamous cell cancer developing later in life.

Radiation induces many pathologic changes to the bowel lumen that result in acute toxic reactions and late effects. When the gastrointestinal mucosa is involved in the radiation field, it is not quickly replaced because of damage to the stem cells. The bowel mucosa becomes denuded, and this has several implications. The patient is at increased risk for swelling and bleeding of the bowel, as well as infection. Multiple other cellular changes lead to diarrhea, malabsorption, dehydration, and electrolyte imbalances. In addition, patients with a colonic J pouch have more frequent pouch-related problems that have an effect on continence and evacuation (Gervaz et al, 2001). Care of the patient with diarrhea includes a bland, low-residue, and low-lactose diet, a bulking agent such as psyllium fiber, antidiarrheals such as loperamide or diphenoxylate hydrochloride with atropine sulfate, hydration, and electrolyte replacement.

Proctitis may also occur. Acute proctitis causes tenesmus, bloody mucus discharge, and rectal pain. This usually resolves in a few weeks. Interventions include perianal hygiene procedures, sitz baths, and the use of hemorrhoidal preparations, sucralfate enemas, and belladonna-and-opium suppositories. In chronic proctitis, patients do not experience symptoms until about 1 year after treatment. Symptoms can be mild to severe and can have a great impact on the patient's quality of life. Ulceration, bleeding, perforation, fistula formation, and stenosis can occur. It is important to rule out other possible causes of these problems such as tumor recurrence or other conditions, so a good physical examination would be necessary, along with radiographic studies and an endosonography.

Cystitis is another potential side effect. Symptoms are dysuria, frequency, hesitancy, obstructive symptoms, and hematuria.

Sexual dysfunction is a frequent occurrence. Symptoms in men are erectile dysfunction, and women may experience vaginal dryness, vaginal stenosis, and dyspareunia. Management of erectile dysfunction might include medications or mechanical devices such as a penile implant or vacuum devices. Water-based lubricants for women are recommended, and estrogen creams may be prescribed. Management of vaginal stenosis includes vaginal sexual intercourse three times a week and the use of a vaginal dilator.

Late effects seen in some patients are the result of injury to the vasculature that leads to ischemia and fibrosis. This can cause necrosis or ulceration. Shallow erosions are commonly seen and may involve the vessels, which can lead to bleeding. Some patients experience perforation, abscess formation, or peritonitis. Fibrosis can lead to other problems such as adhesions and obstruction. Other late effects or long-term complications are persistent diarrhea, fibrosis and stricture, proctitis, urinary incontinence, bladder atrophy or bleeding, and sexual dysfunction.

Complications with Postoperative Radiation

There are several complications to postoperative radiotherapy in patients with rectal cancer. These include radiation skin reactions, fatigue, nausea, diarrhea, small bowel obstruction, delay in starting radiation due to delayed wound healing, fatigue, and other problems that are dose-limiting. The addition of 5-FU to radiation therapy increases the occurrence of acute toxicities. Patients experience an increased amount of diarrhea (Onaitis et al, 2001). Bone marrow suppression is seen, and the patient's blood counts must be monitored.

Adjuvant Therapy: Quality of Life

When evaluating efficacy of adjuvant therapy, it is equally important to evaluate improvement in patients' quality of life. Morbidity related to treatment may be significant in some patients. Radiation may have long-lasting effects on bowel function. Chemotherapy has side effects that affect the GI system, as well as effects on bone marrow functioning. Side effects are magnified when chemotherapy and radiation therapy are combined. Compliance with a combined modality regimen may be affected because of the morbidity. Risks and benefits of treatments must be evaluated both by the clinician and the patient. The benefit of the decreased risk of local recurrence should outweigh the risks of side effects.

Metastatic Rectal Cancer

Stage IV rectal cancer is metastatic cancer. The most common site of metastasis is the liver. If the malignancy is deemed to be unresectable, medical interventions might include systemic chemotherapy, hepatic intraarterial chemotherapy by means of an implantable pump, cryosurgery, embolization, or radiation therapy. Radiation may be given to palliate symptoms of advanced rectal cancer. Pain reduction may be achieved in approximately 80% of patients.

ANAL CANCER

Cancers of the anus are infrequent. They account for approximately 2% to 3% of all gastrointestinal carcinomas (Coia, Ellenborn, and Ayoub, 2000). In the year 2002, approximately 3900 new cases and 500 deaths from anal cancers were expected (American Cancer Society, 2002; Jemal et al, 2002). Cancer of the anus can be divided into two categories: cancer of the anal canal, which includes squamous cell carcinoma; and adenocarcinoma and related types. The squamous cell cancers of the anal canal are treated with a combined radiation and chemotherapy protocol. The prototypical radiochemotherapy schedule was developed by Nigro and colleagues and published in 1974, hence it is referred to as the Nigro protocol. The treatment includes a combination of low dose radiation therapy combined with cytotoxic chemotherapy agents (Cummings, 1995).

The adenocarcinoma anal cancers behave like the adenocarcinoma of the rectum, and their treatment is similar to that for rectal adenocarcinoma. The anal margin cancers located distal to the anal verge are considered skin cancers and are treated accordingly. An example of the anal margin cancer is the squamous cell carcinoma. These cancers occur most commonly in individuals with a prior history of chronic anal skin irritation. Such irritation may result from infection with human papillomavirus in the presence of condylomata accuminata lesions. The treatment of these cancers depends on the size of the tumor and the depth of invasion. The treatment may involve excisional therapy, use of topical creams (e.g., Aldara [Imiquimod] 5% cream) and at times combined radiation and chemotherapy (Coia, Ellenborn, and Ayoub, 2000; Corman, 1998; Hull, 2002).

NURSING CONSIDERATIONS

Nursing care of the patient with colorectal cancer requires an understanding of the pathophysiology of this disease, treatment regimens, complications, toxicities reactions, and symptom management. Toxicity of chemotherapy depends on the drugs administered, the routes of delivery, and the doses. This toxicity ranges from mild to severe. Mucositis frequently occurs in patients receiving 5-FU and is also seen with other chemotherapeutic agents. Mucositis can involve the lips, oral cavity, and the entire sequence of the GI tract down to the anus. Patients may complain of discomfort or pain in these areas about 5 days after receiving the drug, with potential worsening of symptoms in 10 to 14 days. Mucositis can progress to erythema, ulceration, and swelling of the mucosa. Pain can be mild to severe. Potential complications of mucositis are infection, which can disseminate into the bloodstream, poor oral intake, and taste changes. Mucositis can be a dose-limiting toxicity, which means that the chemotherapy may be interrupted or delayed, and a dose reduction may be required for the next treatment cycle. A thorough assessment of the oral cavity should be done, looking for erythema, dry mucous membranes, sores or ulcerations, swelling, and infection. The nurse should ask the patient about pain anywhere along the GI tract and provide analgesics as needed per physician order. Oral hygiene is important in these patients and should be started when chemotherapy is begun. Commercial mouthwashes should be avoided, since they contain alcohol, which dries the mucous membranes. Saline mouth rinses are good for oral cleaning. Physician-prescribed mouth rinses such as an antifungal medication may be needed if the patient is experiencing moderate to severe stomatitis. These are used to prevent or treat infection. Oral topical anesthetics are available for severe oral pain. The desired outcomes of interventions for mucositis are prevention of infection, maintenance of adequate fluid and food intake, and pain management.

Other gastrointestinal side effects are nausea, vomiting, and diarrhea. Although many chemotherapy drugs have the potential to cause some degree of nausea and/or vomiting, most of these drugs used in colorectal cancer usually do not cause severe nausea and vomiting. However, irinotecan and oxiliplatin are moderately emetogenic and require premedication with an antiemetic. Antiemetics such as prochlorperazine can be used as needed for patients receiving chemotherapy. When indicated, the 5-HT-3 antagonists may be used. These antiemetics act on the different receptors that trigger vomiting. It is important that nausea and vomiting be prevented or controlled beginning with the first treatment. Another strategy to prevent nausea and vomiting is to have the patient stay away from strong odors such as perfumes or cooking odors. Distraction may be used if the patient feels nauseated.

Diarrhea is another potential side effect of therapy. The agents 5-FU, irinotecan, and oxiliplatin are known to cause diarrhea, and it can be severe, particularly with irinotecan. Diarrhea caused by irinotecan is classified as early onset, occurring within 24 hours of administration, or diarrhea that occurs after that time. Early onset diarrhea and other associated symptoms are a cholinergic effect and should be treated with atropine. Later diarrhea is treated with aggressive antidiarrheals. Patients who experience diarrhea related to chemotherapy need a good assessment. It is important to obtain a good history regarding onset, frequency of stools, appearance, consistency, and accompanying symptoms such as crampy abdominal pain or incontinence. Other causes such as *Clostridium difficile* infection and lactose intolerance should be ruled out. Severe diarrhea can lead to fluid and electrolyte abnormalities, fatigue, skin excoriation, and perineal fungal infections. Interventions for patients experiencing diarrhea include fluid and electrolyte repletion. Oral fluids to consider are water, sports drinks, or Pedialyte. Antidiarrheal medications may be indicated. Dietary changes should include eliminating greasy and spicy foods, limiting gas-forming foods such as broccoli and cauliflower, and limiting milk and milk products. Patients need to be instructed on skin care of the perineal area. Other challenges include bowel alterations due to surgery, such as patients with a colostomy or ileostomy, and patients who are taking opioids for pain.

Bone marrow functioning is affected by chemotherapy. Patients will experience myelosuppression, which ranges from mild to severe. The degree of myelosuppression depends upon the chemotherapeutic agent used, the dose, and whether the patient received abdominal radiation. A decrease in white blood cells increases the patient's risk of infection. This risk is directly related to the degree of reduction in the white blood cells, specifically the neutrophils. Irinotecan can cause a significant decrease in the white blood cells. All patients need to have their blood counts monitored. Neutropenia is a dose-limiting complication of irinotecan administration, and doses must be reduced if the patient becomes neutropenic. If the patient experiences neutropenia, he or she should be educated about protective measures against infection and when to report a fever. Other decreases may be seen in the platelet count and hematocrit but are usually mild and do not require intervention.

Skin reactions are a side effect of some chemotherapy drugs. Photosensitivity can be caused by 5-FU, and patients need to be instructed to protect their skin from the sun. Hyperpigmentation may be seen as a darkening of the vein where 5-FU was administered and surrounding veins. This effect may be distressing to some people. Wearing long-sleeved clothing covers the arms and hides the hyperpigmentation.

Another side effect seen with 5-FU and capecitabine is hand-and-foot syndrome (palmar-plantar erythrodysesthesia). This is a cutaneous syndrome causing erythema of the palms of the hands and the soles of the feet. As it progresses in severity, other signs and symptoms are reported: swelling, discomfort, moist desquamation, ulceration, blistering, or severe pain that causes great difficulty in performing activities of daily living. This side effect occurs more commonly with prolonged continuous infusion of 5-FU versus bolus administration, and is a very common side effect with capecitabine. Hand-and-foot syndrome can be a dose-limiting reaction. Keeping the affected areas lubricated with ointments is important. Other interventions will depend on the severity of this side effect.

Alopecia is usually mild in patients being treated for colorectal cancer unless they are receiving irinotecan, capecitabine, or prolonged courses of 5-FU. The hair loss is usually mild to moderate, although irinotecan can cause moderate to total scalp hair loss. Patients should be educated about this possibility so that they have an opportunity to purchase a wig if they choose. Hair growth occurs when the chemotherapy is completed, although occasionally it starts growing back between cycles.

Peripheral neuropathies are frequently seen with oxiliplatin and occasionally with 5-FU administration. Paresthesias occur in the hands and the feet in a stocking-glove distribution. In the case of oxiliplatin, the paresthesias and dysesthesias may decrease in intensity between cycles of chemotherapy, but are of longer duration with subsequent administrations. Oxiliplatin can induce an acute transient neurotoxicity or a delayed cumulative sensory neurotoxicity (Gamelin et al, 2002). Oxiliplatin treatment is unique in that the acute peripheral, sensory neuropathies that many patients experience are exacerbated by exposure to cold temperatures and cold objects. These symptoms are accompanied by muscular contractions. Patient education must include a discussion about this phenomenon and the measures patients can take that help prevent its occurrence. Impaired proprioception commonly occurs with the administration of oxiliplatin and can have a profound impact on activities of daily living. Peripheral neuropathies usually resolve several months after treatment is completed (Willett et al, 1995).

CLINICAL RESEARCH TRIALS

Ongoing clinical trials are evaluating multiple agents in the treatment of colorectal cancer. One agent of interest is the combination of uracil-ftorafur (UFT). This is an oral fluoropyrimidine that has been studied in several countries. Sulkes and co-workers (1998) reviewed several published clinical trials of UFT in colorectal malignancies. They conclude that these trials' results indicate that UFT shows

antitumor activity in colorectal cancer. In multicentered phase III trials comparing UFT plus leucovorin to 5-FU plus leucovorin, the investigators concluded that the UFT and leucovorin combination yielded a safer administration than 5-FU plus leucovorin. An additional benefit is that since this is an oral regimen, it is more appealing to the patients. There was no survival benefit to either regimen (Douillard et al, 2002). UFT is still in clinical trials in the United States and at this writing does not have FDA approval. There are many early phase clinical trials evaluating dose-limiting toxic effects and efficacy of chemotherapeutic drugs.

In addition to chemotherapy clinical research trials, novel approaches to tumor cell kill are being investigated that include a focus on immunotherapy. Two such approaches include monoclonal antibodies and vaccines. Monoclonal antibodies target a specific receptor on the surface of a cell. Researchers have identified specific tumor-associated antigens for several malignancies. The development and administration of monoclonal antibodies is a promising area of research. A few monoclonal antibodies in other tumor types have received FDA approval due to their antitumor efficacy. One antigen that investigators have discovered on a colon cancer cell line is called EpCAM. A monoclonal antibody that has been developed and is in clinical trials is called edrecolomab (also known as monoclonal antibody 17-1A). It has shown some promising results as single-agent therapy and together with chemotherapy (Schwartzberg, 2001).

Vaccines are in early phase clinical trials but are of interest, since they treat tumors by way of a different mechanism. A tumor vaccine acts on the immune system to induce a cell-mediated immune response against the tumor. Hanna and colleagues evaluated the use of OncoVAX as an adjuvant treatment in stage II and stage III colon cancer (Hanna et al, 2001). This study demonstrated a clinical benefit in recurrence-free survival in stage II colon cancer. There are many vaccines in clinical trials. It is not yet known if they will be effective in the treatment of colorectal cancer.

The field of molecular and cancer biology has taken great strides in identifying a number of abnormal pathways in cancer cells that represent potential targets for cancer drug development. Novel approaches are being developed that target these pathways. Examples of these agents include epidermal growth factor receptor (EGFR) and angiogenesis inhibitors. EGFR is a receptor that is overexpressed in a variety of malignancies including colon cancer. Therapies are being studied that would inhibit EGFR overexpression with the result of inhibiting tumor growth. Examples of some of these therapeutic agents are cetuximab, ZD1839 (Iressa), and OSI-774 (NIH Consensus Conference, 1990).

Another intensely studied therapeutic approach in clinical trials is antiangiogenesis factors. Angiogenesis refers to new blood vessel growth. Tumors require nutrients that are supplied by blood vessels, and to grow they create their own blood vessels from existing blood vessels. A variety of agents that target this process are currently under investigation. Bevacizumab, a recombinant human monoclonal antibody, is showing promising results in clinical trials (NIH Consensus Conference, 1990).

Targeted therapies are being intensely studied in colorectal cancer as well as in other cancers. Ongoing research in this disease offers realistic hope that further improvements in survival will be seen.

CONCLUSION

Care of the patient with an intestinal cancer requires the skills of a health care team that are expert in the field. Although surgical resection remains the predominant therapy, chemotherapy and radiation therapy may also play an important role in the management of these patients. As with some other types of cancer, the principles of treatment depend upon an accurate diagnosis and the identified goals for the patient.

SELF-ASSESSMENT EXERCISES

Questions

1. Which of the following is true of small bowel cancer?
   a. It is directly related to a high-fat, low-fiber diet.
   b. It is a squamous cell tumor and is best treated with radiation therapy.
   c. It is an adenocarcinoma and is generally treated by surgical resection.
   d. It is a common tumor easily picked up on a screening test.
2. List two epidemiology factors that are associated with the development of colorectal cancer.
3. Name the two inherited genetic defects that colorectal cancers are related to.
4. In what section of the intestinal tract do the majority of colorectal cancers occur?
5. Evidence strongly suggests that the majority of sporadic colorectal cancers arise from:
   a. Severely ulcerated areas.
   b. Previously benign adenomatous polyps.
   c. Scar tissue.
   d. The chronic use of laxatives.
6. Name two risk factors for colorectal cancer.
7. Screening for adenomatous polyps should start at what age?
8. Which of the following bowel-cleansing preparations is known to cause electrolyte imbalance and dehydration and cannot be used in patients with renal or hepatic impairment?
   a. Polyethelene glycol (PEG) solution (GoLytely)
   b. Sodium phosphage (NaP) solution (Fleet Phospho-Soda)
9. What is the gold standard adjuvant chemotherapy agent used in the treatment of colorectal cancer?
10. Name the principal site of colorectal cancer metastases.
    a. Lung
    b. Liver
    c. Kidney
    d. Spine
11. The primary treatment for rectal cancer is:
    a. Watchful waiting.
    b. Surgical resection.
    c. Immunomodulators.
    d. Intraluminal radiation.
12. Name two possible benefits to preoperative radiation and chemotherapy in the treatment of rectal cancers.

13. In what instance is adjuvant radiation therapy used for patients with rectal cancer?
14. Name two skin reactions that are common with radiation therapy.
15. Explain what manifestations can be present when the gastrointestinal mucosa is involved in radiation.
16. What are the two types of anal cancer?
17. Discuss the treatment of mucositis.
18. Name two side effects of 5-FU.

Answers

1. c
2. Epidemiology factors include: 90% cases occurring after age 50; western industrialized countries have the highest incidence of colorectal cancer; a moderately higher incidence of colorectal cancer is noted for urban dwellers.
3. Familial adenomatous polyposis and hereditary nonpolyposis colorectal cancer
4. Highest incidence in the sigmoid and right colons.
5. b
6. Genetic predisposition, family history, personal prior colorectal cancer, history of polyps before age 60, persons with inflammatory bowel disease
7. Age 50
8. b
9. 5-FU
10. b
11. b
12. Possible benefits: potential for sphincter preservation because of tumor reduction, decreased seeding of tumor, no postoperative small bowel fixation in the pelvis, better oxygenation within the tumor area, which increases radiosensitivity, and decreased occurrence of complications
13. It is used for patients at high risk for local recurrence.
14. Tissue erythema, dry skin, and dry to moist desquamation
15. Gastrointestinal manifestations include: denuded mucosa, bleeding from the bowel tissue, infection, diarrhea, malabsorption, dehydration and electrolyte imbalances, and proctitis.
16. Adenocarcinoma and squamous cell carcinoma
17. Start oral hygiene as soon as chemotherapy is started. Avoid commercial mouthwashes, consider physician-prescribed mouth rinses such as antifungal medications. Consider the use of oral topical anesthetics.
18. Photosensitivity, hyperpigmentation in the area of administration, hand-and-foot syndrome, and occasionally peripheral neuropathies

REFERENCES

American Cancer Society: *Cancer facts and figures 2002,* Atlanta, GA, 2002, American Cancer Society.

Baquet CR, Hunter CP: Patterns of minorities and special populations. In Greenwald P, Kramer BS, Weed DL, editors, *Cancer prevention and control,* New York, 1995, Dekker.

Barrett MW: Chemoradiation for rectal cancer: current methods, *Semin Surg Oncol* 15:114-119, 1998.

Berg D, Lilienfeld C: Therapeutic options for treating advanced colorectal cancer, *Clin J Oncol Nurs* 4(5):209-216, 2000.

Bertagnolli MM, Mahmound NN: Surgical aspects of colorectal carcinoma, *Hematol Oncol Clin North Am* 11:855-877, 1997.

Bleiberg H: New agents in the treatment of advanced colorectal cancer: irinotecan, tomudex and oxaliplatin. In Bleiberg H, Rougier P, Wilke, HJ editors, *Management of colorectal cancer,* St Louis, 1998, Mosby.

Bond JH: Colon polyps and cancer, *Endoscopy* 33(1):46-54, 2001.

Cascini S, Wadler S: Chemo-embolization in the treatment of liver metastases from colorectal cancer, *Cancer Treat Rev* 22:355-363, 1996.

Church J et al: Practice parameters for the identification and testing of patients at risk for dominantly inherited colorectal cancer—supporting documentation, *Dis Colon Rectum* 44(10):1403-1412, 2001.

Cohen LB: Colorectal cancer: a primary care approach to screening, *Genetics* 51:45-49, 1996.

Coia LR, Ellenborn J, Ayoub JP: Colorectal and anal cancers. In Pazdur R et al, editors, *Cancer management: a multidiciplinary approach,* Melville, NY, 2000, PRP.

Corman ML: In Cormon ML, editor: *Colon and rectal surgery,* ed 4, Philadelphia, 1998, Lippincott-Raven.

Cummings BJ: Anal cancer: Radiation with and without chemotherapy. In Cohen AM et al: *Cancer of the colon, rectum, and anus,* New York, 1995, McGraw-Hill.

Davidson S et al: Alternating floxuridine and 5-fluorouracil hepatic arterial chemotherapy for colorectal liver metastases minimizes biliary toxicity, *Am J Surg* 172:244-247, 1996.

De Bree E et al: Intraperitoneal chemotherapy for colorectal cancer, *J Surg Oncol* 79:46-61, 2002.

de Gramont A et al: Leucovorin and fluorouracil with or without oxaliplatin as first-line treatment in advanced colorectal cancer, *J Clin Oncol* 17(16):2938-2947, 2000.

Donegan WL: New screening guidelines for colorectal cancer, *J Surg Oncol* 58:2-4, 1998.

Douglass HO et al: Survival after postoperative combination treatment of rectal cancer, *N Engl J Med* 315(20):1294-1299, 1986.

Douillard JY et al: Irinotecan combined with fluorouracil compared with fluorouracil alone as first-line treatment for metastatic colorectal cancer: a multicentre randomized trial, *Lancet* 355(9209):1041-1047, 2000.

Douillard JY et al: Multicenter phase III study of uracil/tegafur and oral leucovorin versus fluorouracil and leucovorin in patients with previously untreated metastatic colorectal cancer, *J Clin Oncol* 20(17):3605-3616, 2002.

Duffy MJ: Carcinoembryonic antigen as a marker for colorectal cancer: is it clinically useful? *Clinical Chemistry* 47(4):624-630, 2001.

Dunst J et al: Phase I trial evaluating the concurrent combination of radiotherapy and capecitabine in rectal cancer, *J Clin Oncol* 1(20):3983-3991, 2002.

Fisher B et al: Postoperative adjuvant chemotherapy or radiation therapy for rectal cancer: Results from NSABP Protocol R-01, *J Natl Cancer Inst* 80(1):21-29, 1998.

Frazee RC et al: Prospective randomized trial of inpatient vs. outpatient bowel preparation for elective colorectal surgery, *Dis Colon Rectum* 35(3):223-226, March 1992.

Gamelin E et al: Clinical aspects and molecular basis of oxaliplatin neurotoxicity: current management and development of preventive measures, *Semin Oncol* 29(suppl 5): 21-33, 2002.

Gastrointestinal Tumor Study Group: Prolongation of the disease-free interval in surgically treated rectal carcinoma, *N Engl J Med* 312(23):1465-1472, 1985.

Gervaz P et al: Colonic J pouch function in rectal cancer patients: impact of adjuvant chemoradiotherapy, *Dis Colon Rectum* 44(11):1667-1675, 2001.

Giacchetti S et al: Phase III multicenter randomized trial of oxaliplatin added to chronomodulated fluorouracil-leucovorin as first-line treatment of metastatic colorectal cancer, *J Clin Oncol* 18:136-147, 2000.

Goodman AA: Polypoid disease. In Corman ML, editor, *Colon and rectal surgery*, ed 4, Philadelphia, 1998, Lippincott-Raven.

Grann A et al: Preoperative combined modality therapy for clinically resectable uT3 rectal carcinoma, *Int J Radiat Oncol Biol Phys* 49(4):987-995, 2001.

Greenlee RT, et al: Cancer statistics 2001, *CA Cancer J Clin* 51(1):15-36, 2001.

Haller DG et al: Fluorouracil, leucovorin, and levamisole adjuvant therapy for colon cancer: five year final report of INT-0089, *Proc Am Soc Clin Oncol* (abstract 982) 17:265A, 1998.

Hanna M et al: Adjuvant active specific immunotherapy of stage II and stage III colon cancer with an autologous tumor cell vaccine: first randomized phase III trials show promise, *Vaccine* 19:2576-2582, 2001.

Hearn K et al: Reduce costs and improve patient satisfaction with home pre-operative bowel preparations, *Nurs Case Manage* 5(1):13-24, 2000.

Hidebrant U, Feifel G: Preoperative staging of rectal cancer by intrarectal ultrasound, *Dis Colon Rectum* 28:42-46, 1985.

Hoff PM et al: Comparison of oral capecitabine versus intravenous fluorouracil plus leucovorin as first-line treatment in 605 patients with metastatic colorectal cancer: results of a randomized phase III study, *J Clin Oncol* 19(8):2282-2292, 2001.

Hu K, Harrison L: Adjuvant therapy for resectable rectal adenocarcinoma, *Semin Surg Oncol* 19:336-349, 2000.

Hull T: Examination and diseases of the anorectum. In Feldman M, Friedman LS, Sleisenger MH editors, *Sleisenger and Fordtran's gastrointestinal and liver disease: pathophysiology, diagnoses, management*, Philadelphia, 2002, WB Saunders.

International Multicentre Pooled Analysis of B2 Colon Cancer Trials (IMPACT B2) Investigators: Efficacy of adjuvant fluorouracil and folinic acid in B2 colon cancer, *J Clin Oncol* 17(5):1356-1363, 1999.

Jemal A et al: Cancer statistics, 2002, *CA Cancer J Clin* 52(1):23-47, 2002.

Kachnic L, Willett C: Radiation therapy in the management of rectal cancer, *Curr Opin Oncol* 13(4):300-306, 2001.

Kalenberg MS: Surgical management of colorectal cancer, *Gen Surg News* 5:23-27, May 2002.

Kemeny N et al: Hepatic arterial infusion of chemotherapy after resection of hepatic metastases from colorectal cancer, *N Engl J Med* 341(27):2039-2048, 1999.

Kronborg O: Colon polyps and cancer, *Endoscopy* 34(1):69-72, 2002.

Krook JE et al: Effective surgical adjuvant therapy for high-risk rectal carcinoma, *N Engl J Med* 324(11):709-715, 1991.

Kroser JA, Bachwich DR, Lichtenstein GR: Risk factors for the development of colorectal carcinoma and their modification, *Hematol Oncol Clin North Am* 11(4):544-577, 1997.

Landis SH, et al: Cancer statistics 1999, *CA Cancer J Clin.* 49:8-32, 1999.

Laurie JA et al: Surgical adjuvant therapy of large-bowel carcinoma: an evaluation of levamisole and the combination of levamisole and fluorouracil, *J Clin Oncol* 7:1447-1456, 1989.

Liver Infusion Meta-analysis Group: Portal vein chemotherapy for colorectal cancer: a meta-analysis of 4000 patients in 10 studies, *J Natl Cancer Inst* 89(7):497-505, 1997.

Mamounas E et al: Comparative efficacy of adjuvant chemotherapy in patients with Dukes' B versus Dukes' C colon cancer: results from four National Surgical

Adjuvant Breast and Bowel Project Adjuvant Studies (C-01, C-02, C-03, and C-04), *J Clin Oncol* 17(5):1349-1355, 1999.

Markham M: Intraperitoneal chemotherapy in the management of colon cancer, *Semin Oncol* 26(5):536-539, 1999.

Mayberry RM, et al: Determinants of black/white differences in colon cancer survival, *J Natl Cancer Inst* 87:1685-1693, 1995.

Minsky BD: Multidisciplinary management of resectable rectal cancer, *Oncology* 10:1701-1708, 1998.

Minsky B: Adjuvant therapy of resectable rectal cancer, *Cancer Treat Rev* 28(4):181-188, 2002.

Moertel CG et al: Levamisole and fluorouracil for adjuvant therapy of resected colon carcinoma, *N Engl J Med* 322:352-358, 1990.

Mulcahy MF, Benson AB: New agents for colorectal cancer, *JNCCN* 1:125-136, 2003.

NIH Consensus Conference: Adjuvant therapy for patients with colon and rectal cancer, *JAMA* 264:1444-1450, 1990.

Nordlinger B, Rougier P: Liver metastases from colorectal cancer: the turning point, *J Clin Oncol* 20(6):1442-1445, 2002a.

Nordlinger B, Rougier P: Nonsurgical methods for liver metastases including cryotherapy, radiofrequency ablation, and infusional treatment: what's new in 2001? *Curr Opin Oncol* 14(4):420-423, 2002b.

Nuyttens JJ et al: The position and volume of the small bowel during adjuvant radiation therapy for rectal cancer, *Int J Radiat Oncol Biol Phys* 51(5):1271-1280, 2001.

O'Brien B: Advances in the treatment of colorectal cancer, *Oncol Nurs* 9(2):1-16, 2002.

O'Brien MJ: Colorectal polyps. In Cohen AM et al, editors, *Cancer of the colon, rectum, and anus*, New York, 1995, McGraw-Hill.

O'Dwyer P: Biochemical modulation strategies for management of advanced colon cancer. In Willson JKV, editor: *Cancer: concept to clinic*, Fair Lawn, NJ, 1992, Medical Publishing Enterprises.

Oliveira L et al: Mechanical bowel preparation for elective colorectal surgery, *Dis Colon Rectum* 40(5):585-591, May 1997.

Onaitis MW et al: Neoadjuvant chemoradiation for rectal cancer: analysis of clinical outcomes from a 13-year institutional experience, *Ann Surg* 233(6):778-785, 2001.

Ries L et al: *SEER cancer statistics review, 1973-1997*, Bethesda, Md, 2000, National Cancer Institute.

Rustgi R: Small intestinal neoplasms. In Feldman M, Friedman LS, Sleisenger MH, editors: *Sleisenger and Fordtran's gastrointestinal and liver disease: pathophysiology, diagnoses, management*, Philadelphia, 2002, WB Saunders.

Saddler DA, Ellis C: Colorectal cancer, *Semin Oncol Nurs* 15(1):58-69, 1999.

Saltz LB et al: Irinotecan plus fluorouracil and leucovorin for metastatic colorectal cancer, *N Engl J Med* 343(13):905-914, 2000.

Schwartzberg LS: Clinical experience with edrecolomab: a monoclonal antibody therapy for colorectal carcinoma, *Crit Rev Oncol Hemat* 40(1):17-24, 2001.

Sotsky TK, Ravikumar T: Cryotherapy in the treatment of liver metastases from colorectal cancer, *Semin Oncol* 29(2):183-191, 2002.

Story JA, Savaiano DA: Dietary fiber and colorectal cancer: what is appropriate advice, *Nutr Rev* 59(3pt2):84-86, 2001.

Stotland BR et al: Preoperative and postoperative imaging for colorectal cancer, *Hematol Oncol Clin North Am* 11(4):635-651, 1997.

Sulkes A et al: Uracil-ftorafur: an oral fluoropyrimidine active in colorectal cancer, *J Clin Oncol* 16(10):3461-3475, 1998.

Swedish Rectal Cancer Trial: Improved survival with preoperative radiotherapy in resectable rectal cancer, *N Engl J Med* 336(14):980-987, 1997.

Tepper JE et al: Adjuvant therapy in rectal cancer: analysis of stage, sex, and local control: final report of Intergroup 0114, *J Clin Oncol* 20(7):1744-1750, 2002.

van Geldere D, et al: Complications after colorectal surgery without mechanical bowel preparation, *J Am Coll Surg* 194(1):40-47, 2002.

Vaughn D, Haller D: The role of adjuvant chemotherapy in the treatment of colorectal cancer, *Hematol Oncol Clin North Am* 11(4):699-719, 1997.

Wakefield SE et al: The incidence and Dukes' staging of colorectal cancer over 3 decades, *Eur J Surg Oncol* 24:525-27, 1998.

Wilkes G: New Therapeutic Options in colon cancer: focus on oxaliplatin, *Clin J Oncol Nurs* 6(3):131-137, 2002.

Willett CG et al: Tumor proliferation in rectal cancer following preoperative irradiation, *J Clin Oncol* 13:1417-1424, 1995.

Winawer SJ et al: Colorectal cancer screening: clinical guidelines and rationale, *Gastroenterology* 112(2):594-642, 1997.

Wolmark N et al: Postoperative adjuvant chemotherapy or BCG for colon cancer: results from NSABP protocol C-01, *J Natl Cancer Inst* 80:30-36, 1988.

Wolmark N et al: Randomized trial of postoperative adjuvant chemotherapy with or without radiotherapy for carcinoma of the rectum: National Surgical Adjuvant Breast and Bowel Project Protocol R-02, *J Natl Cancer Inst* 92(5):388-396, 2000.

Yanagi H et al: Preoperative detection of distal intramural spread of lower carcinoma using transrectal ultrasonography, *Dis Colon Rectum* 39(11):1210-4, 1996.

Zmora O, Pikarsky AJ, Wexner SD: Bowel preparation for colorectal surgery, *Dis Colon Rectum* 44(10):1537-1549, 2001.

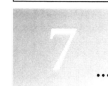

CHAPTER

7

Gastrointestinal Cancers: Surgical Management

CAROL-ANN VASILEVSKY and PHILIP H. GORDON

OBJECTIVES

1. Relate the influencing factors that must be considered when deciding whether a sphincter-preserving or sphincter-sacrificing procedure will be done in the management of a person with colorectal cancer.
2. Describe the preoperative stoma marking considerations in the patient undergoing resection of a colorectal cancer.
3. Distinguish between the following operative procedures: low anterior resection, abdominoperineal resection, and the coloanal anastomosis.
4. Discuss the oncologic results of sphincter-saving procedures.
5. Describe the quality of life issues related to the surgical procedures used to treat colorectal cancers.

INTRODUCTION

With the advent of improved surgical techniques for sphincter preservation in the management of low rectal cancers, the frequency of permanent intestinal stomas has decreased. However, the more frequent use of preoperative radiotherapy to facilitate resection of bulky rectal tumors, as well as the increase in sphincter-saving ultralow anastomoses, has led to an increase in the employment of temporary diverting ileostomies.

This chapter covers the management of patients with rectal cancer in light of one of the focuses of this book, namely disease processes that may necessitate a temporary or permanent stoma. The preop-

erative considerations involved in planning a stoma are described; the chapter also explores the criteria used in the selection of operative procedures for rectal cancers, as well as their functional and oncologic results and the various types of stomas that can be created.

PREOPERATIVE CONSIDERATIONS

Preoperative counseling and stoma site selection are critical in the preparation of a patient for surgery. This entails a meeting with a wound, ostomy, and continence/enterostomal therapy (WOC/ET) nurse to provide information about the stoma and to dispel concerns about body habitus, hygiene, and the effect of the stoma on social or athletic activities and intimate relationships. Many difficulties encountered with stomas relate to their improper placement. This can be eliminated with a preoperative planning session, which includes the surgeon, the WOC/ET nurse, and the patient. Improperly placed stomas can result in leakage of intestinal contents, peristomal skin problems, and emotional stress.

When the procedure is elective, marking of the stoma site must be done before the patient reaches the operating room. This may not always be possible when emergency surgery is needed. The stoma should be placed within the rectus muscle (to avoid a peristomal hernia or prolapse), below the belt line (to avoid direct trauma to the stoma and allow it to be better concealed), on a flat surface, and where it can be easily visualized by the patient (to permit patient self-management). The patient should be examined in the supine, sitting, and standing positions to optimize the location of the stoma so that it is visible to the patient. When standing, obese patients may not be able to see a stoma located inferior to the umbilicus. Abdominal wall thickness is usually greater in this area, making delivery of the bowel through the skin aperture more difficult. Thus the stoma site is usually placed in a more superior position in the obese person. When a stoma site is being selected, care should be taken to avoid skin creases, bony prominences, and scars, since these may interfere with adherence of the appliance to the skin. The stoma site can be marked with a marking pen or tattooed with an intradermal injection of methylene blue, or the skin can be lacerated with a needle or scalpel. The latter technique should be discouraged, since it may result in infection. An occlusive transparent dressing may be placed over the site until surgery. Often patients who are being operated on for low rectal cancers are marked for two stomas, a diverting ileostomy should a coloanal anastomosis be performed, and an end colostomy if an abdominoperineal procedure is to be done. The reasoning behind this is that the ultimate decision as to whether a sphincter-saving procedure will be technically feasible is made only at the time of surgical exploration. See Chapter 11 for additional information on stoma marking.

SELECTION OF THE APPROPRIATE OPERATIVE PROCEDURE

The most important goal in surgical resection of a rectal cancer is to obtain clear margins of resection following extirpation of the malignancy. This involves performance of a wide anatomic resection and total mesorectal excision for lower lesions, with the hope of decreasing the incidence of local recurrence. The distal resection margin (i.e., the distance distal to the carcinoma beyond which the rectum has been transected) has long been the subject of considerable controversy. Most authorities would at present accept a distal margin of 2 cm to contain both intramural and retrograde lymphatic spread (Grinnell, 1966).

A myriad of factors influence whether a sphincter-preserving or a sphincter-sacrificing procedure

is appropriate for a given patient. Careful selection is vital to ensure good oncologic and functional results. These factors include the level of the lesion, body build, sex, obesity, the degree of local spread, the presence of complicating features such as perforation or abscess, size and degree of fixation of the lesion, histologic grade of the carcinoma, preoperative incontinence, and overall general health of the patient.

Certainly the most important factor involved in the decision is the level of the lesion. Anatomically the rectum is divided into thirds (see Figure 3-7). The lower third extends from the anorectal ring (3 to 4 cm from the anal verge) to 7 cm from the anal verge, the middle third spans the segment 7 to 11 cm from the anal verge, and the upper third is the segment 11 to 15 cm from the anal verge.

Low Anterior Resection

The term *low anterior resection* (LAR) is applied when the operation necessitates full mobilization of the rectum and an anastomosis is performed below the peritoneal reflection. It is generally accepted that LAR is the treatment of choice for carcinomas located in the upper and middle third of the rectum.

Abdominoperineal Resection

An abdominoperineal resection (APR) involves the surgical extirpation of the rectum (proctectomy), in which the rectum, anus, and sphincter mechanism are removed, and a permanent end colostomy of sigmoid colon is placed through an aperture in a previously marked left lower quadrant marking. The APR has been viewed as the gold standard in the treatment of low-lying rectal cancers. However, advances in surgical expertise and the advent of mechanical stapling devices have facilitated the creation of ultralow anastomoses, reserving APR for the low rectal cancer where anastomosis is not oncologically sound.

Coloanal Anastomosis

A coloanal anastomosis (CAA) entails full mobilization of the rectum and placement of the anastomosis at or just above the levator ani muscles. Although a 2-cm distal margin has been advocated, a 1-cm distal margin is considered oncologically safe provided that the carcinoma has no adverse histologic features; it is favored especially if it means the difference between sphincter sacrifice or preservation (Nelson et al, 2001). This recommendation is based on several studies, which demonstrated that distal intramural spread of a carcinoma is found beyond 1 cm only in 4% to 10% of rectal malignancies (Pollet and Nicholls, 1983; Williams, Dixon, and Johnston, 1983). In the latter circumstances the prognosis is poor, regardless of the length of the distal margin. A comparison of the operative procedures is depicted in Figure 7-1.

Patients with large, bulky carcinoma tumors, poorly differentiated lesions, or histologically unfavorable malignancies should undergo an APR if the distal margin that will be obtained is less than 2 cm. Preservation of intestinal continuity is questionable in patients with poor preoperative anorectal function, since patients with incontinence will

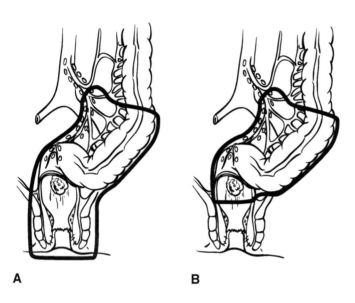

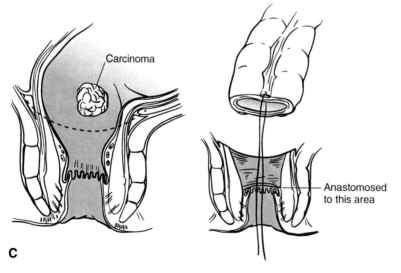

Figure 7-1 Comparison of amount of tissue excised with **A,** abdominoperineal resection, **B,** low anterior resection and **C,** coloanal anastomosis. (From Quality Medical Publishing, St Louis.)

suffer a poor result. Often the decision as to whether a CAA or APR is performed is based on technical factors encountered in the operating room. A sphincter-preserving procedure is more easily accomplished in a woman with a gynecoid pelvis, as well as in a nonobese individual without any intervening complicating features such as local spread or perforation.

Low Anterior Resection and Coloanal Anastomosis with Temporary Diversion

Protection of the ultralow anterior resection and CAA with a diverting stoma, be it a loop ileostomy or colostomy, is strongly advised, since the incidence of anastomotic leakage increases the more distally the anastomosis is created (Karanjia et al, 1994). Male gender and absence of a protective stoma to divert the fecal stream have also been suggested as risk factors for anastomotic dehiscence (Dehni et al, 1998). Anastomotic leaks have been shown to result in significant local complications that prevent stoma takedown and restoration of intestinal continuity in as many as one third of patients. Moreover, functional results in patients with an anastomotic leak are worse once the stoma is closed than in patients who do not suffer an anastomotic dehiscence (Nesbukken, Nygaard, and Lunde, 2001). This is probably secondary to sepsis and perirectal fibrosis, which affect rectal motility and capacity.

There is some controversy as to whether a policy of using diversion with a CAA should be routine. Many of the studies that advocated diversion were retrospective in nature and contained a mixture of diagnoses and varying surgical techniques (Karanjia et al, 1994; Dehni et al, 1998, Rullier et al, 1998). A recent randomized trial comparing outcomes between diverted and nondiverted patients undergoing LAR with colonic pouch showed that there was no difference in the rate of pelvic sepsis between the two groups (Machado et al, 2002). That being said, it is the authors' practice to routinely employ diversion with CAA, especially if the patient has undergone preoperative radiotherapy.

Another point of controversy is whether a loop colostomy or an ileostomy should be used for diversion. Three out of four randomized controlled trials have recommended the use of a loop ileostomy (Williams et al, 1986; Khoury et al, 1997; Gooszen et al, 1998; Edwards et al, 2001). Loop ileostomy was found to be less odorous, required fewer appliance changes, and was associated with fewer overall problems than a colostomy (Williams et al, 1986). Stoma-related complications such as fecal fistula, prolapse, and incisional hernia were more frequent in the loop transverse colostomy group compared to the loop ileostomy patients (Edwards et al, 2001). Others have reported on an increased incidence of postoperative bowel obstruction and other complications after ileostomy closure (Altomare et al, 1990).

FUNCTIONAL RESULTS WITH LOW ANTERIOR RESECTION AND COLOANAL ANASTOMOSIS

Although sphincter preservation decreases the psychologic impact associated with a stoma, reestablishment of intestinal continuity often results in disorders of continence ranging from uncontrollable flatus to frank leakage of stool. Urgency and increased frequency of evacuation, or the anterior resection syndrome, may ensue. This is especially prevalent as the anastomosis is constructed lower in the pelvis.

Anterior Resection Syndrome

Impaired functional results have been reported in up to 50% of patients following LAR or CAA (Kim et al, 2001). Anterior resection syndrome is characterized by frequency of bowel movements with fragmentation (piecemeal stool), urgency of defecation, and varying degrees of incontinence. This impairment is greatest in patients with postoperative anastomotic complications (Hallbook and Sjodahl, 1996; Fichera and Michelassi, 2001) and in those receiving postoperative radiation therapy (Paty et al, 1994a). There may be multiple factors responsible for occurrence of this syndrome. Damage to the sphincter complex may occur as a result of inserting the stapling device, or there may be damage to its innervation at the time of rectal mobilization. Rectal resection may induce loss of normal residual rectal or neorectal sensation, or reduced rectal capacity and compliance, resulting in increased intraluminal pressures that lead to leakage or incontinence. Reduction in length of the large intestine may result in a more liquid effluent reaching the anal canal. Moreover, the addition of radiation therapy, whether it is preoperative or postoperative, may contribute further to anorectal dysfunction. The ensuing skin problems caused by continuous leakage of stool often pose a challenge to the WOC/ET nurse.

In an effort to improve these functional results, the use of a colonic J pouch as a rectal substitute has been reported (Lazorthes et al, 1986; Parc et al, 1986). Several randomized and nonrandomized studies have shown that the pouch is more compliant and can store a higher volume of stool than can the colon following straight CAA, thereby reducing stool frequency and improving continence. This functional superiority remains for 1 to 2 years after surgery, by which time the straight coloanal neorectum has been found to adapt (Ho, Seow-Choen, and Tan, 2000). Evacuation difficulties and constipation have been reported as a drawback of pouch formation (Parc et al, 1986). Formation of a J pouch may also reduce the incidence of anastomotic leak, according to several studies (Ho, Seow-Choen, and Tan, 2000; Hallbook et al, 1996), although this has been disputed by others (Ortiz et al, 1995). However, this procedure may not always be possible because of the presence of a fatty or foreshortened mesentery, which may result in major difficulty in having the pouch reach the level of distal transection.

Another technique, simpler to perform, may have similar functional advantages to the colonic J pouch without the drawback of impaired evacuation: it is the transverse coloplasty (Z'graggen, Maurer, and Buchler, 1999). A coloplasty is created by making an 8- to 10-cm longitudinal incision in the colon just proximal to the area of CAA. The incision is closed transversely, thereby resulting in the formation of a small colonic pouch. This provides a small anterior reservoir, thereby decreasing the incidence of impaired evacuation. A randomized controlled trial comparing the results of using a J pouch or coloplasty with a CAA found that coloplasty resulted in more anastomotic leaks with minimal differences in bowel function after 1 year (Ho et al, 2002).

ONCOLOGIC RESULTS OF SPHINCTER-SAVING PROCEDURES

Several studies have evaluated the oncologic results of LAR and CAA with and without a pouch. Local recurrence rates ranging from 4% to 18% have been reported and 5-year survival rates have been reported to be between 70% to 80% (Kim et al, 2001; Paty et al, 1994b; Nymann et al, 1995; Berger et al, 1999; Kohler et al, 2000; Leo et al, 2000). Nonrandomized retrospective studies have demonstrated no advantage to APR in terms of survival or prevention of local recurrence when compared to sphincter-saving procedures (Nelson et al, 2001; Heald et al, 1997; Wolmark and Fisher, 1986; Amato, Pescatori, and Butti, 1991; Dixon, Maxwell, and Holmes, 1991; Gamagami et al, 1999).

Nerve-Sparing Procedures

An all-important consideration for any pelvic operation in a man is nerve preservation. Surgeons make an effort to prevent injury to the hypogastric nerves by dissection in a plane anterior to them. The pelvic nerves originating from S2, S3, and S4 can be spared by continuing in the plane adjacent to the visceral mesentery of the rectum. Injury is most likely to occur when the carcinoma is low on the anterior rectal wall, jeopardizing the nerves on the posterolateral aspect of the prostate just anterior to Denonvilliers' fascia. Care is therefore taken to ensure, when possible, that Denonvilliers' fascia remains intact on the prostate and the seminal vesicles.

STOMA CONSTRUCTION
Ileostomy
Loop Ileostomy

A loop of terminal ileum as distal as possible and close to the ileocecal valve is delivered through an aperture made previously in the abdominal wall. If there is no tension on the loop and the abdominal wall is not overly thick, there is no need for a supporting rod to be placed. The loop is opened or matured to allow the afferent limb to be the larger of the two openings and the functional limb. It is everted to assume the appearance of an end ileostomy (Figure 7-2).

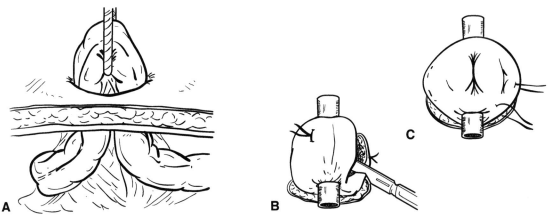

Figure 7-2 Loop ileostomy construction. **A,** Loop of bowel exteriorized. **B,** Support rod placed to maintain position of bowel on abdominal surface. Distal ileum is incised. **C,** Loop ileostomy matured. (From Hampton BG, Bryant RA: *Ostomies and continent diversions: nursing management,* St Louis, 1992, Mosby.)

End-Loop Ileostomy

An alternative to the conventional loop ileostomy is the end-loop stoma in which the ileum is divided by a linear stapler, a short segment of mesentery is divided, and the stapled proximal end is matured like an end ileostomy. The antimesenteric corner of the distal limb is excised and matured at skin level (Figure 7-3) and to the untrained eye resembles a fistula. A variation of this technique is occasionally used in which the efferent limb remains closed and is tacked to the afferent limb at fascial level.

Loop-End Ileostomy

A loop-end ileostomy is used when the abdominal wall is too thick or the mesentery is too short, so that the ileum cannot be elevated to the anterior abdominal wall without tension. It is constructed by dividing the ileum with a linear stapler and elevating a loop of ileum at a point where the bowel can be elevated above the abdominal wall (Figure 7-4).

Colostomy

End Colostomy

An end colostomy may be temporary or permanent. It is regarded as permanent with the performance of an APR and if the carcinoma is assessed to be fixed to bony structures in the pelvis, thus rendering it unresectable. In the latter case the carcinoma is left in place, the portion of colon immediately proximal to the lesion is transected with a linear stapler, and a portion of colon proximal to the lesion is brought to the surface of the abdominal wall. An end colostomy may be performed as a temporary procedure following resection of the rectosigmoid for malignant disease that is complicated by perforation or in circumstances that render the performance of a primary anastomosis unsafe. In this case, the carcinoma is resected, the remaining distal end colon/rectum is transected with a linear stapler (Hartmann's pouch) and the end colostomy fashioned with the remaining portion of proximal colon. In the case of a permanent stoma, the stoma may be fashioned through an extraperitoneal tunnel or intraperitoneally in the standard approach. It is thought that the former may result in a reduced rate of peristomal hernia or prolapse. Recurrence of carcinoma at the stoma site is extremely uncommon; however, if it should occur, resection of the stoma is indicated.

Loop Colostomy

The loop transverse colostomy is still the most frequently used method to achieve temporary or

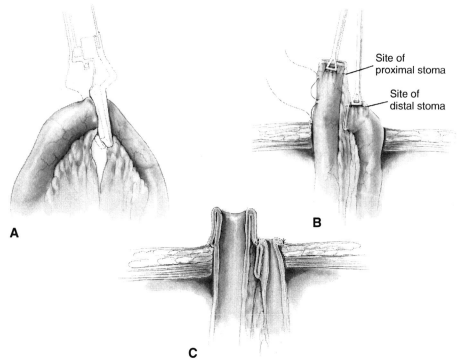

Figure 7-3   End-loop ileostomy. **A,** Ileostomy loop is divided between staples. **B,** Proximal end is elevated above skin level and everted. **C,** Both ends are sutured to skin. (From Quality Medical Publishing, St Louis)

short-term fecal diversion whether necessitated by obstruction or low anastomosis. In the case of the obstructed colon, this type of colostomy is most likely to prolapse once the distention has subsided, since the skin aperture is created quite large to accommodate the distended colon. Loop colostomy is constructed in a similar fashion as was described previously for the loop ileostomy. In contrast, however, a loop colostomy may be constructed over a fascial bridge or with the use of a supporting rod.

End-Loop Colostomy

When dealing with an obstructed colon, the distended colon is less likely to reach the anterior abdominal wall without tension, which can cause compressive venous obstruction. In this situation, the end-loop colostomy may be advantageous. The end-loop colostomy is analogous to the end-loop

ileostomy previously described. The advantage of this type of colostomy over the preceding one with rods and bridges is that it may result in improved patient stoma care by allowing a more secure pouching system application.

Hidden Colostomy

Another type of colostomy, called a hidden colostomy, may be more suitable in a patient found to have an unresectable carcinoma of the rectum or colon with extensive metastases or carcinomatosis. If the lesion is not causing complete or partial obstruction, the surgeon must decide between doing nothing and creating a colostomy, knowing that the patient may never need it. With this type of colostomy, the colon is buried in the subcutaneous fat where it can be identified at a later date. If obstruction occurs, this stoma can be opened under local anesthesia. Although the resulting

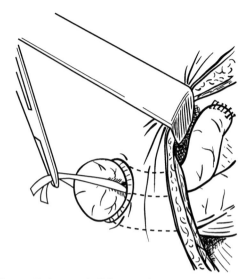

Figure 7-4 Turnball loop-end stoma. Distal portion of bowel segment is brought to abdominal surface as loop. Anterior wall of bowel segment is opened and matured to form functional and nonfunctional limbs characteristic of loop stomas. (From Hampton BG, Bryant RA: *Ostomies and continent diversions: nursing management,* St Louis, 1992, Mosby.)

stoma is not ideal, it is usually opened when the patient is terminal or near terminal.

QUALITY OF LIFE ISSUES

In a recent review of 17 cross-sectional studies (Sprangers et al, 1995), a sizable percentage of patients treated with either a permanent stoma or sphincter-preserving procedures reported limitations in their quality of life. Both patient groups were troubled by frequent bowel movements. Stoma patients reported higher degrees of psychologic distress and restrictions with respect to their social and sexual functioning. The majority of studies included in this review used nonstandardized study-specific questionnaires, and none looked at patients with ultralow anastomoses.

Another review of 54 papers (Camillieri-Brennan and Steele, 1998) found that patients suffer from both short- and long-term sequelae after treatment for rectal cancer, but global quality of life improved after surgery in most patients. In one study comparing quality of life in patients with an APR to those with an LAR, overall quality of life seemed to be better for patients who underwent APR rather than ultralow resection (Grumann et al, 2001). The differences were significant for diarrhea, constipation, and sleeping problems. They also evaluated whether the level of anastomosis affected quality of life and found that patients with lower anastomoses reported poorer quality of life than those with higher anastomoses. Patients with low anastomoses reported poorer social function and body image and had significantly increased gastrointestinal and defecation-related symptoms, which severely disrupted their social life. However, it must be emphasized that quality of life tools are subjective. Personal and cultural factors can easily introduce confounding results. For example, some patients may tolerate symptoms of stool frequency and urgency in exchange for the absence of a stoma, and this may inadvertently influence the outcome of a study. In the one above (Grumann et al, 2001), the levels of anastomosis (very low and high anterior resections) were lumped together. Other investigators did not find that patients with LAR had a worse quality of life than those with APR (Kerr et al, 2002). They also noted quality of life scores improved over time for LAR patients, whereas they did not for APR patients. They noted that for patients with temporary stomas, quality of life scores improved with stoma closure. Considering these factors, Kerr and colleagues (2002) believe that colostomies are more likely to be associated with a worse quality of life than poor bowel function.

CONCLUSION

Although avoidance of a permanent colostomy is one of the major goals in surgery for rectal cancer, it is vital that surgeons and their patients be cognizant of the fact that, following ultralow anterior resection and CAA, functional results may be suboptimal and these functional results may be further compromised by radiation therapy.

SELF-ASSESSMENT EXERCISES

Questions

1. What is the most important goal of surgical resection of a rectal cancer?
   a. Avoidance of a permanent stoma
   b. Removal of the tumor and salvage of as much colon and rectum as possible
   c. Clear margins of resection following removal of the tumor
   d. Return to normal bowel function after recovery
2. What is the acceptable distal resection margin when surgically removing a colorectal cancer?
3. Define the three anatomic sections of the rectum.
4. The surgical treatment of choice for a carcinoma in the upper and middle third of the rectum is:
   a. APR.
   b. LAR.
   c. CAA.
5. What is the gold standard surgical procedure for treatment of low-lying rectal cancers?
6. Explain what is mobilized in the performance of the CAA.
7. Discuss why it is strongly advised that a protecting stoma be created when a patient undergoes an LAR and/or a CAA.
8. The results reporting oncologic results of the LAR and CAA range between:
   a. Local recurrence: 4% and 18%, 5-year survival rate: 70% to 80%.
   b. Local recurrence: 20% to 25%, 5-year survival rate: 60% to 70%.
   c. Local recurrence: 30% to 35%, 5-year survival rate: 50%.
9. Discuss the quality of life issues reported for patients with rectal cancers treated with surgical interventions.

Answers

1. c
2. A distal margin of 2 cm, to contain both intramural and retrograde lymphatic spread, is the acceptable margin.
3. The three anatomic sections of the rectum are the lower third, which extends from the anorectal ring (3 to 4 cm from the anal verge) to 7 cm from the anal verge; the middle third, which is 7 to 11 cm from the anal verge; and the upper third, which is 11 to 15 cm from the anal verge.
4. b
5. APR
6. The surgical mobilization of the rectum and performance of the anastomosis at or just above the levator ani muscles
7. It is strongly advised that protection of the ultralow anterior resection and CAA be accomplished with a diverting stoma, since the incidence of anastomotic leakage increases the more distally the anastomosis is created.
8. a
9. A sizable percentage of patients with a permanent stoma or with sphincter-preserving procedures report limitations in their quality of life. In one study comparing quality of life in patients with an APR to those with an LAR, overall quality of life seemed to be better for patients who underwent APR rather than ultralow resection. One study noted that the level of anastomosis affected the quality of life, and that patients with lower anastomoses reported poorer quality of life than those with higher anastomoses.

REFERENCES

Altomare DF et al: Protective colostomy closure: the hazards of a "minor" operation, *Int J Colorectal Dis* 5:73-78, 1990.

Amato A, Pescatori M, Butti A: Local recurrence following abdominoperineal excision and anterior resection for rectal carcinoma, *Dis Colon Rectum* 34:317-322, 1991.

Berger A et al: Rectal excision and colonic pouch-anal anastomosis for rectal cancer oncologic results at five years, *Dis Colon Rectum* 42:1265-1271, 1999.

Camillieri-Brennan J, Steele JC: Quality of life after treatment of rectal cancer, *Br J Surg* 85:1036-1043, 1998.

Dehni N et al: Influence of a defunctioning stoma on leakage rates after low colorectal anastomosis and colonic pouch-anal anastomosis, *Br J Surg* 85:1114-1117, 1998.

Dixon AR, Maxwell W, Holmes J: Carcinoma of the rectum: a 10-year experience, *Br J Surg* 78:308-311, 1991.

Edwards D et al: Stoma-related complications are more frequent after transverse colostomy than loop ileostomy: a prospective randomized clinical trial, *Br J Surg* 88:360-363, 2001.

Fichera A, Michelassi F: Long-term prospective assessment of functional results after proctectomy with coloanal anastomosis, *J Gastrointest Surg* 5:153-157, 2001.

Gamagami R et al: Coloanal anastomosis for distal third rectal cancer: prospective study of oncological results, *Dis Colon Rectum* 42:1272-1275, 1999.

Gooszen A et al: Temporary decompression after colorectal surgery: randomized comparison of loop ileostomy and loop colostomy, *Br J Surg* 85:76-79, 1998.

Grinnell RS: Lymphatic block with atypical and retrograde lymphatic metastases and spread in carcinoma of the colon and rectum, *Ann Surg* 163:272-280, 1966.

Grumann MM et al: Comparison of quality of life in patients undergoing abdominoperineal extirpation or anterior resection for rectal cancer, *Ann Surg* 233:149-156, 2001.

Hallbook O et al: Randomized comparison of straight and colonic J-pouch anastomosis after low anterior resection, *Ann Surg* 224:58-65, 1996.

Hallbook O, Sjodahl R: Anastomotic leakage and functional outcome after anterior resection of the rectum, *Br J Surg* 83:60-62, 1996.

Heald R et al: Abdominoperineal excision of the rectum—an endangered operation, *Dis Colon Rectum* 40:747-751, 1997.

Ho YH et al: Comparison of J pouch and coloplasty pouch for low rectal cancers. A randomized, controlled trial investigating functional results and comparative anastomotic leak rates, *Ann Surg* 236:49-55, 2002.

Ho YH, Seow-Choen F, Tan M: Colonic J pouch function no longer better at 2 years—randomized controlled study with clinical, manometric and barostat follow-up (abstract), *Aust NZ J Surg* 70:A51, 2000.

Karanjia N et al: Leakage from stapled low anastomosis after total mesorectal excision for carcinoma of the rectum, *Br J Surg* 81:1224-1226, 1994.

Kerr J et al: Colostomies may influence patient quality of life more than poor sphincter function: letter to editor, *J Clin Oncol* 20:3930-3931, 2002.

Khoury G et al: Colostomy or ileostomy after colorectal anastomosis? A randomized trial, *Ann R Coll Surg Engl* 69:5-7, 1997.

Kim N et al: Ultralow anterior resection and coloanal anastomosis for distal rectal cancer: functional and oncological results, *Int J Colorectal Dis* 16:234-237, 2001.

Kohler A et al: Long-term results of low anterior resection with intersphincteric anastomosis in carcinoma of the lower rectum: analysis of 31 patients, *Dis Colon Rectum* 43:843-850, 2000.

Lazorthes F et al: Resection of the rectum with construction of a colonic reservoir and coloanal anastomosis for carcinoma of the rectum, *Br J Surg* 73:136-138, 1986.

Leo E et al: Total rectal resection and complete mesorectum excision followed by coloendoanal anastomosis as the optimal treatment for low rectal cancer: the experience of the National Cancer Institute of Milano, *Ann Surg Oncol* 7:125-132, 2000.

Machado M et al: Defunctioning stoma in low anterior resection with colonic pouch for rectal cancer, *Dis Colon Rectum* 45:940-945, 2002.

Nelson H et al: Guidelines 2000 for colon and rectal cancer surgery, *J Natl Cancer Inst* 93:583-596, 2001.

Nesbukken AA, Nygaard K, Lunde O: Outcome and late functional results after anastomotic leakage following mesorectal excision for rectal cancer, *Br J Surg* 88:400-404, 2001.

Nymann T et al: Rate and treatment of pelvic recurrence after abdominoperineal resection and low anterior resection for rectal cancer, *Dis Colon Rectum* 38:799-802, 1995.

Ortiz H et al: Coloanal anastomosis: are functional results better with a pouch? *Dis Colon Rectum* 38:375-377, 1995.

Parc R et al: Resection and coloanal anastomosis with colonic reservoir for rectal carcinoma, *Br J Surg* 73(2):139-141, 1986.

Paty P et al: Long-term functional results of coloanal anastomosis for rectal cancer, *Am J Surg* 167:90-95, 1994a.

Paty P et al: Treatment of rectal cancer by low anterior resection with coloanal anastomosis, *Ann Surg* 219:365-373, 1994b.

Pollet W, Nicholls R: The relationship between the extent of distal clearance and survival and local recurrence rates after curative anterior resection for carcinoma of the rectum, *Ann Surg* 198:159-163, 1983.

Rullier E et al: Risk factors for anastomotic leakage after resection of rectal cancer, *Br J Surg* 85:355-358, 1998.

Sprangers MAG et al: Quality of life in colorectal cancer: stoma vs. nonstoma patients, *Dis Colon Rectum* 38:361-369, 1995.

Williams N, Dixon M, Johnston D: Reappraisal of the 5 centimetre rule of distal excision for carcinoma of the rectum: a study of distal intramural spread and of patients' survival, *Br J Surg* 70:150-154, 1983.

Williams N et al: Defunctioning stomas: a prospective controlled trial comparing loop ileostomy with loop transverse colostomy, *Br J Surg* 73:566-570, 1986.

Wolmark N, Fisher B: An analysis of survival and treatment failure following abdominoperineal resection and sphincter-saving resection in Dukes' B and C rectal carcinoma: a report of the NSABP clinical trials, *Ann Surg* 24:480-489, 1986.

Z'graggen K, Maurer C, Buchler M: Transverse coloplasty pouch. A novel neorectal reservoir, *Dig Surg* 16:363-366, 1999.

CHAPTER

8

Gastrointestinal Etiologies Leading to a Fecal Diversion

JANICE M. BEITZ

OBJECTIVES

1. Describe the historical perspectives, epidemiology, and risk factors for the following disorders: diverticular disease, radiation enteritis, ischemic colitis, infectious enteritis, intestinal obstruction (dynamic and adynamic), and gastrointestinal trauma.

2. Explain the pathophysiology, clinical presentation, differential diagnosis, and diagnostic studies for the following disorders: diverticular disease, radiation enteritis, ischemic colitis, infectious enteritis, intestinal obstruction (dynamic and adynamic), and gastrointestinal trauma.

3. Delineate medical and surgical treatment of the following disorders: diverticular disease, radiation enteritis, ischemic colitis, infectious enteritis, intestinal obstruction (dynamic and adynamic), and gastrointestinal trauma.

4. Describe selected nongastrointestinal etiologies that may necessitate fecal diversion: spinal cord injury, ovarian cancer, and prostate cancer.

INTRODUCTION

Multiple gastrointestinal etiologies may necessitate the creation of a fecal diversion (i.e., ileostomy, colostomy). Some of the causes may include diseases that are inflammatory or neoplastic in nature, whereas other precipitating events are trauma-related, iatrogenic, or infectious. This chapter focuses on six major etiologies: diverticular disease, radiation enteritis, ischemic colitis, infectious enteritis, intestinal obstruction, and gastrointestinal trauma. Brief discussions of ovarian cancer, prostate cancer, and spinal cord injury (SCI) are also included as nongastrointestinal precipitating etiologies for fecal diversion. For discussions of inflammatory bowel disease (IBD) and colon cancer, the reader is referred to Chapters 4 to 7 in the text.

GASTROINTESTINAL ETIOLOGIES
Diverticular Disease

Diverticular disease of the colon is commonly described as a malady of Western civilization; that is, it is most prevalent in developed nations. To describe the condition as a disease is partially a misnomer because over two thirds of the persons affected (e.g., the elderly) will remain entirely asymptomatic. However, 20% to 25% of affected people will eventually manifest clinical symptoms. The purpose of this discussion is to describe the nature of diverticular disease and associated terminology, epidemiology, risk factors, pathophysiology, clinical presentation, differential diagnosis, diagnostic studies, and medical and surgical treatments.

Historical Perspectives

Diverticular disease is a problem of the twentieth century that is likely related to the greater lifespan of the population and major changes in dietary habits, especially decreases in the fiber content of daily food intake. The initial description of the condition was made by a French surgeon, Alexis Littre, in 1700 (Stollman and Raskin, 2002). The disorder was later described in the nineteenth century by

Cruveilhier and Graser, but most publications and research on diverticular disease occurred in the twentieth century, especially from the 1960s onward (Rodkey and Welch, 1998).

Associated Terminology

Diverticular disease represents the spectrum of the disorder from an asymptomatic state to severe inflammation and colonic rupture. In 1909, Terrill first proposed the use of the terms *diverticulosis* and *diverticulitis* (Rodkey and Welch, 1998). Diverticulosis is a condition in which pouches of intestinal lining balloon out through weakened areas of intestinal wall (Figure 8-1). The pouches are called diverticula (one is called a diverticulum).

Diverticulosis generally is asymptomatic or has mild symptoms (i.e., cramps, bloating).

Diverticulitis occurs when diverticula become inflamed and/or infected. A likely cause of this infectious-inflammatory process is stool or food particles becoming trapped in the pouches (Diverticular Disease, 2002). Modern descriptions of the disorder have specified additional terminology for further clarification (Box 8-1).

Epidemiology/Risk Factors

The exact prevalence of colonic diverticulosis is challenging to measure, given that up to 80% of patients are asymptomatic. However, certain patterns of disease occurrence are well elucidated. The

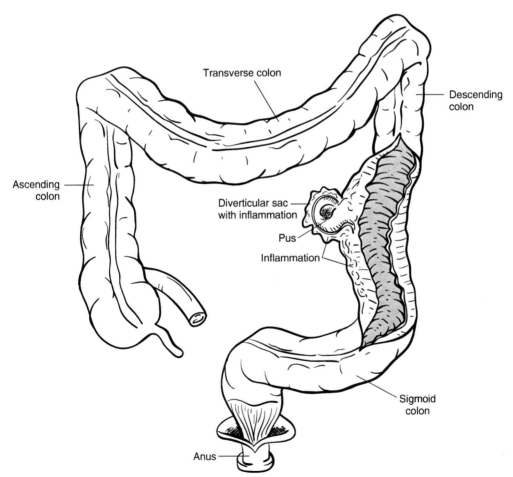

Figure 8-1 Diverticulitis. (From Doughty DB, Broadwell-Jackson: *Gastrointestinal disorders*, St Louis, 1993, Mosby.)

BOX 8-1   Basic Diverticular Disease Terminology

••

Diverticular Disease
Disease spectrum encompassing both diverticulosis and diverticulitis

Diverticulosis
Condition of having diverticula present in bowel

Diverticulitis
Condition of having inflamed diverticula

Uncomplicated diverticulitis
Inflammation of diverticula confined to local area with walling off of inflammatory response (phlegmon)

Complicated diverticulitis
Inflammation of diverticula leading to abscess, obstruction, fistula formation, or colonic perforation

Symptomatic uncomplicated diverticular disease (SUDD)
Condition of having nonspecific symptoms like pain, bloating, and/or altered bowel habits that may be attributed to diverticular disease

---

incidence of diverticular disease clearly increases with age; an estimated 60% to 70% of persons older than 80 years are affected. Conversely, diverticular disease is rare in those younger than 40 years (Kazzi and Kazzi, 2002). For example, only 1% to 2% of the population has diverticular disease by age 25 (Carter and Whelan, 2000). No apparent sex bias occurs; both men and women are equally affected (Stollman and Raskin, 1999; Stollman and Raskin, 2002).

Geographically a clear tendency exists. Diverticular disease is common in industrialized nations, particularly the United States, Northern Europe, England, and Australia (i.e., where low-fiber diets are eaten) and rare in countries of Asia and Africa (i.e., where high-fiber diets are the norm) (Hyde, 2000; Kazzi and Kazzi, 2002; Rodkey and Welch, 1998; Stollman and Raskin, 2002).

Sociocultural factors likely play a role. Research suggests that diverticular disease is more common among lower-income people than in higher socio-economic groups. Lack of awareness and lack of access to sources of dietary fiber, such as fruit and vegetables, are possible factors (Hyde, 2000). Relocation to a higher incidence area also plays a factor in altering bowel function. Japanese living in the United States and Arabs living in Israel have higher rates of diverticulosis than their counterparts in their native countries (Stollman and Raskin, 2002).

Although environmental issues (i.e., diet) affect the prevalence of diverticular disease, race and genetic factors are linked to its anatomic distribution. In contrast to Western patients, diverticular disease among Asians demonstrates predominance for the right colon, whereas persons from the West have disease that is mostly found in the left colon, especially the sigmoid segment (Kazzi and Kazzi, 2002).

Pathophysiology

Although diverticular disease may affect any part of the gastrointestinal (GI) tract, diverticulum formation usually occurs in the colon, particularly the sigmoid segment where 95% to 98% of all diverticula occur. Diverticular disease is usually acquired over time, but it also may be congenital, for example in the rare Meckel's diverticulum (Kazzi and Kazzi, 2002).

Diverticula are herniations of the mucosa, the submucosa, or of the entire thickness of the colon wall through the muscularis layer. They have been called "the bulges you never see" (Diverticulosis, 2002). Almost all diverticula are acquired and are considered "false diverticula" because they involve only the mucosal layer (Carter and Whelan, 2000). The precise etiology of the disorder is unknown, but it is proposed to be related to colonic motility issues (i.e., high pressures inside the bowel) and the anatomical structure of the blood supply to the colon.

Fiber, that component of dietary intake that the body cannot digest, helps stool to be soft and easy to pass and acts as a constipation deterrent. Intraluminal pressures increase when stools are not easy to pass. The increased pressure resulting from straining causes weak spots in the colon wall to bulge outward. The weak spots have been demonstrated to be where small arterial blood vessels, the vasa recta, penetrate the bowel wall. The weakness of the muscular bowel wall at these areas of vascular penetration allows herniation of the mucosa and submucosa, leading to diverticulum formation. Most often, diverticula form between a single mesenteric taenia and one of the antimesenteric taenia. Diverticula classically occur in two or four parallel rows (Kazzi and Kazzi, 2002; Rodkey and Welch, 1998; Stollman and Raskin, 1999; Stollman and Raskin, 2002). The number of diverticula may range from a single lesion to hundreds of lesions. Usually they are from 5 to 10 mm in diameter, but they can exceed 2 cm. One effect of the anatomic structure of diverticula is worth noting. Diverticula are surrounded by a rich arterial plexus; thus, bleeding that occurs from a diverticulum is usually arterial, and the amount may be significant.

Clinical Presentation/Differential Diagnosis/Diagnostic Studies

Differential diagnosis of diverticular disease is challenging, especially in its diverticulitis phase, since the disorder mimics other conditions including irritable bowel syndrome, IBD, ischemic colitis, and colonic neoplasms (Carter and Whelan, 2000). Initial workup of the patient includes a complete history and physical (especially rectal, pelvic, and abdominal assessments).

Characteristic signs and symptoms of diverticulitis include left lower quadrant pain, fever, nausea, vomiting, and sometimes a change in bowel patterns. Dysuria, rebound tenderness, and a palpable mass in the left lower quadrant may also be present. Laboratory evaluations include urinalysis, complete blood count, and liver function tests. Usually, leukocytosis is present, and urinalysis and liver enzymes are normal (Oliviera and Wexner, 1998).

Diagnostic tests can include plain abdominal x-rays or computed tomography (CT) scans. CT with oral contrast is the diagnostic modality of choice (Carter and Whelan, 2000). Patients with diverticulitis usually show colonic inflammatory changes, thickening of the bowel wall, paracolic fat streaking, and phlegmon (microperforation). Because CT scanning visualizes other abdominal organs, other diagnoses can be ruled out.

Contrast enemas have been used to document the presence of diverticula and muscle wall hypertrophy. However, the instillation of contrast material may result in the rupture of a diverticulum, so this approach is used with great caution in diverticulitis. Colonoscopy and flexible sigmoidoscopy are contraindicated in the presence of diverticulitis (Carter and Whelan, 2000). When diverticulitis is *not* present, the full spectrum of diagnostic modalities can be used including contrast enemas, fiberoptic endoscopy, and CT scanning.

Medical Treatment

The medical treatment of diverticular disease depends upon whether the patient is actively suffering from diverticulitis. In asymptomatic diverticulosis or in symptomatic but uncomplicated diverticular disease, treatment has two major emphases: increasing dietary fiber and medication therapy. Although the literature suggests that increasing dietary fiber will not ameliorate symptoms of diverticulosis immediately (Stollman and Raskin, 2002), a consensus exists that increased dietary fiber intake will eventually improve symptoms and bowel function in persons with uncomplicated disease. The linkage is so strong that some authors have called diverticulosis a "deficiency disease" that can be prevented by increasing fiber in the diet (Painter and Burkitt, 1971). The American Dietetic Association recommends a daily intake of 20 to 35 grams of fiber. A fiber product such as Citrucel or Metamucil (psyllium) may also be used once daily. These products provide 4 to 6 g of fiber per dose (Diverticulosis and Diverticulitis, 2002). Ideally, fiber intake should be increased over a period of 6 to 8 weeks. Increased fluid intake is also necessary; 2 to 3 L of water per day is recommended.

Medical treatment for diverticulitis focuses on three areas: clearing up the inflammation and infection, resting the colon, and preventing or minimizing complications. Many antibiotics have been used to treat infection, including amoxicillin plus clavulanic acid, sulfamethoxazole-trimethoprim with metronidazole, or a quinolone class drug with metronidazole. Symptoms should improve within 2 to 3 days if complications do not ensue. Antibiotic therapy should continue for 7 to 10 days.

Bowel rest approaches are determined by the intensity of the patient's condition. For outpatients, clear liquids with no or low fiber intake is recommended. For the more acutely ill person, hospitalization may be necessary. These patients should be kept on clear liquids or remain on nothing-by-mouth status, or NPO. Intravenous therapy may be necessary for hydration.

Medications used in the more acutely ill person are different, being more broad-spectrum (i.e., covering both aerobic and anaerobic bacteria). Common regimens include either an aminoglycoside and metronidazole or a second- or third-generation cephalosporin. Most patients (more than 70%) will improve with medical therapy (Carter and Whelan, 2000).

Surgical Treatment

Surgical treatment is recommended for both recurrent diverticulitis and for acute, first-time diverticulitis that does not respond to medical therapy. The chance of successful medical management of diverticulitis decreases with each recurrence. Most authorities agree that elective resection of the diseased portion of bowel should be proposed to affected persons after the second confirmed episode of diverticulitis (Carter and Whelan, 2000).

The course of diverticulitis becomes complicated and unresponsive to medical therapy with the occurrence of abscess, full perforation, fistula, or obstruction. Sometimes abscesses can be drained by CT-guided percutaneous drainage; if this approach is ineffective, colonic resection may be necessary.

Immediate surgery should be undertaken in patients whose condition fails to respond to percutaneous drainage, patients who have large, fecal-containing abscesses, or severely debilitated patients. Potential procedures include drainage of the abscess with proximal diversion and creation of a Hartmann's pouch; disease segment resection and abscess drainage with proximal diversion and creation of a Hartmann's pouch; or abscess drainage, resection of the diseased bowel, and

colorectal anastomosis with or without a temporary diversion.

Fistula formation is a complication of diverticulitis that almost always requires surgical intervention, since fistulas rarely close. Most fistulas are colovesical and result in persistent urinary tract symptoms (i.e., dysuria, fecaluria, urinary tract infection). Fistulas must be surgically removed for definitive treatment.

Chronic diverticulitis often results in a thickened and fibrotic colon wall with associated narrowing of the bowel lumen. Over time, the narrowing of the colon, especially the sigmoid, can result in complete or partial obstruction. Surgical resection of the narrowed segment usually relieves the problem (Alapati and Mihas, 1999).

Radiation Enteritis

Radiation enteritis is not a disease process per se but a response of the body to iatrogenic damage, or that which occurs during treatment for another disease or disorder. Radiation enteritis is malfunction of the large and small bowel that arises during or after radiation therapy to the abdomen, pelvis, or rectum. When attempting to destroy cancer deep in the body, radiation therapy may also damage the surrounding healthy tissue. Disorders that are commonly treated with radiotherapy are colon, ovarian, and prostate cancers.

Historical Perspectives

Radiation-induced damage to the large intestine was first described in 1987 (Colwell and Goldberg, 2000; Walsh, 1987). Since that time, the occurrence of radiation enteritis and associated proctitis has increased with the generation of super-voltage radiation machines using computerized delivery.

Treatment-related bowel injury has now become a well-recognized sequela of external beam radiation therapy, especially when it is combined with chemotherapy (Macheta et al, 2001). When the condition affects the small bowel or proximal colon, it is termed enterocolitis or enteritis. When the rectum is affected, it is called radiation proctitis. Radiation enteritis is particularly associated with treatment of pelvic area cancers, which are mostly carcinomas; most carcinomas respond well to radiotherapy.

Epidemiology/Risk Factors

Radiation enteritis occurs in both early-acute and late-chronic forms. As many as 5% of patients treated with a pelvic radiation dose of 4500 rads may develop acute transient damage (Karnam and Barkin, 2002).

The chronic form of radiation enteritis, with significant intestinal radiation damage and sequelae, will develop in approximately 1% to 25% of patients (Base-Smith, 2002; Karnam and Barkin, 2002). The most serious consequences can be fatal: intestinal failure with severe malabsorption or mechanical bowel obstructions from radiation strictures. Affected persons may require surgery or long-term parenteral nutrition (Scolapio et al, 2002).

Risk factors associated with small and large bowel damage may include previous abdominal surgery, diabetes, low-lying small intestine loops, thin body build, cardiovascular problems like hypertension or heart failure, concomitant chemotherapy, dose of radiation, tumor size and spread, use of radiation implants, pelvic inflammatory disease, or poor nutrition (Karnam and Barkin, 2002; Radiation Enteritis, 2002b). On the other hand, reports note that hypertension, diabetes, and heart failure are not risk factors (Noyer and Brandt, 2002).

Interestingly, radiation enteritis damage does not necessarily correlate with symptoms. Radiation enterocolitis can remain clinically silent and resolve completely a few weeks after the radiotherapy (Leupin et al, 2002).

Pathophysiology

The cytotoxic effect of radiotherapy is mainly on proliferating epithelial cells such as those comprising the small and large bowel. Necrosis of crypt cell walls can be observed in as little as 12 to 24 hours after a dose of 150 to 300 cGy (Radiation Enteritis, 2002a).

Radiation enteritis has an acute and a chronic form. Acute damage affects 5% to 50% of patients during radiotherapy. It occurs within the treatment period and resolves usually 4 to 6 weeks later. Microscopic analysis reveals mucosal cell loss, endothelial swelling of the arterioles, and crypt abscesses. The damage leads to diminished caloric function, impaired fluid absorption, and watery or mucoid discharge.

Chronic enteritis occurs in a smaller number of patients, usually several months to years later. A recent study suggests an occurrence rate of 17% to 18% (Miller et al, 1999). Endoscopy reveals friable mucosa, spontaneous oozing, pallor, and angiectasis (i.e., blood vessel dilation). Microscopic scrutiny reveals progressive vasculitis and ischemia of the bowel wall leading to bleeding and ulceration, stricture formation, obstruction, fibrosis, and fistula development to the bladder, vagina, or bowel. The fibrotic damage can become so severe that a so-called frozen pelvis can ensue (Colwell and Goldberg, 2000). The rectosigmoid is at particular risk of injury because it is fixed in the pelvis and therefore receives more radiation in pelvic radiotherapy (Noyer and Brandt, 2002).

The short- and long-term consequences of pelvic radiation therapy can be devastating. There may be a significant decrease in quality of life, or patients may suffer malabsorption and compromised nutrition. Radiation-induced diarrhea is an effect of the damage to the bowel lining that may resolve or continue to be problematic (Murphy, 2000).

It should be noted that external beam radiation is commonly used to treat prostate cancer. The radiotherapy may cause not only gastrointestinal symptoms such as nausea, vomiting, and diarrhea, but also urinary side effects: urinary frequency, impotence, urethral stricture, and urinary stress incontinence. The symptoms of enteritis, proctitis, and altered urinary function negatively affect the quality of life of prostate cancer patients treated with radiation (Colwell and Goldberg, 2000).

Clinical Presentation/Differential Diagnosis/Diagnostic Studies

The clinical manifestations of acute radiation-induced colitis or enteritis are well known and include nausea, vomiting, diarrhea, abdominal cramping, incomplete evacuation, and tenesmus. Symptoms of an inflamed rectum, including mucus-like discharge, rectal pain, and rectal bleeding, may result from radiation damage to the rectum (radiation proctitis). A comprehensive history and physical examination elicits the history of radiotherapy treatments. Differential diagnosis of radiation enteritis depends on a comprehensive history and physical and endoscopic-histologic review. Conditions such as infections, collagenous and ischemic colitis, IBD, and colitis associated with nonsteroidal antiinflammatory drugs (NSAIDs) must be ruled out. These conditions have different appearances in the bowel lumen and on the microscopic cell level (Leupin et al, 2002). Recurrent tumors must also be ruled out. Diagnostic criteria for radiation enteritis include endoscopic and histopathology changes such as intestinal mucosal inflammation or fibrosis, microvascular ischemia, friable mucosa, and prominent vascular pattern in the absence of recurrent malignancy (Miller et al, 1999).

Medical Treatment

The treatment of radiation-induced enteritis is challenging, because radiotherapy-associated pathophysiologic changes can generate an array of symptoms caused by malabsorption of bile salts, adhesive disease, and stricture formation. The major focus in the treatment of radiation-induced enteritis is the prevention and limitation of small bowel exposure. Surgical approaches to prevention are discussed in the next section. Medical approaches to prevention and treatment include use of elemental diets, replacement of lost fluids, and sucralfate and other pharmacotherapy. Two experimental agents, ribosecysteine and WR 2721, have been demonstrated to lower the incidence of bowel toxicity in both the small and large intestine (Karnam and Barkin, 2002). Decreasing the radiation dose by 10% may improve symptoms of acute enteritis without decreasing tumor destruction. In addition, nausea, vomiting, and diarrhea will usually respond to therapy with antiemetics and antidiarrheals (i.e., Kaopectate, Lomotil, Paregoric, Imodium, and Donnatal).

Bile-salt problems may be controlled with the use of cholestyramine (a bile-sequestering agent). On occasion, narcotics may be required to relieve pain, and steroid foams may be used to relieve rectal inflammation and irritation (Radiation

Enteritis, 2002c). Diarrhea may also be relieved by the use of a psyllium bulkage agent. Fatty acid enema treatments have decreased the symptoms of radiation proctitis. Laser and heat probes have been used to stop chronic rectal bleeding (Murphy, 2000; Noyer and Brandt, 2002).

Nutrition may also play a role in acute enteritis. Radiation-damaged intestines do not produce enzymes well, particularly lactase. A lactose-free, low-fat, and low-fiber diet may help control symptoms of enteritis (Radiation Enteritis, 2002b). Foods that should be avoided are milk and milk products, whole bran bread and cereal, nuts, seeds, fried and greasy foods, raw vegetables, rich pastries, strong spices and herbs, chocolate, coffee, tea, and alcohol. (Use of tobacco should also be avoided.) Foods that may help control enteritis include bananas, applesauce, white bread, macaroni and noodles, potatoes, cooked vegetables, eggs, and mild processed cheese (Radiation Enteritis, 2002b). Medical treatment of chronic radiation enteritis symptoms is approached in the same way as symptoms of acute radiation enteritis.

A new noninvasive approach to radiation enteritis is hyperbaric oxygen therapy. French researchers studied 36 patients with chronic radiation enteritis. Nineteen of the patients improved significantly in condition or were cured (Gouello et al, 1999).

Surgical Treatment

A surgical method by which radiation enteritis can be *prevented* is the creation of internal slings, using either synthetic or omental tissue, that act to keep the small bowel away from the radiated field (Karnam and Barkin, 2002; Kouraklis, 2002). This approach has proven to be largely successful.

Surgical treatment of extant radiation enteritis is usually associated with the manifestations of late changes. Complete or partial bowel obstructions, necrosis, strictures, or perforation can occur. Most often, severe radiation enteropathy requires a bowel resection rather than a diverting ostomy. However, complete bowel obstruction may necessitate a temporary stoma. Any operative repair is fraught with difficulties, since compromised blood supply, adhesive disease, and poor nutritional status make all surgical interventions risky in this patient population (Karnam and Barkin, 2002).

Parenteral nutrition (hyperalimentation) is an adjunct in the care of those who develop severe intestinal problems with radiation enteritis. Parenteral nutrition can be used before or after surgery to improve nutritional status. It has even been used effectively in home care for patients with radiation enteritis (Girvent et al, 2000; Scolapio et al, 2002).

The literature suggests strongly that, when necessary, complete resection of the diseased segment is preferred over intestinal bypass. Bypassed segments of bowel may develop bacterial overgrowth, fistula formation, and perforation (Karnam and Barkin, 2002). Surgery should only be considered and undertaken after thorough assessment of the patient's clinical condition and the full extent of radiation damage is revealed. When the diseased bowel is resected, a temporary stoma may be used (Noyer and Brandt, 2002).

Ischemic Colitis

Ischemic colitis is an unusual condition of the bowel that results from hypoperfusion. Although it may affect persons of all ages, the condition is usually seen in the elderly. Ischemic colitis is the most common ischemic injury of the gastrointestinal tract, and one of the most common disorders of the large intestine in older persons (Alapati and Mihas, 1999). The problem occurs when inadequate mesenteric blood flow causes an imbalance between metabolic demands of the colon and available oxygen, resulting in cellular injury. Although all segments of the bowel can be affected, ischemic colitis most often affects the left colon, especially the splenic flexure and sigmoid areas. Colon ischemia encompasses a wide clinical spectrum from mild, reversible disease to severe, irreversible damage.

Historical Perspectives

The spectrum of colon injury as a result of low blood flow was first definitively described by Boley and Marston in the 1960s (Arnott, Ghosh, and Ferguson, 1999; Greenwald and Brandt, 1998; MacDonald, 2002). They described it as a reversible

vascular occlusion and detailed the gangrenous, structural and transient forms; until that time the only clearly recognized form of colon ischemia had been bowel gangrene. The "classic" patient was identified as an older individual with concomitant cardiovascular disease, hypertension, diabetes mellitus, and chronic renal failure. More recently, young adult patients are being identified who have ischemic colitis related to use of oral contraceptives, vasopressin analogs, and use of oral decongestants containing pseudoephedrine (Ryan, Reamy, and Rochester, 2002; Shibata et al, 2002).

Epidemiology/Risk Factors

The true incidence of ischemic colitis remains elusive. Estimates suggest that ischemic colitis is the most common form of all gastrointestinal ischemic disease and generates roughly 1 in 2000 acute admissions to the hospital (Brandt and Boley, 1992). The exact amount of ischemic colitis is difficult to quantify, since many cases are never diagnosed or are misdiagnosed. Because of its relative rarity and the problem of misdiagnosis, no controlled clinical trials are available to help guide diagnosis and treatment (MacDonald, 2002).

Existing studies suggest there is no gender predilection for its occurrence, and more than 90% of affected persons are in their 70s or older. Many elderly persons have concomitant atherosclerosis that may contribute to the ischemia. Occasionally, specific etiologies for the ischemic episode become evident, but usually no clear cause for the ischemia is identified. Recent studies suggest there *is* a gender difference in younger patients. Preventza, Lazarides, and Sawyer (2001) found an almost 2:1 female to male ratio in their study of ischemic colitis in young adults.

Pathophysiology

Ischemic colitis is a consequence of a low perfusion state in the colon and is commonly classified as occlusive or nonocclusive disease. In occlusive disease, an actual obstruction in the mesenteric arterial blood supply is the culprit. In nonocclusive disease, the trigger is not intravascular obstruction but a low-flow or vasoconstrictive state. The end result of both forms is inadequate blood supply to the gut.

Causes of occlusive colon ischemia include thromboembolic phenomena, postaortic reparative surgery, trauma, vasculitis, radiation injury, hypercoagulable states, and pancreatitis. Nonocclusive ischemic colitis can result from various forms of shock, congestive heart failure, colonic obstruction, and from the use of some medications or other drugs (e.g., digitalis, catecholamines, estrogens, NSAIDs, sumatriptan, and crack cocaine) (Mason, 1999; Muniz and Evans, 2001; Sumatriptan and Ischemic Colitis, 2002). Much of the pharmacologic effect on the bowel is related to the agents' strong vasoconstrictive effect (Boghdadi and Henning, 1997).

Other, more unusual, causes have also been reported. Ischemic colitis has been associated with use of herbal products and severe dieting practices (Ryan, Reamy, and Rochester, 2002; Shibata et al, 2002). A recent research study suggests that young adult ischemic colitis sufferers experienced two or more etiologic contributing factors (e.g., hormone usage, cigarette smoking, hypertension), none of which would alone be sufficient to cause the disorder (Zauber and Sinha, 2002).

Although most colonic ischemia cases have no clearly identifiable cause, two contributing factors have frequently been identified: distal colon obstruction and aortic surgery. Colon obstruction, in the form of colon cancer, volvulus, fecal impaction, or postoperative stricture, acts to decrease blood flow to the affected segment. Aortic surgery also predisposes to decreased mesenteric blood supply in some people. Ischemic colitis is an outcome in up to 10% of elective aortic surgery patients and up to 60% in persons with a ruptured abdominal aortic aneurysm (Greenwald and Brandt, 1998).

The nature of the mesenteric blood supply structure may contribute to the problem. The superior mesenteric artery, the inferior mesenteric artery, and their branches supply blood to various segments of the colon. The splenic flexure, the descending colon, and the sigmoid colon are regions where the two circulations meet (the so-called "watershed area"), and ischemic damage is more common in these areas than in others

(Greenwald and Brandt, 1998). In addition to these anatomic features, the sensitivity of the colonic blood supply to autonomic stimulation, and the high intraabdominal pressure generated at times, render the colon extremely vulnerable to ischemia (Alapati and Mihas, 1999).

The tissue changes seen in the colon after ischemia depend on the duration and severity of the injury. Today ischemic colitis is categorized into six subsets, based on the degree and transience of the damage: (1) reversible ischemic colopathy (submucosal or intramural hemorrhage); (2) transient ischemic colitis; (3) chronic ulcerating ischemic colitis; (4) ischemic colonic stricture; (5) colonic gangrene; and (6) fulminant universal ischemic colitis (Noyer and Brandt, 2002). Because the lining of the bowel is the most metabolically active, it is most susceptible to damage. Mild changes like mucosal and submucosal hemorrhages or necrosis are mostly reversible. When more damage occurs, granulation tissue develops in the mucosa and submucosa layers. Abundant fibrous tissue deposits in the colon, and chronic ulcerations develop. Severely damaged mucosa may develop strictures (usually 3 to 4 weeks after the acute event). With the most severe form, transmural infarctions occur and lead to gangrene, perforation, and potential death. Rare complications include inflammatory polyposis, pyocolon (collection of pus within the colon), and toxic megacolon.

Ischemic tissue damage to the colon is not caused solely by hypoxia. Reperfusion injury occurs when the blood flow is subsequently restored (i.e., when increased amounts of oxygen cause free radicals and other toxic by-products to be released). In addition, ischemic colitis leads to the systemic release of inflammatory cytokines and other inflammatory response mediators (Toursarkissian and Thompson, 1997). All these substances serve to cause changes in bowel tissue, some of which may be permanent.

Clinical Presentation/Differential Diagnosis/Diagnostic Studies

Ischemic colitis in older patients usually has an insidious onset with left-sided abdominal pain, distention, urgency to defecate, and diarrhea. Nausea and vomiting may also occur. These symptoms progress steadily and are eventually joined by lower gastrointestinal hemorrhage (loose stool with dark clots or bright red blood). The most severe form of ischemic colitis is characterized by transmural gangrenous necrosis lending rapidly to peritonitis with peritoneal signs.

In contrast, younger patients with ischemic colitis often are first seen with symptoms that develop in a relatively acute manner. They demonstrate more rectal bleeding, report more acute constipation prior to onset, and usually have a more self-limiting, transient course (Toursarkissian and Thompson, 1997).

Differential diagnosis of ischemic colitis depends upon comprehensive history and physical assessment, endoscopy, abdominal plain films, and pathologic tissue examination. No specific symptom or pathognomonic sign exists for the disease. No specific chemical or enzymatic markers occur in intestinal ischemia. Differential diagnosis must rule out other conditions such as IBD, infectious colitis, pseudomembranous colitis, diverticulitis, pancreatitis, appendicitis, toxic megacolon, and colon obstruction. Definitive diagnosis of ischemic colitis is usually obtained by endoscopy. The colon mucosa is usually pale, with petechial hemorrhage in the mild form of the condition. More severe disease is marked by progressively darker tissue (e.g., blue to black) and increasing ulceration. However, barium enema and colonoscopy are contraindicated when the patient's condition is severe and there is the risk of perforation (Marti et al, 2001; Noyer and Brandt, 2002).

Biopsy of the colonic tissue is very helpful with differential diagnosis. Ischemic colitis is characterized by crypt destruction, epithelial cell sloughing, edema, capillary thrombosis, and the presence of fewer inflammatory cells than normal.

Angiography of the mesenteric vessels is rarely helpful, because major visceral vessels are usually patent. Ultrasonography may be used to facilitate ruling out of other disorders, although it is rarely diagnostic of ischemic colitis. CT scanning is only partially helpful, since it may remain normal even in the presence of actual ischemic colitis. Barium enemas (BE) are rarely used in the acute phase because of their poor diagnostic capability and the danger of perforation and other problems. However, BE can be done in the subacute or chronic phases; "thumbprinting" due to submucosal edema and hemorrhage is the classic radiologic finding associated with ischemic colitis (Noyer and Brandt, 2002).

Medical Treatment

The medical management of ischemic colitis patients is guided by the intensity and duration of hypoxia at the colon wall (Marti et al, 2001). In general the literature suggests that symptoms in up to two thirds of patients with ischemic colitis will resolve with conservative medical therapy (MacDonald, 2002). Patients without peritoneal signs are managed nonsurgically by stopping oral intake, instituting vigorous intravenous hydration, administering broad-spectrum antibiotics, monitoring vital signs intensively, and stopping the administration of medications or agents known to be associated with the condition (e.g., decongestants, oral estrogens, and crack cocaine). Vasodilators like glucagon and papaverine hydrochloride have been tried but with dubious success (Alapati and Mihas, 1999). In mild ischemia, symptoms usually respond to the treatment regimen within 1 week. Repeat endoscopy is performed to assess for sequelae like permanent tissue damage.

Early diagnosis of ischemic colitis is often tentative. Investigations into other possible causes of the abdominal pain should continue until diagnosis is confirmed. Stool should be cultured for pathogens and assayed for *Clostridium difficile* toxin.

Surgical Treatment

If patients demonstrate signs suggestive of peritonitis (e.g., fever, marked leukocytosis, and tense, painful abdomen), or if x-rays show pneumoperitoneum, they usually require surgical intervention. Bowel perforation is the most common indication for surgery (Preventza, Lazarides, and Sawyer, 2001). The ischemic section of the colon is resected, including areas of dubious viability. An ileostomy or colostomy is performed; primary anastomosis is *not* recommended in the acute phase, especially with colonic ischemia on the left side. The distal segment can be matured as a mucous fistula or simply oversewn and left in the abdomen as a Hartmann's pouch. The reason for diversion is the high risk of suture dehiscence and anastomosis failure.

What determines who will progress to requiring surgical therapy? The literature suggests that coexisting diabetes, profound hypotension, initial hemodynamic instability, and prolonged ileus are predictors of the more serious forms of ischemic colitis that require bowel resection (MacDonald, 2002).

Surgery may also become necessary in patients with chronic (segmental) colitis or formation of severe strictures after injury. Primary anastomosis is not considered unless colonic tissues are verifiably viable (Alapati and Mihas, 1999).

Infectious Enteritis

Infectious enteritis is a GI tract disorder that can be caused by many enteric pathogens. Infectious enteritis is sometimes also called gastroenteritis. Enteric infections are a relatively rare cause of GI diversions. More commonly, people with stomas may develop an infection of the bowel and experience the symptoms associated with the disorder. If diarrhea is severe, fluid loss can cause significant dehydration, especially in persons with a small bowel stoma.

Almost all infectious enteritis disorders are transmitted by the fecal-oral route or from contaminated food or water. Some forms can be sexually transmitted. The nature of the setting also affects the type of microorganism responsible for the GI infection. For example, children in a day care center are more likely to have food-related disorders (Marsh, 2000). Elderly persons in intensive care units who have received extensive antibiotic therapy are more likely to develop *C. difficile* infection.

Historical Perspectives

Infections of the GI tract have been described for centuries, although their causes may not always have been known. Today, acute infectious diarrhea disease is a major, worldwide health problem and results in enormous morbidity and mortality. In the United States, acute diarrhea is also a common cause of morbidity, though rarely a life-threatening event.

Past decades have brought increased hospitalizations for infectious enteritis. From 1985 to 1994, a 2½-fold increase in hospitalization rates for viral enteritis occurred, at the same time a fourfold increase in hospitalization rates for bacterial enteritis emerged (Frost, Craun, and Calderon, 1998).

Although antibiotics have been causing diarrhea for decades, pseudomembranous colitis was first described in 1893, and the role of *C. difficile* as an agent of diarrhea was only elucidated in the approximate period of 1978 to 1980. It is now recognized as a major nosocomial infection (Boriello, 1995).

Epidemiology/Risk Factors

There are almost 100 million cases of acute infectious enteritis (gastroenteritis) annually in the United States. Environmental factors play a part in the incidence of infectious enteritis. Contaminated water and food and poor personal hygiene can contribute to the spread of enteric pathogens. At high risk for infectious enteritis are groups like children in day care centers, travelers to tropical and subtopical regions, homosexual men, those living in unsanitary conditions, and debilitated or immunosuppressed persons.

Most acute diarrhea episodes in the United States are self-limited viral infections. Disease due to fungi, protozoa, and helminthes (parasitic worms) are present, but are much more likely in patients from the developing world. Enteric pathogens are estimated to cause 25 to 99 million episodes of diarrhea each year in the United States, generating over 2 million physician visits (Frost, Craun, and Calderon, 1998).

C. difficile–associated disease (CDAD) remains a leading cause of nosocomial illness. It is the most common bacterial cause that is identifiable of nosocomial diarrhea (Boriello, 1995). The prevalence of CDAD ranges from 0.15% to 10% for hospitalized patients during nonoutbreak times and from 16% to 29% during hospital outbreaks (McFarland et al, 1999). Interestingly, epidemiologic data show that *C. difficile* occurs both in the community and in hospitals, but *C. difficile* spores appear in much greater concentrations in hospitals, with a predilection for the acute care setting (Silva, 2001).

Risk factors for infectious enteritis include a history of recent travel (within 6 months), contact with individuals who are ill (e.g., day care centers or schools), recent antibiotic usage, and dietary ingestion during foodborne outbreaks (Infectious Enteritis, 2002). For *C. difficile* infection, risk factors include older age, prolonged hospital stay, antibiotic administration, admission to the intensive care exist, tube feedings, endoscopy, exposure to antineoplastic medications, and malignancy (Yip et al, 2001).

The epidemiologic implications associated with these at-risk groups are significant. Increasing rates of worldwide travel and high-risk health behaviors and more elderly, debilitated populations suggest that acute infectious enteritis cases are likely to increase for the foreseeable future.

Pathophysiology

Because the GI tract is continuously exposed to the dangers of the environment, the tract has several mechanisms by which it defends itself. These include mechanical barriers, chemical defenses, colonization resistance, and acquired immunity. The gut mucosa, the first line of defense, is also supported by chemical changes. Gastric acidity reduces the burden of coliform organisms that are ingested by 99%. Fibronectins, a type of protein, prevent colonization of the oropharynx by pathogens. Normal flora of the bowel promotes gut health. Finally, GI-associated lymphoid tissue is present in the lamina propria, intraepithelial lymphocytes, and Peyer's patches of the bowel, and fights organisms by phagocytosis (Baden and Maguire, 2001).

Many pathogens are associated with infectious enteritis. They infect by overcoming the natural defenses of the gut. Bacterial causes include *Shigella, Salmonella, Yersinia, Campylobacter, Escherichia coli,* and *C. difficile.* Viral causes include cytomegalovirus, herpes simplex virus, Norwalk virus, rotavirus, and astrovirus. Fungal causes include *Histoplasma capsulatum* and *Blastomyces.*

Parasitic causes include *Entamoeba histolytica* (Taylor and DiPalma, 1998).

The pathophysiologic effects of the pathogenic microorganism differ with the infecting agent, though signs and symptoms exhibited by patients may be similar. Bacterial agents cause vomiting and diarrhea by three general mechanisms: (1) production of toxins; (2) direct invasion of the bowel with resultant inflammation; and (3) a combination of toxin production and invasion. *C. difficile,* an anaerobic organism, has been likened to a "protein factory." Under favorable circumstances (when antibiotic therapy alters the natural balance of colonic flora), *C. difficile* produces an array of proteinases that markedly affect mucosal cells and physiologic systems of the bowel. Toxins A and B, for example, bind to mucosal cells; they induce fluid secretion and disrupt cell integrity, leading to cell death. Focal lesions occur in the colon and there is an inflammatory response accompanied by possible pseudomembrane development and extensive fluid losses.

All antibiotics can induce *C. difficile* infection, which is alternatively called antimicrobial agent–associated colitis. Common agents include ampicillin, amoxicillin, cephalosporin, and clindamycin (Pothoulakis, 2002; Silva, 2001).

Clinical Presentation/Differential Diagnosis/Diagnostic Studies

A number of disorders have features similar to enteritis or colitis and must be considered in the differential diagnosis. These include chronic lymphocytic leukemia, vasculitis or connective tissue disease, lymphoma, hemolytic-uremia syndrome, and immune deficiency syndromes (e.g., acquired immunodeficiency syndrome, or AIDS) (Taylor and DiPalma, 1998).

The clinical presentation of infectious enteritis may be similar despite differing causative agents. Depending on severity, signs and symptoms may include profuse, watery diarrhea accompanied by dehydration, increase in liquid consistency and number of stools in 24 hours, fever, abdominal discomfort, and possibly dysentery (multiple small-volume stools containing blood and mucus). *C. difficile* infection usually presents with watery diarrhea containing excessive mucus but not blood. Sometimes stool odor becomes more foul (Chutkan and Balba, 2002; Pothoulakis, 2002).

The identification of infectious enteritis should be gleaned from history, presenting symptoms, and associated epidemiologic factors. More definitive diagnosis is associated with analyzing a sample of feces. Stool should be tested for occult blood, checked for ova and parasites, and cultured for organisms. A fecal smear should be examined for white blood cells. Some infecting agents are best observed under the microscope after they have been stained. Viral agents may not be identifiable by commercial tests, since some pathogens have no diagnostic tests available. It is crucial to note that at least three stool samples should be sent for testing because some agents (e.g., *Giardia*) are shed intermittently (Marsh, 2000).

Endoscopy offers added diagnostic strengths. Endoscopic evaluation allows direct visualization of the bowel lumen as well as histopathologic eval-uation. Culture of biopsies, as well as tissue scrutiny, can help differentiate infection from IBD. In the case of *C. difficile* infection, pseudomembranes can be visualized and this information added to that needed for correct differential diagnosis.

Medical Treatment

Diarrhea of 2 to 3 days' duration is seldom worked up unless fever, bloody diarrhea, and/or severe abdominal pain are present. If these signs or complications are present, it is hoped that diagnostic testing will establish the definitive cause.

Whatever the underlying problem, the primary therapy for all patients with infectious colitis is oral hydration (i.e., replacement of both fluids and electrolytes). Viral infections eventually resolve spontaneously. Other infections may require antibiotic therapy. A common approach is to treat with a quinolone antibiotic such as ciprofloxacin (Cipro). Other infectious agents are commonly treated by various antibiotics (Table 8-1).

TABLE 8-1   Antibiotic Therapy for Common Infectious Enteritis Pathogens

ORGANISM	PHARMACOTHERAPY
Amebiasis	Metronidazole (Flagyl) 500 mg PO
	Dehydroemetine 1-1.5 mg/kg/d IM
	Both agents plus a luminal amebicide (iodoquinol [Yodoxin]), 650 mg PO; paromomycin, 500 mg PO for invasive intestinal infection and hepatic abscesses: cyst passers without symptoms require luminicidal agent only
Campylobacter jejuni colitis	Ciprofloxacin (Cipro) 500 mg PO (norfloxacin, 400 mg; ofloxacin, 400 mg; ciprofloxacin, 500 mg, all PO)
	Erythromycin 500 mg, or azithromycin 500 mg daily
	Vibramycin 100 mg bid
Cryptosporidium	Paromomycin (Humatin), 500 mg PO
	Azithromycin
	Hyperimmune bovine colostrum
	Nitazoxanide
	Benefit and duration of any therapy unclear; spontaneous resolution without specific therapy in immunocompetent hosts and in HIV-infected individuals with CD4 counts >150 cells/mm^3
Cyclospora	TMP-SMX double strength TMP-SMX 1 DS PO

Continued

TABLE 8-1   Antibiotic Therapy for Common Infectious Enteritis Pathogens—cont'd

Enterotoxic *Escherichia coli* diarrhea	Oral ciprofloxacin (Cipro) 500 mg
	TMP-SMX
	Doxycycline 100 mg bid
	Furazolidone
Giardiasis	Metronidazole (Flagyl) 250 mg PO
	Tinidazole
	Quinacrine hydrochloride
	Furazolidone (Furoxone)
	Relapses may occur
Isospora	TMP-SMX 1 DS PO
	Pyrimethamine + folinic acid
	Maintenance therapy required in patients with AIDS
Microsporidium	Albendazole 200-400 mg PO
	Albendazole more effective for *Encephalitozoon intestinalis* than for *Enterocytozoon bieneusi*; available for compassionate use only
Salmonella gastroenteritis	Rx usually not required
	Oral ciprofloxacin (Cipro) 500 mg (norfloxacin, 400 mg; ofloxacin, 400 mg; ciprofloxacin, 500 mg PO)
Shigellosis	Ciprofloxacin (Cipro) 500 mg PO (norfloxacin, 400 mg; ofloxacin, 400 mg)
	Septra-DS bid (recent resistant strains noted)
	Amoxicillin 500 mg (recent resistant strains noted)
Vibrio cholerae	Doxycycline 100 mg
	TMP-SMX or
	Ampicillin
Yersinia-induced diarrhea	Oral ciprofloxacin (Cipro) 500 mg (norfloxacin, 400 mg; ofloxacin, 400 mg; ciprofloxacin, 500 mg PO)
	TMP-SMX or doxycycline
	Antibiotic therapy only in severe (systemic) cases

Compiled from Baden LR, Maguire JH: Gastrointestinal infections in the immunocompromised host, *Infect Dis Clin North Am* 15(2):639-670, 2001; Chutkan RK, Balba NH: Infectious disease of the colon. In DiMarino AJ, Benjamin SB, editors: *Gastrointestinal disease: an endoscopic approach*, Thorofare, NJ, 2002, Slack; Infectious enteritis: website: www.members.tripod.com, accessed 9/13/02; and Marsh WW: Infectious diseases of the gastrointestinal tract, *Adolescent Med* 11(2):263-278, 2000.
TMP-SMX, Trimethoprin-sulfamethoxazole.

C. difficile most often responds well to special antibiotic therapy accompanied by ceased administration of the triggering antibiotic. Oral metronidazole (Flagyl) in dosages of 250 mg qid to 500 mg tid or oral vancomycin in dosages of 125 to 500 mg qid for 10 to 14 days is recommended. However, some patients will have recurrence and require additional therapy. Recurrence is associated with older age and sicker overall status (Baden and Maguire, 2001; Infectious enteritis, 2002; McFarland et al, 1999).

A special note should be made about infectious enteritis treatment. Antidiarrhea agents should *not* be used in infectious enteritis because the organisms become retained in the bowel and cause more reaction. Antidiarrheals should be withheld until infectious enteritis has been definitively ruled out (Silva, 2001).

An important subgroup of patients with infectious enteritis will develop a long-term complication: postinfectious irritable bowel syndrome (IBS). Although most infectious enteritis patients recover fully, research suggests that persons with enteritis infections run a nearly 12% risk of new-onset IBS (Spiller, 2002). Most of these postinfectious IBS patients will eventually recover normal bowel function but may need transient IBS therapy (low-lactose diet, and administration of loperamide and codeine to control diarrhea).

Surgical Treatment

Surgical intervention for treatment of infectious enteritis is rarely necessary. In the case of *C. difficile* infection, more severe complications like fulminant colitis can occur. This condition is associated with severe abdominal pain, diarrhea, high fever, chills, and tachycardia. If the patient's condition does not improve with therapy, surgical intervention (i.e., bowel resection, colectomy) may be necessary (Pothoulakis, 2002).

Other serious complications can occur from infectious enteritis, especially depending on the pathogen. For example, *Shigella* and *E. coli* can cause bowel perforation necessitating emergency surgery with a diverting stoma (Marsh, 2000).

Patient condition is another issue to consider. When surgery is needed, it is more often seen in immunocompromised hosts. When the severe complications occur that necessitate surgery (e.g., intestinal perforation), the presentation of signs and symptoms in other organ systems may be more subtle because of an impaired immune response (Baden and Maguire, 2001; Lopez and Sanders, 2001).

Intestinal Obstruction

Intestinal obstruction is a disorder that is associated with significant morbidity and possible death. Defined as a partial or complete obstruction of the large or small intestine that impedes the natural progression of digestion and assimilation (Shelton, 1999), intestinal obstruction can be classified according to various aspects of the process.

Bowel obstruction is most commonly classified as mechanical (i.e., dynamic) or nonmechanical (i.e., paralytic or adynamic). In the former, some physical mass is fully or partially blocking the bowel lumen. Nonmechanical obstruction is due to some form of ileus. Common causes of adynamic obstruction are accidental or surgical trauma (e.g., laparotomy), electrolyte imbalances (e.g., hypokalemia), and infectious or inflammatory processes (e.g., appendicitis, pneumonia, pelvic inflammatory disease). Causes of dynamic obstruction include adhesions, hernia, neoplasms, colonic polyps, intussusception, congenital anomalies, strictures, volvulus, and idiopathic pseudoobstruction (Ogilvie's syndrome) (Arnott, Ghosh, and Ferguson, 1999; Intestinal Obstruction, 2002).

Historical Perspectives

Bowel obstructions have been recognized since antiquity, although patients in early days did not usually survive obstruction. Volvulus of the colon was described in the Egyptian Papyrus Ebers and in the writings of ancient Greek and Roman physicians. Hippocrates, the father of medicine, described using anal air insufflation to untwist sigmoid volvulus (Chiao and Rex, 2002). In more recent times, physicians have been able to intervene and have learned techniques that promote better healing and long-term GI function.

One of the first recorded "ostomy" patients in 1784 was Margaret White of England, who had an umbilical hernia that perforated the abdominal wall. Her surgeon, William Chiselden, performed a colostomy by removing the dead bowel and leaving Margaret with a transverse colostomy (Black, 2000).

Epidemiology/Risk Factors

Obstruction of the bowel is a common cause of acute abdominal pain, which is the presenting symptom accounting for one fifth of all emergency admissions to surgical services (Shelton, 1999). Mortality differs but logically it is higher in compromised hosts. For example, the rate ranges from 7% to 14% in elderly patients (Shelton, 1999).

The epidemiology of selected mechanical obstructions is well delineated. In Western nations, intestinal volvulus (abnormal rotation or twisting of the bowel around its mesentery) is an uncommon cause of obstruction (1% to 3% of all bowel obstructions). In Africa, the Middle East, India, and areas of Russia, volvulus of the colon is one of the most common causes of intestinal obstruction (up to 54%) (Chiao and Rex, 2002). When volvulus occurs in persons in the United States, it most commonly occurs in the sigmoid colon. A major association appears to be chronic constipation.

Risk factors for bowel obstruction are clearly age related. Certain disorders are more common in neonates, children, or adults. In children and neonates, hernias and Hirschsprung's disease are the more common causes. Tumors and diverticulitis are more commonly implicated in the elderly. Across all age groups, abdominal adhesions are the greatest risk factor, accounting for up to 60% of all obstruction cases. Most often, adhesions occur after abdominal surgery. Other risk factors for intestinal obstruction include Crohn's disease, abdominal trauma, ulcerative colitis, Meckel's diverticulum, endometriosis, tumors of the small or large bowel, infectious disorders like cytomegalovirus or tuberculosis of the intestine, bowel ischemia, multiple sclerosis, or myasthenia gravis (Shelton, 1999).

Cancer of the colon is discussed more fully elsewhere in this book (Chapter 6). However, it should be noted that malignant bowel obstruction is a frequent clinical complication in patients with advanced abdominal or pelvic cancers and metastases to the peritoneal cavity. Incidence of bowel obstruction ranges up to 42% in ovarian cancer and 28% in colorectal cancer (Platt, 2001; Rawlinson, 2001).

Pathophysiology

The pathophysiology of bowel obstruction derives from three processes: neurologic or vascular incompetence of the GI tract or alterations in the intestinal wall. Impaired nerve and/or blood supply usually acts to decrease peristalsis. Bowel wall alterations such as inflammation, compression, or strangulation decrease the bowel lumen size, slowing the passage of bowel contents.

The damage that occurs depends on several factors: whether the obstruction is complete or partial, whether a large amount of functional bowel is lost, and the pressure in the bowel lumen. Sufferers of narrow lumens can develop malabsorption syndromes, and complete obstructions can generate life-threatening situations. Whatever their cause, bowel obstructions bring about retained intestinal contents, buildup of gas and fluids, and electrolyte imbalances. Fluid and electrolyte changes occur because they leak out of the bowel into the peritoneum. Common findings include hypokalemia, hypocalcemia, and hypomagnesemia.

Clinical Presentation/Differential Diagnosis/Diagnostic Studies

Bowel obstruction signs and symptoms are related to the underlying pathophysiologic events. Primary effects include altered bowel sounds, distention, and abdominal discomfort. Stool output will likely decrease, and the gastric drainage possibly change. Other effects may include vomiting, malnutrition, fever, and hypotension. Onset can be quick or insidious. Pain associated with intestinal obstruction depends on the location and the completeness of obstruction. Incomplete obstruction is associated with an alternation of pain that occurs after eating and periods with no pain. Full obstruction, especially of the small intestine, is associated with more frequent, and more severe, pain (Chiao and Rex, 2002).

Several diagnostic tests can be used to identify intestinal obstruction, including laboratory and radiologic studies. The CT scan is the most useful test in differentiating specific causes and location of mechanical obstructions. Magnetic resonance imaging has also been used with success. Ultrasound testing has proven to be somewhat effective. Peristaltic markers that are radiopaque have been used to determine intestinal transit time and the site of obstruction. Laboratory tests normally include complete blood count (CBC), electrolyte levels, and liver and pancreatic function tests. Laparoscopy offers the greatest sensitivity in identifying the pathologic condition, since obstructed areas can be directly visualized (Chiao and Rex, 2002).

Medical Treatment

Medical management focuses primarily on identifying potential risk factors. Determining whether obstruction is complete or partial is important in the development of a treatment plan. Conservative medical therapy includes intestinal rest with tube decompression. Nasogastric or nasointestinal tubes drain fluids and gas, thus decreasing pressure in the gut. The tube may pass through a partial obstruction and keep it partially open. A rectal tube may be used to reduce large bowel dilation.

For terminal patients, the approach may be altered. Intravenous fluids, pain relief, and drugs altering GI motility are administered. When the obstruction is complete, the highest goal of care is maintenance of fluid and electrolyte balance. Extravasation of fluid may result in hypovolemia and electrolyte abnormalities. Ringer's lactate or saline is usually used to balance values that are out of normal range.

Another medical technique that has been used to relieve obstruction is endoscopic therapy. Air enema (air inserted through a scope) has been used to reduce intussusception.

In cases of intestinal pseudoobstruction (Ogilvie's syndrome), the problem is caused by problems in the muscle and nerves of the intestine. Since no physical blockage occurs, the main treatment is nutritional support (intravenous feeding) and the use of antibiotics to treat infections. Medications like opiates and antidepressants are discontinued because they can affect intestinal motility (Chiao and Rex, 2002; Intestinal Pseudo-Obstruction, 2002).

Surgical Treatment

Surgical treatment of bowel obstruction is usually reserved for two situations: when the risk of perforation is strong, or when bowel rupture has occurred. Common criteria according to which surgery is indicated include tachycardia, fever, leukocytosis, increasing pain, and no improvement following tube decompression (Shelton, 1999).

A newer set of approaches has improved care in recent years. Laparoscopic approaches have allowed lysis of adhesions without a large incision. Instead of performance of a colostomy, intestinal stents have been placed successfully, especially in situations calling for palliative care.

If possible a bowel resection is performed to relieve the obstruction. If extensive bowel damage or ischemia is present, a temporary or permanent colostomy may be necessary.

Gastrointestinal Trauma

Trauma to the GI tract generally occurs in two forms: blunt or penetrating. Blunt trauma is the most common mechanism of injury to the bowel. In many cases of blunt abdominal trauma, internal damage may occur, but the patient may be successfully managed conservatively by bowel rest and the monitoring of vital signs and laboratory studies of fluid and electrolyte levels. Penetrating GI trauma almost always requires some surgical intervention, whether on an emergency basis or delayed.

In contemporary society the rate of trauma-related injuries is increasing as a result of mechanization of the workplace, use of motor vehicles, falls, fire, and, most recently, terrorist acts. The rising incidence and severity of injuries has led to the proportional expansion of the knowledge base and progress toward multidisciplinary treatment of all trauma, including GI trauma. A medical subspecialty, traumatology, has arisen as a consequence of the rapid growth of knowledge and need for treatment (Base-Smith, 2002).

Historical Perspectives

Trauma to the GI tract has been recorded for centuries, especially in descriptions of combat. From ancient references in the Bible to abdominal penetrating trauma (in the Book of Judges) to descriptions of the fatal wounding of the Byzantine Emperor Julian "the Apostate" by bowel trauma, to more modern descriptions by Heister in the eighteenth century on perfecting enterostomies in battlefield victims (Black, 2000; Uppot, Wills, and Gheyi, 2002), ostomies and intestinal trauma as consequences of injury have been targeted. However, the greatest increases in surgical techniques and patient survival after trauma did not occur until the late nineteenth and twentieth centuries.

The contemporary surgical management of penetrating colon injuries grew out of World War II experiences. For years, diverting colostomy for all penetrating colon injuries was the standard of care. More recent literature and research suggests that the vast majority of penetrating colon injuries do *not* require diversion but can be managed with primary repair (Gonzalez et al, 2000). Because of better diagnostics, antibiotics, and management techniques, from World War II to the Vietnam War, mortality from penetrating abdominal gunshot wounds decreased from 42% to 9% (Uppot, Wills, and Gheyi, 2002).

Epidemiology/Risk Factors

Trauma kills more people from 1 to 44 years of age in the United States than does disease. At least 100,000 deaths per year can be attributed to trauma (Base-Smith, 2002). Trauma has its greatest impact on children and young adults because of its age-related bias. Motor vehicle accidents, falls, and firearm-related injuries are the most common causes of trauma (Intestinal Trauma, 2002). The abdomen is the third most commonly injured body region. Abdominal injuries account for 10% of trauma deaths. In general, more males experience traumatic injuries than females (Uppot, Wills, and Gheyi, 2002). Sadly, in 2001 homicide was the thirteenth cause of death in the United States (Centers for Disease Control and Prevention, 2001).

Pathophysiology

The pathophysiologic consequences of GI trauma are related to the nature and the severity of the injury. Blunt trauma is, as mentioned, the most common mechanism of injury to the bowel. Of those with blunt abdominal trauma, 5% will have intestinal and/or mesenteric injury. Blunt trauma can result from falls, assaults, or vehicular accidents. Penetrating trauma to the bowel is typically secondary to knife or gunshot wounds.

Blunt bowel injury occurs from two mechanisms: compression forces and deceleration forces. By increasing intraluminal pressure in the bowel and/or compressing it against solid organs, compression forces can overstretch the bowel or create a full-thickness perforation by way of a "burst" injury. Deceleration forces tear the bowel loops at points of fixation like the ileocecal valve or the ligament of Treitz. The consequences can include a torn bowel wall, shearing of the mesentery, and loss of blood supply to colonic segments (Dauterive, Flancbaum, and Cox, 1985; Kushimoto et al, 2001).

Penetrating trauma can range from a mild abrasion of the serosa to severe mesenteric, vascular, and bowel wall injury (Uppot, Wills, and Gheyi, 2002).

Each anatomic region of the GI tract is associated with characteristic patterns of injury. The most common site of gastric rupture following blunt trauma (often after a full meal) is the anterior wall, followed by the greater curvature. Duodenal injuries are usually due to penetrating trauma. Common injuries include duodenal wall hematoma or duodenal wall rupture. Colonic injury can occur from both penetrating and blunt trauma. Frequently damaged areas include the transverse and sigmoid colon or the cecum (Uppot, Wills, and Gheyi, 2002).

The consequences of penetrating GI trauma are related to the nature of the injuring agent and the resultant internal damage. Stab wounds penetrating the abdominal wall are usually more predictable. Gunshot damage is related to its degree of energy transfer (high velocity compared to low velocity) and the secondary missile effect of bone fragments or bullet fragments. Shotguns and hunting rifles, especially at close range, usually result in massive tissue damage (Komar and Patel, 2002).

Other factors affecting patient response are patient age, the degree of injury, the necessity for transfusion, and fluid requirements. Older age, greater severity of trauma, and greater administration of blood and intravenous fluids is closely correlated with mortality (Tornetta et al, 1999).

One of the "nicer" aspects of penetrating or blunt abdominal injuries to the GI tract is that the GI organs are redundant; large segments of the tract and its accessory organs can be removed, and yet good quality of life can still occur (Orenstein, 2002).

Clinical Presentation/Differential Diagnosis/Diagnostic Studies

Clinical presentation of GI trauma is clearly related to the nature and agent of the traumatic event and the resultant tissue injury. Patients may have very mild symptoms or be profoundly ill. Prompt assessment of the situation is vital.

Diagnosis of the degree of trauma depends heavily on a good history (including trauma event history), physical examination, and diagnostic testing. Abdominal trauma patients will likely receive the following studies if they are hemodynamically stable: CT scan of the abdomen, ultrasound, chest x-ray, and laboratory studies such as complete blood count and chemistries, prothrombin time, partial thromboplastin time, arterial blood gases, urinalysis, and dip stick. Typing and cross-matching for blood transfusion is usually performed. Usually patients will have nasogastric intubation and urinary bladder catheterization. They may also have diagnostic peritoneal lavage (Komar and Patel, 2002).

Patients with massive tissue trauma may require a newer approach to trauma care called "damage control" (Johnson et al, 2001; Porter, Ivatury, and Nassoura, 1997). This approach involves rapid, temporary measures to control bleeding and bowel contamination, followed by rapid closure of the abdomen. The second step includes correction of acidosis, hypothermia, and coagulopathy in the intensive care unit. The third step is planned reoperation for definitive repair of injuries.

Medical Treatment

Medical treatment of GI trauma involves watchful waiting and is more likely to be used in blunt trauma. Multiple diagnostic studies are conducted to evaluate for severe organ damage or perforation of the intestines. CT scan with contrast has proven enormously helpful in evaluating the integrity of traumatized organs (Kushimoto et al, 2001; Uppot, Wills, and Gheyi, 2002).

Surgical Treatment

In the traumatized patient, surgery is no longer a given unless the evidence from diagnostic testing is unequivocal that organ damage has occurred, or if the patient is exsanguinating. Particularly for blunt abdominal trauma the research suggests that delayed laparotomy (greater than 4-hour wait time) is being used appropriately; that is, when GI tract damage has truly occurred or if medical management has failed (Sorensen, Mikhail, and Karmy-Jones, 2002).

Surgical approaches to treatment of GI trauma have changed significantly in the last two decades. From the Second World War through the 1970s, GI trauma with bowel damage and perforation was treated with repair and diversion of the fecal stream. More recent research suggests that colostomy is not always necessary except in rectal trauma. In fact, in penetrating colon trauma including injuries to the left colon, the preferred method of treatment is primary repair, including resection, without colostomy (Demetriades et al, 2001; Eshragi et al, 1998; Murray et al, 1999).

Even in the situation of open pelvic fractures, colostomy may not be necessary for all patients (Pell, Flynn, and Seibel, 1998). Multiple investigations support the theory that fecal diversion does not protect high-risk trauma patients from infection (Dente et al, 2000; Gonzalez and Turk, 2002; Woods et al, 1998). In addition, primary repair of GI trauma (e.g., anastomoses) should be done by handsewing rather than stapling, since the latter is associated with more anastomotic leaks and intraabdominal abscesses (Brundage et al, 2001).

When fecal diversion is used in the GI trauma patient, the most common technique is a loop colostomy. A Hartmann's procedure (i.e., resection, with oversewing of distal end and an end stoma) may be used in the hemodynamically unstable patient who requires diversion.

Although primary repair of colon injuries is now more commonly accepted than fecal diversion, the management of severe rectal injuries is unchanged. Diversion of the fecal stream and drainage of the presacral space to avoid large hematoma formation is still the accepted approach. Colostomy formation is increasingly reserved for rectal injuries and destructive colon injuries with extenuating circumstances, such as hemodynamic instability and multiple associated injuries (Gonzalez and Turk, 2002).

COMMON NONGASTROINTESTINAL CAUSES FOR FECAL DIVERSION

Several other nongastrointestinal etiologies are notably associated with creation of a fecal diversion. These include spinal cord injury (SCI) ovarian cancer, and prostate cancer. They are briefly discussed here. The reader is referred to specialized texts and other chapters of this book for more in-depth discussions of the topics.

GI problems rank seventh as the cause of death in persons with SCI. The loss of bowel and bladder control in SCI patients is consistently listed as one of the most significant aspects of functional loss, even more important than loss of use of the legs (Frost, 1998). SCI patients are prone to ileus, gastric ulcer, and fecal impaction. Intestinal obstruction frequently occurs as a complicating factor after acute SCI. Adynamic (i.e., nonmechanical) obstruction will usually respond slowly to restoration of fluid and electrolyte balance and supportive therapy. When mechanical obstruction occurs after SCI, the treatment is almost always surgical. Common causes for the mechanical obstruction include adhesions, hernias, and tumors. Fecal impaction that is severe and chronic may actually benefit from a fecal diversion for greater ease of care and prevention of impaction. A related issue is the healing of pressure ulcers in the perineal and ischial areas of SCI patients with recurrent damage. Healing of these ulcers is often hastened with a diverting colostomy (Arnott, Ghosh, and Ferguson, 1999).

Ovarian cancer is a common cause for fecal diversion though it is not a GI etiology. Ovarian cancer is renowned for its metastatic spread and remains the number one gynecologic killer in the United States and the Western world (Ozols, 2002). It usually moves along the peritoneal surfaces of the abdomen, invades organs, and commonly affects the bowel. GI surgery for ovarian cancer, especially recurrent disease, is almost always tumor reductive surgery (tumor debulking). Reparative surgery on the GI tract may include removal of an impending obstruction or creation of a diversion to promote better quality of life in a palliative situation. A recent study from the Mayo clinic suggests that GI surgery is often necessary at three times in the disease course: during the primary surgery, in "second-look" procedures, and later for palliative purposes. In 364 patients with ovarian cancer, rectosigmoid resec-tion was the most common bowel operation over-all (65%) in the primary surgery group. In 30% of these resections, colostomy surgery was performed (Tamussino et al, 2001).

Prostate cancer is the fourth most commonly diagnosed malignancy in men worldwide. It is also the second most common cause of male cancer death (after lung cancer) (Brawley and Barnes, 2001). It is especially deadly in men of African heritage. For example, African-Americans have the highest incidence and mortality of any group for which clear data are available. The disease process of prostate cancer or its accompanying therapy can result in the creation of a diversion. For example, metastases can generate a bowel obstruction. Conversely, local radiation therapy may create chronic enteritis side effects that may require the construction of a stoma.

CONCLUSION

There is a wide variety of disorders that can result in a fecal diversion. This chapter has focused on six etiologies associated with stoma formation. Comprehensive understanding of the precipitating disorder(s) is a major component of good care and must be a part of the health care provider's repertoire of skills.

SELF-ASSESSMENT EXERCISES

Questions

1. Diverticulosis differs from diverticulitis in that the latter involves:
   a. Formation of a blind pouch.
   b. High intraluminal pressures.
   c. Inflammation caused by trapped stool.
   d. Weakening of the bowel wall.
2. A wound, ostomy, and continence nurse accompanies a patient to the endoscopy laboratory. The nurse explains to the patient that diverticula, if present, will likely be found in the:
   a. Distal ileum.
   b. Cecum.
   c. Sigmoid colon.
   d. Anal canal.

3. Which of the following signs or symptoms is *not* usually associated with diverticulitis?
   a. Fever and malaise
   b. Nausea and vomiting
   c. Right upper quadrant pain
   d. Dysuria
4. In contemporary health care, the most definitive diagnostic test for diverticulitis is:
   a. Ultrasound.
   b. Positron emission tomography scan.
   c. CT scan.
   d. Colonoscopy.
5. In asymptomatic diverticulosis, treatment has two major emphases:
   a. Purgative enemas and oral cathartics.
   b. Bowel rest and fluid restoration.
   c. Antibiotic therapy and clear liquid diet.
   d. Dietary modification and medication therapy.
6. A complication of diverticular disease that almost always requires surgical intervention is:
   a. Intestinal inflammation.
   b. Microperforation.
   c. Abscess formation.
   d. Fistula formation.
7. A factor that is not commonly associated with radiation enteritis is:
   a. Previous abdominal surgery.
   b. Pelvic inflammatory disease.
   c. Concomitant chemotherapy.
   d. Obese body frame.
8. Acute radiation enteritis differs from chronic radiation enteritis in which of the following factors?
   a. Timing
   b. Occurrence rate
   c. Nature of intestinal sequelae
   d. All of the above
9. Patients with acute radiation-induced colitis would likely not demonstrate the following symptom:
   a. Abdominal cramping
   b. Diarrhea
   c. Rectal pain
   d. Constipation
10. Surgical approaches to prevention of radiation enteritis includes:
    a. Bowel resection.
    b. Lysis of adhesions.
    c. Fecal diversion.
    d. Omental sling.
11. Whether older or younger patients are affected, a common pathophysiologic factor in all ischemic colitis patients is:
    a. Severe hypertension.
    b. Intestinal hypoperfusion.
    c. Abdominal surgery.
    d. Systemic infection.
12. A young woman is admitted to a stepdown intensive care unit with a diagnosis of suspected ischemic colitis. A risk factor in her history includes:
    a. IBD.
    b. Asymptomatic low blood pressure.
    c. Contraceptive hormone use.
    d. Chronic constipation.
13. The most common bacterial cause of nosocomial diarrhea is:
    a. *Shigella.*
    b. Cytomegalovirus.
    c. *Histoplasma.*
    d. *C. difficile.*
14. High-risk groups for infectious enteritis include all of the following, *except:*
    a. Home care patients.
    b. Children in day care.
    c. Travelers to foreign countries.
    d. Homosexual men.
15. The major difference between dynamic and adynamic bowel obstruction is that the latter involves:
    a. A blocking physical mass.
    b. Intussusception or volvulus.
    c. Adhesions in the abdomen.
    d. Some form of ileus.
16. Across all age groups, the greatest risk factor for bowel obstruction is:
    a. Abdominal adhesions.
    b. Crohn's disease.
    c. Hernias.
    d. Diverticulitis.

17. Blunt abdominal trauma can result in "burst injury" to the GI tract because:
    a. Points of fixation for the GI tract are torn.
    b. The blood supply is lost.
    c. The mesentery is sheared off.
    d. Compression raised the intraluminal pressure.
18. The pathophysiologic consequences of damage to the GI tract are affected by:
    a. The velocity of the missile.
    b. The location of the damage.
    c. Secondary damage effect from bone and bullet fragments.
    d. All of the above.
19. A major change in the treatment of penetrating abdominal trauma with GI tract damage is the recognition that:
    a. Primary repair is not recommended.
    b. Stapled GI tract anastomosis is preferred.
    c. Fecal diversion lowers postoperative infection rates.
    d. Diverting colostomy is not always necessary.
20. Fecal diversion of the GI tract is highly recommended for trauma of the:
    a. Ascending colon.
    b. Duoderm.
    c. Splenic flexure.
    d. Rectum.

Answers

1. c
2. c
3. c
4. c
5. d
6. d
7. d
8. d
9. d
10. d
11. b
12. c
13. d
14. a
15. d
16. a
17. d
18. d
19. d
20. d

REFERENCES

Alapati SV, Mihas AA: When to suspect ischemic colitis? *Postgrad Med* 105(4):177-187, 1999.

Arnott I, Ghosh S, Ferguson A: The spectrum of ischemic colitis, *Eur J Gastroenterol Hepatol* 11:295-303, 1999.

Baden LR, Maguire JH: Gastrointestinal infections in the immunocompromised host, *Infect Dis Clin North Am* 15(2):639-670, 2001.

Base-Smith V: Trauma in the 21st century, *Perspectives: Recovery strategies from OR to Home* 3(4):1, 4, 5, 2002.

Black PK: *Holistic stoma care*, London, 2000, Bailliere Tindall.

Boghdadi MS, Henning R: Cocaine: pathophysiology and clinical toxicology, *Heart Lung* 26:466-483, 1997.

Boriello SP: Clostridial disease of the gut, *Clin Infect Dis* 20(Suppl 2):S242-S250, 1995.

Brandt L, Boley ST: Colonic ischemia, *Surg Clin North Am* 72:203-229, 1992.

Brawley OW, Barnes S: The epidemiology of prostate cancer in the United States, *Semin Oncol Nurs* 17(2):72-77, 2001.

Brundage SI et al for the WTA Multi-Institutional study group: Stapled versus sutured gastrointestinal anastamoses in the trauma patient: a multicenter trial, *J Trauma* 51:1054-1061, 2001.

Carter JJ, Whelan RL: Evaluation and medical management of diverticular disease, *Semin Colon Rectal Surg* 11(4):196-205, 2000.

Centers for Disease Control and Prevention, National Center for Injury Prevention and Control: *20 Leading causes of death, United States, 2001, all races, all sexes,* website: webapp.cdc.gov/cgi-bin/broker.exe, accessed 1/2/04.

Chiao GZ, Rex DK: Motor disorders of the colon. In DiMarino AJ, Benjamin SB, editors: *Gastrointestinal disease: an endoscopic approach,* Thorofare, NJ, 2002, Slack.

Chutkan RK, Balba NH: Infectious disease of the colon. In DiMarino AJ, Benjamin SB, editors: *Gastrointestinal disease: an endoscopic approach,* Thorofare, NJ, 2002, Slack.

Colwell JC, Goldberg M: A review of radiation proctitis in the treatment of prostate cancer, *JWOCN* 27(3):179-187, 2000.

Dauterive AH, Flancbaum L, Cox EF: Blunt intestinal trauma: a modern day review, *Ann Surg* 201(2):198-203, 1985.

Demetriades D et al: Penetrating colon injuries requiring resection: diversion or primary anastamosis: an AAST prospective multicenter study, *J Trauma* 50(5):765-774, 2001.

Dente CJ et al: Ostomy as a risk factor for posttraumatic infection in penetrating colonic injuries: univariate and multivariate analyses, *J Trauma* 49:628-637, 2000.

Diverticular disease: website: www.intestinalfoundation.org/library/diverticular.shtml, accessed 9/11/02.

Diverticulosis: website: www.hopkinsafter50.com, accessed 9/11/02.

Diverticulosis and diverticulitis: website: www.atlgastro.com/divertic.htm, accessed 9/14/02.

Eshragi N et al: Surveyed opinion of American trauma surgeons in management of colon injuries, *J Trauma* 44(1):93-97, 1998.

Frost F: Spinal cord injury: gastrointestinal implications and management, *Top Spinal Cord Inj Rehab* 4(2):56-80, 1998.

Frost F, Craun GF, Calderon RL: Increasing hospitalization and death possibly due to *Clostridium difficile* diarrheal disease, *Emerg Infect Dis* 4(4). Website: www.csc.gov/ncidod/eid/vol4no4/frost.htm, updated 6/26/1999, 1998, accessed 9/14/02.

Girvent M et al: Intestinal failure after surgery for complicated radiation enteritis, *Ann R Coll Surg Engl* 82(3):198-201, 2000.

Gonzalez RP, Turk B: Surgical options in colorectal injuries, *Scand J Surg* 91(1):87-91, 2002.

Gonzalez RP et al: Further evaluation of colostomy in penetrating colon injury, *Am Surg* 66(4):342-347, 2000.

Gouello JP et al: The role of hyperbaric oxygen in radiation induced digestive disorders 36 cases, *Presse Med* 28(20):1053-1057, 1999.

Greenwald DA, Brandt LJ: Colonic ischemia, *J Clin Gastroenterol* 27(2):122-128, 1998.

Hyde C: Diverticular disease, *Nurs Standard* 14(51):38-43, 2000.

Infectious enteritis: website: www.members.tripod.com, accessed 9/13/02.

Intestinal obstruction: websitewww.fpnotebook.com/sur52.htm, accessed 9/11/02.

Intestinal pseudo-obstruction: National digestive diseases information clearinghouse, website: www.niddk.nih.gov/health/digest/summary/intpseud/intpseud.htm, accessed 9/13/02.

Intestinal trauma: www.lifetractech.com/product_info_trauma_stats.htm, accessed 11/5/02.

Johnson JW et al: Evolution in damage control for exsanguinating penetrating abdominal injury, *J Trauma* 51:261-271, 2001.

Karnam US, Barkin JS: Congenital, inflammatory, iatrogenic, and systemic disorders of the small intestine. In DiMarino AJ, Benjamin SB, editors: *Gastrointestinal disease: an endoscopic approach* (pp 757-772), Thorofare, NJ, 2002, Slack.

Kazzi AA, Kazzi Z: Diverticular disease, Emedicine, website: www.emedicine.com/EMERG/topic152.htm, accessed 9/11/02, updated 6/20/01, 2001.

Kouraklis G: Reconstruction of the pelvic floor using the rectus abdominis muscles after radical pelvic surgery, *Dis Colon Rectum* 45(6):836-839, 2002.

Kushimoto S et al: Duodenal mucosal injury caused by blunt abdominal trauma, *J Trauma* 51:591-593, 2001.

Leupin N et al: Acute radiation colitis in patients treated with short-term preoperative radiotherapy for rectal cancer, *Am J Surg Pathol* 26(4):498-504, 2002.

Lopez F, Sanders CV: Dermatologic infection in the immunocompromised (non-HIV) host, *Infect Dis Clin North Am* 15(2):671-690, 2001.

MacDonald PH: Ischaemic colitis: best practice and research, *Clin Gastroenterol* 16(1):51-61, 2002.

Macheta M et al: Chemotherapy for leukemia following previous pelvic radiotherapy is associated with severe enteritis and hemorrhagic cystitis, *Ann Hematol* 80(8):485-487, 2001.

Marsh WW: Infectious diseases of the gastrointestinal tract, *Adolescent Med* 11(2):263-278, 2000.

Marti VP et al: Experience and results on the surgical and medical treatment of ischaemic colitis, *Revista Espa Nola De Enfermedades Digestivas* 93(8):505-508, 2001.

Mason MG: The "crack belly": newly recognized bowel sequelae after crack cocaine intoxication, *J Emerg Nurs* 25(5):373-376, 1999.

McFarland LV et al: Recurrent *Clostridium difficile* disease: epidemiology and clinical characteristics, *Infect Control Hosp Epidemiol* 20(1):43-50, 1999.

Miller AR et al: The incidence and clinical consequences of treatment-related bowel injury, *Int J Radiat Oncol Biol Phys* 43(4):817-825, 1999.

Muniz AE, Evans T: Acute gastrointestinal manifestations associated with use of crack, *Am J Emerg Med* 19(1):61-63, 2001.

Murphy J: Testing control of radiation-induced diarrhea with a psyllium bulking agent: a pilot study, *Canad Oncol Nurs J* 10(3):96-100, 2000.

Murray JA et al: Colonic resection in trauma: colostomy vs. anastamosis, *J Trauma* 46(2):250-253, 1999.

Noyer CM, Brandt LJ: Systemic, iatrogenic, and unusual disorders of the colon. In DiMarino AJ, Benjamin SB, editors: *Gastrointestinal disease: an endoscopic approach* (pp 915-940), Thorofare, NJ, 2002, Slack.

Oliviera L, Wexner S: Abdominal pain and diverticulosis. In Welch J et al, editors: *Diverticular disease – management of the difficult surgical case* (pp 33-54), Philadelphia, 1998, Williams & Wilkins.

Orenstein JB: Talking trauma: a laymen's guide to the grisly details. *The Washington Post* October 15, website: Proquest.umi.com, accessed 11/5/2002.

Ozols RF: Update on the management of ovarian cancer, *Cancer J* 8(suppl 1):522-530, 2002.

Painter NS, Burkitt DP: Diverticular disease of the colon: a deficiency disease of western civilization, *BMJ* 1:450-454, 1971.

Pell M, Flynn WJ, Seibel R: Is colostomy always necessary in the treatment of open pelvic fractures? *J Trauma* 45(2):371-373, 1998.

Platt V: Malignant bowel obstruction: so much more than symptom control, *Int J Palliative Nurs* 7(11):547-554, 2001.

Porter JM, Ivatury RR, Nassoura ZE: Extending the horizons of "damage control" in unstable trauma patients beyond the abdomen and gastrointestinal tract, *J Trauma* 42(3):559-561, 1997.

Pothoulakis C: *Clostridium difficile* infection. About irritable bowel syndrome: website:

www.aboutibs.org/publications/cdifficile.html, updated 8/4/02, accessed 9/14/02.

Preventza OA, Lazarides K, Sawyer MD: Ischemic colitis in young adults: a single-institution experience, *J Gastrointestinal Surg* 5(4):388-392, 2001.

Radiation enteritis: website: www.acor.org, accessed 11/5/02, 2002a.

Radiation enteritis: website: www.mednets.com, accessed 9/14/02, 2002b.

Radiation enteritis: website: www.my.wedmd.com, accessed 11/5/02, 2002c.

Rawlinson F: Malignant bowel obstruction, *Eur J Palliative Care* 8(4):137-140, 2001.

Rodkey GV, Welch JP: An overview. In Welch J et al, editors: *Diverticular disease – management of the difficult surgical case* (pp 1-31), Philadelphia, 1998, Williams & Wilkins.

Ryan CK, Reamy B, Rochester JA: Ischemic colitis associated with herbal product use in a young woman, *J Am Board Fam Pract* 45(3):309-312, 2002.

Scolapio JS et al: Outcome of patients with radiation enteritis treated with home parenteral nutrition, *Am J Gastroenterol* 97(3):662-666, 2002.

Shelton BK: Intestinal obstruction, *AACN Clinical Issues* 10(4):478-491, 1999.

Shibata M et al: Ischemic colitis caused by strict dieting in an 18-year-old female, *Dis Colon Rectum* 45:425-428, 2002.

Silva J: Antibiotic-associated diarrhea and colitis, *Emerg Med* 33(3):13-14, 2001.

Sorensen VJ, Mikhail JN, Karmy-Jones R: Is delayed laparotomy for blunt abdominal trauma a valid quality improvement measure in the era of nonoperative management of abdominal injuries? *J Trauma* 52:426-433, 2002.

Spiller RC: Post infectious irritable bowel syndrome, website: www.med.unc.edu/wrkunits/2depts/medicine/fgidc/post-infestious.htm, accessed 9/14/02.

Stollman NH, Raskin JB: Diagnosis and management of diverticular disease of the colon in adults, *Am J Gastroenterol* 94(11):3110-3121, 1999.

Stollman N, Raskin JB: Diverticular disease. In DiMarino AJ, Benjamin SB, editors: *Gastrointestinal disease: an endoscopic approach* (pp 859-880), Thorofare, NJ, 2002, Slack.

Sumatriptan and ischemic colitis, *Nurse's Drug Alert* 24(5):38, 2000.

Tamussino KF et al: Gastrointestinal surgery in patients with ovarian cancer. *Gynecol Oncol* 80:79-84, 2001.

Taylor BA, DiPalma JA: Colitis: Key components of the evaluation, *Consultant* 38(2):375-378, 1998.

Tornetta P et al:. Mortality and morbidity in elderly trauma patients, *J Trauma* 46(4):702-706, 1999.

Toursarkissian B, Thompson RW: Ischemic colitis, *Surg Clin North Am* 77(2):461-470, 1997.

Uppot RN, Wills J, Gheyi VK: Bowel trauma, website: www.emedicine.com/radio/topic89.htm, accessed 11/5/02, 2001.

Walsh D: Dead tissue traumatism from roentgen ray exposure, *BMJ* 3:272-273, 1987.

Woods RK et al: Open pelvic fracture and fecal diversion, *Arch Surg* 133:281-286, 1998.

Yip C et al: Quinolone use as a risk factor for nosocomial *Clostridium difficile*–associated diarrhea, *Infect Control Hosp Epidemiol* 22:572-575, 2001.

Zauber NP, Sinha S: Ischemic colitis in young healthy adults not associated with inherited hypercoagulable conditions, *J Applied Res Clin Exper Therapeutics,* website: www.jrnlappliedresearch.com/articles/vol2Iss2/Zauberspr02.htm, accessed 9/13/2002.

BIBLIOGRAPHY

Ball SK, Groley GG: Blunt abdominal trauma: a review of 637 patients, *J Mississippi State Med Assoc*, 37(2):465-468, 1996.

Baqar S et al: *Campylobacter jejuni* enteritis, *Clin Infect Dis* 33:901-905, 2001.

Beyer FL: Gastrointestinal disorders: roles of nutrition and the dietetics practitioner, *J Am Dietetic Assoc* 98(3):272-277, 1998.

Bonadio WA: Acute infectious enteritis in children – emergency department diagnosis and management, *Emerg Med Clin North Am* 13(2):457-472, 1995.

Borum ML: Irritable bowel syndrome, *Prim Care Clin Office Pract* 28(3):523-538, 2001.

Ciftci AD: Gastrointestinal tract perforation due to blunt abdominal trauma, *Ped Surg Int* 13(4):259-264, 1998.

Clayton J: Changing trends in the laboratory diagnosis of gastroenteritic infections, *Nurs Standard* 14(11):42-46, 1999.

Cohen M et al: Staged reconstruction after gunshot wounds to the abdomen, *Plast Reconstr Surg* 108(1):83-92, 2001.

D'Agostino J: Common abdominal emergencies in children, *Emerg Med Clin North Am* 20(1):139-153, 2002.

Fabian JC: Infection in penetrating abdominal trauma: risk factors and preventive antibiotics, *Am Surg* 68(1):29-35, 2002.

Falcone RE et al: Colorectal trauma: primary repair or anastomosis with intracolonic bypass vs. ostomy, *Dis Colon Rectum* 35:957-963, 1992.

Friedel D, Thomas R, Fisher RS: Ischemic colitis during treatment with alosetron. *Gastroenterology* 120:557-560, 2001.

Freiler JF, Durning SJ, Ender PT: *Clostridium difficile* small bowel enteritis occurring after total colectomy *Clin Infect Dis* 33:1429-1431, 2001.

Green PH, Rosenberg RM: Infectious diseases of the small intestine. In DiMarino AJ, Benjamin SB, editors: *Gastrointestinal disease: an endoscopic approach* (pp 683-696), Thorofare, NJ, 2002, Slack.

Guin PR: Advances in spinal cord injury care, *Crit Care Nurs Clin North Am* 13(3):399-409, 2001.

Hamm L: Pediatric pharmacotherapy: *Clostridium difficile*, website: www.hsc.virginia.edu/cmc/pedpharm/v6n6.htm, accessed 9/14/02, last updated 8/9/2000.

Head G et al: Intramural hematoma of the descending colon after blunt abdominal trauma *Clin Ped* 39(6):373-374, 2000.

Heitkemper M, Jarrett M: Irritable bowel syndrome: causes and treatment, *Gastroenterol Nurs* 23(6):256-263, 2000.

Hirshberg A, Wall M, Mattox KL: Planned reoperation for trauma: a two-year experience with 124 consecutive patients, *J Trauma* 37(3):365-369, 1994.

Klausner JM, Rozin RR: Late abdominal complications in war wounded, *J Trauma*, 38(2):313-317, 1995.

Levine CD: Toxic megacolon: diagnosis and treatment challenges, *AACN Clinical Issues* 10(4):492-499, 1999.

Lewis BS: Vascular diseases of the small intestine. In DiMarino AJ, Benjamin SB, editors: *Gastrointestinal disease: an endoscopic approach* (pp 727-740), Thorofare, NJ, 2002, Slack.

Nichols RL, Smith JW: Risk or infection, infecting flora and treatment considerations in penetrating abdominal trauma, *Surg Gynecol Obstet* 177:50-54, 65-70, 1993.

Ong CL, Png DJ, Chan ST: Abdominal trauma: a review. *Singapore Med J* 35(3):269-270, 1994.

Richard CS, Hiruki T, McLeod RS: Differentiation of inflammatory bowel disease from diverticulitis. In Welch J et al, editors: *Diverticular disease: management of the difficult surgical case* (pp 67-75), Philadelphia, 1998, Williams & Wilkins.

Sawyer MA, Sawyer EM: Short-bowel syndrome, Emedicine, website: www.emedicine.com/med/topic2746.htm, accessed 9/13/02, last updated 9/16/2002.

Stevens P: Management of traumatic wounds: a nursing perspective, *World Council Enterostomal Ther J* 16(2):10-11, 14-16, 1996.

Talan DA: New concepts in antimicrobial therapy for emergency department infections, *Ann Emerg Med* 34(4):503-516, 1999.

Waldman AR: Bowel obstruction, *Clin J Oncol Nurs* 5(6):281-286, 2001.

Welch JP et al, editors: *Diverticular disease management of the difficult surgical case,* Baltimore, 1998, Williams & Wilkins.

Yarbro CH, Ferrans CE: Quality of life of patients with prostate cancer treated with surgery or radiation therapy, *Oncol Nurs Forum* 25(4):685-693, 1998.

Zimmerman HM, Curfman KL: Acute gastrointestinal bleeding, *AACN Clinical Issues* 8(3):449-458, 1997.

ONLINE RESOURCES

Intestinal obstruction, Adam: website: www.besthealth.com/surgery/intestobstruct_5.html.

Intestinal obstruction: Texas Pediatric Surgical Associates: website:www.pedisurg.com/ptEduc/Intestinal_obstruction.html.

Radiation enteritis: National Cancer Institute: website: www.nci.nih.gov/cancer_information/doc, accessed 9/13/02, last updated 9/2002.

Radiation enteritis: Gastrolab Image Gallery: website: www.gastrolab.net/g2g01.htm.

Radiation enteritis: Discovery Health Channel: website: www.health.discovery.com/diseasesandcond/encyclopedia/2575.html.

PART

III *Urinary Diversions*

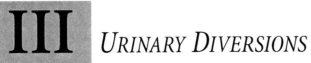

Anatomy and Physiology of the Urinary System

MIKEL GRAY

OBJECTIVES

1. Explain the structures and functions of the upper and lower urinary tract.
2. Identify the role of the kidneys in maintaining homeostasis.
3. Discuss the process of urine formation in the kidney.
4. Compare the pelvic support structure for the female and male.
5. Compare the urethra in the male and the female.
6. Explain the significance of normal bladder wall compliance.
7. Identify factors responsible for urinary continence.
8. Describe the micturition process.
9. Discuss the metabolic implications of isolating a section of the colon for urinary reconstruction.
10. Explain why the surgeon detubularizes the bowel when creating a urinary reservoir.

INTRODUCTION

Management of a urinary ostomy is based on fundamental knowledge of the urinary system, including the paired upper urinary tracts (i.e., kidneys, renal pelves, and ureters); the lower urinary tract (i.e., urinary bladder, urethra, and pelvic floor support structures); and the changes in urinary filling, storage, and evacuation associated with reconstruction of the urinary system. This chapter will review the coverings of the urinary system including the abdominal wall and flank, its major organs and their function, and alterations in function associated with urinary diversion or reconstruction, particularly when one or more segments of bowel are incorporated into the urinary tract.

UPPER URINARY TRACTS

The principal organs of the urinary system, the paired kidneys, the renal pelves, and proximal ureters, comprise the upper urinary tract. They are primarily responsible for urine formation and transportation, whereas the lower urinary tracts are mainly responsible for urine storage and elimination.

Retroperitoneum

The upper urinary tracts are housed primarily within the retroperitoneum (Figure 9-1) (Kabalin, 1998; McDougal, 2002a). The retroperitoneum is bounded posteriorly by the lower thoracic and the upper sacral vertebrae and the posterolateral abdominal wall (i.e., the flank). Its roof is formed by the fascia of the diaphragm, and its anterior border is the peritoneal sac and the overlying abdominal wall.

The lower thoracic and the lumbar vertebrae form a central landmark for the retroperitoneum; the vertebral bodies and their processes serve as the origin for the principal fascia and muscles visualized when surgical reconstruction and stoma formation involves the upper urinary tracts (Kabalin, 1998). Anteriorly the eleventh and twelfth ribs (and the tenth rib in some persons) extend into the retroperitoneum.

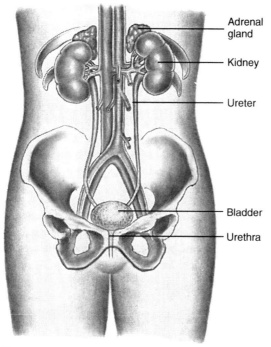

Figure 9-1   Components of the urinary system. (From Thompson JM et al: *Mosby's clinical nursing*, ed 5, St Louis, 2002, Mosby.)

The flank (i.e., posterolateral abdominal wall) contains dense fascia that originates from the lumbar vertebrae and travels superficially to the back muscles to cover the posterior aspect of the sacrospinous muscle. Latissimus dorsi muscles originate from the lumbar spine to cover the superior and medial muscles of the flank. Middle and anterior fascial planes originate from the lumbar vertebrae to separate the sacrospinous muscle from the quadratus lumborum, just as a superficial fascial plane separates this muscle from the abdominal wall. All of these fascial layers merge to form a tough, dense structure that serves as a landmark for surgical approach to the upper urinary tracts and make it unnecessary to cut through the muscles of the anterior abdomen or flank. In addition a costovertebral ligament attaches the L1 and L2 vertebrae to the twelfth rib; this dense ligament may require incision to increase mobility of this rib, if

the kidney is approached surgically from a posterior perspective.

Three muscles of the flank are of greatest surgical significance: the external obliques, the internal obliques, and the transverse abdominis. The external oblique muscles are the most superficial; they originate at the lower ribs and insert along the iliac crests. The external obliques can be retracted for specific urinary system procedures without the need for cutting. The internal oblique muscles originate at the iliac crest and extend in a superior and oblique direction to insert on the lower ribs. The deeper transverse abdominis muscle originates within the dorsal lumbar fascia and runs posteriorly to the lateral border of the rectus sheath.

The psoas muscle, whose shadow is visible on a plain abdominal radiograph, lies in the groove between the thoracolumbar vertebral bodies and their transverse processes (Kabalin, 1998; McDougal, 2002a). It originates between T12 and L5 and runs inferiorly while tapering to join the iliacus muscle. At this point, it is usually referred to as the iliopsoas muscle, and it continues its downward course to insert on the femur. The psoas muscles are covered by the psoas sheath, an extension of the transversalis fascia.

Several fascial and fatty structures lie immediately adjacent to the kidneys. Dense connective tissue adheres to the renal cortex and is surrounded by perirenal fascia. These fascial planes are enclosed within a layer of perinephric fat that serves as a shock absorber when there is a blow to the abdomen or kidney. In addition to these structures, the kidney and adrenal gland are covered by Gerota's fascia, which comprises a significant landmark when the upper urinary tracts are approached surgically.

Adjacent Organs

Several organs lie in close proximity to the kidneys and must be carefully identified and protected during surgical reconstruction and diversion (Kabalin, 1998). The duodenum runs vertically and anterior to the hilum of the right kidney, right renal vessels, ureteropelvic junction (UPJ), and right proximal ureter. The tail of the pancreas lies close to the left adrenal gland and the upper pole of the left kidney. This relationship is particularly significant, because the pancreatic and splenic vessels are at risk for injury when the left kidney is manipulated surgically. Whereas the majority of the colon is located far from the paired kidneys, the hepatic flexure courses close to the lower pole of the right kidney, the ascending colon courses just behind the right ureter, and the descending and sigmoid colon traverse near the left ureter. Because of these relationships, the colon may be moved medially when the upper urinary tracts are approached from an abdominal surgical incision.

Adrenals

Although aspects of the pancreas, duodenum, and colon lie in close proximity to the kidneys, none lie as close as the adrenal glands. The paired adrenal glands lie superior to each kidney. They are 3 to 5 cm in height, and 2 to 3 cm in width (Rosol et al, 2001). The adrenals are surrounded by Gerota's fascia, but they are anatomically and functionally distinct from the kidneys. Although the right kidney is usually located slightly lower within the retroperitoneum owing to the presence of the liver, the right adrenal is slightly higher.

The microscopic anatomy of the adrenal glands consists of two principal regions: the cortex and medulla. The adrenal cortex is the larger, outer histologic region and contains three histologic layers: the zona glomerulus, the zona fasciculata, and the zona reticularis. The zona glomerulus comprises cells that are arranged in round balls or arched loops and manufacture the mineralocorticoid hormone aldosterone. Aldosterone acts to maintain sodium and potassium levels; its absence leads to fluid and electrolyte imbalance and death. A middle layer, the zona fasciculata, synthesizes the glucocorticoids (primarily cortisol), which are critical for carbohydrate and protein metabolism. The zona reticularis produces adrenocortical androgens and estrogens. However, only a relatively small portion of the body's androgenic hormones are produced by the adrenals. The larger portion is synthesized by the testes or ovaries.

The microscopic anatomy of the smaller, inner medulla contains chromaffin cells that synthesize epinephrine and norepinephrine. Chromaffin cells respond to stimuli from the autonomic nervous system. As a result, norepinephrine and epinephrine can be released rapidly, allowing the body to respond promptly to physical or emotional challenges.

The blood supply of the adrenal glands arises from numerous small arteries that branch from the aorta, the inferior phrenic artery, and the ipsilateral renal artery. A single adrenal vein exits the organ; the right adrenal vein is short and drains directly into the abdominal aorta, whereas the left vein joins the left inferior phrenic vein before draining into the left renal vein. Lymph nodes drain into the paraaortic nodes. The nervous supply of the adrenal is intimately related to the autonomic nervous system; multiple sympathetic fibers from the splanchnic nerve enter the adrenal by way of the course of the adrenal vein. These nerves synapse in the chromaffin cells of the medulla to provide the close physiologic relationship of the adrenal medulla and the autonomic nervous system.

KIDNEYS

The kidneys are found in the retroperitoneum parallel to spinal levels T12 to L3 (Figure 9-2) (Kabalin, 1998; McDougal, 2002a). They have a characteristic bean shape whose convex surface is oriented toward the lateral aspect of the retroperitoneum; its concave surface faces toward the vertebral bodies (Figure 9-3). The concave renal hilum is the point where the renal artery, veins, and ureter enter or exit from the kidney. The normal adult kidney is 11 cm long and about 5 to 7 cm wide. Women's kidneys tend to be typically slimmer than those of men. The kidneys are roughly equal in size, but because of the liver the right kidney lies lower than the left.

Gross visualization of a bisected kidney reveals two regions, the pelvis and the parenchyma. The parenchyma (the meat of the kidney) is subdivided into a cortex and a medulla that, like those of the adrenal gland, are visible to the unaided eye. The renal medulla contains pyramids whose bases are oriented toward its convex periphery, whereas their apices approach the hilum. The surrounding cortex

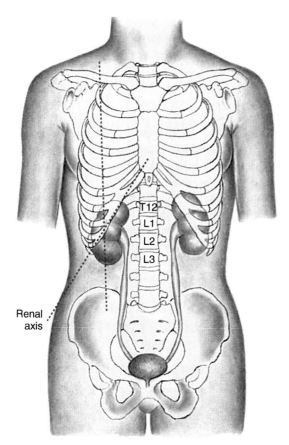

T12
L1
L2
L3

Renal axis

Figure 9-2   Anatomic relationships of paired kidneys to the spinal column and lower rib cage. (From Thompson JM et al: *Mosby's clinical nursing*, ed 5, St Louis, 2002, Mosby.)

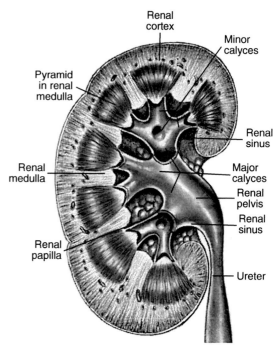

Renal cortex

Minor calyces

Pyramid in renal medulla

Renal sinus

Renal medulla

Major calyces

Renal pelvis

Renal sinus

Renal papilla

Ureter

Figure 9-3   Cross-section anatomy of the kidney demonstrates the cortex and medulla of the renal parenchyma, pyramids, and pelvicaliceal system. (From Thompson JM et al: *Mosby's clinical nursing*, ed 5, St Louis, 2002, Mosby.)

is characterized by columns and lobules that surround and fill the space between pyramids.

Renal arteries branch directly from the abdominal aorta to supply blood to the kidneys. A single renal artery is normal, but pairing can occur. The renal arteries split into segmental, lobar, interlobar, and interlobular arteries, then divide into the afferent arterioles for individual nephrons. The approximately 90-degree angle of these bifurcations slows flow for filtration in the nephron. The postglomerular capillaries merge into interlobular veins, which combine into arcuate, interlobar, lobar, and segmental veins. Venous blood drains into the shorter, right renal vein, which enters directly into the vena cava, or into the left renal vein, which is 3 times as long as the right and crosses anterior to the aorta to drain into the inferior vena cava. The lymphatic channels drain into paraaortic and paravena caval node chains.

The kidneys receive far more blood flow than is necessary to meet the metabolic needs of local tissues. A large volume entering the kidney is filtered of its water and small molecules (solutes); the kidneys then resorb selected portions of this filtrate and excrete waste materials via the urine. Although arterial blood enters the kidneys at a relatively high pressure, the process of renal filtration, excretion, and resorption occurs within a low-pressure environment.

Microscopic Anatomy

The nephron is a tubular structure that begins with a cuplike glomerulus and continues with a proximal convoluted (i.e., twisted) tubule, the loop of Henle, the distal convoluted tubule, and the collecting duct (Valtin, 1995; Vander, 1995; Noland, 1997). Afferent and efferent arterioles are located at the corresponding end of Bowman's capsule; the vasa recta and peritubular are found immediately adjacent to the tubules of the nephron. The proximity of the nephron and adjacent vessels is critical to renal filtration and urine formation.

The collecting duct of each nephron combines with other collecting ducts to drain into an apex of a renal pyramid. From this point, the fluid drains into the papillae, of which there are seven to nine within each kidney. The papillae contain valvular mechanisms that allow antegrade flow (i.e., efflux) from nephron to renal pelvis and prevent retrograde flow (i.e., reflux) from pelvis to parenchyma. These are the first of two valves designed to promote efflux while preventing reflux; the second is the UPJ, which joins the upper and lower urinary tracts. The papillae extend laterally toward the abdominal wall and posteriorly toward the flank. The papillae join with a minor calyx, which has a cupped appearance on intravenous urography. They empty into major calices and the renal pelvis.

The kidneys contain two types of nephrons, cortical and juxtamedullary. Juxtamedullary nephrons have long loops of Henle and extend deep into the parenchyma. They are adapted to resorb and thus preserve water and sodium, when intake of these essential substances is low. Cortical nephrons have shorter loops of Henle that extend only a short distance into the renal cortex (Tisher and Madsen, 2000).

Physiology of the Kidney

The kidneys perform a number of functions that are essential to life, including filtration of metabolic waste and toxins from the blood, and maintenance of internal homeostasis. They also have endocrine and paracrine functions, influencing blood pressure, vascular volume, red blood cell production and apoptosis, and bone growth and maintenance.

Urine Formation

The kidneys form urine to maintain internal homeostasis and rid the body of waste products and toxins (Valtin, 1995; Vander, 1995; Noland, 1997). The efficiency of blood flow to the kidneys in normal adults is such that roughly 1200 ml of blood (25% of cardiac output) reaches the kidneys each minute. However, the percentage of cardiac output reaching the kidneys can vary from 30%, to 12% during intense exertion. Acute physical distress may reduce blood flow to the kidneys even further, bringing about the risk of acute renal insufficiency or renal failure unless flow is restored quickly.

The porous walls of the glomerular capillaries filter approximately 180 L of fluid per day. All but 1 to 2 L of this fluid is resorbed, roughly four times as much fluid as all the other capillary beds in the body combined. The glomerular capillary membrane filters blood without excessive fluid loss thanks to several histologic adaptations. Three layers of epithelial cells line the glomerular capillaries: the inner capillary endothelium, the basement membrane, and the outer epithelial layer of specialized cells called podocytes. The inner epithelium has slitlike openings called fenestrae. The basement membrane is negatively charged and highly permeable to small molecules. The podocytes of the glomerular epithelium have footlike processes adhering to the negatively charged basement membrane. These interlock into a network of intercellular clefts or filtration slits. As a result the glomerular capillaries are 100 to 500 times more permeable than other capillary beds, but they remain highly selective as to the substances they filter. Water, electrolytes, urea, and other waste products filter readily from the blood, and larger molecules (e.g., proteins) and blood cells do not. The filtrate in Bowman's capsule is similar to plasma except that it lacks the blood cells and proteins characteristic of the bloodstream.

The glomerular filtration rate (GFR) is the volume filtered by the kidneys in a given period of time (Guyton, 1996). The GFR is affected by three forces: hydrostatic pressure, filtration pressure, and plasma oncotic pressure. Hydrostatic pressure reflects blood flow in the glomerular capillaries; it promotes filtration. Filtration pressure is the pressure within Bowman's capsule; it restricts the GFR. Plasma oncotic pressure reflects movement of water and solutes from high concentrations to lower until equilibrium is achieved. This promotes filtration because the filtrate has fewer large molecules than the blood in the glomerular capillaries. Normally hydrostatic pressure and plasma oncotic pressure exceed the pressure in Bowman's space, which favors blood filtration and toxin removal, along with unneeded fluid and electrolytes.

Several factors can alter hydrostatic pressure or the pressure inside Bowman's capsule, thus altering the GFR and affecting urine formation (Valtin, 1995; Vander, 1995; Noland, 1997; Tisher and Madsen, 2000). Dilation of afferent and efferent arterioles increases renal blood flow and GFR; constriction reduces both. Another factor that affects renal blood flow and GFR is sympathetic nervous system tone. Sympathetic nerve stimulation constricts the afferent arteriole, reducing blood flow to the nephron and lowering the GFR. Radical stimulation such as severe physical distress can drop the GFR to 0 ml/min for 10 minutes or more. However, changes in systemic blood pressure are less likely to affect renal blood flow, since the kidney autoregulates blood flow even if systemic blood pressure is fluctuating.

The initial filtrate collects in the glomerulus before moving into the proximal convoluted tubule (Tisher and Madsen, 2000). Brush border cells line the proximal convoluted tubule and resorb most of the filtrate by osmotic (i.e., passive) as well as active mechanisms. Sodium, chloride, and some urea are actively resorbed by the proximal tubule, and water is resorbed along its osmotic gradient. The proximal tubule actively resorbs glucose, bicarbonate, potassium, calcium, phosphate, uric acid, and amino acids. When the filtrate reaches the loop of Henle, 60% to 70% of the filtered sodium and water and half of the urea have been resorbed, along with >90% of the potassium, glucose, bicarbonate, calcium, and phosphate. These substances are resorbed in the proximal convoluted tubule according to their transport maximum, the highest volume of a substance that can be resorbed by active transport in a fixed time. If the amount of a particular substance is exceeds its TM, the rest remains in the filtrate for ultimate excretion. This is particularly significant in diabetes mellitus; plasma glucose of 180 mg/dl or greater exceeds the TM for glucose, resulting in glucosuria detectable by dipstick urinalysis.

Along with most water and solutes filtered by the glomerulus, the proximal tubule exchanges hydrogen ions for sodium. Similar secretory pathways exist for creatinine and other organic bases, and exogenous organic acids including drugs. This allows the body to clear itself of metabolic waste products and drugs, and regulate pH.

Sodium and water are selectively excreted and resorbed as the filtrate enters the loop of Henle, determining urine concentration and the body's hydration (Marunka, 1997; Giebisch and Klein-Robbenhaar, 1993). Fluid entering the loop of Henle has much the same osmotic pressure as plasma. Once in the loop, sodium and water are secreted or resorbed to allow the dilution level of the urine to be greater or lower than that of plasma; this capability is affected by the length of the loop and by the variable permeability of the loop cells to sodium and water. The process involves constant interaction between the loop and the adjacent vasa recta, and is called the countercurrent exchange system.

When the concentration of water in the filtrate is adjusted to the homeostatic requirements of the body, more water may be added when the filtrate enters the distal convoluted tubule and collecting duct (Tisher and Madsen, 2000). Specialized epithelial cells in the distal convoluted tubule and collecting duct are impermeable to urea, favoring excretion of urea in the urine, but they are able to resorb large amounts of sodium. This allows further urine concentration and water preservation. However, unlike in the loop of Henle, sodium resorption in this part of the nephron is regulated by aldosterone and antidiuretic hormone. After the filtrate passes from the collecting duct into the calyx it can properly be considered urine. From there it enters the pelvicaliceal system, the ureters, and the bladder relatively unchanged.

In summary, the process of ridding the body of water-soluble waste products and toxins while maintaining homeostasis requires that most of the filtrate that enters the glomerulus be resorbed, and most of the urea and nitrogenous, water-soluble waste be excreted with the urine.

Homeostasis and the Kidney

By filtering blood and forming urine, the kidneys regulate the body's internal environment, specifically the proper concentrations of water and electrolytes, including hydrogen, to maintain pH. Water-soluble metabolic products and toxic substances are excreted.

Water and Hydration

Water accounts for 57% to 75% of the human body (Vander, 1995). Most of the water, about 25 L, is found in the intracellular space. Fifteen liters is contained in the extracellular space, 3 L of which is in the plasma. Over 2 L of water is lost daily from the lungs and skin, or in feces and urine. As mentioned, the kidneys filter 180 L of plasma a day. Without efficient resorption, the loss of fluids and solutes would soon lead to dehydration and death. Water resorption starts in the proximal tubule and continues in the loop of Henle. These processes resorb most of the water required for internal homeostasis. The kidneys are also influenced by antidiuretic hormone (ADH), a pituitary hormone affecting the volume of water in the urine and the thirst reflex. As total water volume drops, plasma becomes hyperosmotic. The rise in concentration of solutes stimulates ADH release from the posterior pituitary gland, increasing resorption of water. However, if the individual drinks enough water to make the plasma slightly hypoosmotic, ADH secretion is inhibited. This reduces thirst and increases water excretion to restore internal homeostasis. Diuretic medications affect the mechanisms of water resorption and excretion (Wilcox, 2000). The kidneys also regulate electrolytes essential to metabolic function, including sodium, chloride, potassium, bicarbonate, calcium, and magnesium.

Sodium

Sodium is the most abundant positively charged ion in the body (Valtin, 1995; Vander, 1995). Most sodium is found in the extracellular fluid space, 135 to 145 mEq/L, whereas just 10 to 14 mEq/L is found in the intracellular fluid compartment. Excretion and resorption are regulated by the kidneys primarily in response to fluid volume and sodium concentrations in the plasma. The sympathetic nervous system, the renin-angiotensin aldosterone hormone mechanism, and atrial natriuretic peptide, which is released from cells in the atria of the heart in response to atrial stretch, also affect sodium regulation. Like water, sodium is resorbed both passively and actively. The proximal tubule resorbs sodium as $NaHCO_3$ or $NaCl$. The loop of Henle actively uses sodium to concentrate urine and preserve water. The distal tubule and collecting duct, under the influence of aldosterone, also resorbs sodium.

Potassium

The proximal convoluted tubule also resorbs most of the potassium in the glomerular filtrate. The ascending loop of Henle then resorbs additional potassium (Giebisch, Malnic, and Berliner, 2000). The late distal tubule and collecting duct later actively adjust the potassium concentration, according to the metabolic needs of cardiac muscle and other cells. Dietary intake, serum levels of adrenal mineralocorticoids (i.e., aldosterone), hydrogen ion balance, and diuretics primarily regulate potassium balance. In renal failure, the nephrons initially increase potassium excretion in response to reduced GFR, until the GFR drops below 5 ml/minute, indicating end-stage renal failure and potentially fatal hyperkalemia.

Calcium, Phosphate, and Magnesium

The proximal convoluted tubule passively resorbs most of the calcium, phosphate, and magnesium (i.e., 60% to 65%). Henle's loop resorbs another 20%. The distal convoluted tubule actively readjusts the final proportion under the influence of the hormones parathormone, calcitonin, and glucagon. Diet, hydrogen ion (i.e., acid-base) balance, and metabolic vitamin D or cholecalciferol also influence calcium, phosphate, and magnesium balance (Suki, Lederer, and Rouse, 2000). Diuretics affecting the loop of Henle decrease calcium resorption (Giebisch and Klein-Robbenhaar, 1993).

Acid-Base Balance

Serum pH normally ranges from 7.37 to 7.42, a balance affected by CO_2 production, consumption of inorganic acids, and production of naturally occurring acidic substances. If the body's pH fell below a mildly alkaline balance, metabolic processes would be interrupted and death would rapidly ensue. The lungs act as short-term regulators of pH by respiring excess CO_2, binding hydrogen ions entering the blood by hemoglobin buffering with bicarbonate ions. Long-term regulation is afforded by the kidneys, which excrete excessive hydrogen ions in exchange for bicarbonate, thus helping provide the necessary bicarbonate for buffering. The kidneys also excrete ammonium ions and dietary acids (Hayashi, 1998).

Endocrine Functions of the Kidney

Paracrine or endocrine substances including erythropoietin, renin, angiotensin, and cholecalciferol are secreted by the kidneys, affecting both adjacent tissues and distant organs.

Erythropoietin

Cells lining the capillaries adjacent to the renal tubules produce the hormone erythropoietin (Noland, 1997), which stimulates the bone marrow to produce red blood cells (i.e., erythrocytes). The kidneys produce 90% to 95% of the body's erythropoietin. Hypoxia or reduction in renal blood flow enhances erythropoietin secretion. In renal failure, erythropoietin production is compromised, leading to a decline in hematocrit and profound anemia. Recombinant human erythropoietin can stimulate the bone marrow and restore an adequate hematocrit level (Ludat et al, 2000).

Renin-Angiotensin

The juxtaglomerular apparatus (JGA), a group of specialized cells adjacent to the glomerulus, produces the enzyme renin (Guyton, 1996). Renin is released in response to stimuli including decreased plasma sodium concentration, systemic blood pressure, and stimulation of β-adrenergic nerve receptors in the JGA. Renin secretion converts angiotensinogen to angiotensin I. Angiotensin I interacts with angiotensin-converting enzyme, primarily in the small blood vessels of the lung, to form angiotensin II. Angiotensin II is a powerful vasopressor, constricting the afferent arteriole of the glomerulus and stimulating sodium resorption by decreasing GFR and slowing sodium filtration. Activation of the renin-angiotensin system leads to aldosterone secretion in the adrenal glands.

Aldosterone

The adrenal cortex is stimulated to secrete aldosterone by angiotensin II, an increase in the serum concentration of potassium, a decrease in the concentration of sodium in the extracellular fluid, or the secretion of adrenocorticotropin hormone, or ACTH (Rosol et al, 2001). Aldosterone increases sodium resorption within the distal convoluted tubule along with angiotensin II. Aldosterone, however, increases the elimination of potassium.

Cholecalciferol

The kidneys also regulate the production of bioavailable vitamin D (Feldman, 1999). Whether vitamin D is obtained by way of the diet or as a vitamin supplement, it must be converted into a metabolically active form (1,25-dihydroxycholecalciferol) for use by the human body. Exogenous vitamin D is converted into 1,25-dihydroxycholecalciferol, initially in the liver and finally in the kidneys. This essential vitamin affects increases intestinal absorption of calcium and promotes ossification of bones and teeth.

RENAL PELVIS AND URETER

Urine is transported from the paired renal pelves to the bladder by means of an active process called peristalsis (Gray and Brown, 2002). The renal pelvis is a funnel-shaped extension of the ureter whose wider end attaches to the renal hilum before tapering to a 6 Fr diameter at the UPJ. The ureter is a 24- to 30-cm tube that connects the UPJ to the bladder by way of the ureterovesical junction (UVJ). The left ureter is typically longer than the right because of the slightly inferior location of the right kidney. After tapering into the UPJ, the ureter runs in a medial fashion, passes over the psoas muscle and approaches the sacroiliac joint of the pelvic bone. It then turns laterally before curving back toward the base of the urinary bladder, where it terminates as the UVJ. The diameter of the ureter is narrowest in three locations: at the UPJ, near the iliac arteries, and at the UVJ.

The microscopic anatomy of the ureter is characterized by an inner mucosa, submucosa, a layer of smooth muscle, and outer adventitia. The ureteral mucosa comprises transitional-cell epithelium that is resistant to secretion or resorption of urinary constituents, including water and sodium. The submucosa houses motor and sensory nerves, local vascular structures, and a lymphatic drainage system. The smooth muscle of the ureter is arranged into a complex network containing an outer layer of longitudinal smooth muscles, a middle circular layer, and inner longitudinal layers.

Arterial blood reaches the ureter from a variety of sources. The upper ureteral segments may receive blood from branches of the renal, gonadal, or adrenal arteries. The lower ureter is supplied by branches of the obturator artery. In men the ureter may receive blood from branches of the deferential artery, and the uterine artery may supply the lower ureter of women. Venous drainage reflects the arterial supply, as do lymphatic drainage channels. Lymphatic channels from the upper ureter drain into paraaortic or renal nodes, and channels from the lower ureter usually drain into the common or external iliac nodes.

URETERAL FUNCTION

Peristaltic contractions, originating in pacemaker cells located in the calyces or the renal pelvis, push a bolus of urine through the ureter and into the bladder through the ureterovesical junction (Weiss, 1998). The renal pelvis stores only 15 to 20 ml of urine before propagating a peristaltic wave that opens the UPJ. The resting intraluminal pressure is raised by the peristaltic contraction from 0-5 cm H_2O to 20-80 cm H_2O, pushing the urine bolus ahead of it. Gap junctions, which allow electrochemical communication between muscle cells and the smooth muscle of the ureters, act as a single unit. By this means, a single peristaltic wave contraction continuously pushes the urine through the entire ureter and to the bladder, even in denervated or transplanted ureters.

Mechanical distention is not the only source of ureteral peristalsis. Neurologic, endocrine, and pharmacologic factors also mediate ureteral peristalsis. The number and the amplitude of contractions are increased by stimulation of α-adrenergic receptors in the ureteral wall. Stimulation of β-adrenergic receptors causes ureteral relaxation. Administration of epinephrine or catecholamines causes vigorous ureteral peristalsis by the release of catecholamines that stimulate cholinergic receptors. Other neurotransmitters in the ureter include tachykinins and calcitonin gene-related peptide (CGRP). CGRP inhibits peristalsis, and tachykinins stimulate it. The tachykinins substance P, neurokinin A, and neuropeptide K are particularly abundant in the sensory nerves of the renal pelvis. The distal ureter includes abundant inhibitory nerves containing CGRP.

Ureterovesical Junction

The UVJ consists of the distal ureter, the adjacent bladder wall, and the trigone (Figure 9-4) (Gray and Brown, 2002; Kramer, 1992). Its primary purpose is to allow antegrade flow of urine from upper to lower urinary tract (efflux) while preventing retrograde urine flow from lower to upper tract (reflux). Three principal factors, the distal ureter and its fascia, the trigone, and the adjacent bladder wall, interact to accomplish this goal. Rather than entering the ureter at a sharp angle, the distal ureter tunnels through the bladder wall and the trigone at a gentle angle over a length of nearly 1.5 cm. Tunneling of the distal (i.e., intramural) ureter helps to prevent reflux by sealing the ureter in response to contraction of the trigone or smooth muscle within the adjacent bladder wall. Waldeyer's sheath is a trilayered fascial casing that attaches the ureter to the bladder and limits the mobility of the distal ureter. Smooth muscle within the adjacent bladder wall provides additional anatomic integrity, and it promotes closure of the UVJ during micturition. The final factor, the trigone, is a triangular smooth muscle located in the base of the bladder. Its superficial segment joins the trigone to the intramural ureter, and its deep segment is contiguous with Waldeyer's sheath.

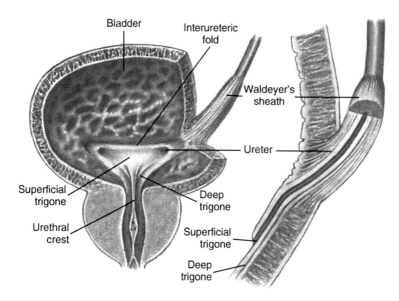

Figure 9-4   The ureterovesical junction. (From Thompson JM et al: *Mosby's clinical nursing*, ed 5, St Louis, 2002, Mosby.)

During bladder filling and urine storage, relaxation of the trigone and detrusor muscles allow urine to pass through the UVJ in response to a peristaltic contraction, whereas passive pressures (including abdominal forces created by physical exertion, coughing, or sneezing) maintain UVJ closure between peristaltic waves. In contrast, contraction of the detrusor and the trigone with micturition prevents reflux into the upper urinary tracts by raising closure pressure within the intramural ureter well beyond that created by ureteral peristalsis. The risk of reflux is further lessened because the trigone contracts for approximately 20 seconds after voiding is completed.

LOWER URINARY TRACT

The lower urinary tract consists of the urinary bladder, the urethra, and the pelvic floor support structures (Brooks, 1998). Although the bladder is initially located in the lower abdomen, it assumes its position in the abdominopelvic area as the child matures and the pelvic bone grows and widens.

Pelvis and Pelvic Floor Support Structures

The pelvic bone comprises the sacrum and the paired innominate bones formed by fusion of the iliac, ischial, and pubic bones (Figure 9-5) (Brooks,

1998). The abdominal wall forms the anterior border of the pelvic cavity. Just beneath the skin are Camper's fascia and a loose layer of subcutaneous fat and superficial vessels. Scarpa's fascia is found underneath these layers; it fuses with Camper's fascia laterally, Coille's fascia (a reflection of peritoneal fascia) medially, and the deep fascia of the thigh inferiorly.

The abdominal muscles lie just below Scarpa's fascia (Brooks, 1998). The external and internal obliques and the transverse abdominis muscles were described earlier. However, the principal muscle of the anterior abdominal wall that extends to the abdominopelvic cavity is the rectus abdominis. The rectus abdominis originates from the pubic tubercles and medius and inserts at the xiphoid process and the nearby costal cartilage. It is also distinguished by three to four tendinous bands that are attached to the anterior rectus fascial sheath, allowing the surgeon to divide the muscle when approaching organs of the urinary and gastrointestinal tracts without significantly retracting the entire muscle. However, because the rectus abdominis is enervated by approximately six thoracic nerves, paramedial incisions lateral to the rectus may cause atrophy or ventral hernias and are to be avoided. The pyramidalis muscles are superficial to

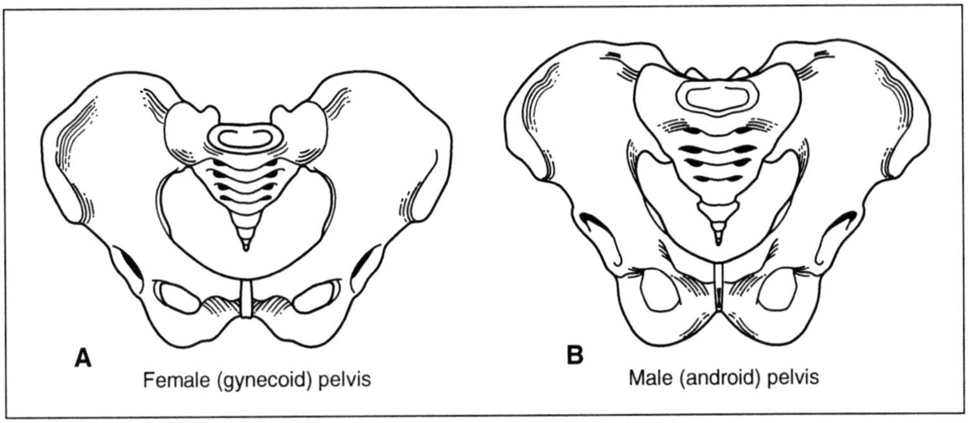

Figure 9-5   Pelvic bone of female (**A**) and male (**B**) pelvis. (From Doughty DB: *Urinary and fecal incontinence: nursing management*, ed 2, St Louis, 2000, Mosby.)

the rectus and lie within its fascial plane. They originate at the pubic crest and insert into the linea alba.

Pelvic Floor

The description of pelvic floor support structures provided in this chapter is limited to endopelvic fascia, pelvic floor muscles, and true ligaments that provide support for the lower urinary tract and contribute to urethral sphincter mechanism competence. The reader should refer to Chapter 3 for a more detailed description of the rectum and rectal sphincters.

Female Pelvic Floor

The endopelvic fascia, the levator ani, the perineal membrane, and the external anal sphincter comprise the primary support structures within the pelvic floor in women (Ashton-Miller, Howard, and DeLancey, 2001; Sampselle, Delancey, 1998). Pelvic organs connect to the bony pelvis by the endopelvic fascia, which contains collagen, elastin, and smooth muscle. Elements of the endopelvic fascia are sometimes referred to surgically as if they were distinct ligaments, which has a certain practical relevance; however, the endopelvic fascia is a functional unit of the pelvic floor rather than a network of ligaments (Table 9-1).

The levator ani, a U-shaped muscle that attaches anteriorly to the paired pubic bones and laterally to the ischial spines and the arcus tendineus muscle, is the primary support structure of the female pelvic floor. It can be anatomized into smaller muscles such as the ileococcygeus and the pubococcygeus, but for continence nursing purposes it is regarded as if it were a single muscle. The levator ani supports the bladder base and the urethra. It is best represented as a floor that remains firm under the pressure of the viscera in a standing position of the body.

The lower urinary tract is also supported by the anal sphincter and the perineal membrane. The perineal membrane, a triangular fibrous structure, attaches the perineal body to the pubic bones to restrain descent of the pelvic viscera. The triangular perineal membrane spans the anterior pelvis except for a passage for the vagina and urethra.

Male Pelvic Floor

The endopelvic fascia, the levator ani, and the anal sphincter are also support features of the male pelvic floor and contribute to continence (Myers et al, 1998; Mikuma et al, 1998). In men, as in women, the endopelvic fascia contains collagen, elastin, and smooth muscle. In addition, in men this structure includes a reflection of retroperitoneal fascia with

TABLE 9-1   Condensations of the Female Endopelvic Fascia

LIGAMENT	DESCRIPTION
Pubourethral ligaments	Condensations of endopelvic fascia that bridge lower, inner surface of symphysis pubis and middle of urethra
Urethropelvic ligaments	Endopelvic fascia providing support for bladder neck and proximal urethra
Vesicopelvic ligaments	Fascial condensations that attach to pelvic side walls, providing lateral support to bladder base and pelvic side wall; loss of this fascial support creates a paravaginal wall defect
Cooper's ligament	Condensation of connective tissue at the top of the crural arch from the inferior iliac to the pubic bone; provides support and structure for the floor of the inguinal canal
Broad ligament	Triangular fold of the peritoneum; supports uterus and fallopian tube
Round ligament	Passes from superior lateral angle of the uterus to the internal inguinal ring and supports uterus and fallopian tube
Uterosacral ligament (sacrouterine ligament, or cardinal-uterosacral complex)	Two short cords that pass from cervix toward the sacrum; holds the cervix upward and backward and provides forward slant of uterus
Mackenrodt's ligament (cardinal ligament)	Condensation of uterosacral fascial complex; contributes to support of upper vagina, cervix, and uterus
Sacrospinous ligaments	Attaches ischial spine to lateral aspect of sacrum and coccyx; used for repair of severe uterine prolapse
Arcus tendineus fasciae pelvis—"white line"	Linear condensation extending from the pubic bone to the ischial spine; acts as important surgical landmark

an outer stratum enfolding the inner surface of the pelvic muscles, an intermediate stratum embedding the pelvic organs in a protective layer of compressible fat, and an inner stratum enfolding the bladder dome and part of the gastrointestinal tract. In men the levator ani, often subdivided into pubococcygeus and ileococcygeus, is the primary support for the lower urinary tract. Its U shape is similar to that seen in women, but larger and thicker, to meet the different physiologic demands on the male pelvis. Pelvic support also includes the anal sphincter and the perineal membrane, but there is some question as to whether the male anatomy includes a urogenital diaphragm as such.

Urinary Bladder

The urinary bladder is a hollow, muscular organ with a fixed base and a highly distensible body (also referred to as the detrusor muscle) (Figure 9-6) (Gray and Brown, 2002; Dixon and Gosling, 1987;

Elbadawi, 1996). It is further characterized by two inlets—the ureteral orifices of the paired UVJ and the urethral outlet. When empty, the distensible bladder walls collapse against its fixed base; as it fills, the bladder assumes a more ovoid or spheric shape as it rises toward the umbilicus. The bladder is anchored to the abdominal wall by the urachus, and the superior portion of the bladder body is covered by peritoneal fascia. In women this fascia also covers the uterus. Similar to the kidneys, the bladder is cushioned by surrounding retropubic and perivesical fat and connective tissue (Kabalin, 1998).

Arterial blood reaches the bladder by way of branches of the vesical and internal iliac arteries. Two vascular structures are encountered when a patient undergoes a cystectomy, the lateral and posterior pedicles. The pedicles are formed by the lateral and posterior vesical ligaments in men and the cardinal and uterosacral ligaments in women. They

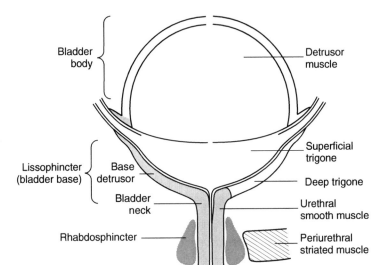

Figure 9-6 Urinary bladder with its fixed base and distensible body (detrusor muscle). (From Doughty DB: *Urinary and fecal incontinence: nursing management,* ed 2, St Louis, 2000, Mosby.)

contain a venous plexus that ultimately drains into the internal iliac vein. Lymphatic channels in the bladder drain into external iliac nodes, although some channels may empty into the obturator or internal iliac nodes. In addition, lymphatics from the bladder base and the trigone muscle drain into the internal and common iliac nodes.

Microscopically, the bladder wall is composed of four histologic layers. The lumen is lined with a transitional cell epithelium or uroepithelium that prevents the resorption of urine and is arranged in a manner whereby the cells thin out as the bladder fills, from a thickness of from five to seven deep to a single cell depth. The uroepithelium also manufactures a covering of glycosaminoglycan-rich mucus that protects the mucosa from irritants in the urine. Beneath the uroepithelium, the lamina propria contains connective tissues, arteries, and veins. The lamina propria is loosely connected to the uroepithelium but tightly attached to the muscular tunic of the bladder. The smooth muscle bundles of the detrusor are arranged in a characteristic, complex meshwork arrangement, unlike the longitudinal or circular layers typical of the bowel. Detrusor smooth muscle contains collagen and elastin, providing the structural integrity or memory needed for effective micturition. Excessive collagen deposition is one characteristic of some lower

urinary tract disorders, such as denervation. This leads to bladder trabeculation and compromised contractility. The resulting comparative rigidity of the bladder wall can adversely affect upper urinary tract urine production and drainage. The exterior layer of the bladder is composed of fibroelastic connective tissues forming an adventitia.

Arterial blood reaches the bladder from the superior, inferior, and medial vesical arteries, and branches of the obturator, inferior gluteal, or internal iliac arteries. In the female, branches of the uterine and vaginal arteries also provide arterial blood to the bladder. In contradistinction to the upper tract, the venous drainage of the bladder does not mirror arterial supply. The bladder veins drain into the plexus of Santorini and thence into the inferior hypogastric vein. The lymphatic channels of the bladder drain into the external iliac, hypogastric, and common iliac nodes.

Urethra

The female urethra follows a short, straight course compared to the male (Ashton-Miller, Howard, and DeLancey, 2001; Sampselle and DeLancey, 1998), originating at the bladder neck and running at an approximately 16-degree angle for 3.5 to 5.5 cm, and terminating above the vaginal vestibule. The urethral lumen, like the bladder, is lined with epithelium that secretes protective mucus. A rich network of arteries, veins, and lymphatics, as well as layers of striated and smooth muscle that is densest at the middle third, characterizes the urethral submucosa. The lower two thirds are contiguous with the vagina, which shares the striated and smooth muscle in this area with the urethral submucosa. The entire length of the female urethra acts as a sphincter mechanism, providing continence during bladder filling as well as a urine conduit for micturition.

The male urethra is divided into proximal and distal portions, with a combined length of approximately 23 cm (Myers et al, 1998). The proximal urethra functions as a sphincter mechanism, not unlike the whole length of the female urethra. The distal urethra has no continence role; it is a conduit for urine and semen. The proximal urethra originates at the bladder neck and is surrounded by the prostate. The verumontanum elevates the floor of the prostatic urethra before it tapers into a membranous segment 2 to 2.5 cm in length, extending from the prostatic apex through the pelvic floor at a point sometimes referred to as the urogenital diaphragm. At the termination of the membranous urethra, the distal urethra begins. It comprises the bulbous urethra, the pendulous urethra, the fossa navicularis and the meatus. Anatomically, the male urethra is composed of an epithelial lining, submucosal vascular and lymphatic networks (lamina propria), and outer adventitia. Striated and smooth muscle in the proximal urethral wall contributes to the male sphincter mechanism. The wall of the distal urethra does not contain such muscle.

Branches of the pudendal artery in men and the vaginal artery in women supply arterial blood to the urethra (Gray and Brown, 2002). The deep dorsal vein drains venous blood in men. The pelvic venous plexus drains venous blood in women. The urethra's lymphatic channels drain into the superficial and deep inguinal nodes and the hypogastric, the obturator, and the internal and external iliac nodes.

Continence Physiology

Three factors are primarily responsible for urinary continence: anatomic integrity of the urinary sys-

tem, control of the detrusor muscle, and competence of the urethral sphincter mechanism (Gray and Brown, 2002; Gray, 2000). A particularly common cause of the urinary incontinence seen by the wound, ostomy, and continence (WOC) nurse is an interruption of the anatomic integrity of the urinary system due to surgical intention, congenital ectopia, or fistulas.

The anatomy of the urinary system may be conceptualized as a single tube, originating in the nephron and extending to the urethral meatus. Urinary continence relies on this tube or tract maintaining its anatomic integrity so that urine entering the collecting duct within the renal parenchyma is delivered to the bladder through a single, antegrade pathway. Refer to Chapter 10 for detailed descriptions of the causes and the pathophysiology of surgically created urinary diversion, or fistulas associated with interruption of this anatomic integrity and the subsequent extraurethral urinary incontinence.

Urinary continence also requires volitional control of the detrusor muscle (Steers, 1998). This control is the result of the complex coordination between multiple centers within the brain, brainstem, spinal cord, and peripheral nerves, and also the unique characteristics of the detrusor muscle itself.

Bladder function is modulated by several areas of the brain (DeGroat, 2000). A detrusor motor area is found in the superomedial area of each frontal lobe. Areas of the brain modulating detrusor function include the thalamus, the extrapyramidal nervous system in the basal ganglia and cerebellum, and the hypothalamus. Together these areas mediate inhibition of the detrusor reflex to forestall premature or overactive detrusor contractions until voluntary urination. The ability to inhibit detrusor contractions is compromised by injury to any of these areas, resulting in detrusor hyperreflexia and the potential for urge incontinence.

Three areas in the brainstem are particularly significant to bladder function (Steers, 1998). The periaqueductal gray matter serves as a central coordinating center for messages between the brain and the spinal cord. In addition, a micturition center in the pons coordinates detrusor and striated sphincter responses to bladder filling and micturition. Under the influence of this center, the urethral sphincter relaxes during micturition and contracts during bladder filling. Finally a collection of neurons in the dorsolateral tegmentum of the brainstem (the l region) facilitates bladder filling and storage.

Neurons in the sympathetic and parasympathetic nervous systems affect detrusor control through the spinal cord (Steers, 1998). Bladder storage is promoted by sympathetic neurons at spinal levels T10 to L2. Under the influence of modulatory centers in the brainstem and brain, β_3-adrenergic receptors in the detrusor muscle are stimulated by these nerves, promoting relaxation, filling, and storage. Excitation of α-adrenergic receptors in the proximal urethra and bladder neck causes urethral closure and is postulated to inhibit detrusor contractions by reflex pathways in the spine. Micturition is promoted by stimulation of the parasympathetic nervous system. Parasympathetic neurons are located within sacral spinal segments S_{2-4}. The stimulation of these neurons under the influence of modulatory areas in the brain and brainstem causes detrusor contraction and sphincter relaxation. Damage to these neurons causes paralysis or areflexia of the detrusor muscle and urinary retention.

The peripheral nerves relay messages from the spinal cord to the bladder. The lumbar sympathetic nerves primarily provide sympathetic stimuli to the bladder. Parasympathetic stimuli reach the bladder by way of the pelvic plexus. These nerves contain afferent (i.e., sensory) and efferent (i.e., motor) axons communicating with the central nervous system regarding urine volume in the bladder and bladder wall status. Neurotransmitters relay messages from bladder to brain by way of the spinal cord and the brainstem (Steers, 1998; DeGroat, 2000), providing the continuous communication needed for conscious control over voiding. The influence on bladder function of neurotransmitters in the brain is not thoroughly understood. Animal research suggests that the primary neurotransmitter in the brain may be glutamic acid. Serotonin, gamma amino butyric acid, dopamine, acetylcholine, adenosine triphosphate (ATP), and nitric oxide are also thought to be involved. In the spinal cord and the peripheral nerves, preganglionic nerve synapses respond to acetylcholine, with receptors characterized as nicotinic rather than muscarinic like those of the bladder wall.

Characteristics of the detrusor muscle itself also contribute to continence (Gray, 2000; Steers, 1998). For example the smooth muscle of the bladder wall contains many more nerve receptors than smooth muscle bundles within the ureter or gastrointestinal system. They also lack the gap junctions characteristic of the gastrointestinal tract. Gap junctions allow communication between smooth muscle cells that are independent of the nervous input that is critical for peristalsis, whereas neurological regulation of smooth muscle is critical to the infrequent, voluntary detrusor contractions needed for urinary continence.

Neurotransmitters within the bladder wall also regulate continence (Steers, 1998; DeGroat, 2000; Hegde and Eglen, 1999). The primary excitatory neurotransmitter of the detrusor is acetylcholine, which acts upon specific receptors within the bladder wall to cause muscle contraction under nervous control. Five types of muscarinic receptor have been identified. The detrusor muscle contains only two types: M_2 and M_3. M_3 receptors account for about 20% of the cholinergic receptors within the bladder wall, but they are directly responsible for the volitional detrusor contraction critical to micturition. In contrast, M_2 receptors account for 80% of the cholinergic receptors in the bladder wall; they influence detrusor muscle tone by inhibiting the relaxing effects of adrenergic receptor stimulation. Norepinephrine acts on β_3-adrenergic receptors in the bladder wall to promote detrusor relaxation and bladder filling. ATP is found in nonadrenergic, non-cholinergic receptors. ATP facilitates detrusor muscle contraction, but its role is secondary to acetylcholine. Additional neurotransmitters also influence bladder filling and micturition; they include vasoactive intestinal polypeptide, substance P, CGRP, and nitric oxide synthase. These neurotransmitters control afferent signals such as urgency, pressure, or pain.

Sphincter Mechanism Competence

Typically the urethral sphincter is defined only by its muscular components (Gray and Brown, 2002; Gray, 2000; Staskin et al, 1985), with an internal sphincter at the bladder neck and an external sphincter in the mid- and distal urethra in women and the membranous urethra in men. This view overlooks the important compressive elements of the sphincter, and the rhabdosphincter. The urethral sphincter is best conceptualized as a single mechanism with elements of compression and tension and support structures.

The compressive elements of the sphincter include a soft urethral mucosa, mucus produced by this epithelium, and the vascular cushion formed by the lamina propria (Staskin et al, 1985; Zinner, Sterling, and Ritter, 1980). Flexibility in the epithelial mucosa of the urethra is needed to maintain a watertight seal for continence. The flexibility of this mucosa is shown by the way it prevents urine leakage around a catheter, even though the catheter deforms the urethra and allows passage of urine. Mucosal secretions increase the surface tension of the urethral wall, filling the gaps when the epithelium closes after urination, thus adding to sphincter compression. The contribution of mucus to surface tension is significant. The vascular cushion of the lamina propria is another compressive element of the urethral sphincter. The lamina propria, with its network of arteries and veins, is a noncompressible cushion of blood that transmits closing forces on the urethra, including abdominal pressure and tension from the muscular elements of the sphincter.

However, urethral compression by itself does not prevent urinary leakage during exertion or in an upright position. Sphincter closure under stress requires active contraction of smooth and striated muscle in the urethral wall. In men, smooth muscle bundles surround the bladder neck, comprising the internal sphincter (see Figure 9-6) (Steers, 1998). In addition to continence, this mechanism prevents retrograde ejaculation of semen into the bladder.

Other smooth muscle bundles arranged longitudinally extend into the prostatic urethra and contribute to sphincter closure. Located within the membranous urethra, the rhabdosphincter is a set of specialized C-shaped skeletal muscle fibers (Pannek and Senge, 1998), exclusively slow twitch (type 1) in nature, that maintain for prolonged periods the tone needed for continence between episodes of urination. Periurethral striated muscle also contributes to urethral closure in both men and women (Mostwin and Burnett, 1997). The periurethral striated muscles combine both slow and rapid twitch fibers to provide further protection in response to intense physical exertion or sudden increase in abdominal pressure.

Tension elements of the female urethral sphincter are combined from smooth and skeletal muscle (Ashton-Miller, Howard, and DeLancey, 2001; Sampselle and Delancey, 1998; Staskin et al, 1985). Longitudinal smooth muscle bundles starting at the base of the bladder extend nearly the entire urethral length. There is also circularly arranged smooth muscle at the bladder neck, and a rhabdosphincter is located in the middle third of the female urethra. Sometimes this structure is called the sphincter urethrae. The compressor urethrae, originating at the perineal membrane, and the urethrovaginal sphincter, encircling the vaginal wall, contain mainly slow twitch fibers with some fast twitch elements and are also part of the female sphincter mechanism.

Support of the urethra and the bladder base is vital for continence, especially in women (Ashton-Miller, Howard, and DeLancey, 2001; Sampselle and DeLancey, 1998). The levator ani, the endopelvic fascia, the perineal membrane, and the anal sphincter provide support to bladder base and urethra, in particular keeping the bladder base in the optimal intraabdominal position for urethral closure, under muscular control by the sphincter mechanism, and with transmission of abdominal forces to the urethral lumen. Descent of the bladder base can result in stress incontinence (sphincter incompetence) even if the intrinsic muscular elements of the sphincter are functional (Staskin et al, 1985).

Urethral smooth muscle is under neurologic control. Individual muscle cells respond to excitation from local nerve receptors (Steers, 1998), α-adrenergic receptors found in the smooth muscle of the bladder neck and proximal urethra in both men and women. Unlike detrusor smooth muscle, stimulation of receptors in urethral smooth muscle contracts the muscle bundles and results in urethral sphincter closure. The cholinergic innervation of urethral smooth muscle possibly aids urethral funneling during micturition. The rhabdosphincter, or sphincter urethrae in women, is dually innervated, with somatic innervation from the pudendal nerve and sympathetic receptors from the inferior hypogastric plexus. The pudendal nerve, arising in the sacral spinal cord at levels S_{2-4}, provides somatic innervation to the periurethral and pelvic floor muscles, including the levator ani. Contraction during bladder filling and relaxation during urination are reflexive responses occurring under the influence of the brainstem micturition center, which can be overridden, for instance by abrupt interruption of micturition caused by pelvic floor and periurethral striated muscle contraction that takes place if a person is startled during urination. The sensorimotor nucleus of the brain mediates voluntary control of the periurethral and the pelvic floor muscle, signaling the pelvic muscles through the pyramidal tracts of the spine.

Summary of Bladder Filling and Micturition

From the factors reviewed above, it is possible to briefly summarize the process of bladder filling and storage, as well as micturition. Bladder filling is characterized by detrusor muscle relaxation and closure of the sphincter mechanism. Several areas in the brain and brainstem modulate detrusor muscle relaxation, and this neural input is expressed at the level of the spinal cord as sympathetic predominance communicated to the bladder by way of the inferior hypogastric and pudendal nerves. At the level of the detrusor muscle, muscarinic receptors remain quiet, while norepinephrine acts at β_3-adrenergic receptors promoting bladder filling and storage. At the level of the sphincter mechanism, norepinephrine acts prima-

rily at a-1 receptors within the urethral smooth muscle and the rhabdosphincter to increase tone and urethral closure, and acetylcholine acts at nicotinic receptors within the rhabdosphincter and the periurethral striated muscles to increase muscle tone and oppose urine loss.

During micturition, the brain and brainstem release their inhibitory influence over the bladder by means of unknown mechanisms, and the pontine micturition center ensures coordination between detrusor muscle contraction and sphincter mechanism relaxation. When the detrusor contraction achieves an adequate intravesical pressure, the urethra opens and urinary flow begins. This contraction typically persists for some seconds after micturition ceases, and ideally after urine is completely evacuated from the vesicle. The sphincter mechanism again closes, the detrusor muscle returns to a relaxed state, and the cycle begins anew.

PHYSIOLOGY OF URINARY DIVERSION AND RECONSTRUCTION

As discussed previously, the urinary system is capable of transporting and storing urine over a prolonged period of time, and of evacuating urine under voluntary control (Gray and Brown, 2002; Gray, 2000; Steers, 1998). Reconstructive surgery of the urinary system, whether its purpose is to create an incontinent urinary conduit, a continent diversion, or an orthotopic neobladder, typically adds or substitutes a segment of the gastrointestinal tract to the lower urinary tract, permanently altering function of both organ systems. While the character and magnitude of this alteration varies based on the segment of bowel or stomach selected for incorporation into the urinary stream, and on the disease process leading to surgery, a review of known physiologic alterations associated with incorporation of segments of the gastrointestinal tract into the urinary system will aid the WOC nurse who routinely manages patients who have undergone augmentation, diversion, or substitution procedures.

Smooth Muscle Contractility

The smooth muscle of the lower urinary tract possesses several properties that allow volitional control over micturition, including a nearly 1:1 ratio of nerves to muscle cells and the absence of gap junctions allowing the peristaltic type of contractions (Gray and Brown, 2002; Gray, 2000; Steers 1998). However, the smooth muscle of the stomach, as well as of the large and small bowel, differs significantly from the detrusor. For example, the large and small bowels are cylindrical in shape and lined with multi-unit smooth muscle cells that produce peristaltic contractions in response to distention. As a result, reconstruction using a cylindrical segment of small or large bowel results in bolus contractions as it fills with urine. In order to avoid this outcome, surgeons detubularize the bowel whenever they seek to create a reservoir for urine (see Chapter 10) (Pannek and Senge, 1998; McDougal, 2002b). Specifically, they reconstruct the bowel so that it approximates an ovoid or spherical reservoir rather than a cylinder. This maneuver allows an increase in reservoir volume that is nearly half again as large as that achieved by attaching a cylindrical bowel segment. Although detubularization does increase reservoir capacity, it does not override the bowel segment's ability to mount and propagate a peristaltic contraction. In order to minimize the efficiency of these contractions, surgeons will split the bowel along its antimesenteric border. Initially this interrupts peristaltic contractions, although low-pressure contractions recur in some patients (Pope et al, 1998).

The selection of bowel also influences smooth muscle contractility (McDougal, 2002b). The smooth muscle of the colon is capable of very high-pressure bolus contractions, whereas the smooth muscle of the ileum typically mounts lower-pressure contractions. Selection of a segment of the stomach avoids bolus contractions, but a pattern of recurring low-pressure contractions is observed, reflecting its role as the "pacemaker" of the gastrointestinal tract.

Metabolic Implications

Because of its essential role in nutrition, isolation of the bowel from the fecal stream alters metabolism in several relevant ways. The most common metabolic sequelae associated with urinary system reconstruction are metabolic acidosis, electrolyte abnormalities, altered sensorium, bone demineralization or growth retardation, frequency-dysuria syndrome, vitamin deficiency, and altered absorption of specific drugs.

When exposed to urine, both the colon and small bowel secrete sodium and bicarbonate and resorb ammonia, ammonium, and hydrogen and chloride ions (Mundy, 1999; Stein et al, 1998). The ileum also resorbs potassium, and the colon absorbs a smaller amount. As a result, mild metabolic acidosis affects approximately 50% of all patients undergoing augmentation enterocystoplasty, continent urinary diversion, or orthoptic neobladder surgery. Although mild, chronic metabolic acidosis is considered clinically relevant because it is associated with osteomalacia or bone demineralization.

The mechanisms leading to osteomalacia are not entirely understood, but it is hypothesized that ammonium ion and/or potassium may play important roles (Mundy, 1999; Stein et al, 1998). Several mechanisms contribute to demineralization:

- Loss of calcium from the bones in an attempt to buffer serum pH
- Increased sulphate absorption from the gut leading to further calcium loss
- Impaired hydroxylation of the metabolically active form of vitamin D (1,25 dihydroxycholecalciferol)
- Activation of osteoclasts, increasing bone resorption

The effects of osteomalacia are particularly relevant in children, since it is associated with growth retardation (Mundy, 1999), and they may be particularly undesirable for adult women with osteoporosis. Fortunately they can be reversed by early treatment of acidosis by alkalinizing agents such as sodium bicarbonate (Stein et al, 1998).

In contrast to the bowel, incorporation of the stomach into a urinary diversion or augmentation enterocystoplasty is associated with hypochloremic, hypokalemic alkalosis. Alkalosis is rarely a problem for patients with normal renal function, but it may be severe in children with renal insufficiency and may lead to respiratory depression, altered mentation, and seizures. The condition is reversed by administration of sodium chloride, arginine hydrochloride, and potassium chloride.

Gastrocystoplasty, or augmentation of the bladder with a segment of stomach, has been associated with a hematuria-dysuria syndrome characterized by painful bladder spasm, urgency, suprapubic or periurethral pain, gross hematuria varying from bright red to dark brown and without underlying infection, erosion and irritation of the perineal skin, and dysuria. The reported occurrence of the syndrome following gastrocystoplasty varies from 6% to 36% (Chadwick et al, 2000; Nguyen et al, 1993), but its etiology and pathophysiology remain unknown.

Incorporation of the jejunum is associated with electrolyte imbalances including hyponatremia, hypochloremia, azotemia, and metabolic acidosis (McDougal, 2002b). Imbalances are more severe when the proximal jejunum is incorporated into urinary reconstruction and may lead to nausea, vomiting, diarrhea, weakness, and fever. The incidence of clinically relevant electrolyte imbalances varies from 25% to 75%, leading most surgeons to avoid using this segment altogether (McDougal, 2002b).

Vitamin B_{12} is absorbed from the terminal ileum and stored in the liver for up to 24 months. Incorporation of the ileum in reconstructive urologic surgery may impair the body's ability to absorb and maintain adequate levels of vitamin B_{12}, leading to anemia and neurologic abnormalities. It has been postulated that the magnitude of risk is related to the total length of terminal ileum isolated from the fecal stream (McDougal, 2002b), but length of ileum alone (Ganesan et al, 2002) or preservation of the terminal 15 cm of ileum (Fujisawa et al, 2000) do not prevent this significant sequela. Because of the liver's ability to store vitamin B_{12} over a prolonged period, it is important to monitor patients for deficiency for at least 2 years following surgery, and to supplement by means of monthly injections when indicated.

Magnesium deficiencies, drug intoxication or altered ammonia metabolism may lead to an altered sensorium (McDougal, 2002b). In severe cases, an ammoniagenic coma may occur, particularly in patients with underlying liver disease such as cirrhosis. The metabolism and actions of drugs also may be altered, particularly agents that are absorbed from the gastrointestinal tract and excreted in their original formulation by the kidney. Examples include phenytoin, cisplatin, methotrexate, and vinblastine.

CONCLUSION

Basic knowledge of the urinary system is important for the clinician when caring for and managing the person with urinary system disorders that may lead to a urinary diversion. The urinary system is complex, and an understanding of structure and function will provide necessary information to provide care to the patient with a urinary diversion.

SELF-ASSESSMENT EXERCISES

Questions

1. Kidneys are influenced by a hormone that affects the volume of water in urine and the thirst reflex. This hormone is:
   a. Aldosterone.
   b. Adrenaline.
   c. ADH.
   d. Estrogen.
2. What is the active process called in which urine is transported from the kidneys to the bladder?
3. The primary neurotransmitter of the detrusor that acts on specific receptors within the bladder wall to cause muscle contraction is:
   a. Acetylcholine.
   b. Norepinephrine.
   c. Dopamine.
   d. Serotonin.
4. Neurotransmitters relay messages from the bladder to the brain by way of _____ and _____.
5. A common metabolic complication that can occur with urinary system reconstruction is:
   a. Metabolic alkalosis.
   b. Vitamin D absorption.
   c. Urinary retention.
   d. Metabolic acidosis.

6. What is the hormone that stimulates bone marrow to produce red blood cells?

7. Name the three forces that affect the GFR.

8. The glomerular capillaries filter approximately 180 L of fluid per day.
   True _____ False _____

9. List the three factors responsible for urinary continence.

10. Osteomalacia is associated with chronic metabolic acidosis.
    True _____ False _____

11. Detublarization of the bowel is primarily done to decrease peristaltic contractions in the reservoir for urine.
    True _____ False _____

12. The entire length of the female urethra functions as a sphincter mechanism to provide continence, whereas the male urethra has two functions: the proximal urethra functions as a sphincter mechanism, but the distal portion has no continence role.
    True _____ False _____

13. What is the function of the distal urethra of the male?

Answers

1. c
2. Peristalsis
3. a
4. Spinal cord and brainstem
5. d
6. Erythropoietin
7. Hydrostatic, filtration, and plasma oncotic pressure
8. True
9. Anatomic integrity of the urinary system, control of the detrusor, and compliance of the urethral sphincter mechanism
10. True
11. False; detubularization of the bowel is done to increase the capacity in the reservoir for urine.
12. True
13. The distal urethra of the male acts as a conduit for urine and semen.

REFERENCES

Ashton-Miller JA, Howard D, DeLancey JO: The functional anatomy of the female pelvic floor and stress continence control system, *Scand J Urol Nephrol* 207:1-7, 2001.

Brooks JD: Anatomy of the lower urinary tract and male genitalia. In Walsh PC et al, editors: *Campbell's urology*, Philadelphia, 1998, WB Saunders.

Chadwick PJ et al: Long-term follow-up of the hematuria-dysuria syndrome, *J Urol* 164(3 Pt 2):921-923, 2000.

DeGroat WC: Innervation of the lower urinary tract: an overview, 20th Annual Meeting of the Society for Urodynamics and Female Urology, Dallas, Tx, May 1, 2000.

Dixon J, Gosling J: Structure and innervation in the human. In Torrens M, Morrison JFB, editors: *The physiology of the lower urinary tract*, London 1987, Springer-Verlag.

Elbadawi A: Functional anatomy of the organs of micturition, *Urol Clin North Am* 23:177-210, 1996.

Feldman D: Vitamin D, parathyroid hormone, and calcium: a complex regulatory network, *Am J Med* 107:637-639, 1999.

Fujisawa M et al: Long-term assessment of serum vitamin B_{12} concentrations in patients with various types of orthotopic intestinal neobladder, *Urology* 56(2):236-240, 2000.

Ganesan T et al: Vitamin B_{12} malabsorption following bladder reconstruction or diversion with bowel segments, *ANZ J Surg* 72(7):479-482, 2002.

Giebisch G, Klein-Robbenhaar G: Recent studies on the characterization of loop diuretics, *J Cardiovasc Pharmacol* 22(Suppl 3):S1-10, 1993.

Giebisch G, Malnic G, Berliner RW: Control of renal potassium excretion. In Brenner BM, editor: *The kidney*, ed 6, Philadelphia, 2000, WB Saunders.

Gray ML, Brown KC: Genitourinary system. In Thompson JT et al, editors: *Mosby's clinical nursing*, ed 5, St Louis, 2002, Mosby.

Gray M: Physiology of voiding. In Doughty DB, editor: *Urinary and fecal incontinence: nursing management*, ed 2, St Louis, 2000, Mosby.

Guyton AC: *Medical physiology*, Philadelphia, 1996, WB Saunders.

Hayashi M: Physiology and pathophysiology of acid-base homeostasis in the kidney, *Intern Med* 37:221-225, 1998.

Hegde SS, Eglen RM: Muscarinic receptor subtypes modulating smooth muscle contractility in the urinary bladder, *Life Sci* 64:419-428, 1999.

Kabalin JN: Anatomy of the retroperitoneum, kidneys and ureters. In Walsh PC et al, editors: *Campbell's urology*, Philadelphia, 1998, WB Saunders.

Kramer SA: Vesicoureteral reflux. In Kelalis PP, King LR, Belman AB, editors: *Clinical pediatric urology*, Philadelphia, 1992, WB Saunders.

Ludat K et al: Complete correction of renal anemia by recombinant human erythropoietin, *Clin Nephrol* 53 (Suppl):S42-49, 2000.

Marunka Y: Hormonal and osmotic regulation of NaCl transport in renal distal nephron epithelium, *Jpn J Physiol* 47:499-511, 1997.

McDougal WS: The kidney. In Gillenwater JY et al: *Adult pediatric urology*, ed 4, Philadelphia, 2002a, Lippincott, Williams & Wilkins.

McDougal WS: Use of intestinal segments and urinary diversion. In Walsh PC et al, editors: *Campbell's urology*, ed 5, Philadelphia, 2002b, WB Saunders.

Mikuma N et al: Magnetic resonance imaging of the male pelvic floor: the anatomical configuration and dynamic movement in healthy men, *Neurol Urodynamics* 17:591-597, 1998.

Mostwin JL, Burnett AL: Anatomic aspects of urinary incontinence. In O'Donnell PD: *Urinary incontinence*, St Louis, 1997, Mosby.

Mundy AR: Metabolic complications of urinary diversion, *Lancet* 353(9167):1813-1814, 1999.

Myers RP et al: Anatomy of radical prostatectomy as defined by magnetic resonance imaging, *J Urol* 159:2148-2158, 1998.

Noland LR: Renal system. In Thompson JT et al: *Mosby's clinical nursing*, ed 5, St Louis, 1997, Mosby.

Nguyen DH et al: The syndrome of dysuria and hematuria in pediatric urinary reconstruction with stomach, *J Urol* 150:707, 1993.

Pannek J, Senge T: History of urinary diversion, *Urol Int* 60(1):1-10, 1998.

Pope JC IV et al: Augmenting the augmented bladder: treatment of the contractile bowel segment, *J Urol* 160(3 Pt 1):854-857, 1998.

Rosol TJ et al: Adrenal gland: structure, function, and mechanisms of toxicity, *Toxicol Pathol* 29:41-48, 2001.

Sampselle CA, Delancey JOL: Anatomy of female continence, *JWOCN* 25:63-74, 1998.

Staskin DR et al: Pathophysiology of stress incontinence, *Clin Obstet Gynecol* 12:357-388, 1985.

Steers WD: Physiology and pharmacology of the bladder and urethra. In Walsh PC et al, editors: *Campbell's urology*, ed 7, Philadelphia, 1998, WB Saunders.

Stein R et al: Whole-body potassium and bone mineral density up to 30 years after urinary diversion, *Br J Urol* 82(6):798-803, 1998.

Suki WN, Lederer ED, Rouse D: Renal transport of calcium, magnesium and phosphate. In Brenner BM, editor: *The kidney*, ed 6, Philadelphia, 2000, WB Saunders.

Tisher CG, Madsen KM: Anatomy of the kidney. In Brenner BM, editor: *The kidney*, ed 6, Philadelphia, 2000, WB Saunders.

Valtin H: *Renal function: mechanisms preserving fluid and solute balance in health*, ed 3, Boston, 1995, Little-Brown.

Vander AJ: *Renal physiology*, ed 5, New York, 1995, McGraw-Hill.

Weiss RM: Physiology and pharmacology of the renal pelvis and ureter. In Walsh PC et al, editors: *Campbell's urology*, Philadelphia, 1998, WB Saunders.

Wilcox CS: Diuretics. In Brenner BM, editor: *The kidney*, ed 6, Philadelphia, 2000, WB Saunders.

Zinner NR, Sterling AM, Ritter R: Role of inner urethral softness in urinary incontinence, *Urology* 16:115-117, 1980.

Urinary Diversions: Surgical Interventions

NANCY TOMASELLI and DAVID E. MCGINNIS

OBJECTIVES

1. List the risk factors for bladder cancer.
2. Describe the indications for urinary diversions.
3. Explain the methods of treating superficial and invasive bladder cancer.
4. Discuss the indications for urinary diversion in patients with prostate cancer, interstitial cystitis, refractory radiation cystitis, and neurogenic bladder.
5. Discuss the indications, surgical procedures, and postoperative care of the patient undergoing the following procedures: nephrostomy, ureteral diversion, ureteroenterocutaneous diversions (ileal conduit, colon conduit), and bladder level diversions (cystotomy tube, vesicostomy).
6. Describe the indications, surgical procedure, and postoperative care for the patient receiving an Indiana pouch and a neobladder.
7. List complications related to ureteroenterocutaneous and continent diversions.

INTRODUCTION

Urinary diversions have been performed since the mid-1800s. They are created to divert the urine out of the body through an alternative route and are named for the structure that is used to create the diversion. For example, an ileal conduit is named for the ileum used to form the passageway for urine to exit from the body. Initially, urinary diversions involved bringing the urinary drainage system (ureter, bladder) to the skin (i.e., ureterostomy, vesicostomy), or internally to the sigmoid colon (i.e., ureterosigmoidostomy). Ureterostomy and vesicostomy are no longer considered procedures of choice because of the difficulties in creating a budded stoma, stenosis of the stoma, and problems with stoma location and pouch application. Ureterosigmoidostomy is rarely performed because of the high incidence of pyelonephritis and colon cancer associated with it.

Using a segment of bowel to improve the quality of the stoma, the ileal conduit, was popularized in the 1950s by Bricker. This procedure, which allowed for a budded stoma on a flat abdominal plane, became the procedure of choice and enhanced patients' quality of life.

Early experience with continent diversions in the 1950s by Gilchrist and the 1960s by Koch were somewhat unsuccessful as a result of metabolic and continence issues. Modifications of the Gilchrist procedure, leading to the creation of an Indiana pouch and other variations, began in 1985. Interest in continent diversion procedures increased in the 1980s and 1990s, and has made continent diversion a commonly used technique in many hospitals. This renewed interest is attributed to improved surgical techniques and acceptance of clean intermittent catheterization and long-term complications of the ileal conduit. Continent diversions aim to improve cosmesis by either providing a small continent stoma (requiring catheterization instead of an external appliance), or anastomosing a reservoir to the urethra and allowing the patient to void by way of the urethra without any stoma at all (i.e., neobladder).

INDICATIONS FOR A URINARY DIVERSION

Diversion of the urine is required when the bladder must be bypassed or removed because of fistulous leakage of the urinary tract (often a temporary condition), or as a temporary measure after urologic procedures. Overall, it is rare for a permanent urinary diversion to be necessary when the bladder is being left in place.

The most common indication for a urinary diversion is bladder cancer. Other, less common, indications are prostate cancer, interstitial cystitis, neurogenic bladder, and refractory radiation cystitis. Occasionally a diversion is required because of exenteration for the treatment of adjacent cancers, such as rectal or cervical cancer.

Bladder Cancer

Incidence. Bladder cancer is the fourth most common cause of cancer death in American men. It is about three times more common in men than it is in women.

Risk Factors. There are several factors that increase the risk for bladder cancer. As far back as 1895, workers exposed to aniline dye developed bladder cancer years or decades after exposure. Aromatic amines have also been identified as causative agents for bladder cancer.

Cigarette smoking poses an even greater risk of bladder cancer. The increasing incidence of bladder cancer in women can be attributed to the fact that more women are smoking and working in environments where they are exposed to causative agents.

Artificial sweeteners, such as saccharine and cyclamates, have been implicated as carcinogens in animal studies. However, there is no significant evidence that they act as carcinogens in humans. Schistosomiasis has also been found to be a causative agent. The parasites lay eggs in the muscle wall of the bladder and intestine. In turn, the irritation the ova create on the bladder wall leads to squamous cell carcinoma. This infection is endemic to the Nile river valley and rarely seen in the United States.

Chronic irritation of the bladder can also cause squamous cell cancer. Patients with chronic indwelling Foley catheters as well as those whose bladders have been left in place along with creation of a urinary diversion are at greater risk for bladder cancer. This typically has a delayed onset of 10 to 15 years or more.

Large doses of phenacetin over a 10-year or greater period may cause a higher incidence of transitional cell carcinoma. The cancer usually occurs in the renal pelvis and ureters. Other analgesics have not been implicated. Cyclophosphamide has been identified as another causative agent. Patients treated with pelvic radiation have a higher incidence of transitional cell carcinoma of the bladder.

Bladder cancer has been noted to occur in familial clusters. However, it is unclear if this is due to the same environmental exposures or to some genetic predisposition.

Natural History. The course of transitional cell carcinoma of the bladder can have wide variability. The main issues with implications for bladder cancer are recurrences within the bladder or other parts of the urinary tract, and progression to metastasis. At one end of the spectrum are the superficial, low-grade cancers that are very indolent, and at the other end are high-grade, invasive cancers that are extremely lethal.

All cancers are categorized by histologic type, grade, and stage. About 95% of all bladder cancers are transitional cell carcinoma; the rest are either adenocarcinoma or squamous cell carcinoma. Transitional cell carcinomas are usually graded 1, 2, or 3. Grade is a description of the microscopic appearance of the cancer, but correlates with its potential for rapid growth, invasion, metastasis, and recurrence. Stage refers to the location of the cancer and a tumor, nodes, and metastasis, or TNM, system is usually used to describe it. The T stage is crucial for bladder cancer: T_0 and T_{cis} refer to superficial disease; T_1 means disease is borderline; and T_2, T_3, and T_4, mean disease has invaded into or through the bladder musculature.

Superficial bladder cancers mainly pose a problem of recurrence. About 70% of superficial cancers recur within the bladder if treated with biopsy alone. Progression to invasive disease only occurs in 10% to 15% of cases. Factors that increase the risk of recurrence and invasion include higher grade, larger tumors, multiple tumors, and nearby carcinoma in situ (Gillenwater et al, 1996).

Invasive bladder cancers pose a risk of progression. About 50% of invasive cancers already have metastatic disease at the time of diagnosis. Patients with metastatic bladder cancer have a dismal prognosis: the vast majority die of their cancers within 2 years.

Diagnosis. Bladder cancer is most commonly found during the evaluation of hematuria, either grossly visible or microscopic. When observed grossly, it is typically painless and "total," meaning that it is seen equally at the start to the end of each void. The standard urologic evaluation of hematuria includes an imaging study (i.e., computed tomography scan, renal/bladder ultrasound, or intravenous pyelogram), cystoscopy, and urinary cytology studies. Bladder cancer is usually identified by cystoscopy as a solid or polypoid lesion, or occasionally as a flat red patch in the bladder. Cytology studies are commonly not diagnostic, but occasionally may give the only sign of bladder cancer. Sometimes, bladder cancer is found in the evaluation of urinary tract infections or voiding symptoms, such as frequency and urgency.

When found with cystoscopy, the diagnosis must be established by biopsy, which is usually performed under anesthesia. The pathologic analysis of the biopsy will confirm the histologic type (typically transitional cell carcinoma). The pathology will also indicate the grade of the tumor and the depth of invasion, which are extremely important for management.

Management. The treatment of superficial bladder cancer is focused on monitoring for recurrences and the unusual case where the cancer progresses to invasive disease. Radical cystectomy and urinary diversion is rarely required for superficial disease; occasionally it is needed for diffuse, unresectable disease or cancer that does not respond to intravesical treatment (i.e., the placement of agents into the bladder with a catheter to treat the cancer and prevent recurrences). Carcinoma in situ is a more dangerous form of superficial cancer that can have a high risk of progression; disease that does not respond to intravesical therapy may necessitate cystectomy and diversion. Radical cystectomy and urinary diversion is the current standard of care for invasive bladder cancer. Alternatives to radical surgery, such as external beam radiation or combined chemotherapy and radiation, have not been shown to be as effective as radical surgery.

Prostate Cancer

Prostate cancer does not usually require a urinary diversion. However, if prostate cancer progresses, ureteral obstruction may occur as a result of lymph node involvement or local extension of the tumor into the base of the bladder. This may require management with a percutaneous nephrostomy or ureteral stent placement. Also, prostate cancer patients initially treated with radiation whose cancer recurs locally may, in rare cases, opt for surgical resection. Most postradiation surgery involves a radical prostatectomy, but sometimes cystoprostatectomy and urinary diversion are required. The cure rate of such salvage surgery is generally low.

Interstitial Cystitis

Interstitial cystitis is a painful disorder of unknown etiology affecting the bladder, the urethra, and the adjacent pelvic floor muscles. It is characterized by moderate to severe bladder and pelvic pain, nocturia, diurnal urinary frequency, and urgency. Ulceration or petechial hemorrhage may be present on endoscopic examination. Surgery is rarely indicated and is limited to patients with severe, debilitating symptoms that have failed to respond to all other available treatment options. Options for surgery include continent or incontinent urinary diversions, bladder augmentation, and orthotopic neobladder. There is some evidence that the same inflammatory process can later involve the urinary conduit. After surgery, patients may experience residual pelvic pain (Gray, Albo, and Huffstutler, 2002). For this reason, most urologists are reluctant to perform diversions for patients with interstitial cystitis.

Neurogenic Bladder

Neurogenic bladder is characterized by bladder dysfunction caused by lesions of the central or peripheral nervous systems. Conditions that may be present with neurogenic bladder include cerebrovascular accidents, multiple sclerosis, diabetic neuropathy, postsurgical (i.e., after such procedures as low anterior resection or radical hysterectomy) malignancy, infection (e.g., Lyme disease or encephalopathy), and trauma (i.e., head or spinal cord injury). If conservative therapies such as intermittent catheterization fail, a urinary diversion may be considered but is only rarely required. Most urologists would consider this the option of last resort, since it typically involves major surgery in a debilitated patient.

Refractory Radiation Cystitis

Individuals with incapacitating symptoms from radiation-induced damage to the bladder may require surgical intervention if they do not respond to conservative therapy. Radiation can damage sphincter or bladder muscular function and cause severe incontinence or urinary fistulas. A cystectomy and urinary diversion may be performed in some patients. Usually a simple conduit is performed rather than a continent diversion because of the higher risks in operating on radiated bowel. Many urologists use a section of bowel for the conduit that is most likely out of the field of radiation, such as transverse colon. In most cases, the bladder is removed at the time of surgery unless it seems excessively risky. If the bladder is not removed, it must be capable of draining any secretions; otherwise it requires catheterization to prevent infections (called pyocystis in a defunctionalized bladder and discussed later in this chapter).

TYPES OF URINARY DIVERSIONS

Diversion of urine can be performed by several techniques. A tube can be placed in the kidney (i.e., nephrostomy tube) or the bladder (i.e., suprapubic tube). Part of the urinary system can be brought out to the skin by creating a cutaneous diversion such as a pyelostomy, ureterostomy, or vesicostomy. The urinary system can also be diverted cutaneously by using a segment of the bowel (ileal or colon conduit, continent Indiana pouch, or orthotopic neobladder). Suprapubic and nephrostomy tubes can be used for either a temporary or a permanent diversion. Creating them is typically a low-risk procedure, but as permanent diversions they require high maintenance and have significant infectious risks. Pyelostomy, ureterostomy, and vesicostomy are rarely used in adults because they generally provide poor-quality stomas. In selected pediatric patients these procedures may be appropriate for temporary urinary diversion but are rarely intended for lifelong management of the urinary tract. The most common method of establishing a permanent urinary diversion involves the interposition of a segment of bowel to fashion the stoma. In incontinent diversions, an external appliance must constantly be worn to collect urine. In continent diversions a pouch is made of the bowel segment that can store urine as a substitute for the bladder.

Patients and their doctors often face a choice, among the permanent diversions, between an ileal conduit, a continent pouch, or a neobladder. The continent diversions require that there be sufficient healthy bowel and good renal function. The patient must be in good health, since the continent diversion typically requires a longer operative time. Continent diversions are more complex and therefore have a higher risk both of complications and of reoperation. The benefit of continent diversions is the improved cosmesis and, in the case of a neobladder, almost normal voiding function. Continent diversions require more maintenance by the patient, so good candidates must be highly motivated, have good manual dexterity and normal mental capacity, and be willing to do regular self-catheterization (Table 10-1).

Diversion of the Renal Pelvis: Nephrostomy Indications

A nephrostomy is most often performed because of ureteral obstruction such as a stone, a stricture,

TABLE 10-1   URINARY DIVERSIONS

Incontinent Urinary Diversions

TYPE	PROCEDURE	INDICATIONS	ADVANTAGES	CONTRAINDICATIONS/ DISADVANTAGES
General Issues				Requires external collection device
Cystostomy (suprapubic tube)	Tube/Foley placed directly into urinary bladder	Chronic bladder drainage Difficult urethral catheterization Contraindication to urethral catheterization	Smaller length of bowel required than continent ostomy, less surgery time Avoids urethral catheterization Decreases risk of urethral strictures, and urethral erosion	Urinary tract infections, stones Clogged catheters Increased risk of bladder cancer
Nephrostomy	Tube inserted percutaneously through the flank into renal pelvis	Urethral obstruction (stones, stricture, or malignancy) Diversion of urine from urinary fistulas Percutaneous treatment (temporary) of large renal calculi	Relieves obstruction Easily inserted under local anesthesia	Hemorrhage can occur during placement Obstruction can result from mineral encrustations inside tube Pain and infection can arise secondary to obstruction of nephrostomy tube
Ureterostomy	Ureters mobilized and brought to skin surface	Poor candidates for intestinal diversions		Difficult stoma creation and location Stomal stenosis
Ileal conduit	Segment of small intestine isolated, the proximal end closed, and the distal end brought out through an opening in the abdomen and used to create a stoma Ureters implanted into the segment	Invasive bladder cancer Congenital anomalies Neurogenic bladder Refractory interstitial cystitis Inability to manage a continent urostomy or a neobladder	Less prone to stenosis than the ureterostomy	Renal deterioration

	Description	Indications	Advantages	Disadvantages / Considerations
Colon conduit	Same as ileal conduit; the colon is used in place of the small intestine	Bladder cancer Neurogenic bladder Refractory interstitial cystitis Preexisting small bowel disease Small bowel damage by pelvic radiation		Renal deterioration Metabolic abnormalities
Uretero-sigmoidostomy	Ureters implanted into the intact sigmoid colon	Rarely indicated	Elimination of both stool and urine controlled by anal sphincter	Metabolic abnormalities Ureteral obstruction Pyelonephritis Malignancy
Vesicostomy	Bladder mucosa sutured to abdominal opening	Temporary bladder drainage for infants and young children	Easy access to bladder in infants	Poor-quality stoma Peristomal dermatitis Stomal stenosis Infection Stone formation

Continent Urinary Diversions

	Description	Indications	Advantages	Disadvantages / Considerations
General issues	A urinary reservoir is created from isolated intestinal segments, anastomosed to the ureters and a continent, catheterizable stoma attached to the abdominal wall.		No pouching system needed	Considerations: Requires increased surgery time Not appropriate for patients with: Significant renal insufficiency Bowel disease Prior bowel resections Bowel malignancy Inflammatory bowel disease Requires appropriate patient selection criteria Patient must be capable of self-intermittent catheterization Contraindications: Ulcerative colitis Pelvic radiation Colon cancer Progressive neurologic disorder Morbid obesity Stomal incontinence Possibility of difficult catheterization
Continent cutaneous diversion (Indiana, Florida, Miami, Mainz pouches)	Isolated, detubularized bowel segment is used to create reservoir; ureters implanted; a continent catheterizable channel created	Patients with: Bladder cancer Neurogenic bladder Refractory interstitial cystitis Children with: epispadias, cloacal exstrophy Physically able to undergo a lengthy surgery Adequate renal function	Presevation of continence No need for externally applied pouching system Discrete flush stoma	

Continued

TABLE 10-1   URINARY DIVERSIONS—cont'd

TYPE	PROCEDURE	INDICATIONS	ADVANTAGES	CONTRAINDICATIONS/ DISADVANTAGES
Continent Urinary Diversions—cont'd				
Mitrofanoff	Appendix is separated from the cecum, reversed and anastomosed to the reservoir in a non-refluxing fashion to create a reservoir; valve is constructed to attach reservoir to skin	Children with spina bifida, prune belly, exstrophy	Low complication rate Easy access for catheterization	Patient must be capable of self-catheterization
Kock pouch	Urine reservoir is created using small bowel with a proximal nipple and a distal nipple attached to the abdominal wall via a stoma. Urine is drained via stoma with intermittent catheterization.	Careful patient selection	No external pouching system	High (25%) nipple failure rate Complex surgical procedure Metabolic acidosis
Orthotopic neobladder	Reservoir made from segment of detubularized intestine attached to the urethra	Patients with: A cancer-free trigone and urethra A competent, unobstructed sphincter	No stoma Patient voids independently using native sphincter	Bladder tumors that extend into the trigone or proximal urethra Metabolic acidosis in 50% of patients Urinary calculi Stenosis of ureteral anastomosis Possible urinary retention

or malignancy. Occasionally one is used to divert urine away from a urinary fistula. Nephrostomies are also placed temporarily for the percutaneous treatment of large renal calculi.

Surgical Procedure. A nephrostomy tube is inserted through the flank into the renal pelvis and is performed percutaneously with radiologic guidance under local anesthesia. Urologists or interventional radiologists may place these tubes. There are a variety of tubes used for this procedure, including Foleys, Malecots, and locking catheters (e.g., Cope loop). Foleys and Malecots are usually large (18 to 24 Fr) and are typically used after percutaneous lithotripsy for large renal stones; their larger caliber is useful to allow evacuation of any residual stone fragments. When serving only for diversion, a small locking catheter (8 to 12 Fr) is used. This catheter has an internal string that runs from its tip to its hub. At the time of placement, the string is pulled to form a loop at the end of the catheter, and the string is tied at the hub to "lock" the loop in place. The string must be cut before such a locking catheter can be removed.

Postoperative Care. Immediately after placement of the nephrostomy tube, the patient should be monitored for hematuria and internal bleeding (i.e., perinephric hematoma). The tube should also be observed routinely for encrustation, which can be dislodged by rolling the tube between the fingers. Fluid intake (oral or intravenous) must be instituted to prevent obstruction from blood or encrustation, and tubes must be checked for patency when repositioning the patient. The tubes may be anchored in place with sutures, although this is not absolutely necessary for locking catheters, and secured with tape. Using proper technique with leg-bag and bedside drainage systems can reduce infection risks. Occasionally nephrostomy tubes require irrigation to wash out clots or ensure patency. The renal pelvis typically has a capacity of 5 to 15 ml, so only 5 to 10 ml should be used for irrigation. Irrigation should also be performed at low pressure; at high pressures there is extravasation of irrigant into the renal hilum or retroperitoneum, and the fluid is absorbed intravenously or by lymphatics.

Results. Nephrostomy tubes are a reliable method of relieving obstruction, and can easily be placed under local anesthesia even in seriously ill patients. By comparison, internal ureteral stents can be less reliable in relieving obstruction from malignancy, and their placement requires administration of a general anesthetic. The disadvantages of nephrostomy tubes are the need for external drainage and tube changes at 6- to 8-week intervals, as well as the complications listed in the following paragraph.

Complications. Hemorrhage can occur during nephrostomy placement because of the vascularity of the renal parenchyma. Although hematuria is common, significant bleeding from a chronic nephrostomy tube is rare. Obstruction may result from compression or angulation of the tube, or from mineral encrustations inside the tube. Pain and infection may occur secondary to obstruction of the nephrostomy tube.

Ureteral Diversions

Ureterostomy

Ureterostomies may still be considered for patients who are poor candidates for an ureteroenterocutaneous diversion. However, they are no longer considered the procedure of choice because of the difficulty in creating a bud stoma in a good location and the high incidence of stenosis. Although still rare, they are most frequently used as a temporary measure in pediatric patients.

Ureteroenterocutaneous Diversions

Ileal Conduit

Indications. Several factors must be considered when deciding between a continent and incontinent urinary diversion. This process can be challenging not only for the physician but for the patient as well. Benefits and risks must be weighed regarding the patient's malignancy, comorbidities, functional status, and personal preferences. Patient education is imperative to the success of either procedure.

Physician Considerations. Urinary conduits require that a section of bowel be "borrowed" to make a stoma and either a conduit or a pouch. Less bowel is needed to create an incontinent diversion. Therefore, for patients with decreased small bowel length from multiple bowel resections, congenital anomalies, or bowel diseases, incontinent diversions are the procedure of choice.

Bowel segments outside the irradiated bowel should be used, if possible, for patients who have had pelvic or abdominal radiation. However, even if irradiated bowel must be used, results have been encouraging for incontinent and continent diversions (Link and Lerner, 2001).

Continent diversions also entail more complex operations, requiring a longer time under anesthesia; they also have an increased risk of postoperative complications compared with ileal conduit procedures. In particular, the reoperation rate after continent diversion is significantly higher than after an ileal conduit.

Contraindications to continent diversion include significant renal insufficiency, and prior bowel resections or bowel disease such as bowel malignancy or inflammatory bowel disease.

Patient Considerations. Many patients with cancer suffer from situational depression that may impair their ability to make decisions regarding surgical options. It is unclear whether the depression makes the postoperative recovery more difficult (Eisenberger et al, 1999).

An incontinent diversion requires the use of an external collection device or appliance as opposed to a continent diversion, which requires a less costly dressing over the stoma. A change in body image occurs in both operations. To date, the literature is unclear as to how these diversions affect quality of life. However, studies have shown there is not a significant difference in overall satisfaction with body image or physical or sexual relations with incontinent and continent diversions (Krupski and Theodorescu, 2001).

Patients most often choose to have a continent diversion because of improved cosmesis: there is no need to wear an external appliance. In the case of neobladders there is not even a stoma, and the patient is able to void independently. Both of these factors contribute to an improved quality of life.

However, patients must accept the increased work that is required to maintain a continent diversion, including the need for clean intermittent catheterization.

In addition, patients' motivation and ability to master the skills required to manage the continent urostomy must be evaluated. Manual dexterity and mental status must be determined to be adequate if patients are to be candidates for intermittent self-catheterization. Patients who are unmotivated, or lacking in the mental capacity or manual dexterity to perform self-catheterization faithfully, should have an ileal conduit instead of a continent diversion.

Preoperative Considerations. The preoperative visit by the wound, ostomy, and continence/enterostomal therapy (WOC/ET) nurse is a critical component to the outcome for the patient. This visit provides the opportunity to educate the patient regarding the role of the WOC/ET nurse, assess physical and psychologic aspects, initiate patient teaching, and determine stoma site selection.

All patients undergoing a diversion will need preoperative bowel preparation. Most urologists will employ a 1- or 2-day regimen with a low residue diet, mechanical cleansing (e.g., with GoLytely, Fleet Phospho-soda, or the equivalent), and antibiotic cleansing (i.e., with neomycin and/or erythromycin).

Surgical Procedure. An ileal conduit is fashioned with a segment of ileum close to the ileocecal valve with an intact mesentery. The 12 to15 cm segment of ileum closest to the ileocecal valve are generally preserved, because of its importance in bile and vitamin B_{12} absorption. A 10- to 12-cm section of ileum is selected by palpating and transilluminating the mesentery of the ileum to confirm the presence of a good blood supply. Surgical staplers are used to divide and rejoin the bowel. The gap in the mesentery where the ileum is harvested is closed to prevent internal herniation. The proximal end of the ileal conduit is stapled closed and then sutured, so that the staples do not come in contact with urine. The distal end of the conduit is brought out onto the abdominal wall as the stoma, and any staples removed. The ureters are anastomosed to the ileum in a refluxing fashion. The stoma is constructed as an end or loop stoma. Usually an end stoma is employed. At the time of surgery, the stoma is created so that it protrudes out from the abdominal wall in a "rosebud" appearance (Figure 1-2). This facilitates fitting an external pouching system, providing protection to the skin from urine contact. For patients who are obese, the loop stoma or Turnbull loop (see Figure 8-4) is used, because the conduit is under tension as it brings the stoma out to the skin level. A Turnbull loop stoma preserves the blood supply to the stoma even though it is under tension, since there is intact mesentery both proximal and distal to the stoma, which is not under tension. The ureters are transplanted into the loop end conduit.

Postoperative Care. Ureteral stents are placed to maintain patency to protect the anastomoses of the ureters to the bowel segment. These stents exit the stoma and may be different lengths or colors to identify which tube is in which ureter. Typically they are left in place for 5 to 7 days. Care must be taken not to dislodge the stents when changing the ostomy appliance. A Foley catheter or closed suction drains may be used to drain the area of the ureteral anastomoses and pelvis. All tubes should be clearly labeled with separate drainage systems to monitor output.

The postoperative hospital course mainly involves return to normal bowel function and normal ambulation. A nasogastric tube is typically placed at the time of surgery and removed in 1 to 3 days when there are signs of the return of bowel motility (bowel sounds, flatus, or bowel movement). Ambulation begins the day after surgery, or as soon as the patient is able. Generally the hospital stay after urinary diversion is 5 to 10 days.

Education regarding the care of the pouching system must begin in the hospital and continue on an outpatient basis with home care as needed. Support systems such as access to supplies and financial and family support must also be considered, in addition to routine follow-up with the physician and the WOC/ET nurse.

Results. Mortality from radical cystectomy and ileal conduit is reported to be 1% to 3%. Early complications include bleeding, need for transfusion, wound infection, pelvic abscess, bowel obstruction, prolonged ileus, urine leak, and ureteral obstruction (Marshall, 1990).

Complications. Stomal complications are the most common problem after urinary diversion. These include stomal stenosis, bowel necrosis, parastomal hernia, prolapse, and stomal retraction. Some of these complications require repeat surgery to correct, and others can be managed with proper stomal care alone.

Complications related to the ureterointestinal anastomoses can occur. These include leakage (i.e., urinary fistula), stricture, and pyelonephritis. There has been controversy about the need to anastomose

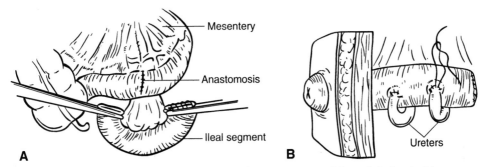

Figure 10-1 Surgical construction of ileal conduit. **A,** Segment of ileum is isolated with mesentery intact. Bowel continuity is reestablished; proximal ileal segment is closed. **B,** Distal end of ileal segment is brought to abdominal surface as stoma; ureters are anastomosed to ileal segment. (From Broadwell DC, Jackson BS: *Principles of ostomy care*, St Louis, 1982, Mosby.)

the ureter to the bowel in a refluxing as opposed to a nonrefluxing fashion. Some medical literature suggests that nonrefluxing ureteral anastomoses have a lower risk of infection and long-term renal deterioration, but other studies have refuted that claim (Walsh et al, 1998). However, nonrefluxing anastomoses have a higher risk of ureteral stricture and are difficult to perform in a small bowel conduit. Most urologists perform refluxing ureteral anastomoses for nearly all diversions.

Up to 80% of patients with incontinent diversions will have asymptomatic bacteriuria. Although this puts these patients at a higher risk of pyelonephritis than the general population, bacteriuria does not require antibiotic therapy (Link and Lerner, 2001).

Progressive renal deterioration is common after urinary diversion, but typically is observed after many years (10 to 20). Most likely this is due to infections, chronic bacterial colonization, ureteral reflux, and, in some cases, chronic obstruction.

The development of cancer in ileal and colon conduits is rare with only a few reported cases, and those generally 10 or more years after surgery (Link and Lerner, 2001). The incidence is much less common than in ureterosigmoidostomies.

Stones are more common after urinary diversion than in the general population. Stone formation occurs as a result of the increased risk of urinary tract infection and colonization. The most common stone type is the typical "infection stone": magnesium ammonium phosphate. Stones may also be formed on any foreign body left in the urinary tract. Care is taken at surgery to use sutures that dissolve, rather than permanent sutures, and to remove any staples or exclude them from contact with urine.

Colon Conduit

Indications. The use of the colon for construction of a conduit may be more appropriate for patients with preexisting small bowel disease such as Crohn's disease with ileal involvement, or small bowel damage from pelvic radiation. Most urologists do not use colon for routine diversions because the colon is a little more difficult to work with than the ileum.

Surgical Procedure. The sigmoid or transverse colon is most often used to create a colon conduit. The procedure is similar to an ileal conduit. Some surgeons will create nonrefluxing anastomoses between the ureters and the colon so that urine cannot reflux from the conduit to the kidneys.

Postoperative Care. The postoperative care results and complications are basically the same as with ileal conduits. Stomal complications are slightly less common because of the larger size of the colon. If nonrefluxing ureteral anastomoses are performed, then there is a higher incidence of ureteral obstruction with colon conduits.

Ureterosigmoidostomy

In the early twentieth century, the ureterosigmoidostomy was recognized as the first continent urinary diversion. At that time, it was considered the standard method of urinary diversion. It is performed by placing the ureters into the sigmoid colon in a nonrefluxing fashion. However, the procedure is no longer performed in developed countries because of the high incidence of pyelonephritis and colon cancer associated with it. It is still performed in some parts of the world because indigent patients would not be able to afford ostomy supplies.

Diversions at the Bladder Level

Cystotomy Tube (Suprapubic Tube)

Indications. This procedure is performed as an alternative to Foley catheter drainage by way of the urethra. Suprapubic tubes may be indicated in patients who need chronic bladder drainage, who are not candidates for intermittent catheterization, and who have difficult urethras to catheterize or have a contraindication to urethral catheterization.

Surgical Procedure. There are several variations in surgical technique; most involve placement under local anesthesia. The bladder is filled (either by means of a urethral catheter or percutaneously with a needle) to provide a large target and push the bowel out of harm's way. Local anesthesia is infiltrated in the skin and the bladder wall. Some suprapubic tube kits come with a trochar and sheath, which are placed in the bladder. Then the trochar is removed, and a catheter is placed through the sheath and the sheath removed. Other kits come with a catheter and a trochar inside the catheter, and the trochar is removed after catheter placement. In complex cases, cystoscopy or ultrasound may be used to guide placement, or placement may require an open procedure and general anesthesia.

Postoperative Care. Suprapubic tube placement is done as an outpatient procedure. The initial tube that has been placed may be sutured to the skin or affixed to the skin by an adhesive dressing. Chronic tubes are typically Foley catheters and are not sutured to the skin. Usual catheter care is required.

Results. Suprapubic tubes carry the same long-term risks as urethral catheterization, such as urinary tract infections, stones, and clogged catheters. They avoid the discomfort and difficulty of urethral catheterization (usually minor), the risk of urethral strictures, and the risk of urethral erosion (catheter pressure on the urethra can damage the tissue and open the urethra ventrally on the penis, causing hypospadias), which is fortunately unusual. Suprapubic tubes and urethral catheterization carry a risk of bladder cancer, if kept chronically for more than 10 years, and an extremely low risk of death from urosepsis.

Complications. In addition to those mentioned in previous paragraphs, there could be accidental entry into the peritoneum and intraperitoneal urine leakage, or accidental injury to the bowel. Both of these complications are extremely rare.

Vesicostomy

Indications. A vesicostomy is most often performed in infants and young children to provide temporary bladder drainage. It is usually closed before toilet-training age. This procedure is rarely done in the adult.

Surgical Procedure. A small transverse incision is made midway between the umbilicus and the symphysis pubis. After the dome of the bladder is mobilized and the wall of the bladder is sutured to the rectus fascia, a small transverse incision is made in the bladder. The bladder mucosa is then sutured to the opening in the abdominal skin.

Postoperative Care. Care must be taken to protect the skin while managing the urine with dia-

pers. The family should be instructed in daily care, the need for adequate fluid intake, and signs of infection, stones, or stenosis.

Results. Although requiring general anesthesia, vesicostomies are minor procedures, well tolerated, and usually performed on an outpatient basis.

Complications. Peristomal dermatitis, stomal stenosis, stomal prolapse, infection, and stone formation can occur with a vesicostomy.

Continent Diversions

Continent diversions have followed two different courses: continent cutaneous diversion in which a catheterizable stoma is created, such as the Indiana pouch, and orthotopic bladder replacement or "neobladder" in which an internal pouch is attached to the urethra.

Indiana Pouch

Indications. The overall indications for a continent as opposed to an incontinent urinary diversion are reviewed in the ileal conduit section above. When choosing between a neobladder and an Indiana pouch, there are several issues to consider. The neobladder is generally considered to have a superior cosmetic outcome (no stoma at all). However, the patient must be willing to self-catheterize per urethra. A neobladder may be performed when a malignancy does not involve the urethra. Some urologists will not perform a neobladder if the prostate is involved with cancer, there is carcinoma in situ, or the bladder neck is involved with cancer in women. However a neobladder can have a particular advantage for obese patients, since the thickness of their abdominal wall can make creation and management of a cutaneous stoma more difficult.

The surgery is no longer considered unsuitable for women. However, more women than men require daily self-catheterization to manage chronic urinary retention, and women experience more incontinence both day and night (Link and Lerner 2001). Currently very few urologists have experience with performing neobladders in women.

In summary, most urologists would consider the neobladder the ideal continent diversion for men, and probably in the future it will become so for women as well. Currently, unless the urologist has extensive experience with neobladders in women, the Indiana pouch would be the preferred form of continent diversion for them.

Preoperative Considerations. Patients are often overwhelmed with their postoperative care unless meticulously prepared before surgery. Several issues should be reviewed before surgery: intermittent catheterization, stoma marking and stoma care, and the postoperative course and the need for temporary drains.

Before surgery, patients should be taught the technique of intermittent self-catheterization. This is also an opportunity to evaluate the patient's motivation and capability to catheterize.

Stoma site selection must also be determined. All patients are informed that intraoperative findings may necessitate an incontinent rather than a continent diversion. A standard right lower quadrant stoma site should be marked, with the usual consideration for location of belt line, skin folds and a flat surface for an external appliance. Some urologists use this site for the stoma of an Indiana pouch, and others use the umbilicus, considering that this may be more aesthetically pleasing. Additional factors in the placement of a continent stoma are that it must be visible for the patient to catheterize, and an external appliance may be required if the continence mechanism fails.

Patients must also be informed of the purpose of all the postoperative tubes and drains, since patients are routinely discharged with several of these tubes. All of the tubes will require intermittent irrigation to prevent blockage from mucus.

Emotional challenges must also be addressed with the patient. They may grieve the loss of a body part and will experience a change in body image related to the incision and stoma.

Surgical Procedure. This procedure is a modification of the original Gilchrist procedure dating back to the 1950s. There are several variations of this procedure that involve using the ileocecal segment for a reservoir, and use either the ileum or the appendix for a catheterizable limb. All these variations depend on some common principles: detubularization of the bowel, using a sufficient amount of

bowel to create a pouch capacity of 400 to 800 ml, and using flap-valve mechanisms to prevent ureteral reflux and create a continent stoma limb. Detubularization of the bowel involves opening the bowel along its length to disrupt the muscular contractions of the bowel, which can lead to high pouch pressures and postoperative incontinence. A flap valve is formed when a channel, having entered the lumen of a storage space, naturally closes when there is no flow through it, like a cloth firehose. The channel can easily open when there is urine flow, but the flap closes when there is no flow, and pressure from the storage space cannot cause flow back up the channel.

The Indiana pouch is created from the ascending and transverse colon and 10 to 12 cm of terminal ileum. Bowel continuity is reestablished by anastomosing the distal ileum to the colon. This is typically accomplished with bowel staplers. The ureters are brought through the back of the cecum. Instead of being directly sewn to the pouch in a refluxing fashion, the ureters are brought into the pouch for a short distance (1 to 2 cm), spatulated, and tacked to the inside of the pouch. This arrangement creates a nonrefluxing flap-valve mechanism. The entire cecum and transverse colon are opened anteriorly (i.e., away from the mesentery) and closed in a "clam shell" fashion. This detubularizes the bowel used for the pouch. The catheterizable limb is fashioned from the ileum. The diameter of the ileum is reduced to the size of a catheter by stapling along the antimesenteric border to excise excess ileum. The ileocecal valve is plicated, and this acts as a continence mechanism. When the ileum is brought to the skin as a stoma, care is taken to make sure the channel is straight and easy to catheterize (Figure 10-2). The urologist will always catheterize the pouch repeatedly in the operating room to confirm that catheterization is easy.

Postoperative Care. Ureteral catheters are placed in the renal pelves so that they extend through the ureters, the reservoir, and out to external drainage. These protect the anastomoses of the ureters to the intestinal pouch and maintain patency of the ureters. Care should be taken to stabilize all tubes to prevent dislodgement, and

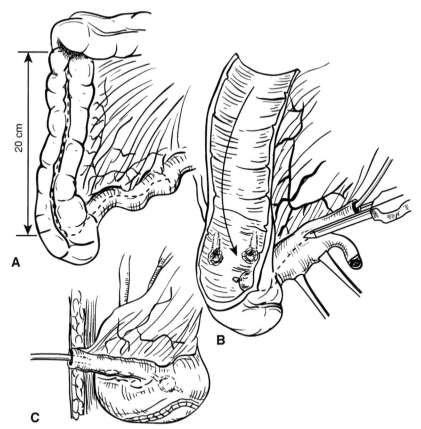

Figure 10-2 Modified Indiana pouch. **A,** The right colon and segment of terminal ileum are isolated. **B,** The right colon is opened anteriorly. The ureters are sewn to the posterior wall of the colon. The antimesenteric aspect of the ileum is removed with a stapler to provide a catheter-sized channel. **C,** The colon is reclosed in a "clamshell" fashion. The ileum (the catheterizable limb) is brought through the abdominal wall to make the stoma. (From Gillenwater JY et al: *Adult and pediatric urology,* ed 3, St Louis, 1996, Mosby.)

typically they are sutured to the skin at the time of surgery. Ureteral catheters are usually removed 5 to 10 days after surgery.

To maintain unobstructed drainage from the reservoir, a large catheter is brought out from the reservoir to the skin. Most urologists use a 24 Fr. Foley or Malecot catheter. Internally the pouch is sewn to the underside of the abdominal wall at this location to prevent urine leakage. This catheter drains urine and mucus from the pouch and is attached to dependent drainage. Irrigation of the

tubes is required to remove mucus to ensure free flow of urine. Typically this irrigation is required quite frequently the first few days after surgery (i.e., every 3 to 4 hours) and is tapered to a lower frequency as the pouch heals and as mucus becomes more manageable.

The catheter should be gently irrigated; 60 ml of normal saline is put in and allowed to drain, a procedure that is repeated until clear returns are observed. The catheter remains in place for about 3 weeks after surgery. Before discharge from the hospital, patients must be taught how to irrigate the catheter and to keep the catheter connected to dependent drainage.

In addition, patients will have several closed suction drains (Jackson-Pratt, Hemovac, or the equivalent). These drain any temporary leakage of urine or lymphatic fluid. These are usually removed prior to hospital discharge. Also, a 14 or 16 Fr. catheter is placed in the stoma at the time of surgery. Most surgeons just cap this tube: its purpose is mainly to help keep the catheterizable channel straight as it heals, so it will be easy to catheterize in the future.

Approximately 3 weeks after discharge from the hospital, the patient returns. The catheter in the stoma is removed. A "pouchogram" is performed by way of the percutaneous catheter to test the reservoir for anastomotic leaks, pouch capacity, and the antireflux mechanism.

Once the integrity of the pouch is found to be satisfactory, intermittent self-catheterization can be taught. The patient is instructed to catheterize the stoma with a 16 or 18 Fr. red rubber catheter or a Coudé catheter. Intubation of the stoma may be an emotionally frightening experience for the patient. Several sessions may be needed to increase his or her comfort level. Once the patient is comfortable with catheterization, then the Foley catheter is removed. See Box 10-1 for a suggested catheterization schedule.

Proper cleaning, storage, and purchase of the catheters must also be learned by the patient. Used catheters should be washed with a mild detergent, rinsed well, and allowed to dry before they are stored in a clean, plastic bag. Catheters are replaced once every 3 months. Patients who are prone to infection should replace the catheter weekly or biweekly (see Box 10-1).

A small dressing or a large Band-Aid can be placed over the stoma for protection. The patient should carry medical information and wear identification to inform others about the continent urinary reservoir.

Over time, the reservoir will expand to a capacity of 600 to 1000 ml. As the pouch expands, the time between catheterizations lengthens. During this interval, spasms of the pouch may occur, caus-

ing incontinence. The patient will need to know how to apply a pouch or how to contact a WOC/ET nurse for assistance in pouch application, until the incontinence ceases to occur.

As patients proceed through the rehabilitation period, they achieve increased independence. The catheterization schedule can be adapted to meet their individual lifestyles and intake habits. In time, they learn the feeling of a full reservoir and are eventually able to empty before going to bed, sleep through the entire night, and empty first thing in the morning. However, intake patterns and capacity vary, and some patients may have to set an alarm at night to avoid over-distention or leakage.

Experienced caregivers and other persons with such diversions can be an immense help to the patient in mastering the skills required to manage a continent diversion.

Results. The goal of all continent diversions is to maintain a continent reservoir with low pressure that collects and stores urine, allowing urine to exit conveniently under voluntary control. Incontinence occurs in 7% of cases and generally requires revision to correct. Difficulty with catheterization can also require surgical revision of the pouch, as occurs in 2% of cases. Although reflux of the ureteric anastomoses occurs in about 7% of cases, most times this is not treated. Ureteric stricture or obstruction occurs in 5% of cases and usually requires endoscopic or open surgical revision to correct (Walsh et al, 1998). Several other pouch procedures that incorporate the use of the large bowel include the Florida, Miami, and Mainz pouches.

Complications. The most catastrophic postoperative complication is failure to catheterize at appropriate intervals and subsequent pouch rupture. This requires emergency surgery and can be fatal. The other postoperative complications are similar to those seen with ileal conduits. The main difference in complication rates with continent diversions compared with incontinent diversions is a higher reoperation rate (about 20% vs. 10%) (Gillenwater et al, 1996).

Neobladder
Indications. Good candidates for the creation of a neobladder are healthy with early stage invasive

BOX 10-1   Continent Urostomy Catheterization

1. Gather equipment:
   Red rubber catheter
   Water-soluble lubricant (Surgilube or K-Y Jelly)
   Syringe and saline
   Band-Aid or dressing
2. Wash hands.
3. Remove the dressing or Band-Aid.
4. Sit on the toilet, sit on a chair facing the toilet, or stand.
5. Lubricate the catheter with water-soluble lubricant.
6. Gently insert the catheter into the stoma until urine begins to flow from the catheter. When the urine flow stops, insert the catheter a few more inches to see if any more urine will drain. To be sure you have drained all the urine out of the pouch, massage your abdomen, cough, and then pull the catheter out slowly.
7. If the catheter does not drain, it may be clogged with mucus. Draw up 30 ml of saline into the syringe and irrigate the catheter. You can also remove the catheter from your stoma, rinse with hot water, lubricate, and reinsert it.
8. Remove the catheter when the urine stops flowing.
9. Replace the dressing or Band-Aid over the stoma.
10. Wash the catheter with a mild soap and water, rinse with water, dry with a paper towel, and allow the catheter to fully dry before storing it in a zip-lock type of bag. Use a new bag each time you use the catheter.
NOTE: The catheters can become very soft and should be replaced about every 3 months. Carry a catheter at all times in a clean zip-lock type of bag.

Catheterization Schedule
Check with your doctor to see how often you should catheterize your stoma when you go home. The schedule below is a guide. The goal is to gradually work up to catheterizing 4 to 5 times a day and to sleep for 6 to 7 hours at night without waking up to empty the pouch. The size of the pouch and how much fluid you drink will affect how often you need to catheterize the pouch. You will need to set an alarm to get up at night to catheterize.

	Day	**Night**
Week One	Every 2 hours	Every 3 hours
Week Two	Every 3 hours	Every 4 hours
Week Three	Every 4 hours	Every 5 hours
Week Four	Every 5 hours	Every 6 hours

CAUTION: It is a good idea to wear a Medic Alert bracelet that says "Continent Urinary Diversion."

---

disease. Patients with visual impairment or obesity are more suited for a neobladder than other types of diversions. Other indications are discussed with the indications for an Indiana pouch elsewhere in this chapter.

Surgical Procedure. A neobladder is an internal urinary reservoir constructed from a portion of the ileum or colon in which the urethra is anastomosed to the reservoir. Most commonly a long segment of ileum is used (about 60 cm) and detubularized; the edge of the bowel away from the

mesentery is opened along its length and sewn back together as a spherical pouch. Detubularization disrupts the normal peristaltic contractions of the bowel and prevents those contractions from raising the pressure within the pouch. The ureters are sewn into the pouch in a refluxing fashion, because of the technical difficulty of making a nonrefluxing anastomosis in the small bowel. Many urologists use a short limb of small bowel for the ureteral anastomoses; this configuration is called a Studer pouch (Figure 10-3). This makes it easy to attach short ureters, and easy to convert a neobladder to a standard ileal conduit should this be required later on. Continence depends on the urethra and external sphincter. Most urologists are well versed in preserving these structures from extensive experience with radical prostatectomy. The pouch is sewn to the urethra to complete the procedure.

Postoperative Care. A catheter is placed in the urethra and serves not only as a stent for the anastomosis between the urethra and neobladder but also as an outlet for urine. Most urologists place a suprapubic tube as well, and the patient is discharged from the hospital with both a urethral catheter and a suprapubic tube. Patients immediately after

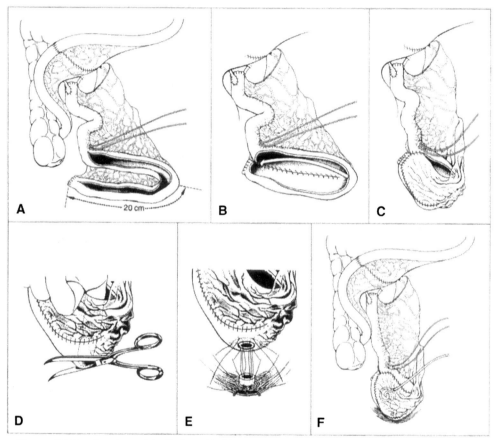

Figure 10-3 Creation of the ileal neobladder (Studer pouch) with an isoperistaltic afferent ileal limb. **A,** A 60- to 65-cm distal ileal segment is isolated (approximately 25 cm proximal to the ileocecal valve) and folded into a ∪ configuration. Note that the distal 40 cm of ileum constitutes the ∪ shape and is opened on the antimesenteric border, whereas the more proximal 20 to 25 cm of ileum remains intact (afferent limb). **B,** The posterior plate of the reservoir is formed by joining the medial borders of the limbs with a continuous, running suture. The ureteroileal anastomoses are performed in a standard end-to-side technique to the proximal portion (afferent limb) of the ileum. Ureteral stents are used and brought out anteriorly through separate stab wounds. **C,** The reservoir is folded and oversewn (anterior wall). **D,** Before complete closure, a buttonhole opening is made in the most dependent (caudal) portion of the reservoir. **E,** The ureteroenteric anastomosis is performed. **F,** A cystostomy tube is placed, and the reservoir is closed completely. (From Walsh PC et al: *Campbell's urology*, ed 8, vol 4, Philadelphia, 2002, WB Saunders.)

surgery have ureteral catheters and several closed suction drains, but all these tubes are generally removed before discharge. The patient goes home with a Foley catheter via the urethra, which remains for about 3 weeks; the patient must be taught how to irrigate the catheter with a syringe with 60 ml of saline 4 times a day. Before the tubes are removed, a "pouchogram" is performed by injecting contrast material into the pouch to check for leaks. If the pouch is healed, the Foley catheter is removed. The patient must now relearn how to void. It is important that the neobladder be regularly emptied to prevent stasis of urine. Drainage of urine from the neobladder is dependent upon passive emptying when the external sphincter is relaxed, and on abdominal straining to compress the pouch. The patient may have to perform intermittent self-catheterization if these techniques are not sufficient. Some patients will need to perform self-catheterization either short- or long-term to help evacuate the mucus that the neobladder will continue to produce. The patient may also have to learn how to perform pelvic floor exercises to maintain continence (Box 10-2). Patient satisfaction with this procedure remains high, because the normal anatomy is preserved.

Results. A common postoperative problem for patients with neobladders is nocturnal enuresis. Most patients with neobladders will have a sensation of bladder fullness, but typically this is not enough to wake them. Depending on the capacity of the neobladder and the sleep pattern of each

---

BOX 10-2   Neobladder Instructions

Schedule for Urination

After the Foley catheter is removed, you will learn how to train your bladder to regain control over urination. When urinating, you must relax and bear down. It is important to carefully follow the schedule (see below) to urinate and also to do the pelvic floor exercises faithfully. The goal is to empty your bladder every 6 hours. Your schedule may be different, depending on the size of the pouch and the amount of fluid you drink. Leakage at night may occur in the beginning. An alarm clock can be set to be sure you get up at night to urinate. You may need to use disposable absorbent products. This improves after the training period.

	Day	**Night**
Week One	Every 2 hours	Every 3 hours
Week Two	Every 3 hours	Every 4 hours
Week Three	Every 4 hours	Every 5 hours
Week Four	Every 5 hours	Every 6 hours
Week Five	Every 6 hours	

Schedule for Pelvic Floor Muscle Exercises

Do the following exercises three times a day. Before getting out of bed in the morning and before going to sleep, lie flat with your knees bent. At lunchtime, sit in a chair with a hard surface. You will do a total of 60 exercises a day: 20 in the morning, 20 at lunch time, and 20 before going to sleep at night.

1. Squeeze for 1 second and relax for 5 seconds. Do this 10 times.
2. Then squeeze for 5 seconds and relax for 10 seconds. Do this 10 times.
3. After 2 weeks, increase the squeeze from 5 to 8 seconds.
4. Two weeks after that, increase the squeeze from 8 seconds to 10 seconds.

Imagine you are stopping your urine stream in the middle of urinating. When you do this, you will be squeezing your pelvic floor muscles.

Do not hold your breath or squeeze your abdomen or buttocks.

Do not skip exercises or do more than what your health care provider has prescribed.

CAUTION: It is a good idea to wear a Medic Alert bracelet that says "Continent Internal Urinary Diversion."

patient, nighttime continence can be achieved by setting an alarm clock to ring once or twice a night to wake the patient to void.

Not all patients achieve daytime continence. About 10% have some incontinence, ranging from stress to total incontinence. The reason for these excellent results is that most urologists have become quite skilled at preservation of the urethral continence mechanism as a result of extensive experience with this during radical prostatectomy. Patients older than 65 years may have a lower rate of continence, similar to that noted with radical prostatectomy, and patients in whom nerve sparing was not performed have a lower rate of continence as well. Continence may also be compromised by low-capacity or high-pressure reservoirs; this generally implies failure to use enough bowel for construction of the neobladder, or failure to fully detubularize the bowel.

There is about a 2% mortality rate and a 12% early reoperation rate. Late complications include bowel obstruction, hernia, deep venous thrombosis, and ureteral strictures (2%) (Studer and Zingg, 1999)

Complications. Urinary retention may be a sign of tumor recurrence in the urethra, strictures of the urethra or bladder neck, or mucus plugs. Urologic evaluation with cystoscopy and urodynamics may be required to sort this out. Urethral strictures can be treated with urethral self-dilation or internal urethrotomy. Urethral recurrence of transitional cell carcinoma often requires urethrectomy and conversion to a cutaneous diversion. For unknown reasons, urethral recurrences after creation of a neobladder have been relatively rare (1% or less), compared with cutaneous diversions (about 5%) (Walsh et al, 1998).

Soft-tissue infections of the pouch or pouchitis can occur, resulting in symptoms of fever, bacteriuria, and pouch pain, and may be treated with antibiotic therapy. If febrile urinary tract infections occur after the perioperative period, the patient is examined for pyelonephritis. Persistent bacteriuria may occur in as many as 40% of patients with neobladders or other continent diversions, and is associated with increased risk of upper urinary tract calculus formation, pouchitis, and pyelonephritis (Link and Lerner, 2001).

Stone formation in the diversion can occur if emptying is incomplete, causing urinary stasis, and if staples or permanent sutures are exposed to urine. Kidney stones are also more common in patients after the formation of a neobladder.

COMPLICATIONS RELATED TO URETEROENTEROCUTANEOUS AND CONTINENT DIVERSIONS

Metabolic Complications

Ongoing monitoring of fluid and electrolyte balance is required, since metabolic complications can occur when urine is stored in intestinal reservoirs. The typical electrolyte abnormality seen with colon and ileal segments is hyperchloremic metabolic acidosis. Ileum and colon segments secrete sodium ions in exchange for hydrogen ions, and bicarbonate in exchange for chloride. These phenomena, in addition to ammonium ion absorption, cause an increase in urea and creatinine levels. When the ileocecal valve and ileal segments are removed, decreased digestion and absorption may occur secondary to increased intestinal transit time, resulting in metabolic acidosis and diarrhea.

With resection of small amounts of ileum, malabsorption of bile salts and vitamin B_{12} may occur. If larger portions of the ileum are resected, there may be malabsorption of fat and fat-soluble vitamins. Diarrhea and steatorrhea may occur from the malabsorption of bile acid salts, and may subsequently increase the synthesis of bile acids (Dixon, Wasson, and Johnson, 2001).

The amount of electrolyte absorption depends on the type and length of bowel used, as well as the amount of time urine has contact with the absorptive bowel mucosa (i.e., transit time). Patients with renal and hepatic dysfunction will have more difficulty compensating for metabolic complications. The ileal loop has a low risk of metabolic complications as a result of the small surface area and quick transit time (Link and Lerner, 2001).

COMPLICATONS RELATED TO ALL TYPES OF URINARY DIVERSION

Pyocystis

Pyocystis is the collection of infected fluid in a defunctionalized bladder. Most patients who undergo a urinary diversion will have their bladder removed. Occasionally the bladder is not removed at the time of surgery if it is considered excessively risky or the bladder is deemed otherwise "unresectable." The bladder mucosa will continue to make some secretions that will drain out from time to time. If the bladder outlet is obstructed, then these secretions can collect and may become infected. Treatment generally consists of drainage and administration of antibiotics. The main difficulty with pyocystis is that it can be difficult to recognize.

Urinary Extravasation

A complication common to all types of diversion is urinary extravasation. This typically occurs at the ureterointestinal anastomoses. It is discovered because of excessive drainage from the drains placed at the time of surgery. Prevention of this complication involves careful technique to preserve the blood supply to the ureter and the pouch, and care with the anastomotic technique. Treatment generally involves making sure the leakage is well drained, and almost always it will resolve spontaneously.

CONCLUSION

The role of the WOC/ET nurse is to keep abreast of the specialized knowledge related to urinary diversions, along with preoperative and postoperative management, patient education, and attending to the emotional aspects for patients of such procedures. Selection of the appropriate diversion involves assessment of the individual patient's disease and physical, psychosocial, and financial considerations. Lifelong follow-up and management of complications is imperative for the patient to return to and maintain an optimal lifestyle.

SELF-ASSESSMENT EXERCISES

Questions

1. Risk factors for bladder cancer include all of the following *except*:
   a. Cigarette smoking.
   b. Aromatic amines.
   c. Schistosomiasis.
   d. Artificial sweeteners.
2. What is the current standard of care for invasive bladder cancer?
   a. Radical cystectomy and urinary diversion
   b. Intravesical treatment
   c. Radiation therapy
   d. Watchful waiting
3. About 95% of all bladder cancers are:
   a. Transitional cell carcinoma.
   b. Adenocarcinoma carcinoma.
   c. Squamous cell carcinoma.
   d. Urothecal carcinoma.
4. Permanent, surgically created urinary diversions include all of the following *except*:
   a. Nephrostomy.
   b. Neobladder.
   c. Ileal conduit.
   d. Indiana pouch.
5. Describe the surgical procedure for creation of an ileal conduit.
6. Why is the ureterosigmoidostomy no longer performed in developed countries?
7. Why would the placement of a suprapubic tube be indicated?
8. How is a vesicostomy created?
9. Describe the difference between a continent cutaneous diversion such as the Indiana pouch and neobladder.
10. Postoperative care of the patient with an Indiana Pouch includes:
    a. Pouching of the stoma for collection of periodic leakage.
    b. Irrigation of the catheter to prevent mucus from plugging drainage.

c. Insertion of a red rubber catheter into the stoma every 4 hours.

d. Urethral irrigation twice daily.

11. Define detubularization as it relates to the creation of a neobladder.

12. Components of the neobladder are:
    a. Ureteral catheters placed in the renal pelvis.
    b. Ureters anastomosed to the bowel.
    c. Urethral anastomoses to the reservoir.
    d. Pouch is created from cecum.

13. Complications of ureteroenterocutaneous diversions include all but:
    a. Pouch rupture.
    b. Metabolic abnormalities.
    c. Malabsorption of bile salts and vitamin B_{12}.
    d. Urinary extravasation.

14. Complications associated with neobladders include all but:
    a. Urinary retention.
    b. Pouchitis.
    c. Hernia.
    d. Stone formation.

Answers

1. d
2. a
3. a
4. a
5. An ileal conduit is fashioned with a segment of ileum close to the ileocecal valve with an intact mesentery. A 10- to 12-cm section of ileum is selected and surgical staplers are used to divide and rejoin the bowel. The proximal end of the ileal conduit is stapled closed and then sutured so that the staples do not come in contact with urine. The distal end of the conduit is brought out onto the abdominal wall as the stoma. The ureters are anastomosed to the ileum in a refluxing fashion. The stoma is constructed as an end or loop stoma.

6. The procedure is no longer done because of the high incidence of pyelonephritis and colon cancer.

7. Suprapubic tubes may be indicated in patients who need chronic bladder drainage, who are not candidates for intermittent catheterization and have difficult urethras to catheterize, or have a contraindication to urethral catheterization.

8. A small transverse incision is made midway between the umbilicus and symphysis pubis. The bladder wall is sutured to the rectus fascia, and the bladder mucosa is sutured to the opening in the abdominal skin.

9. In a continent cutaneous urinary diversion, a catheterizable stoma is created (i.e., the Indiana pouch) and the pouch is intubated periodically to drain urine. With the orthotopic bladder replacement (i.e., neobladder), an internal pouch is attached to the urethra, and the orthotopic bladder is emptied by straining the abdominal muscles to void.

10. b

11. Detubularization disrupts the normal peristaltic contractions of the bowel and prevents those contractions from raising the pressure within the continent pouch.

12. b

13. a

14. c

REFERENCES

Dixon L, Wasson, D, Johnson, V: Urinary diversions: a review of nursing care, *Urol Nurs* 21(5):337-346, 2001.

Gillenwater JY et al: *Adult and pediatric urology*, St Louis, 1996, Mosby.

Gray M, Albo M, Huffstutler S: Interstitial cystitis: a guide to recognition, evaluation, and management for nurse practitioners, *JWOCN* 29:93-102, 2002.

Eisenberger CF et al: Orthotopic ileocolic neobladder reconstruction following radical cystectomy: history, technique and results of the Johns Hopkins experience, 1986-1998, *Urol Clin North Am* 26:149-156, 1999.

Krupski T, Theodorescu, D: Orthotopic neobladder following cystectomy: indications, management, and outcomes, *JWOCN* 28:37-46, 2001.

Link RE, Lerner SP: Rebuilding the lower urinary tract after cystectomy: a roadmap for patient selection and counseling, *Semin Urol Oncol* 19(1):24-36, 2001.

Marshall, FF: *Urologic complications: medical and surgical, adult and pediatric*, St Louis, 1990, Mosby.

Studer UE, Zingg EJ Jr: Ileal orthotopic bladder substitutes: what we have learned from 12 years experience with 200 patients, *Urol Clin North Am* 24:781-793, 1999.

Walsh, PC et al, editors: *Campbell's urology*, Philadelphia, 1998, WB Saunders.

FECAL AND URINARY DIVERSION MANAGEMENT

Preoperative and Postoperative Management

JANE E. CARMEL and MARGARET T. GOLDBERG

OBJECTIVES

1. Identify critical elements in the preoperative assessment for a person scheduled for ostomy surgery.
2. Discuss the impact of cultural values and belief systems on teaching self stoma care.
3. Relate the role of the wound, ostomy, and continence/enterostomal therapy nurse in counseling and sexual education.
4. Describe the levels of the *Permission, Limited Information, Specific Suggestions* and *Intensive Therapy* or PLISSIT Model.
5. Identify teaching techniques to apply with the pediatric patient and the elderly patient.
6. Describe assessment criteria for selecting a stoma site.
7. Describe methods used to mark a stoma site.
8. Relate components of the postoperative assessment for the person with a new ostomy.
9. List stoma assessment criteria.
10. Describe the relationship of stoma function to stoma location along the GI tract.
11. Name the requirements for successful colostomy irrigation.
12. Describe the expected condition of the peristomal skin.
13. List the most common early postoperative complications.
14. Identify postoperative pouching principles.
15. Describe the progression of self stoma care instruction.
16. Discuss areas of concern to most people with a new stoma.

INTRODUCTION

The person undergoing ostomy surgery has many challenges to face in adjusting not only to the physical, but also the body image changes that accompany this kind of surgery. In addition, a whole new set of behaviors surrounding caring for the ostomy must be learned. The literature reflects that one of the most important variables in predicting positive adjustment and successful outcomes is ostomy self care.

It is very important that the education that will assist the person about to have an ostomy begin immediately following the decision to perform the surgery. This chapter focuses on some of the ways and means the wound, ostomy, and continence (WOC/ET) nurse can provide educational and emotional support to patients undergoing the creation of a stoma.

PREPARING THE PATIENT UNDERGOING THE CREATION OF A STOMA

Ostomy education is the foundation that assists the person with an ostomy to reach an optimal level of adjustment and return to a productive, satisfying life. Over the years the WOC/ET nurse has provided the essentials for ostomy rehabilitation. Early discharge, no provision for preoperative visits, and reimbursement restraints within insurers' coverage add to the stress on the patient and the WOC/ET nurse in meeting the challenges of a successful recovery from ostomy surgery (Turnbull, 2002).

The primary goal in planning preoperative education strategy is to determine the patient's ability to perform self ostomy care and resume his or her prior life style. A secondary goal is to identify any adverse factors that might be modified to facilitate learning during the recovery time (Smith, 1992).

Patient education begins in the preoperative period. Once the surgeon has made the diagnosis and surgery is scheduled, a person may experience apprehension of the unknown. The important roles of the nurse, specifically the WOC/ET nurse, include not only that of educator but also as clinician and counselor to promote autonomy and self-esteem.

Mowdy (1998) reports that the person facing ostomy surgery experiences fear of pain and mutilation of their body image. The initiation of preoperative education reduces anxiety and stress with the goal of a successful postoperative recovery. Education and counseling during the preoperative time requires sensitivity from the nurse, who must establish a safe, comfortable environment that allows for the patient to express fears and ask questions. The nurse must answer questions clearly, truthfully, and accurately, since there must be a level of trust established between nurse and patient. It is important to know what patients have been told and the understanding of the surgery they bring to the education. One important opening question can be "What has the doctor told you?" Another question to ask is "Have you ever known anyone with an ostomy?" The information obtained from answers to these questions will provide an understanding of the patient's point of view and provide the foundation on which to develop a teaching plan that is specific to that patient's needs and concerns.

Some people know of a family member or a distant acquaintance who has an ostomy and enjoys a very productive life. There is also the possibility of their knowing a person who had a very difficult time managing their ostomy. Adjustment to an ostomy affects more people than the one who undergoes the surgery. Black (2000a) observed that the emotional adjustment of the spouse or partner is often a key to the affected person's adaptation. Mowdy (1998) reports that parents of a child with an ostomy exert profound influence on the emotional adjustment of the child to the new ostomy. Anger, fear, and guilt can affect the adjustment of both the parents and the child.

The following section addresses the preoperative assessment, types of learning styles, developing a teaching plan across the lifespan, preoperative and postoperative information, counseling, and stoma site marking.

PREOPERATIVE PREPARATION
Assessment

Most patients are admitted to the hospital on the morning of the surgery. Therefore the preoperative session is extremely important to help alleviate the patient's anxiety and deal with his or her major concerns. Some facilities have structured preoperative teaching programs for surgical patients. For the person scheduled for ostomy surgery, the WOC/ET nurse has specific topics to address during this visit: explanation of the surgery, stoma appearance and stoma appliances, basic review of stoma care, activities of daily living (ADLs) with an ostomy, and stoma site marking. Areas to assess include the patient's knowledge of the diagnosis and surgical procedure, feelings concerning the surgery, educational level, family support system, previous dietary habits, type of employment, physical activities, sports and hobbies, any physical limitations, medical conditions, previous surgeries, and financial and insurance status (Box 11-1). During the preoperative visit, the WOC/ET nurse should determine whether the patient would find reading material covering ostomy care and seeing an ostomy pouching system helpful.

Redman (1997) explains that learning is most effective when an individual is ready emotionally and has a need to know something. It is important to avoid any barriers during the session, such as unfamiliar medical terminology, in order not to confuse the person and add further stressors. It is helpful when explaining the surgical procedure to draw or show a picture explaining anatomy, and how and where the stoma will be created. There are also teaching models and flip charts that are excellent ways to demonstrate anatomy and resulting stoma type. Videos are available from some ostomy

BOX 11-1 Preoperative Assessment
••
Medical and surgical history
Diagnosis for fecal or urinary diversion
Surgical procedure scheduled
Education level
Support system
Psychosocial support
Cultural and spiritual issues
Language barriers
Activities/hobbies
Vision
Hearing
Hand dexterity and motor skills
Skin sensitivities/allergies
Other physical challenges

---

manufacturers that may be helpful for the person to take home and review.

Part of the initial assessment involves evaluating whether a person is receptive to any teaching or information at the moment. Reactions are varied; some people arrive with a list of questions, whereas others may have already sought information from friends or from the Internet and think they already "know everything." Still others are so overwhelmed that they become almost paralyzed and don't know what to ask. The nurse should never make assumptions about the amount of information patients need. It is important to know if they are "high information seekers" or "low information seekers." Time should be allowed to identify any barriers to teaching so the plan can be modified to accommodate individual needs such as beliefs, cultural norms, and language.

A complete medical and surgical history is a valuable tool that provides information that can assist the WOC/ET nurse in addressing patient needs. Some patients may have had an ostomy in the past, and questions concerning how they managed and accepted it elicit information valuable for planning their teaching. They may have had a negative experience with ostomy complications or pouching problems. They need reassurance that they may not encounter these problems again.

During the preoperative visit the WOC/ET nurse must take time to assess for any limitations or physical disabilities. This would include vision, hearing, dexterity, skin sensitivities and allergies, language, cultural and spiritual beliefs, emotional and mental status, and psychosocial status.

Vision

The ostomy patient who has limited vision or is legally blind presents a challenge for the nurse in developing a teaching plan. A goal to keep in mind is to focus on the blind person's strength and keen sense of touch to accomplish independence in ostomy care (Lemiska and Watterworth, 1994). The visually impaired person is sometimes viewed as not being capable of learning new information because of the disability; however, many visually impaired people lead very independent, productive lives.

When planning the ostomy teaching session for the individual who is visually impaired, it is important to incorporate the tactile approach. Expert opinion supports the use of a two-piece pouching system because it will be easier to center the skin barrier by feeling the stoma by touch. The patient should be taught to change the ostomy system when the ostomy is not actually functioning. The patient with an ileal conduit can be taught to use a tampon, a dental wick, or a plastic bottle, slightly larger than the stoma (the bottle should be filled with cotton balls, Kleenex, or toilet tissue). These devices wick the urine so the peristomal skin remains dry, and also act as a guide for centering the skin barrier (Box 11-2).

When teaching people with poor eyesight, care should be taken to be sure that they are wearing their glasses or using any other modifiers that they would use at home. It is good practice to have favorable lighting in the room, avoid standing in front of windows, and avoid using literature that has small print on glossy paper. The use of blue- or cream-colored paper reduces glare that can be created by direct light (O'Shea, 2001). The patient should always be asked if he or she is able to see what is being demonstrated. The use of magnifying glasses can also be helpful for the person with poor

BOX 11-2   Teaching Plan for the Visually Impaired Person

1. Instruct the patient to place the index finger of the non-dominant hand on the inside of the mouth (this mucous membrane feels similar to the intestinal mucosa of the stoma) and then to touch the skin of the cheek. This will demonstrate the differences between the two textures.
2. Place the patient's same finger to the peristomal skin and then the stoma.
3. Instruct the patient to wash and dry the peristomal skin using this tactile approach.
4. Guide the patient to place the skin barrier of the two-piece system over the stoma.
5. Once the skin barrier is secure, direct the patient to attach the pouch to the barrier by feeling the rim of both and fastening.
6. Direct the patient to test the security of the system by tugging downward on each side of the pouch.
7. The patient should be given time to practice these steps until a two-piece pouching application can successfully be performed.

Adapted from Lemiska L, Watterworth B: Case study: teaching ostomy self-care to a legally blind patient, *Ostomy/Wound Management* 40(2):52-54, 1994.

vision. A booklet written in Braille with a diagram of the intestinal tract and tactile aids to represent the stoma has been developed by Coloplast (Coloplast Corporation, Marietta, GA). There is also an audio tape and a large-print diagram of the intestinal tract is available for the person with limited sight (Flick and Woodward, 2000).

Hearing

It is important to have a quiet environment when teaching regardless of whether the person has a hearing deficit or normal-range hearing. Noises such as overhead paging, fans, and television or radio can be very distracting when trying to keep the patient focused during the teaching session. The person with limited hearing or total hearing loss should not be treated as unable to follow a teaching plan to become self-sufficient in ostomy care because of the hearing deficit alone.

Important points to remember when teaching are to speak slowly in a normal tone while facing the person. If the person wears a hearing aid, the nurse should check that it is on and functioning correctly. The person with a hearing aid should be encouraged to check or replace the battery.

The person who is profoundly deaf requires an interpreter just as the person whose primary language is not English does. The nurse should sit facing the person who reads lips, ensure good lighting, and speak slowly. Helpful teaching tools are videos, illustrations, and educational booklets. The patient should be encouraged to write down any questions or concerns.

Hand Dexterity/Motor Skills

The patient's hand dexterity is important to consider in assessing his or her ability to manage ostomy skills such as applying and removing a clip, cutting a pattern, and emptying a pouch. It is helpful to question patients on the type of work they do or what hobbies and sports they participate in, to help assess their ability to perform the motor skills required for ostomy care. A person may have a history of a cardiovascular accident that has left no function in the dominant hand; some have tremors of the hand or arthritis. The nurse will need to observe how independently each person functions in ADLs.

The nurse should recommend options that simplify the ostomy care, such as precut pouches. There are clips available for those with poor dexterity, and there is also a pouch that has a Velcro-like closure that eliminates the clip altogether (Coloplast, Hollister). A two-piece system is available with the easy application feature that the pouch can be attached to the barrier with only one hand; this alleviates fear of the pouch not being safely attached to the flange.

Various urostomy pouch drainage spouts and tabs may need to be tried by the patient to determine which is the easiest to use. The person with a colostomy may consider a two-piece system with closed-ended pouches that can be disposed of when filled; this would eliminate the need to use a clip.

Consulting with an occupational therapist may be beneficial, since these professionals are an excellent resource in teaching manual skills and know the kind of equipment available to assist the patient with limitations.

Skin Sensitivities/Allergies

General skin condition should be assessed for any dermatologic conditions such as psoriasis, and a history obtained of any topical allergies (e.g., to tape). This is important to know before surgery, since the WOC/ET nurse may need to make special arrangements for a pouching system other than the one routinely used after surgery. The patient must be monitored carefully for any signs of skin reaction to the ostomy product. It may be necessary to test different ostomy systems to identify product sensitivities. Nonadhesive pouching systems are available for the person who cannot wear the adhesive ones.

Language Barriers

A translator is required when the patient does not speak English and the nurse is not familiar with his or her native language. It is helpful to contact the family, since there may be a family member that does speak English. There are also translator phones available that many hospitals have invested in to meet the needs of a multicultural patient population. When working with a nonmedical translator, it is important to remember that this person may need help in understanding the concepts to be translated. Some important points to practice when teaching through a translator are:

- Speak directly to the patient, not the translator.
- Use simple, clear directions.
- Follow each instruction with a demonstration.
- Take time for pauses when working through the translator.
- Have the translator ask the patient to repeat the instructions to evaluate the patient's comprehension of the procedure (O'Shea, 2001).

Several ostomy manufacturers have developed teaching booklets and videos in different languages.

There are websites that provide teaching material in many languages (see Appendix B). Using pictures can also be helpful in teaching ostomy care to the person with a language barrier.

Cultural/Spiritual

One of the challenges the nurse may face when implementing a teaching plan is a person with different culture, beliefs, and spiritual concerns. It is important for the nurse to complete a cultural environment assessment. Zoucha and Zamarripa (1997) states that nurses must remain open and honest to beliefs and values that are different from their own. Imposition of beliefs, practices, and values on a member of another culture compromises care outcomes. Patient may have concerns regarding the impact of the ostomy on their cultural or religious life (Blackley, 1998). It is recommended that the nurse seek advice from a religious or ethnic advisor. Leininger's (1991) Sunrise Model is an assessment tool for evaluating the patient to provide a culturally congruent care plan. The seven cultural values identified there (although not the only ones possible) are:

1. An ideal of optimal health
2. Freedom and democracy
3. Individualism
4. Achieving and doing
5. Cleanliness
6. Goal-oriented "respect of time"
7. Value of technology and automation

Cultural accommodation promotes integration of professional and traditional or folk methods for health care, which may include folk healers, prayer, or family participation (Zoucha and Zamarripa, 1997). It is important to try to maintain a cultural bridge between folk care and professional care. Often the professional care and the folk care do not fit well. The nurse must be sensitive to these differences.

In the Mexican-American culture, the nurse must first seek approval from the male head of the family before working directly with the patient. For the nurse practicing home care, it is important to obtain permission before communicating with the patient (Zoucha and Zamarripa, 1997).

In the Jewish, the Hindu, and the Muslim religions, cleanliness and intact body are prerequisite to the performance of certain religious ceremonies. It is not uncommon for people of these backgrounds to initially refuse ostomy surgery (Blackley, 1998).

Several studies have identified the supportive strategy of faith as being very helpful to those who have spiritual beliefs (Halsted and Fernsler, 1994).

Other Physical Conditions

When meeting patients for the first time, the nurse should observe and question them about limitations in mobility that require use of other devices, such as a brace. Is the patient in a wheelchair, or do other physical limitations play a part, such as those caused by multiple sclerosis? This information will help in selecting the ideal stoma site and the type of ostomy appliance. It is very useful to know previous surgical history and any history of radiation treatments in the pelvic area.

Emotional and Mental Acuity

The initial meeting with the patient should include an observation of mental acuity. This assessment will help in establishing an appropriate teaching plan. The patient may be accompanied by a family member or a caregiver, who may speak for the patient. The nurse needs to ascertain whether the patient will be doing self ostomy care or another person will be responsible for the care.

Psychosocial/Financial Issues

It is important to determine whether the patient has a support system and if others will be with the patient during the hospitalization, as well as on discharge. Support from family and friends provides the patient with physical and mental support and comfort. Insurance coverage information is meaningful for making decisions regarding the ostomy system and other supplies that will be required. Some insurance companies contract exclusively with an approved durable medical products supplier, and the patient and family need this information to plan how to obtain them. As of this writing, if the patient has Medicare and is receiving home care services, the agency also provides the ostomy supplies while the patient is under its care.

Sexuality

Sexuality and body image are closely linked to a person's self-esteem. When a person faces impending ostomy surgery, many anxieties arise concerning body image, social issues, and sexual performance. Sexuality and sexual function have been labeled the "hidden" problem of stoma care (Black, 1994). A stoma creates concerns for a person in three important areas of sexuality: (1) body image, (2) specific sexual dysfunction, and (3) management of the stoma during sexual activity (Weerakoon, 2000).

During the preoperative visit the nurse should ask specific questions and provide information related to sexuality, even if the patient does not ask. The nurse should talk with both partners to provide information and reassurance that not only is this a valid concern, but an ostomy should not interfere with the ability to experience a satisfying intimate relationship (Box 11-3).

The nurse must not assume that the older person does not have an active sexual life. People are living longer, active lives, and maintaining sexuality is as important to the older person as it is to the younger person.

It is helpful to know what the surgeon has already told the male patient regarding any changes in sexual function after surgery. Any type of radical perineal or rectal surgery may affect

---

BOX 11-3 Sexual Assessment

1. Are you sexually active?
2. Do you think your ostomy will affect your sexual activity?
3. Have you discussed your concerns with your partner?
4. Have you noticed any changes in your sexual activity?
5. Have you had any problems with sexual performance: erection, ejaculation, vaginal lubrication, or pain with intercourse?

From Turnbull G: Dealing with sexuality after ostomy surgery, *Progression* 1(1), 1989; Wilson R: The nurses' role in sexual counseling, *O/WM* 41(1):72-82, 1995.

sexual function; male impotency and female dyspareunia are examples.

Special counseling and discussion should take place with the homosexual patient and preferably his or her partner. Careful explanation is needed to ensure the understanding that the stoma cannot be used for sexual activity because of the risks of prolapse and stoma trauma. It may be helpful to offer to make a referral to a gay and lesbian ostomy support group through the United Ostomy Association.

Counseling/Rehabilitation
Sexual Counseling
The WOC/ET nurse needs to provide a safe and comfortable environment in which the person can discuss concerns about sexuality in an open, honest manner. Certain criteria are required for effective counseling: (1) acceptance and comfort with one's own sexuality and that of others; (2) the realization that sexuality and sexual expression are an important component of self-esteem; (3) knowledge of sexuality and sexual function; (4) awareness of one's own values and beliefs regarding sexual function; (5) the ability to be comfortable when discussing sexual matters; (6) ability to accept patients' and partners' lifestyles and sexual activities; and (7) knowledge of when and where to make a referral (Shipes, 1987). The goal of sexual rehabilitation is to restore the capacity for loving and receiving love (Golis, 1996).

The PLISSIT Model for sexual counseling was developed by Annon and consists of four levels: Permission, Limited Information, Specific Suggestions and Intensive Therapy (Box 11-4) (Weerakoon, 2000). This is one method that can be used in counseling. The WOC nurse should refer the patient to a qualified sex therapist if it appears that the patient would benefit from counseling.

Teaching the Ostomy Patient
Types of Learning
When teaching patients, including a person with an ostomy, it is important that the clinician know the basic principles of education. There are three domains or types of learning to consider when

---

BOX 11-4   PLISSIT Model
....

Permission
The patient is given permission to express sexual concerns and anxieties.
The nurse provides a comfort zone for the patient to facilitate open communication.

Limited Information
The nurse clarifies specific fears and misconceptions.
The nurse provides factual information re surgical alterations and effects of surgery on sexuality.

Specific Suggestions
The nurse provides helpful suggestions specific to the patient's problem.
Specific interventions are offered: empty pouch before sexual activity, use pouch covers or special underwear.

Intensive Therapy
The nurse refers the patient to an appropriate source.
Specific individualized therapy may be needed, such as reconstructive surgery and surgical implants.
Psychosocial therapy may be required.

From Sprunk E, Alteneder RR: The impact of an ostomy on sexuality, *Clin J Oncol Nurs* 4(2): 85-88, 2003.
Adapted from Weerakoon P: Meeting participant's needs: description of a sexuality workshop for stomal nurses, *WCET* 20(4):15-21, 2000.

planning patient education: cognitive, affective, and psychomotor. Learners are motivated by being helped to set their own goals and receiving clear feedback about their performance and effective praise (Redman, 1997).

Cognitive Learning. The WOC/ET nurse must be acutely observant in assessing the patient's ability to understand and comprehend the information and instructions being presented. This can be accomplished not only with literate persons, but also with those who may not be able to read or write.

There are successive stages of the cognitive learning process: knowledge (i.e., the person remembers the information), comprehension (i.e., the person understands the information), application (i.e., the person can apply the knowledge to the ostomy procedure), synthesis (i.e., the person can assemble the information), and evaluation (i.e., the person can perform the ostomy care independently and recognizes when to ask for help).

Affective Learning. In this domain patients learn to recognize their attitudes, values, and feelings. This stage has five progressive steps. The first step is receiving; with the ostomy patient this occurs when viewing the stoma for the first time and accepting the need to learn to perform self care. In the second stage, responding, the patient demonstrates his or her response to receiving the information by participating in ostomy care, for example, by applying the clip to the pouch. At the third step, valuing, the ostomy patient realizes that performing and mastering self care will contribute to the return to a normal, independent life. The fourth step, organizing, is when the person realizes that the stoma is a better option than living with poor health, such as rectal cancer or inflammatory bowel disease, and recognizes that it will improve quality of life. The fifth step, internalization, is recognized when the person returns to the former lifestyle and incorporates ostomy care as a part of daily routine. Affective learning is a slower process than cognitive learning.

Psychomotor Learning. The psychomotor process involves mastering motor skills required for performing ostomy care tasks such as changing the pouching system. This learning is acquired in a progressive, organized fashion. It involves perception, readiness, guided response, mechanism, adaptation, and origination (O'Shea, 2001). This is demonstrated by the person's readiness to correctly cut the barrier opening to fit the stoma. The patient is guided by the nurse to complete the process of measuring the stoma, cutting the barrier, and applying the pouching system. Positive reinforcement by the nurse is essential for the person to gain confidence in these skills.

Developing a Teaching Plan across the Lifespan

Once the WOC/ET nurse has done a through assessment of the patient, a teaching plan should be developed based on the person's needs, fears, and concerns. Patient education is a process of diagnosis and intervention. The teaching process can be seen as parallel to the nursing process in that each has a phase of assessment, diagnosis, goals, intervention, and evaluation (Redman, 1997). Table 11-1 describes stages of development and effects of illness that can be incorporated into a teaching plan.

Infant/Pretoddler

When planning a teaching session for the infant or the pediatric ostomy patient, the nurse will need to be very observant in assessing not only the patient's needs but also the parent's needs. Parents of infants may be required to learn many new skills, over and above the ostomy care. The infant may require other skilled care such as tube feedings, administration of medication, and respiratory care. It is important to schedule sessions when the parent is not overwhelmed with other teaching sessions by the health care team.

Parents should be encouraged to spend time touching and holding the baby in order to establish bonding. Instruction should start early to engage the parent in direct care of the infant to overcome fears about hurting the baby. The parent can be taught to employ management techniques when performing ostomy care, for example providing a toy or mobile to distract the baby while changing or emptying the pouch, and dressing the baby in one-piece clothing to prevent exploring hands from dislodging the pouch (Box 11-5).

TABLE 11-1   **Erikson's Eight Stages of Development and Effects of Illness**

AGE	STAGE	EFFECTS
0-1 Years	Trust vs. Mistrust	Withdrawal, separation from family
1-2 Years	Autonomy vs. Shame/doubt	Self-doubt, overprotective parents
3-5 Years	Initiative vs. Guilt	Limited activities, inhibition
6-12 Years	Industry vs. Inferiority	Poor self-esteem, less autonomy
Adolescent	Identity vs. Role confusion	Limited peer relationships, poor body image
Young adult	Intimacy vs. Isolation	Fear of rejection, afraid of commitment
Middle adult	Generativity vs. Stagnation	Fear of role changes, loss of occupation/relationship
Older adult	Integrity vs. Despair	Loneliness, loss of spouse, loss of independence/ living environment

Adapted from Shipes E: Psychosocial issues: the person with an ostomy, *Nurs Clin North Am* 22(2):296, 1987.

BOX 11-5   Teaching Points for the Pediatric Patient

Choose a quiet time to change the pouch.
Provide a small toy/stuffed animal near by to distract the child.
Assemble all necessary supplies.
Empty the pouch into the diaper before changing.
Do not use elastic bands or small clips for pouch closure, as the child may be able to remove the closure and place it in the mouth.
Use one-piece clothing to conceal the pouch from inquisitive hands.

Toddler/Preschool Child

Children between the ages of 6 months and 4 years are vulnerable to illness and the hospital environment because they may interpret these experiences as punitive and self-caused. Preparing children for hospital admissions is critical in helping them adjust and feel secure that they will return to the home environment. Children find comfort in reassurances that one of their parents will stay with them during the hospital admission. Also, children should select a favorite toy or stuffed animal to take to the hospital, since this helps their adjustment to a strange environment. Reassurance from both the family and the nursing staff is essential to assure children that they haven't done something wrong that resulted in a hospital admission.

Children learn best by active participation, rehearsal of skills, and role-playing. Motivation demonstrated by a child is perhaps the most important prediction of success in self care. Children under the age of 5 need to know how procedures will affect them. For example, before changing a child's pouching system the nurse should explain the procedure in simple terms and be honest in describing whether there will be any discomfort in the procedure. The child should be allowed to handle equipment to encourage ostomy acceptance.

Teaching dolls are available (e.g., from Hollister) that can help children feel less frightened of the ostomy (Figure 11-1). Infant-sized pouches can be given to a child to apply to dolls or stuffed animals. Children can undertake more tasks as their motor skills develop. Other ostomy teaching tools for children are coloring books (e.g., from United Ostomy Association). Many of the ostomy equipment companies provide colorful stickers that children enjoy to place on the pouch.

Before children are ready to enter school at 5 to 6 years of age, they should be independent in emptying their pouches. This accomplishment is similar to becoming "potty trained." Children should be praised for their accomplishments. The WOC/ET nurse should observe parent attitudes that may influence the child's progress toward independence.

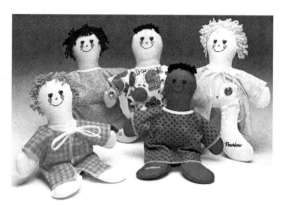

Figure 11-1 Shadow Buddy Dolls. (Courtesy Hollister, Inc., Libertyville, IL.)

School-Age Child

By the age of 6, children should be comfortable with the daily care of their ostomies. They should be independent and able to manage at school with no supervision. Children who view ostomy care as a normal part of the daily toilet routine will be more adept at integrating the ostomy into their self-image (Smith, 1992).

It is advisable to inform the school nurse about a child's ostomy and to keep extra ostomy supplies in the nurse's office. The school nurse should be knowledgeable about the ostomy equipment in case these children should need supervision. By third grade, children develop cognitive abilities and learn social rules that govern their condition and when to seek care or help.

By sixth grade, their abilities are refined and they should be proficient in ostomy self care and basic problem solving. There are conditions that occur in a school-age child when he or she is scheduled for ostomy surgery. The WOC/ET nurse should teach not only the child but the parent during the preoperative and postoperative phases. Simple explanation with understandable terminology and pictures should be used so the child can understand the procedure and ostomy care.

Adolescent/Young Adult

Adolescence can be a stressful time. Erikson describes this psychosocial phase as identity versus role confusion. Adolescents are very aware of changes occurring in their body appearance and the need to be accepted by their peers. Altered body image and body appearance may influence some aspects of their lives, such as social activities and sexuality (Shipes, 1987).

The adolescent may appear to be very angry and uncooperative in learning self care. As with all patients, the nurse must take the time to establish a positive, trusting relationship. Providing privacy for patients is important to help them feel comfortable in addressing their fears and concerns. The WOC nurse should arrange individual time with the parents and encourage them to allow their adolescent child to take responsibility for as many aspects of the ostomy care as possible, and limit the parental role to providing support. Chronic illness such as ulcerative colitis impacts the parent-child relationship. The child may not have assumed steps toward independence and may still be in the role of a dependent child as a result of the chronic illness. Adolescents can require guidance through steps of problem solving and planning. It may be beneficial to arrange an ostomy visitor (through the local United Ostomy Association chapter) who is the same age as the patient; this can provide positive support from a peer who is leading a normal life with an ostomy.

Another important consideration is the type of pouching system; a low-profile, discreet pouch should be selected to increase confidence and to provide reassurance that the pouching system can be concealed.

Middle-Age Adult

Erikson describes the middle-age stage of life as generativity versus stagnation. This age group seeks satisfaction through productivity in career, family, and civic interests. The person who is to undergo a urinary or a fecal diversion will experience the fear of many losses related to ostomy surgery: the loss of income and social status, changes in roles and relationships, and the potential loss of sexual function along with the loss of body part and function (Shipes, 1987).

The ostomy nurse must be sensitive to a person's fears and concerns. The teaching plan should be individualized to the lifestyle. Knowledge of the patients' occupation and lifestyle will help in the identification of practical skills that are necessary to help them feel comfortable returning to their previous lifestyles. The WOC/ET nurse should question the person about type of work, bathroom availability, and privacy. Demonstration of the use of a public bathroom to empty the pouch will reassure them that this can be done discreetly.

The person with a stoma may experience poor psychosocial outcomes that can range from failure to return to work and withdrawal from social and intimate contact, to depression and anxiety (Klopp, 1990). Teaching sessions should include the partner so they both can learn skills, and the partner can provide support once the person is at home. The nurse should carefully monitor the patient's adjustment or lack of it to request counseling appropriately. Rehabilitation of a person with an ostomy requires a concerted effort of not only the health care team but of family, friends, and community as well (Shipes, 1987).

Elderly

The elderly population has increased significantly in the past 10 years. Today's nurse, regardless of the practice setting, is confronted with the increasing needs of this population.

An important challenge for the older individual with an ostomy is coping with physiologic and psychologic changes (Reynaud and Meeker, 2002). The older person who undergoes ostomy surgery will most likely have other medical conditions that the nurse must be sensitive to when developing a teaching plan. There are many medical conditions that require an ostomy, some resulting in a temporary or permanent stoma. The patient facing the diagnosis of cancer and ostomy surgery is overwhelmed not only with the changes in body image and function, but also with the impact of what could be a terminal condition. Nurses should teach and reinforce coping styles such as positive thinking and maintaining a normal routine and not allowing the ostomy to interfere (Reynauld and Meeker, 2002).

The Oncology Nursing Society developed a position statement in 1992 on cancer and the elderly (Smith, 1994). This statement recommends that nurses caring for the elderly patient with an ostomy do the following:

- Recognize and correct biases toward aging
- Act as advocates for quality care for elderly persons
- Be knowledgeable of special needs for patient teaching and facilitating independence
- Integrate gerontology nursing principles into nursing care

When planning an ostomy teaching session with an older person, it is important to provide information in stages so as not to be overwhelming. The sessions should be scheduled when the patient is receptive and motivated. At the beginning of each session it is a good idea to review what has been already taught and see if there is need for clarification. The information should be given in short sessions so as not to tire or confuse the patient with too much information (Table 11-2).

Assumptions about what the patient wants to learn should never be made. It is important to ask the patient what the patient's goals are. The older population may not want to know all the particulars about surgical procedure; these persons may wish to concentrate on what they need to know to live with this condition, since many of this generation were not raised having "to know all the critical information."

Preoperative Information

During the preoperative session it is important to provide information about what the patient should expect after surgery. A review of the function of the gastrointestinal and urinary systems, creation of a stoma, what a stoma looks like, and how and when it functions are important points to cover. During this session it is helpful to show pictures or draw a picture of the involved anatomy and where the stoma will be located. Many ostomy manufacturers have teaching booklets and flip charts that illustrate these points and provide visual reinforcement. It is important to determine if the patient understands the information or has questions. Many people are not aware of the fact that they can live very well without the parts that

TABLE 11-2   Teaching Strategies with Older Adults

PHYSIOLOGIC CHANGE	TEACHING STRATEGY
Eyes	
Reduced color, focus, and discrimination	Remind to wear glasses
	Ensure adequate light
	Never have patient in front of a window producing glare
Decreased glare tolerance	Sit in front of patient
	Double-space all visual aids
	Use oversized lettering
	Use nonglossy paper with black print
	Use primary colors
Hearing	
Decreased ability to hear high frequency sounds	Speak slowly and clearly
	Do not shout
	Lower pitch of voice when speaking
Decreased ability to understand long sentences spoken quickly	Repeat questions asked
	Use short sentences
	Use familiar terms
Touch	
Fine discrimination reduced	Paper for printed materials should be textured or thick to allow for easier handling
Memory	
Memory is better for information heard than seen; changes in mental status result from illness, not age	Provide repeated exposure to same message
	Talk on patient's level
	Use verbal and visual cues
Slowed problem-solving	Relate material to the person's life
Difficulty in remembering new information	Never rush through material
	Provide options for problem solving

are being surgically removed. The insight that they can live well and long without body parts such as the colon or bladder can be the most important knowledge they can be given. The following provides information that addresses the subjects to be covered with the patient before surgery:

1. *How the gastrointestinal and urinary systems work*—The nurse should review the basic function of the gastrointestinal and the urinary systems, including information that will allow the person to understand the new function of their gastrointestinal and urinary tracts after the operative procedure. They should be helped to understand how the alteration will direct the stoma functioning and their overall health.

2. *Stoma appearance*—The facts should be communicated that the stoma has no nerves and, as stool or urine is discharged, no sensation will be felt (hence the requirement of wearing an ostomy pouch) and that the tissue of a stoma is similar to the lining inside the mouth and will always look red and moist. They must understand that the stoma will be swollen after surgery but will shrink over the next 4 to 6 weeks.

3. *No odor should be present when the pouching system is on*—This is usually a big fear of a

person anticipating ostomy surgery and should be addressed early on. This fact can be emphasized that pouching systems are odor-proof and that the only time there should be odor is when the pouch is emptied; even then, with the use of odor-reducing products, there need not be any odor at all.

4. *Pouching system concealment under clothing*—This concept is important; it can provide patients with reassurance that they will not need to alter their appearance or clothing styles and that others will not know they are wearing a pouching system. There should not be any need to buy loose-fitting clothes.

Preoperative education should also include reviewing with the patient and significant other the importance of the bowel preparation, as well as the postoperative problems that can occur when the bowel preparation is not completed. The patient will be given directions for diet restrictions and bowel preparation. The preparation usually consists of drinking 4 L of an electrolyte solution to thoroughly evacuate the colon. However, patients who are fragile and have severe inflammatory bowel disease or other debilitating disease may not be required to follow the routine preoperative bowel preparation.

Stoma Marking

In 1953 Turnbull (Turnbull and Erwin Toth, 1999) identified the need to perform an assessment of the patient's abdomen before surgery to prevent postoperative problems from poor appliance adherence due to the stoma location. Over the past 50 years the procedure for stoma marking has been refined; however, there are few published studies that use outcomes measurement to validate the procedure. Bass et al (1997) studied the impact of stoma site marking and preoperative education on outcomes of ostomy surgery. He concluded that patients who had preoperative education and stoma marking by a WOC nurse experienced fewer ostomy-related complications.

Stoma marking should be done for all patients scheduled for ostomy surgery, even if there is only a possibility for stoma creation. It is important that the surgeon request a WOC/ET nurse consultation during the preoperative period, allowing for stoma siting and preoperative education. Before examining the patient's abdomen, the nurse should take the time to explain the procedure and the reason for siting the stoma. Establishing the ideal location for a stoma will help prevent future stoma complications and pouching problems. The WOC/ET nurse must know the operative procedure that the patient is scheduled for and any conditions that must be considered (e.g., radiated areas), so the best possible area will be chosen. Consultation with the surgical team will determine if more than one stoma site should be marked. The exact surgical procedure may need to be determined after the abdomen has been entered. After the patient understands the significance of the stoma site selection, the abdomen is examined with the patient in lying, sitting, and standing positions. It is important to assess the abdomen in different positions, since the abdomen contours may change from the lying to standing position and abdominal folds and creases are more pronounced in the sitting position (Box 11-6).

The abdominal assessment begins by identifying the rectus muscle. This muscle extends from the xyphoid process to the symphysis pubis. Stoma placement through the rectus muscle may prevent the formation of a parastomal hernia. The rectus muscle is identified by having the person raise the head while in a supine position, or by instructing the patient to cough or stretch the arms over the head. An alternative method to find the edge of the rectus muscle is to follow the nipple line straight down (Doughty, 2003).

A standard accepted practice is to site the abdominal stoma on the apex of the infraumbilical roll. The infraumbilical roll can best be identified with the patient in the sitting position; one crease can usually be noted above the roll (usually at the level at the umbilicus), and another below. The abdominal contours are not expected to change significantly in this area even with a loss or a gain of weight. A finger can be placed into each crease and the area pinched if the person is thin and

BOX 11-6 Selecting a Stoma Site

1. Determine the exact surgical procedure, the anatomic location, and the type of stoma before site selection.
2. Explain the procedure to the patient.
3. Examine the patient in a well-lighted, warm, private room.
4. Locate the belt line and mark with a water-soluble marker.
5. Stand the patient upright. Instruct the patient to look at the abdomen while you move your fingers down the abdomen until the patient can no longer see your fingers.
6. Ask the patient to lie flat and loosen clothing; determine the edge of the rectus muscles. If necessary, mark with a water-soluble marker.
7. With patient in a sitting position, assess the abdomen for creases or folds. Determine the location of the infraumbilical roll by finding the crease at or near the umbilicus and the crease below the roll, usually just above the pubis. Find the apex of the roll and consider this as a potential site.
8. Observe whether there are abdominal folds or creases, and note location.
9. Place the marking disc on an area that avoids scars, creases, bony prominences, costal margin, umbilicus, and areas of radiation therapy.
10. Confirm that the patient can see the proposed spot and that patient approves of the site.
11. Mark the proposed stoma site per protocol.
12. Document the stoma siting procedure.

From Blackley P: *Practical stoma wound and continence management,* Vermont Vic, Australia, 1998, Research Publications.

it is not possible to visualize the apex of the roll (Figure 11-2).

When assessing the abdomen for stoma placement, the WOC/ET nurse should avoid scars, creases, skin folds, bony prominences, the umbilicus, and if possible the waist or belt lines. Uneven scars and deep creases and folds will cause stress on the pouching system adhesive seal and should be avoided. Bony prominences can slope the pouching system seal away from the stoma, again compromising the adhesive seal. The belt line is best located when the person wears typical clothing; the belt line can be marked with a water-based marker. The area below the belt line can then be assessed for a possible stoma site. It is preferable to place the stoma below the belt line in order to conceal and support the pouching system with clothes. At times, because of low abdominal creases and folds it is not possible to site the stoma below the belt line. Men can be challenging to mark, since they may have no waistline and often wear pants well below the umbilicus at the hip level. Frequently the proposed stoma site is above the "normal belt line" for a man and he may express concerns about pants styles, wearing a bathing suit, or going without a shirt, because the pouch will be visible. It is important to explain that if the stoma is placed in a lower quadrant the presence of creases and fold in the groin area will cause pouching seal failure. The male patient whose stoma site is selected above the belt line may need to be advised on alternative styles of clothing and perhaps, in some instances, on the use of suspenders. It may be helpful to demonstrate the principle of the pouch seal so he can understand that choosing the best possible stoma site should provide him with a secure pouching system seal, one of the main principles of successful ostomy management.

The abdomen is also assessed for skin and muscle tone. The skin should be assessed for dryness and preexisting skin disease and allergies (Smith, 1994). The elderly abdominal skin may have wrinkled creases and skin folds. Patients may have undergone previous surgeries that resulted in scars and hernias. A suitable stoma site that is identified with the patient in a supine position may completely disappear in a crease caused by a sitting position, or sag below the patient's visual field when he or she is standing, because of soft skin and flaccid muscle tone.

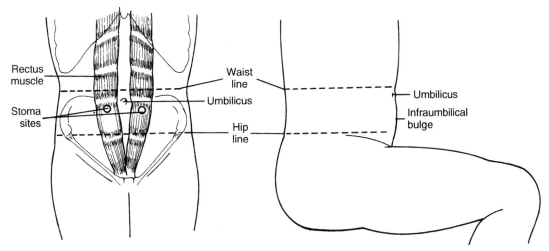

Figure 11-2 **A,** Preferred location of stoma is identified in right and left lower quadrants with patient in supine or standing position. Landmarks such as beltline, umbilicus, and iliac crest are evident. **B,** Preferred location for stoma site with patient in sitting position. (Modified from Schrock TR: Ileostomy and colostomy. In Fromm D, editor: *Gastrointestinal surgery,* vol 2, New York, 1985, Churchill Livingstone.)

It is advisable to use a flat skin barrier or a stoma marking template to assess the amount of flat space needed for pouch adherence. These discs can be placed in several areas on the abdomen to determine the best stoma site. A relatively flat area of approximately 6.55 cm should be chosen.

After the proposed stoma site or sites are selected, a patient should look at them to be sure that the area can be visualized. This is an important consideration for most patients with a stoma because self care is a major postoperative objective. In cases where there is no clear visualization of the selected site, the use of mirrors can be discussed. It is at this time that patients should be provided with the reasons this particular site was selected, and their acceptance for this spot should be elicited.

Stoma Marking Procedure

Several methods have been described: indelible marker with transparent dressing, the tattoo method, and the laceration method.

The *indelible marker method* involves the use of an indelible marking pen. The site is marked with an X or a circle and covered with a transparent dressing. The patient is instructed not to remove the dressing; however, if the letter should fade the patient is instructed to darken the area with the indelible pen and recover it with a new transparent dressing. It is important to send the marking pen and an extra dressing home with the patient. As a rule, sites marked with a surgical marking pen should remain visible for 7 to 21 days.

The *tattoo method* is done by cleaning the desired site with an alcohol prep wipe. A small amount of India ink is dropped on the site and a 25-gauge needle is used to puncture the skin three times through the drop of ink. The ink will be absorbed through the punctures. The residual ink is cleansed from the skin with gauze, and a small adhesive dressing is applied over the mark (Erwin-Toth and Barrett, 1997).

The tattoo method can also be performed by injecting methylene blue (0.01 ml) intradermally with a tuberculin syringe with a 25-gauge needle (Watt, 1982). The advantage of the tattoo method is that it is permanent and the mark easily recognized. However, this is a painful procedure for the patient, who may also object to this permanent mark.

A third reported method, *laceration,* is not recommended because of the risk of infection. The method involves making circular scratches in the epidermis with a 25-gauge needle (Smith, 1992).

The stoma marking, whatever technique is used, must last through the surgical scrub. Many surgeons will scratch the site with a sterile needle before the scrub to ensure identification of the site should the scrub remove the marking. After the stoma site is marked on a child, the site can be covered with a sticker the child has chosen and covered with a transparent dressing.

The principles of stoma site selection include:
- Placement within the borders of the rectus muscle
- Avoidance of skin folds, deep creases, uneven and scarred areas, bony prominences, and the belt line (if possible)
- Provision of approximately 2.5 inches of adhesive surface for the pouching system
- Placement in a location visible to the patient
- Placement acceptable to the patient

Detailed documentation of the stoma site marking is critical. This should include patient's consent to the stoma site and notation of the patient's understanding of the reason for stoma marking. There are recorded litigation cases in which, after surgery, the patient has complained that the stoma was not where it was originally sited. Inadequate or absent notes may cause great difficulty if there is litigation (Black, 2000).

Special Situations

Thin Person

Very thin or cachectic patients may have had a lengthy illness, such as inflammatory bowel disease, that has left them in poor physical condition for surgery. They may have suffered a large weight loss. The abdominal skin turgor may be poor with many skin ripples and pronounced bony prominences. It is important to take time to ask patients about the weight loss: How much weight have they lost? Over what time frame did they lose it? What is their ideal weight? When marking the very thin person the WOC nurse should take into consideration that the patient will gain weight once recovered from the surgery. A method for evaluating a stoma site in this population is to pinch at the umbilical fold and at the fold just above the pubis. Assuming that these two areas may in the future develop creases, the nurse can assess the area between the two supposed creases for a possible stoma site.

Abdominal Distention/Obese Person

The preoperative patient may have large abdominal distention related to medical conditions or obesity. When marking the obese patient with a protruding abdomen, the WOC nurse may not be able to palpate the rectus muscle. In this situation it is best to follow the nipple line down to the abdominal area where the proposed stoma site is to be considered.

In the male patient who is obese, the belt line is frequently in the lower abdominal fold; thus, because there is usually no flat pouching surface below the lower abdominal fold, the stoma site is marked in the upper quadrant where it is visible to the patient. In assessing the proposed stoma site in an obese woman it is important to determine the abdominal topography when she is in a sitting position, since the abdominal girth will change dramatically in this position.

For a woman with pendulous breasts, the abdomen should be viewed with and without the patient wearing her normal bra. Large breasts can cover the stoma if the stoma is placed high on the abdominal wall. A large-breasted woman may need to wear a bra when changing her pouching system. However, if the breasts totally obstruct the entire pouching system, emptying may be an issue; therefore a thorough assessment must be made of the abdomen and consideration given to the visibility of the prospective stoma site.

Physically Challenged Persons

Persons who are physically challenged (e.g., who use a wheelchair or other supportive devices) will need to be assessed and marked while sitting in their own chairs, or using their braces or other orthopedic devices. Wheelchair posture can be far different than that assumed while sitting on an examining table. The same criteria for placement as noted above should be followed; however, it might be necessary to alter some supportive devices to provide access to the pouching system. Contact with the orthotist may be necessary. It can be a problem to mark the person with a kyphosis or lordosis because the body alignment distorts the space for a pouching system. It is helpful to place a pouch over the potential area and have the person wear it for 24 hours to assess adherence issues.

Pediatric Patient

When an infant undergoes stoma surgery it is usually an emergency, and stoma marking cannot be arranged. However, if the opportunity arises for stoma site selection for a newborn, the umbilical cord area should be avoided because once the cord falls off, the surface will be irregular (Boarini, 1989). For the pediatric patient it is helpful to do the procedure when one of the parents is present to eliminate any fears the child will have. An ostomy teaching doll (e.g., from Hollister) should be provided to the patient so the WOC nurse can first demonstrate the procedure on the doll to alleviate the child's fears of the unknown.

Other Considerations

The person who is physically active (e.g., who plays sports, rides a bike, rows) will be concerned about returning to this activity after surgery and recovery. It is helpful to have the person go through the physical movements of their specific sport or activity to identify an area for the stoma that will provide adequate faceplate adherence. In addition, the patient should be asked if special equipment is required on the job; for example, the use of a tool belt or gun holster could raise special considerations in stoma site selection.

Some patients may not tolerate being assessed in the three positions because of pain or limited mobility. The nurse can try raising the head of the bed to simulate the sitting position. The abdomen can then be assessed for any folds or creases. When the patient cannot tolerate having the abdomen palpated for identification of the rectus muscle, the nipple line can be used to find the approximate borders of the rectus muscle, as already noted (Doughty, 2003).

In some situations where the sites available are less than ideal, it may be necessary to mark more than one. The sites can be marked *No. 1*, *No. 2*, and so on, based on the assessment. This should be clearly documented in the patient's record and the surgeon notified about the selections and the site of preference (e.g., No.1).

If the patient has received radiation treatment in the pelvic and abdominal area, the radiated area should be avoided. Narrowing of the capillaries in radiation tissue can increase the risk of mucocutaneous separation after surgery, and the skin can be easily traumatized by the pouch system adhesiveness, since the epidermis will be dry and fragile from radiation treatments (Erwin-Toth and Barrett, 1997).

There are situations where a patient will have to be marked for two stomas, a urinary and a fecal diversion. It is advisable that the two stomas *not* be marked on the same plane if at all possible. The rationale for this is that should a belt be necessary for one of the stoma pouching systems, the belt will ride over the other, affecting the pouching seal. The ileal conduit should be placed higher than the fecal stoma, since the conduit is generally created from the ileum and should in most persons reach the upper right quadrant. For a patient who has an existing stoma and now requires a second stoma, the same considerations should be applied. Allowing adequate adhesive surface between the two stomas for a good pouching system seal is also important. Patients who have undergone numerous surgeries may present a challenge, since they have limited areas for an ideal stoma site. The primary goal in choosing a stoma site is the provision of an adequate pouching seal.

POSTOPERATIVE MANAGEMENT

The creation of an ostomy, whether temporary or permanent, creates the need for multi-faceted adjustments. Radical surgery, coupled with threats to body image and self-esteem and possibly accompanied by a loss of continence, can combine to stress the individual's coping abilities (Colwell, 2001). This has been described as a crisis of both image and function, whereby the person with a fecal or a urinary diversion must adjust to the change in function (i.e., changed elimination) and also begin to incorporate the new (changed) body image. Rehabilitation of the person with an ostomy requires the combined services of a multidisciplinary health care team (Gordon, Rolstad, and Bubrick, 1999) consisting of the medical physician, the surgeon, and the WOC/ET nurse. Efforts should be made to make the patient and family feel part of the team, for example, by collaborative goal setting to further their sense of control. The person with a new ostomy needs a great deal of encouragement and education to accomplish optimal rehabilitation and a return to the former, functional lifestyle. Metcalf (1999) reports that psychologic adjustment may be affected if patients think that they have developed insufficient pouch changing skills or if they have problems with pouch leakage. Pieper, Mikols, and Dawson Grant (1996) describe the primary concerns of a person with a new ostomy as stool leakage and odor, as well as concerns about self stoma care. In a more recent study, Taylor (2003) found that the person with a new ostomy is concerned with "my need to rely on others." These issues are discussed with the patient and family and become the educational goals. Experiences in this period can have a negative or positive effect on the patient's view of life with an ostomy, so it is important that leakage, odor, and pain be under control, as well as reactions to the stoma by health care professionals (Wong and White, 2002).

Overall Patient Assessment

Although the WOC/ET nurse may not perform the overall nursing management of the patient, it is important for this professional to recognize any conditions that will have an impact on the goals for the patient. Information must be gathered regarding the type of procedure and the pathology, and expected outcomes must be identified along with any items requiring care (e.g., tubes, stents). Abdominal assessment includes the inspection of the incision for signs of drainage, redness, or warmth that may indicate dehiscence or wound infection. Bowel sounds are also assessed, and it is normal that these be absent for 24 to 72 hours. It is customary to assess for bowel sounds every 8 hours, since the return of bowel sounds along with flatus indicates the return of bowel function and permits the resumption of oral intake. There may be a closed suction drain in the abdominal space if fluid

accumulation is anticipated. The drain may be attached to a closed suction collection device and is emptied every 8 hours until there is less than 15 ml of output in a 24-hour period (Colwell, 2003).

Pain management has great importance in assisting the patient to comprehend the instructions being given. In addition, Kehlet and Morgensen (1999) report postoperative recovery can be accelerated by effective pain relief. Patient comfort should be the goal; the surgeon and patient should agree on the methods for positioning, medication, and patient-controlled analgesia.

Coping styles can be assessed by asking patients (or significant others) ways in which they have coped with prior stressful situations. Some people cope by requiring much information, whereas others withdraw somewhat and have to be drawn out. Recognizing the coping style helps to identify the most meaningful way of assisting the patient to begin adapting to the changes in body image and function. It should be ascertained whether any prior ostomy instruction has been given to the patient; many times the teaching that was done before surgery may not be fully recalled by the patient in the postoperative period. The patient should be asked to describe any earlier instructions and whether there are any misconceptions that can be corrected. In addition, any prior experiences with ostomies should be discussed; some patients know someone with an ostomy or have a friend or family member who does.

Stoma Assessment

Type

Patients usually leave the operating room with a clear pouch to allow for visualization of the stoma and effluent. The stoma type cannot be ascertained by observation; it should be learned from the patient's record. Further information to be gleaned from the record is whether the stoma is fecal or urinary and whether constructed from large or small bowel, bladder, or ureters, and whether the diversion is incontinent or continent. There may be a rod or bridge present in the case of the loop stoma. Output from an incontinent fecal stoma may not begin for a day or two; however, the incontinent urinary stoma should be expelling urine immediately following stoma construction. Lack of urinary flow from the stoma constitutes a medical emergency, and the surgeon should be notified immediately. The urinary stoma may have one or two stents in place that are inserted during surgery to protect the anastomotic sites between the ureters and the conduit, and maintain patency. These are normally managed at the surgeon's preference but in general are left in place for 5 to 7 days, or until the edema in the ureters subsides and the stents fall out on their own (Black, 2000). Patients discharged earlier than 7 days after surgery may go home with stents in place.

Characteristics

The appearance of the newly created stoma differs with the type of tissue used in the stoma creation. If the stoma is constructed from large or small bowel it will have a dark red, beefy appearance, perhaps with visible sutures at the skin and stoma interface. The stoma created from the ureter or bladder appears pale pink. Most stomas are moist, and if they appear dark brown to black, ischemia should be suspected.

Edema

The majority of stomas have some amount of edema, making the stoma appear shiny and taut and possibly translucent in color, especially in the early postoperative period.

Shape

The shape of the stoma can range from oval to round and can vary with peristalsis; this is important to evaluate for selection of the best pouching system.

Protrusion

The length of the stoma should be assessed, although this may change as postoperative edema resolves. Ideally there will be a degree of protrusion of the stoma, but stoma length can range from flush (below skin level) to moderately protruding (1 to 3 cm) to long (greater than 3 cm) (Erwin-Toth and Doughty, 1992). The flush stoma can create difficulties in maintaining the seal of the pouching system, since the stoma retracts with peristalsis and effluent might pool around or under the pouch faceplate. This can lead to peristomal skin irritation and even odor, as well as leakage. Moderate protrusion of the stoma with a centrally located lumen allows the effluent to be discharged directly into the pouching system (Colwell, Goldberg, and Carmel, 2001). A long stoma may be psychologically offensive to the patient and may not be well disguised under clothing. In addition, the longer stoma is more likely to be injured by trauma, laceration, or being folded or bent over into the pouching system.

Function

The colostomy usually begins to function on an irregular basis with a liquid output that increases over time. In time, the consistency of the output becomes more viscous, and a pattern of evacuation emerges on a more predictable basis. Since a colostomy can be located anywhere along the colon, output consistency and the pattern of elimination will differ depending on whether the stoma is constructed in the proximal (i.e., ascending), medial (i.e., transverse), or distal (i.e., sigmoid) colon. Since the proximal colon primarily mixes the ileal effluent to facilitate water and electrolyte absorption, the consistency of fecal matter passing through an ascending stoma is usually high-volume liquid with a high sodium concentration. Evacuation is both frequent and irregular. Effluent from the medial or middle colon stoma, because of the action of the proximal colon, has less volume and is less liquid; it may appear as pasty to soft or of oatmeal consistency, with irregular evacuation. The distal or sigmoid colostomy, since it is at the end of the colon and thereby retains the majority of the colon's function, has output that is similar to that of the intact colon. Initially this stoma may expel only serous output and flatus; then in 4 to 5 days, stool output begins. This is the only stoma location that allows for regulation of stool elimination through use of irrigation techniques. This is accomplished by the instillation of fluid, which initiates colonic distention that in turn stimulates colonic peristalsis and mass contractions, which leads to stool evacuation (Figure 11-3). Box 11-7 describes the irrigation procedure.

The output of the incontinent ileostomy stoma is usually seen within 24 to 48 hours after surgery and is liquid, bilious, and intermittent. Initially output is

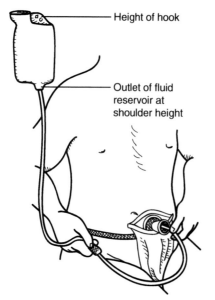

Height of hook

Outlet of fluid reservoir at shoulder height

Figure 11-3 Irrigation procedure. (From Black P: *Holistic stoma care,* London, 2000, Baillière Tindall.)

high, often between 1000 and 1800 ml daily. The effluent thickens as solid food is ingested and adaptation of the small bowel occurs. In the well-established ileostomy, stool volume ranges from 800 to 1000 ml/day (McCann, 2003). Six months after the surgery, the ileostomy output is of oatmeal consistency, and gas and stool are expelled intermittently throughout the 24-hour period. (Grotz and Pemberton, 1993).

As noted previously, the urostomy stoma functions immediately, and for the first 24 to 36 hours the urinary output is blood-tinged and contains mucus threads from the urine's passage through intestinal conduit (Colwell, 2003). After recovery from the surgical procedure, the urostomy pouch will probably require emptying 4 to 6 times daily. The patient may also be offered the option of connecting to continuous nighttime drainage to avoid the need to empty the pouch during sleeping hours (Bryant and Fleischer, 2003). Some patients choose to connect their pouches to a leg bag during the day, depending on their activity level.

Peristomal Skin

The skin around the stoma should be intact, without erosion, rashes, or lacerations. The junction of the stoma and the skin should be examined for any separation between the suture line and the abdominal skin. Any separation that is noted at the mucocutaneous junction should be reported to the surgeon.

Postoperative Complications

Complications occur in 20% to 40% of all patients following the creation of a stoma (Spencer, 2003). Early complications (i.e., in the immediate postoperative period) include ileus and anastomotic leaks, hemorrhage, ischemia, and mucocutaneous separation.

Ileus

An absence of bowel sounds and failure to pass flatus or stool is normal up to 72 hours after surgery. Excessive bowel manipulation, prolonged anesthesia, and pain medications may contribute to prolonged ileus. If there is distention of the proximal bowel, a nasogastric tube may be required to decompress the stomach, relieve nausea, and prevent vomiting until the return of bowel function.

Anastomotic Leak

Intestinal anastomotic leakage is signaled by abdominal distention, signs of peritoneal irritation, high white blood cell count, signs of sepsis, and drainage of feces or urine through drains or incisions. Any signs of anastomotic leakage should be reported to the surgeon, since surgical intervention is frequently required.

Hemorrhage

Minor bleeding from the stoma is common and is usually mucosal and self-limiting or responsive to light pressure. Active bleeding can indicate an open mesenteric vessel and might necessitate surgical intervention (Spencer, 2003).

Ischemia

If the color of the stoma is deep purple, cyanotic, or brown to black, ischemia is suspected. Cause may be related to aggressive stripping of mesentery, a stenotic fascia defect, or excessive tension resulting in devascularization of the stoma. Ischemia ranges from mucosal sloughing to frank necrosis (Spencer, 2003). See Chapter 14 regarding assessment and management of stoma necrosis.

BOX I I-7   Colostomy Irrigation

Personal preferences determine the time of day the person chooses to perform the irrigation. Best results are obtained when the irrigation is performed at the same time each day or every other day (see Figure I I-3).

Equipment
Is usually kept in the same place for use at the same time each day and consists of:
2-L bag: to hold the hypotonic solution (tap water)
Tubing
Cone tip: to conduct the water into the stoma
Large irrigation sleeve: conducts water into the toilet
Clip for the bottom of the sleeve
Lubricant for cone tip

Procedure
1. The irrigation bag is filled with lukewarm tap water and hung at shoulder height. Water is run through the tubing to expel any air in the tubing
2. The patient sits on the toilet and applies the irrigation sleeve to the skin barrier flange or onto the peristomal skin.
3. The end of the sleeve is placed into the toilet.
4. If not previously done, a gloved lubricated finger is gently inserted into the stoma to determine the direction of the colon.
5. The cone is lubricated and placed into the stoma through the top of the irrigation sleeve. The cone is angled to the position of the colon lumen.
6. The clamp on the tubing is opened, and the water is allowed to slowly flow into the colon.
7. If the irrigation fluid runs out around the cone, the cone should be repositioned to ensure it is not up against the colon wall, or advanced slightly into the colon. The amount of fluid used is debatable; many patients use 500 ml and others use as much as 1000 ml. The key is to use enough fluid to cause the return. Most start with 500 ml and evaluate return.
8. Once the fluid is instilled, the abdomen may feel distended.
9. The cone is removed, and there is a rush of fluid and stool that drains down the sleeve into the toilet.
10. When the initial return slows, there is usually a quiet period of 10-15 minutes until further evacuation occurs. This should be done every 24 hours, and generally within about 10 days, the patient can be fairly confident there will be no activity through the stoma until the next irrigation. At that time the interval between irrigation can be increased to 48 hours to test whether results remain the same.
11. A pouch is usually worn to contain gas or any stool that may drain between irrigations.
12. The irrigation sleeve, bag, and cone are rinsed and reused. The bag and cone are usually replaced annually.

Adapted from Erwin Toth P, Doughty D: Principles and procedures of stomal management. In Hampton BG, Bryant RA, editors: *Ostomies and continent diversions: nursing management,* St Louis, 1992, Mosby.

Mucocutaneous Separation

Mucocutaneous separation, which is separation between the suture line and the skin surface, can occur as a result of undue tension, separation of sutures, or in a patient with poor wound healing. A gap between the stoma and the skin will be noted. See Chapter 14 for stomal and peristomal complications.

Pouching Principles

Pouches in the postoperative period are generally clear to allow visualization of the stoma and efflu-ent, as mentioned earlier. The pouch is drainable to permit emptying of flatus or stool without frequent removal or traumatizing the patient's skin. Presized systems are not used at this time, since the stoma is edematous and most likely irregularly shaped, requiring a specific, tailored stomal opening on the pouching system. Convexity is not recommended in the immediate postoperative period because of the need to prevent pressure to the mucocutaneous suture line that could result in a separation.

Self-Stoma Care Instruction

Instruction in ostomy care is given to the patient and any chosen family member before hospital discharge. While the concept of learner readiness is appreciated, there is less time than there used to be to accomplish the amount of education the patient needs in order to begin adaptation to the newly created diversion. In the initial postoperative period as the patient is recovering from the procedure, instruction may be limited to survival skills such as use of the clip for closure and emptying the pouch. The patient should be informed that some ostomy procedures can be managed in a similar manner to prior habits; for instance, the drainable pouch can be emptied directly into the toilet while the person sits back on the toilet seat with legs spread wide. Since this behavior on the toilet is similar to that of the person who does not have an ostomy, it enables the use of public or private toilets and therefore frees the person with an ostomy from only using home toilets. In general, the pouch will be emptied whenever it is one-third to one-half full, but frequency depends on the anatomic location of the stoma and where along the intestinal tract the stoma has been placed. Some people may feel the need to rinse the pouch, although ostomy product manufacturers do not recommend this. Pouches are odorproof, and should any effluent remain in the pouch after emptying, there will be no odor from the pouch that has a clamp firmly in place and the tail clean.

The teaching session is often the moment when the patient finally faces the reality of the stoma, and as such the teaching session can be extremely upsetting to the patient. To lessen the patient's anxiety and maximize the session's usefulness, the pouch-changing procedure is usually taught in small steps, beginning with use of the clamp. This is a non-threatening way to begin; the patient will not look at the stoma or effluent, but will be participating in the beginning of self-stoma care. Teaching progresses to looking at and measuring the stoma, transferring the measurement to the pouching system, and cutting out the actual stoma size. Patients are encouraged to practice emptying the pouch and preparing the pouch system for a pouch change,

thus gaining proficiency while still hospitalized (Bryant and Fleischer, 2003). Instruction continues with cleansing of the peristomal skin with plain soap and water and a paper towel or other disposable cloths. Sterile equipment is not necessary, since neither the stoma nor the pouching system is sterile. Care of the peristomal skin consists of inspection when changing the pouch and noting any changes in the skin such as rashes, irritation, or denuded areas. Should any of these be noticed, the source of irritation should be investigated. Once the cause of the skin irritation is determined, preventive measures should be taken. The WOC/ET nurse will be able to make recommendations for the care of the peristomal skin, and products should be applied as directed. If the abdomen is hirsute, hair removal may be recommended; use of an electric razor is usually best, since depilatories may cause skin irritation and open razors can cause razor burn and also irritate the skin. This will help to decrease the possibility of folliculitis. Instruction should be given in the application of any products used on the peristomal skin such as skin sealants, pastes, and strips.

Box 11-8 and Box 11-9 describe the one- and two-piece pouching systems. Further instruction usually takes place after the patient is discharged, either in the outpatient setting or by visiting nurses in the home. The patient also needs to know when to seek professional help and where to obtain assistance.

Teaching patients with special needs can be challenging. O'Shea (2001) describes some areas to be assessed when teaching the elderly, such as the patient's physiologic and cognitive function, to ascertain whether teaching strategies will require modification. Further, assessment of fine and gross motor skills helps determine if the patient will have difficulty opening packaged equipment, cleansing the skin, and so on. Another challenge is the illiterate patient who cannot be assisted with written materials. O'Shea (2001) suggests the use of color coding or numbering sequences to compensate for inability to read. Video tapes and audio tapes are helpful, and ongoing assessment of the patient's understanding is critical.

BOX 11-8   Pouch Changing Procedure: One-Piece Pouching System

Equipment
One-piece pouch
Scissors
Measuring guide
Ostomy deodorant, room spray deodorant
Paper towels/washcloth
Tape as needed
Plastic bag to dispose of pouching system

Procedure
1. Assemble supplies.
2. Empty pouch into toilet.
3. Gently remove the current pouching system, using both hands to pull the adhesive side of the pouch while pushing away the skin. Save the clamp and place used pouch in plastic bag for disposal.
4. Cleanse skin with water and dry peristomal skin. Shave as necessary.
5. Inspect stoma; a small amount of blood is normally present on cleansing towel.
6. Inspect peristomal skin: no open lesions, erythema, or irritation should be present.
7. Measure stoma with measuring guide or template for up to 6 weeks after surgery. If there has been no change in measurement for 2 to 3 weeks, stomal edema has probably resolved, and the stoma size will remain constant and not require further measuring.
8. For the cut to fit pouch, transfer size to back of faceplate; cut out measured area.
9. Remove paper backing from skin barrier and apply to abdomen. Smooth the skin barrier onto the abdomen as the skin barrier responds to pressure and warmth.
10. If tape is not already part of the adhesive, four pieces of tape may be applied, one to each edge.
11. Before the clamp is applied, ostomy deodorant may be placed into spout of fecal pouch. A room deodorant spray may be used if pouch changing has resulted in release of odor into the room.
12. Urinary pouch has pouch spout and should be closed at this time.

To determine how well the patient has done in acquiring the necessary self care skills, White (2002) recommends that the patient rate his or her self-confidence in performing each of these main tasks at four different stages:

Six Main Tasks
1. Emptying the pouching system
2. Removing the pouching system
3. Washing and drying the skin
4. Measuring the stoma
5. Putting on a new pouching system
6. Getting rid of the used pouching system

Four Stages
1. After trying the main steps of ostomy care before leaving the hospital
2. After 1 week at home
3. After 1 month at home
4. After 3 months at home

General Ostomy Teaching

Ostomy Supplies

The patient and family must be given a written list of all of the supplies that are used in the care of the ostomy, including supply numbers and resources for obtaining those supplies. Insurance and reimbursement details should be sought by the patient, since coverage differs widely; for instance, some suppliers will submit billing to insurance or Medicare whereas others will assist the patient to submit bills. Should a prescription be required for reimbursement, it should be given to the patient before discharge. In addition, a list that includes

BOX 11-9   **Procedure for Changing Two-Piece Pouch System**

Equipment
Skin barrier, pouch, and clamp
Scissors
Measuring guide
Ostomy deodorant, room spray deodorant
Paper towels/washcloth
Plastic bag

Procedure
1. Empty pouch into toilet.
2. Gently remove the current pouching system, using both hands to release the adhesive side of the skin barrier while pushing away the skin. Save the clamp and place the pouching system in a plastic bag for disposal.
3. Cleanse skin with water, dry the peristomal skin, shave if necessary.
4. Inspect stoma; a small amount of blood is normally present on cleansing towel.
5. Inspect peristomal skin: no open lesions, erythema, or irritation should be present
6. Measure stoma with measuring guide for up to 6 weeks after surgery. If there has been no change in measurement for 2 to 3 weeks, stomal edema has probably resolved and the stoma size will remain constant and not require further measuring. If the stoma is round, a precut skin barrier may be used.
7. For the cut to fit skin barrier, transfer measurement size to back of faceplate; cut out.
8. Remove paper backing and apply to abdomen. Smooth the skin barrier onto the abdomen as the skin barrier responds to pressure and warmth.
9. Apply pouch to skin barrier and test for secure seal.
10. If tape is not already part of skin barrier, four pieces of tape may be applied, one to each edge.
11. Before the clamp is applied, ostomy deodorant may be placed into spout of fecal pouch. A room deodorant spray may be used, if pouch changing has resulted in release of odor into the room.
12. Urinary pouch has a pouch spout, and that should be closed.

---

local, online, and mail-order suppliers is helpful to many patients.

Dietary Principles

Postoperative stoma edema may be present up to 6 weeks following surgery. This causes the diameter of the intestine to be narrower, and there may be difficulty in passing high-fiber foods through the stomal lumen. See Appendix C for dietary guidelines for the first 6 weeks following bowel surgery. Also included in Appendix C are lists of foods that thicken stool, loosen stool, or cause gas and odor. The person with a urostomy should be instructed regarding foods that cause odor in the urine, such as asparagus, fish, and various spices.

Gas and Odor Management

The person with a fecal ostomy is usually concerned with the management of flatus, now that the gas will be expelled through the stoma. Although

the ostomy pouch is odor-resistant, meaning there will not be odor until the pouch is emptied, many patients still have concerns. The same foods that contribute to the accumulation of gas and odor (see Appendix C) in the person without an ostomy can cause the same problems in the person with a stoma, except that the gas and odor are now contained in the pouch. Other common causes of intestinal gas are smoking, gum chewing, and the use of straws. Patients report an excessive amount of gas upon waking, related to swallowing air while sleeping. Some patients have reported that fasting for many hours increases the amount of gas from the ileostomy; this is easily managed by eating small, frequent meals rather than allowing 5 to 6 hours to pass between meals. Simethicone can be tried with each meal and before bed. The accumulation of gas and odor is usually more of a problem for the person with a colostomy, since most of the intestinal bacteria which are gas-forming are located in the large bowel (Erwin-Toth and Doughty, 1992). However, a person with a transverse colostomy or ileostomy may also experience odor or gas formation. Careful management of the foods that cause these problems will help, that is, not eating them before occasions that would prove embarrassing; attention should also be paid to any air-swallowing practices. Assessment of self-stoma care practices may be initiated if any odor is discerned in the person with an ostomy. Usually the main cause of odor is a break in the pouching system seal. Should there be no break discovered in the system, the clamping apparatus should be investigated for cleanliness, since this is the only other way odor may escape the pouch.

The use of in-pouch deodorants will help eliminate the escape of any odor when the pouch is emptied. There are also systemic deodorants available that when taken with meals help to eliminate fecal odors. Accessory ostomy products are discussed later in this chapter.

Long-term Management: General

Sexual Function

Any limitations in sexual functioning should be discussed both before and after surgery by the surgeon, since pelvic surgery can disrupt both the nerves and the vascular supply to the genitals. In addition, other treatments such as radiation, chemotherapy, or medications may interfere with sexual function. It is important that the person with a stoma feel able to discuss any concerns and seek further counseling should the need arise. As with any ostomy patient, when engaging in sexual activity the pouch should be empty and the seal checked for intactness. There are clothing options available such as pouch covers and underwear that mask or cover the pouch; there are even mini-pouches to increase the comfort level of the person with a stoma. These options are mostly helpful in the initial sexual encounters after surgery, although some people will choose to use them regularly. Generally patients can be counseled that sexual activity will not be harmful to the stoma; however,

the stoma itself is not to be used as an erogenous area. The female ostomy patient may experience some initial pain on intercourse, and lubrication is recommended. Should pain continue or be problematic, consultation with a gynecologist or sexual counselor should be obtained.

Activities of Daily Living: Water Play

It is possible to continue most ADLs with an ostomy. At a reported ostomy support group meeting, most persons with a stoma were not able to identify any activity that would be adversely affected by the presence of an ostomy, although one woman did note the inability to wear a bikini bathing suit. Most activities merely call for preparation; for instance, before swimming the pouch should be emptied and the edge's adhesive assessed for continuity. Should the edges not be in contact with the skin, or as a routine precaution, tape can be applied to all four sides to assist in keeping the area intact; some people prefer affixing waterproof tape to the area, whereas others report not feeling this to be necessary. Scuba diving, sailing, and other water activities have not been found to be problematic for the person with an ostomy. Should the person with a new stoma doubt the ability to participate in any water activities, soaking in a bathtub while wearing the ostomy equipment that will be used while in the water can increase the confidence level: it can be seen that the pouch will remain intact. This is also true of bathing suits; many new ostomy patients feel awkward or embarrassed, thinking that the pouch will show through the bathing suit. They should be advised to take a long bath in the bathing suit of choice and they will see what the suit looks like when wet and more than likely feel much more comfortable when at the pool or beach. It is also suggested that a bathing suit with a patterned material instead of one in a solid color will help camouflage the pouch. A key precaution, no matter what the activity, is to always have a spare pouching system on hand, whether this is kept in the car or a purse, or at work. Merely having the spare available usually makes the person with an ostomy feel more secure even though the likelihood of needing it may not be very great.

Bathing and Showering

Bathing and showering can be accomplished with or without a pouch; however, the person with an ileostomy will find that the stoma will probably function while the pouch is off. Most people shower or bathe with the pouch on most days and take it off on the day that they will change the pouch. When bathing with the pouch on, the patient should be reminded to dry the area of the skin barrier and under the pouch very well, since fungal rashes in that area as a result of moisture are very common.

Clothing Styles

The great majority of people with an ostomy wear the same clothing styles they did before surgery unless the pouch is above the waistline, in which case they will usually need to wear clothing that is not tucked in at the belt. This is more often the case in men with a short abdomen whose stoma has to be placed on a higher plane. Snugly-fitting underclothes will flatten the pouch, allowing the effluent to be equally distributed in the pouch and helping to provide a flat contour.

Follow-up

The person with an ostomy will require lifelong follow-up, if not with the physician, most certainly with a WOC/ET nurse. To keep current with improved pouching systems, as well as to cope with any stoma care problems that arise, patients should always have a list of resources. In the event that problems arise while traveling, there are worldwide sources of assistance available to the ostomy patient. Aside from a list of resources, it is important that persons with ostomies take an adequate amount of supplies along on journeys, at least twice as much as they think they will need for the trip.

Support Groups

The person with a new ostomy should be given information regarding both a local and the national ostomy support group. As with other support groups, the United Ostomy Association (UOA) consists of people who have experienced similar adjustments and anxieties and serve as role models to assist the person with a new ostomy. Seeing other people who have experienced similar surgeries and have returned to their former lifestyles provides a wonderful example that boosts confidence. In addition, the UOA has a visitation service whereby visitors who are trained by health care professionals can visit the new ostomy patient and share experiences and recovery strategies. Many people report that their experiences as a visitor have greatly assisted in their own rehabilitation.

Quality of Life

The profound effects of an ostomy on the patient's life have been examined in a variety of ways. As long ago as 1983, Olbrisch designed the Ostomy Adjustment Scale to measure patients' subjective responses to an ostomy and the correlation between ostomy adjustment and quality of life (Burckhardt, 1990). A French study of 4739 patients used a stoma care quality of life index to determine the extent of the effects of an ostomy on quality of life. The quality of life scores were significantly higher in patients who were satisfied with the care received than in those who were not satisfied. Those patients who had a good relationship with the "stoma care nurse" and felt confident about changing the appliance had significantly higher scores. This study suggests that access to specialist ostomy (i.e., WOC/ET) nurses is particularly important in the first 3 to 6 months after surgery (Marquis, Marrel, and Jambon, 2003).

McLeod and Baxter (1998) describe quality of life as incorporating not only the physical or functional outcome but also consideration of the emotional and social well-being of the patient. They describe surveys that depict the quality of life as high in patients with ulcerative colitis who have had the continent and incontinent types of surgical procedures performed, and they relate this high quality of life to improvement in physical well-being as the main determinant of outcome. Kohler and Troid (1995) found that patients with ulcerative colitis have a good quality of life after surgery regardless of the nature of reconstruction after proctocolectomy. In a British study of 391 colostomy and ileostomy patients, Nugent et al (1999) used a questionnaire covering preoperative preparation and immediate recovery from surgery, the patient's satisfaction with stoma equipment used, and the effect of the stoma on the patient's life. It was noted that although all patients with a stoma received a visit from a "stoma therapist" before discharge, some patients were dissatisfied with preoperative counseling and postoperative follow-up. It was suggested that even in urgent surgical situations, efforts should be made for a WOC/ET nurse to make a preoperative visit to discuss stoma siting and the practice of ADLs with a stoma. The investigators also related a 30% occurrence of sexual dysfunction (approximately half with impotence and half with dyspareunia). It was observed that patients still obtain the majority of their support from significant others and family members and that these important people must be included in stoma care instruction and counseling. This finding was also reported by Piwonka and Merino (1999), who indicated that successful adjustment to a permanent colostomy is related to self care instruction as well as "appropriate psychological support to integrate the new physical changes into a healthy body image." The authors describe "an inverse relationship between the magnitude of perceived change in body image after colostomy surgery and the patient's psychosocial adaptation." They suggested helping the patient cope with an adjusted body image by teaching self care and rapidly reintegrating the patient into family and social life.

Long-Term Management: Conventional Colostomy

Constipation/Irrigation

Since the person with a colostomy has some amount of functioning colon, constipation is a possibility. A full history of the patient's prior bowel habits should be taken in order to determine the patient's "normal" elimination pattern, along with any history of constipation and relief strategies. The person who has an end colostomy and reports a regular elimination pattern before surgery may be a candidate for irrigation as a management strategy. Irrigation is essentially an enema through the stoma to establish a pattern of elimination. If this strategy interests the patient, instruction is usually

given after the patient is at home, perhaps by the visiting nurse or at a follow-up visit at an ostomy clinic (see Box 11-7). A patient with a history of constipation or fecal impaction needs instruction for managing these, since a stoma does not preclude their occurrence. Constipation should be suspected when the stoma fails to function for more than 24 hours, or conversely when liquid stools, cramping, and swelling abdomen are noted. Whatever the patient has used in the past to prevent or manage constipation will still work, and usually these methods consist of some combination of adequate fluid intake, exercise, and intake of fiber. If symptoms appear and the patient is unsure of what to do, he or she can be advised to increase fluid and fiber intake and contact their physician or the WOC nurse.

Diarrhea

Diarrhea in the person with a fecal ostomy is actually an increase in volume with a more liquid consistency. The patient will note more frequent emptying of their pouching system. If diarrhea is not an unusual event for the patient, prior management methods are discussed. Increasing fluids, dietary manipulation (i.e., more carbohydrates), and fiber intake may help; however, if the diarrhea lasts more than 24 hours, or in the presence of symptoms of dehydration such us cramping, dizziness, or decreased urine output, a physician should be consulted.

Sexual Function/Pregnancy

Sexual functioning may be altered due to surgery or treatments and should be discussed with the physician. Since most ileostomies are performed for inflammatory bowel disease, the patient population is usually younger, and therefore pregnancy may be an issue when sexual activity is resumed. Pregnancy prevention may need to be considered; on the other hand, desired pregnancies have been accomplished in persons with stomas. The physician should be consulted before pregnancy, and WOC/ET nurse included as it progresses, since the pouching system may require modification as the abdomen size increases. Many women with stomas have had successful pregnancies and vaginal deliveries.

Long-Term Management: Conventional Ileostomy

Fluid and Electrolytes/Dehydration

Fluid and electrolyte balance in the person with an ileostomy can be a concern because of the loss of the colon's absorptive function, even though the small bowel will eventually adapt. After the postoperative period, any condition that decreases the body's total fluids, such as vomiting or diarrhea, can lead to dehydration. Symptoms include increased thirst, lethargy, decreased urine output, dry mouth, muscle cramps, and abdominal cramps. As a precaution, patients should drink 10 to 12 8-oz glasses of liquid per day, and in the event of an episode of dehydration, fluid intake must be increased and intravenous fluids given if necessary. Patients need to be aware of signs of dehydration and to contact their health care provider at their first appearance (Bryant and Fleischer, 2003).

Food Blockage

Cramping and abdominal pain along with watery or no stool output in the person with an ileostomy indicates a food blockage or bowel obstruction. Stomal swelling and abdominal distention are further signs of blockage. Foods that cause blockage include high-fiber vegetables such as celery, those in Chinese food, grapes, raisins, pineapple, and popcorn. A warm bath may relax the abdominal muscles to allow the blockage to pass through the stoma, as will drinking warm fluids and assuming positions such as knee-to-chest. If the blockage is not resolved in 24 hours, a health care professional should be contacted. An abdominal x-ray will be obtained. Ileostomy lavage, the instillation of saline into the ileostomy to dislodge any food blockage, may be necessary. Box 11-10 describes the lavage procedure. To prevent food blockages, avoidance of high-fiber foods, chewing foods thoroughly, especially vegetables, and increasing fluid intake are recommended (Bryant and Fleischer, 2003).

High Output Fecal Stomas

Patients who have had several small bowel resections and a proctocolectomy may have a stoma in the upper ileum or jejunum. These patients are at risk for fluid and electrolyte imbalances and nutritional

---

BOX 11-10   Lavage Procedure

Equipment
Catheter-tipped piston syringe
14-16 Fr. catheter
Water-soluble lubricant
Irrigation sleeve
Drainable pouch with clamp
Normal saline warmed to room temperature
Skin cleanser
Soft wash cloth/towels

Procedure
1. Position patient comfortably with knees elevated.
2. Remove pouching system and clean peristomal skin. Apply irrigation sleeve and point into toilet or bed pan.
3. Gently insert a gloved, lubricated finger into stoma to determine the direction of the intestinal lumen.
4. Lubricate catheter and insert approximately 12-15 cm.
5. Using syringe, slowly instill 30-50 ml normal saline and then aspirate the full amount.
6. Repeat step 5 until the blockage is relieved.
7. When blockage is relieved and free drainage is present, measure stoma and apply pouching system (must remeasure as stoma is generally edematous and larger than usual size).
8. Resume usual pouch size after edema resolves.
9. Patient may experience residual abdominal soreness from the increased peristalsis that resulted from attempts to move the obstruction.

deficiencies, since they are unable to absorb enough protein, calories, and vitamins, especially vitamin B_{12}. Vitamin B_{12} should be replaced several times a year by intramuscular injection. It is vital that these patients increase fluid intake to replace that lost in the effluent. Many times, larger pouches such as irrigation sleeves are used to contain large amounts of output, especially at night. Medications to slow transit time may be used and fiber given to thicken stool. The effluent is especially corrosive to the skin, and efforts must be made to contain any leakage onto the skin. Kusuhara et al (1995) suggest the use of somatostatic analogue to reduce the output of the high-output proximal ileostomy.

Long-Term Management: Conventional Urostomy

Fluid and Electrolytes

Prevention of urinary complications involves the intake of adequate fluids, generally 2000 to 2500 ml/day. The fluid flushes the urinary system, dilutes bacteria, and promotes acidic pH of the urine to help prevent bacterial overgrowth. Use of a pouch with an antireflux device, emptying the pouch when one-third full, and use of a night drainage system help to prevent urine from bathing the area around the stoma and contributing to bacterial overgrowth.

Night Drainage System

A night drainage system is a large collection bag that is similar to a catheter drainage bag. The urostomy pouch is attached by a drainage tube to the larger collection bag to ensure that the smaller urostomy pouch is never full and that the patient does not have to wake up in the middle of the night to empty. In addition, keeping the urine away from the stoma prevents the formation of urinary crystals. When alkaline urine bathes the stoma or peristomal skin in an ill-fitting pouching system, crystals will appear as white gritty deposits form. To acidify the urine, vitamin C may be recommended, and the peristomal skin can be treated with vinegar soaks at each appliance change. Another method of treating the crystals is the application of an acidic washer around the stoma on the peristomal skin (Colly seal, Torbot). under the regular faceplate.

CONCLUSION

The challenges of managing a new ostomy are many. The person with a new ostomy needs a great deal of encouragement and education to accomplish optimal rehabilitation and a return to the former, functional lifestyle. The WOC nurse can assist the person to begin the process of adaptation by providing the education necessary to accomplish self stoma care.

SELF-ASSESSMENT EXERCISES

Questions

1. In the adolescent undergoing ostomy surgery, the most important developmental task concerns:
   a. Independence.
   b. Body image and privacy.
   c. Economic issues.
   d. Impact on career.
2. Which of the following preoperative assessment observations would impact the need for the WOC nurse to arrange for a special ostomy system after surgery?
   a. Blind patient
   b. Baseball player
   c. Golfer
   d. History of psoriasis
3. When planning a teaching session for a 3-year-old child with a colostomy and the parents, which of the following would be the most appropriate intervention?
   a. Video
   b. Education booklet
   c. Ostomy visitor
   d. Doll
4. When selecting a colostomy stoma site for a 25-year-old spinal cord-injured woman, which of the following positions is the most important to assess?
   a. Supine
   b. Sitting
   c. Standing
   d. Any position

5. Describe the reason the rectus muscle is identified when selecting a stoma site.

6. List three methods of locating the rectus muscle.

7. Which of the following should be a priority when developing a teaching plan for an elderly person with a colostomy?
   a. Provide a video and education booklet
   b. Arrange for an ostomy visitor
   c. Schedule short teaching sessions
   d. Use a flip chart of the surgical procedure

8. Describe two methods used to mark a stoma site.

9. When teaching a patient who only speaks Spanish and has no family available, which of the following interventions would be the best approach?
   a. Show a video
   b. Arrange a UOA visitor
   c. Arrange to use the services of an interpreter
   d. Provide an education booklet

10. The focus of the PLISSIT model developed by Annon is to:
   a. Provide permission for sexual activities.
   b. Provide sexual rehabilitation to patients.
   c. Encourage a positive self-image.
   d. Encourage individuals with ostomies to resume sexual activities.

11. For the adolescent, which developmental task does chronic illness, such as ulcerative colitis, interfere with? Resolving issues of:
   a. Initiative/guilt
   b. Identity/role confusion
   c. Intimacy/isolation
   d. Industry/inferiority

12. Which ostomy system would be appropriate to recommend for a blind person with an ileostomy?
   a. One piece system
   b. Two piece system
   c. Closed end pouches
   d. Precut, one-piece system

13. The WOC nurse uses principles of affective learning when teaching a postoperative ostomy patient by:
   a. Arranging an ostomy visitor.
   b. Arranging visiting nurse service.
   c. Having the patient empty the pouch with supervision.
   d. Having the patient's wife observe the ostomy system being changed.

14. Information necessary to enhance initial postoperative assessment in a patient with a new fecal or urinary diversion regards:
   a. Procedure, pathology, and expected outcomes.
   b. Stoma location.
   c. Mucocutaneous separation.
   d. Presence of a Jackson Pratt drain.

15. One indication of the return of bowel function is:
   a. Decreased abdominal pain.
   b. Decrease of drainage from the closed suction drain.
   c. Resumption of oral intake.
   d. Presence of flatus.

16. Pain management in the postoperative period is important to:
   a. Assist in patient mobilization.
   b. Assist in pouch change procedure.
   c. Stop patient from being noncompliant.
   d. Hasten bowel function.

17. Identify the most important factors in stoma assessment.

18. How is the type of stoma ascertained?
   a. Visualization
   b. Noting the abdominal location
   c. By examining medical record
   d. Assessing the type and consistency of the output

19. The absence of urinary flow from a newly created urostomy is considered:
   a. Normal.
   b. A temporary issues that will resolve with additional intravenous fluids.
   c. Related to the stents.
   d. A medical emergency.

20. Normal assessment of the newly created stoma includes all of the following *except*:
  a. Stomal edema.
  b. Color of the mucosa.
  c. Stomal necrosis.
  d. Protrusion of the stoma.

21. Ideally the length of the stoma should be:
  a. 5 to 10 cm.
  b. Greater than 4 cm.
  c. At skin level.
  d. 1 to 3 cm.

22. The amount and type of effluent from a newly created fecal stoma is related to:
  a. The time of day.
  b. The amount of parenteral fluids.
  c. The location in the intestinal tract.
  d. Fluid and electrolyte absorption.

23. Output of a newly created incontinent ileostomy should be:
  a. Liquid and bilious.
  b. Solid.
  c. Continuous.
  d. Blood tinged.

24. The skin around the stoma should be:
  a. Denuded because of the shaving and surgical scrub.
  b. Pale as compared to rest of the abdomen.
  c. Erythematous because of the presence of the pouch adhesive.
  d. Intact and healthy.

25. A mucocutaneous separation is thought to be related to:
  a. The presence of acidic effluent from the stoma.
  b. The use of an inappropriate pouching system.
  c. Poor wound, result of undue tension, separation of sutures.
  d. Pouch overfilling and resultant pulling in the area.

26. Early postoperative complications include all of the following *except*:
  a. Ileus.
  b. Anastomotic leak.
  c. Stoma ischemia.
  d. Pyoderma gangrenosum.

27. Describe the pouching principles in the postoperative period.

28. Discuss the adjustments that the person with a new stoma will undergo.

Answers

1. b

2. d

3. d

4. b

5. To avoid potential problems with the development of a parastomal hernia, the stoma is placed through the rectus muscle.

6. The rectus muscle can be identified by instructing the patient to raise their head while in a supine position, or having the patient cough or stretch the arms over the head.

7. c

8. Use a marking pen and cover with a transparent dressing; or use an intradermal injection of methylene blue at the site with a tuberculin syringe.

9. c

10. b

11. b

12. b

13. c

14. a

15. d

16. a

17. Stoma type and stoma characteristics: color, edema, shape, and protrusion

18. c

19. d

20. c

21. d

22. c

23. a

24. d

25. c

26. d

27. Pouching system is clear (to permit visualization of stoma and effluent), drainable, and cut to fit the stoma, and is without convexity.

28. The patient must undergo an alteration in body image, will learn basic stoma care skills, and cope with potential changes in clothing, bathing, and sexual issues.

REFERENCES

Bass EM et al: Does preoperative stoma marking and education by the enterostomal therapists affect outcome? *Dis Colon Rectum* 40(4):440-442, 1997.

Black P: Hidden problems of stoma care, *Br J Nurs* 3(14):707-711, 1994.

Black P: *Holistic stoma care,* Toronto, 2000a, Baillière Tindall, Harcourt Health Sciences.

Blackley P: *Practical stoma wound and continence management,* Vermont Vic, Australia, 1998, Research Publications.

Boarini J: Principles of stoma care for infants, *J Enterostom Ther* 16(1):21, 1989.

Bryant DE, Fleischer IR: Routine management of the patient with an ostomy. In Milne CT, Corbett LQ, Dubuc DL, editors: *Wound, ostomy, and continence nursing secrets,* Philadelphia, 2003, Hanley & Belfus.

Burckhardt CS: The ostomy adjustment scale: further evidence of reliability and validity, *Rehab Psych* 35(3): 149-155, 1990.

Colwell J: Ostomy surgical procedures. In Milne CT, Corbett LQ, Dubuc DL, editors: *Wound, ostomy, and continence nursing secrets,* Philadelphia, 2003, Hanley & Belfus.

Colwell J, Goldberg M, Carmel J: The state of the standard diversion, *JWOCN* 28:6-17, 2001.

Doughty, D: WOCN Ostomy Forum, 2003.

Erwin Toth P, Barrett P: Stoma site marking: a primer, *Ostomy/Wound Management* 43(4):18-25, 1997.

Erwin Toth P, Doughty D: Principles and procedures of stomal management. In Hampton B, Bryant R, *Ostomies and continent diversions: nursing management,* St Louis, 1992, Mosby.

Flick V, Woodward S: Teaching tool for the blind or partially sighted, *WCETJ* 20(3):22-23, 2000.

Golis A: Sexual issues for the person with an ostomy, *JWOCN* 23(1):33-37, 1996.

Gordon PH, Rolstad BS, Bubrick MP: Intestinal stomas. In Gordon PH, Nivatvongs S, editors: *Principles and practice of surgery for the colon, rectum, and anus,* ed 2, St Louis, 1999, Quality Medical Publishing.

Grotzel RL, Pemberton JH: Stoma physiology. In MacKeigom JM, Cataldo PA, editors: *Intestinal stomas: principles, techniques and management,* St Louis, 1993, Quality Medical Publishers.

Halsted M, Fernsler J: Coping strategies of long-term cancer survivors, *Cancer Nurs* 17(2):94-100, 1994.

Kehlet H, Morgensen T: Hospital stay of 2 days after open sigmoidectomy with a multimodal rehabilitation programme, *Br J Surg* 86:227-230, 1999.

Klopp A: Body image and self-concept among individuals with stomas, *J Enterostom Ther* 17(3):98-105, 1990.

Kohler L, Troid LH: Risk-benefit analysis of the ileoanal pouch, *Br J Surg* 82:443-447, 1995.

Kusuhara K et al: Reduction of the effluent volume in high output ileostomy patients by a somatostatic analogue, SMS 201-995 *Int J Colorectal Dis* 7:202, 1995.

Leininger M: *Culture care diversity & university: a theory in nursing,* New York, 1991, National League for Nursing Press.

Lemiska L, Watterworth B: Case study: teaching ostomy self-care to a legally blind patient, *Ostomy/Wound Management* 40(2):52-54, 1994.

Marquis P, Marrel A, Jambon B: Quality of life in patients with stomas: the Montreux study, *Ostomy/Wound Management* 49(2):48-55, 2003.

McCann EM: Routine assessment of the patient with an ostomy. In Milne CT, Corbett LQ, Dubuc DL, editors: *Wound, ostomy, and continence nursing secrets,* Philadelphia, 2003, Hanley & Belfus.

McLeod RS, Baxter NN: Quality of life of patients with inflammatory bowel disease after surgery, *World J Surg* 22:375-381, 1998.

Metcalf C: Stoma care: empowering patients through teaching practical skills, *Br J Nurs* 13-26:8(9):593-600, 1999.

Mowdy S: The role of the WOC nurse in an ostomy support group, *JWOCN* 25(1):51-54, 1998.

Nugent KP et al: Quality of life in stoma patients, *Dis Colon Rectum* 42:1569-1574, 1999.

O'Shea HS: Teaching the adult ostomy patient, *JWOCN* 28(1):47-54, 2001.

Pieper B, Mikols C, Dawson Grant TR: Comparing adjustment to an ostomy for three groups, *JWOCN* 23(4):197-204, 1996.

Piwonka MA, Merino JM: A multidimensional modeling of predictors influencing the adjustment to colostomy, *JWOCN* 26:298-305, 1999.

Redman B: *The practice of patient education,* ed 8, St Louis, 1997, Mosby.

Reynaud S, Meeker B: Coping style of older adults with ostomies, *J Gerontol Nurs* 28(5):30-36, 2002.

Shipes E: Psychosocial issues: the person with an ostomy, *Nurs Clin North Am* 22(2):296, 1987.

Smith D: When the patient with an ostomy is elderly, *Progressions* 6(1):3-11, 1994.

Smith D: Psychosocial adaptation. In Hampton B, Bryant R, editors: *Ostomies and continent diversions: nursing management,* St Louis, 1992, Mosby.

Spencer MP: Ostomies and stomal therapy, *Am Coll Colorectal Surg* 2003: www.fascrs.org/coresubjects/ostomies_stomal_therapy.html.

Taylor D: A comparison of the preoperative and post discharge concerns of the new ostomy patient, Poster presentation at WOCN National Conference, Cincinnati, 2003.

Turnbull G: The importance of coordinating ostomy care and teaching across the settings, *Ostomy/Wound Management* 48(5):12-13, 2002.

Turnbull G, Erwin-Toth P: Ostomy care: Foundation for teaching and practice, *OWM* 45(Suppl):23S-30S, 1999.

Watt R: Stoma placement. In Broadwell D, Jackson B, editors: *Principles of ostomy care,* St Louis, 1982, Mosby.

Weerakoon P: Meeting participant's needs: description of a sexuality workshop for stomal nurses, *WCET* 29(4):15-21, 2000.

White CA: Ostomy routine. In White CA: *Positive options for living with your ostomy,* Almeda, Calif, 2002, Hunter House Books.

Wong VK, White MA: Family dynamic and health: locus of control in adults with ostomies, *JWOCN* 29(1):37-44, 2002.

Zoucha R, Zamarripa C: The significance of culture in the care of the client with an ostomy, *JWOCN* 24(5):270-6, 1997.

12 *Principles of Stoma Management*

··

JANICE C. COLWELL

OBJECTIVES

1. Discuss these assessments, key when considering the choice of a pouching system: stoma characteristics, stoma creation, stoma function, peristomal skin integrity, peristomal plane characteristics, and patient requirements and preferences.
2. State two objectives that must be met when choosing a pouching system.
3. Describe the function of a skin barrier.
4. List the forms of skin barriers and the indications for their usage.
5. Describe the two types of solid skin barriers and compare performance parameters.
6. Describe decision points used when choosing a solid skin barrier: standard- or extended-wear, shape, and fit.
7. Discuss the features of a one-piece versus a two-piece pouching system.
8. Describe the features of drainable and nondrainable pouches.
9. Identify the functions of skin barrier powder, liquid skin barrier, and solvents.
10. Explain reusable pouching systems.

INTRODUCTION

The following principles guide the management of the person with a fecal or urinary diversion:

1. Maintain the pouching seal for a consistent, predictable wear time.
2. Maintain peristomal skin integrity.
3. Support the person with a stoma.

These principles are tailored to each person with a stoma. The plan of care is individualized following a thorough assessment. This assessment includes:

1. Stoma characteristics
   a. Mucosa
   b. Protrusion
   c. Anatomic location
   d. Size and shape
   e. Stoma lumen
2. Stoma construction
3. Stoma function
4. Peristomal skin integrity
5. Peristomal plane characteristics
6. Patient's preferences and requirements
7. Volume and consistency of effluent

STOMA CHARACTERISTICS
Mucosa

The stomal mucosa is assessed for texture and presence of edema. A newly created stoma will have a shiny and tight mucosal appearance (Color Plate 3). The stoma gradually changes shape and size. The fit of the pouching system for this stoma must be reevaluated at frequent intervals. Stomal edema is generally present for up to 6 weeks from creation. A pouching system for the newly created stoma that allows for customization (to accommodate stoma shrinkage) is the most appropriate. A stoma with texture and creases indicates one that is not newly created, and this type of stoma should not have dramatic shifts in size; thus the use of a standard-sized pouching system opening or template can be considered. The mucosa of all stomas should be red, moist, and shiny, and the tissue

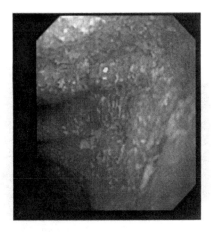

Color Plate 1 Ulcerative colitis.

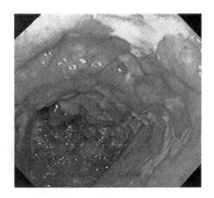

Color Plate 2 Crohn's disease.

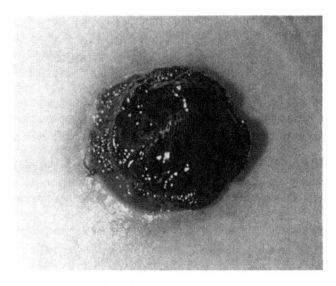

Color Plate 3 Newly created stoma, shiny tight mucosa.

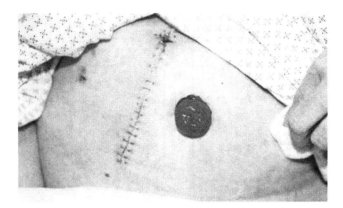

Color Plate 4 Stoma necrosis.

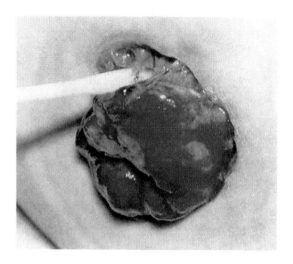

Color Plate 5 Mucocutaneous separation. (Courtesy Cleveland Clinic, Cleveland, Ohio.)

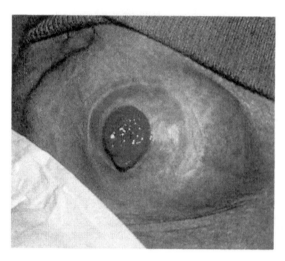

Color Plate 6 Parastomal hernia.

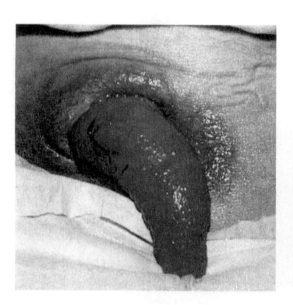

Color Plate 7 Stoma prolapse.

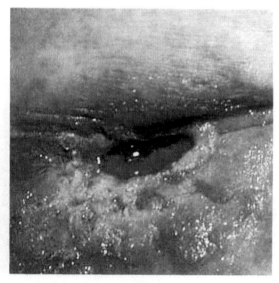

Color Plate 8 Stoma retraction.

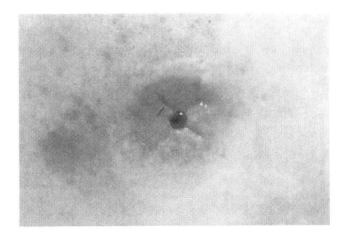

Color Plate 9 Stoma stenosis.

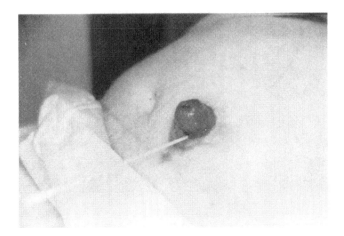

Color Plate 10 Stoma fistula.

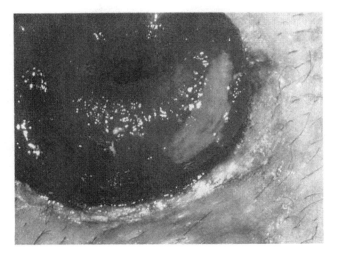

Color Plate 11 Stoma trauma. (Courtesy Cleveland Clinic, Cleveland, Ohio.)

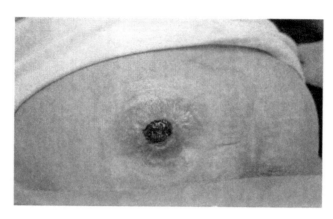

Color Plate 12 Peristomal varices.

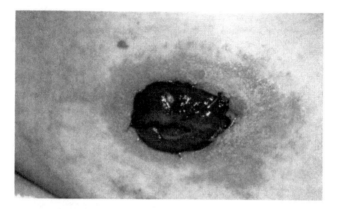

Color Plate 13 Peristomal candidiasis. (Courtesy Nancy McLeese.)

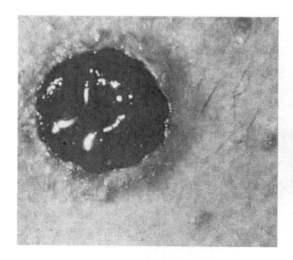

Color Plate 14 Folliculitis.

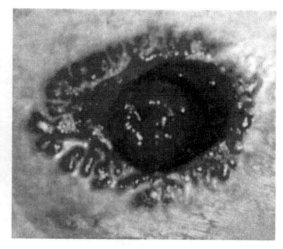

Color Plate 15 Mucosal transplantation. (Courtesy Cleveland Clinic, Cleveland, Ohio.)

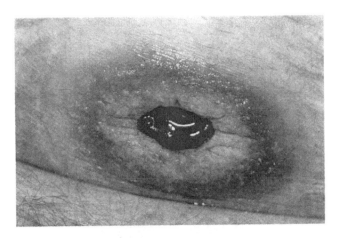

Color Plate 16 Pseudoverrucous lesions.

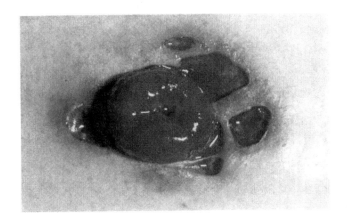

Color Plate 17 Peristomal pyoderma gangrenosum.

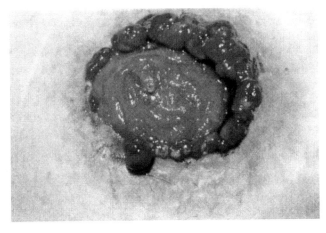

Color Plate 18 Suture granulomas. (Courtesy Cleveland Clinic, Cleveland, Ohio.)

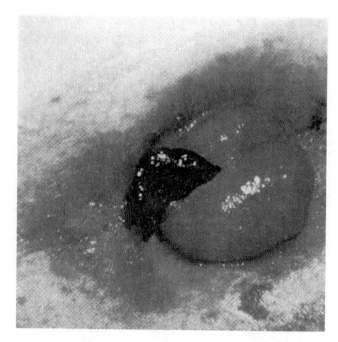

Color Plate 19   Peristomal irritant contact dermatitis

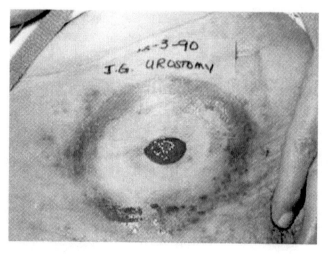

Color Plate 20   Peristomal allergic contact dermatitis. (Courtesy Cleveland Clinic, Cleveland, Ohio.)

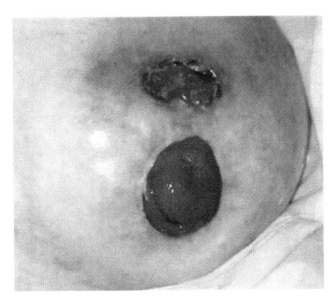

Color Plate 21 Peristomal trauma. (Courtesy Alyce Barnicle.)

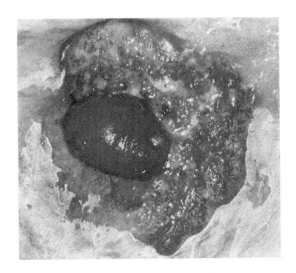

Color Plate 22 Peristomal malignancy.

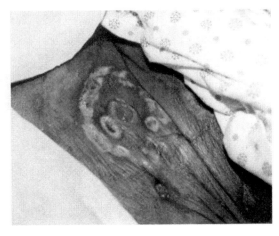

Color Plate 23 Peristomal herpes.

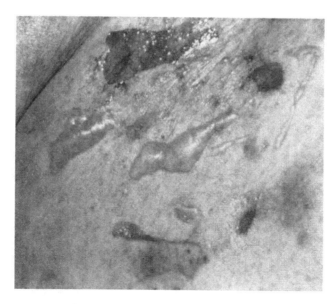

Color Plate 24   Peristomal pemphigus.

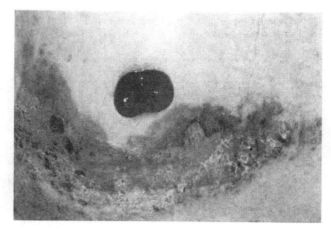

Color Plate 25   Peristomal psoriasis.

should be tense and firm to the touch. A stoma that is brown, black, gray, or flaccid may indicate impaired blood flow (Color Plate 4).

Exceptions to the norm of a red stoma are ureterostomies, which may appear pale pink due to the colse of the ureters. The skin-stoma junction should be closely evaluated in the postoperative period. This connection, referred to as the mucocutaneous junction, should be assessed for separation of the stoma from the skin and for any evidence of skin reaction to the suture material. The normal appearance of the mucocutaneous junction is that of the stoma in apposition to the skin, and in a newly created stoma, sutures will be present at the junction. If a separation between the two is noted, it should be documented by the approximate percentage of separation (e.g., 25% separation) (see Chapter 14 for treatment of a mucocutaneous separation) (Color Plate 5).

Protrusion

The amount of stoma protrusion above the skin level is an important assessment. It is generally agreed that a fecal or a urinary stoma should protrude at least 0.8 inch above the skin. This protrusion allows the stoma output to drain directly into the pouching system. A stoma flush to the skin may allow the effluent to drain under the skin barrier seal and cause pouching system failure. A flush stoma may require the use of a pouching system with convexity to ensure a good pouching system seal. An excessively long stoma can be easily injured when using a flanged pouching system.

Anatomic Location

Stomas typically managed with a pouching system are jejunostomy, ileostomy, colostomy, and urostomy. The anatomic location of the stoma provides information about the amount, consistency, and frequency of the output; this data will be used when choosing the type of skin barrier and, in some cases, the type of pouch.

A jejunostomy is an opening into the jejunum, the midportion of the small intestine. There is a large amount of intestinal secretions from the jejunum, which aid in digestion. Therefore the effluent is watery, clear, and dark green and can be in excess of 2400 ml/24 hours (Erwin Toth and Doughty, 1992).

An ileostomy is an opening into the ileum, which is the third portion of the small intestine. The initial output from a terminal ileostomy after surgical creation is liquid and varies between 800 and 1700 ml/24 hours. As food is introduced into the gastrointestinal tract, the output gains consistency and the amount levels at approximately 500 to 1800 ml/24 hours (Gordon, Rolstad, and Bubrick, 1999). Variations in consistency and volume are governed by the amount of water in the stool (Grotz and Pemberton, 1993).

A colostomy is an opening into a portion of the colon or large intestine. A stoma may be created in any section of the colon: the cecum (rarely created) (Grotz and Pemberton, 1993), the ascending colon, the transverse colon (the largest section of the colon, thus the largest stoma), the descending colon, or the sigmoid colon. The output from the colon varies, depending on the stoma location. The more distal to the ileum the stoma is located, the thicker and less frequent the output. The longer the fecal material is in contact with the colon mucosa, the more liquid is absorbed, and peristalsis decreases as the colon approaches the rectum. Stoma functioning depends on the extent of previous resections, residual disease, medications, types of foods consumed, and concurrent therapies (i.e., chemotherapy and radiation therapy).

Cecostomy output starts out watery and then gains some consistency as the patient eats. Output from an ileostomy begins as liquid and soon develops a consistency described by some as that of thick oatmeal. An ascending colostomy output is very similar in appearance to that of an ileostomy. When located on the left side, a transverse colostomy should have a pasty stool and less water content (Grotz and Pemberton, 1993). The person with a descending or sigmoid colostomy initially has a slightly pasty stool, which may progress to a soft, semiformed stool. Many patients with a left-sided colostomy, when back to normal eating and activity, return to "normal" bowel function of 1 or 2 stools in a 24- or 48-hour period.

A urostomy is an opening into the urinary tract. Commonly created urostomies, which necessitate management with a pouching system, include ileal conduit, sigmoid conduit, ureterostomy, and cutaneous pyleostomy. Although dependent on intake, the normal adult output of urine in 24 hours is about 1500 to 1600 ml (Kilpatrick, 2001).

Location on the abdomen does not necessarily indicate the anatomic location. For example, an ileostomy is usually located on the right side of the abdomen because this allows for easy mobilization (the terminal ileum is located in the lower right abdomen). However, many factors can lead to an alternate physical location of the stoma at the time of surgical creation (e.g., scars, radiation therapy).

Size and Shape

The size and shape of the stoma depends on the reason for its creation, the area of the gastrointestinal or genitourinary tract used, the type of stoma created, and the surgical technique. When a stoma is created proximal to a bowel obstruction or on edematous portion of the bowel, the intestine may be edematous because of the proximity to the involved area. As the postoperative edema subsides, the stoma size decreases, usually over a 6-week period. The small intestine is approximately 2.5 cm wide, whereas the colon varies in width from 2.5 to 6.3 cm. Thus one of the factors that contributes to the size of the stoma is the anatomic location. Loop stomas are generally larger than end stomas because of the use of the "side" rather than the end of the intestine. A ureterostomy is a small stoma because it is created from the ureter, which has a small diameter, as compared to the larger stoma created with an ileal conduit, in which the ileum is used, which has a wider diameter.

The stoma should be measured for size at the site of the stomal attachment to the skin (i.e., mucocutaneous junction), since this measurement will be used to choose the correct pouching system and to monitor stoma progress. Circular measuring guides are available and are convenient to use with a round stoma. An oval stoma can be measured at the longest and widest diameters, or can be sized by using a piece of plastic to trace it. Until edema has subsided, remeasuring at frequent intervals is recommended.

Stoma Lumen

The location of the lumen of the stoma will dictate the direction of the effluent. A stoma lumen that is even with the skin surface may cause the output to drain under the skin barrier on the pouching system. A stoma lumen that is straight up on a stoma with adequate protrusion should discharge the effluent directly into the pouching system, placing less strain on the solid skin barrier. A stoma with a lumen that is at the skin level may cause problems with the pouch seal, because the effluent is directed under the solid skin barrier seal. This type of stoma may require a convex pouching system or use of a skin barrier paste to seal the edge of the solid skin barrier.

Stoma Construction

The type of stoma that is created impacts the choice of a management system. Fecal stoma types can be end or loop. An *end stoma* is created by division of the bowel: the proximal end of the intestine is brought through the abdominal wall, everted, and attached to the skin (see Figure 1-2). Surgical interventions that create an end stoma include total proctocolectomy (i.e., removal of the entire colon and rectum) and an abdominoperineal resection (i.e., removal of the distal colon and rectum). An end stoma does not necessarily mean a permanent diversion. If the distal end of the intestine is closed and left in the abdomen, the distal end is called a Hartmann's pouch (see Figure 1-1). The only opening to the Hartmann's pouch is the rectum; the person with a Hartmann's closure can expect periodic mucous drainage from the rectum. If the colon was not adequately cleansed before the surgical procedure, stool will be expelled from the rectum until the segment is emptied. There are several reasons for creation of a Hartmann's pouch: it obviates the risk for anastomosis under septic conditions (Corman, 1993), decreases the time under anesthesia if the patient is too ill to have a complete proctectomy, and can afford palliation in patients with anorectal disease. The disadvantage is that if a second stage is to be performed, it requires a major abdominal procedure. Occasionally, if the patient is deemed high risk, the Hartmann's procedure may result in a permanent stoma.

A *loop stoma* is created by bringing the bowel through an abdominal wall opening and placing a rod beneath the bowel (see Figure 7-2). A transverse opening is made, and the bowel is everted and matured. The purpose of the rod is to support the loop of intestine. There are several manufactured rods (Figure 12-1); other types of support rods include small pieces of rubber or plastic tubing (see Figure 12-1). A loop stoma can be made in the small or large intestine; however, loop colostomies are performed much less frequently today, because it is believed that that protection of a colonic end anastomosis is better achieved using a loop ileostomy than a loop colostomy. A loop ileostomy does not have the potential to impair the blood supply of the distal colon, is easier to manage, has less odor, and generally is easier to close (Keighley, 1996; Williams et al, 1986). Loop ileostomies are created to protect a distal anastomosis or in the management of a colonic obstruction. A loop colostomy is used for a number of indications: obstructing or perforating lesions of the colon, trauma, anastomotic leak, congenital anomalies, and to protect the anastomosis (Corman, 1993). Loop stomas are generally intended as temporary diversions (see Figure 12-1).

Support rods are left in place until there is no tension on the bowel and healing has taken place. If the support rod extends onto the peristomal skin, the solid skin barrier must fit around or under the

rod to afford protection of the skin from the stoma output.

In some situations the intestine is resected or divided, and both ends are brought out to the abdominal wall. The proximal functional stoma is the end stoma; the distal end is nonfunctioning and referred to as the mucous fistula (see Figure 5-4). The mucous fistula expels mucus at periodic intervals. It is advisable to have at least a 3-inch separation between stomas to allow for pouching of the proximal end stoma. If the distal segment has not been cleansed before the operation, some fecal output can temporarily drain from the mucous fistula, and pouching this stoma may be advisable. After the fecal drainage subsides, a dry dressing to collect mucus and to protect clothing is suggested. Mucous fistulas are created when a primary anastomosis at the time of surgery is not indicated, if a Hartmann's closure is not done, or if there is a distal, unresectable obstruction.

A urostomy can be created along any portion of the urinary tract: a *cutaneous pyelostomy* is an opening into the renal pelvis, a *ureterostomy* (Figure 12-2) is an opening into one or both ureters, and an *ileal* or *sigmoid conduit* (see Figure 10-1) uses the ileum or sigmoid colon to create a passage (i.e., conduit) for the urine to be expelled out through the abdominal wall (see Chapter 10).

Stoma Function

Output is assessed for amount, consistency, and overall appearance. As noted earlier, the amount and consistency of the output depends on the type and anatomic location of the stoma. In the postoperative period, other factors also affect the output. These factors include oral intake, medications, and degree of ambulation. High oral intake of fluid can dilute the fecal and urinary output; therefore, a conscientious effort must be made to record intake, as well as output, to assist in assessment of hydration or dehydration. Certain medications can slow bowel function (i.e., narcotics), whereas others can cause an increase in urinary output (i.e., diuretics).

In addition to the stoma volume measurement, an important assessment for the person with a fecal stoma is the consistency of the output. Pure liquid

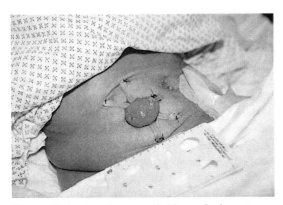

Figure 12-1 Plastic support bridge under loop stoma.

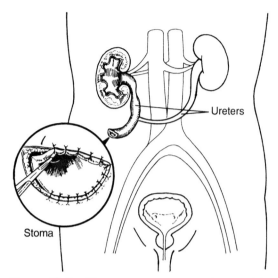

Ureters

Stoma

Figure 12-2 Transureteroureterostomy is created by end-to-side anastomosis of one ureter to the other. (Modified from Cukier J: Ureteral diversions. In Glenn J, editor: *Urologic surgery*, ed 4, Philadelphia, 1991, JB Lippincott.)

output from an ileostomy or colostomy can indicate an alteration in function and is usually accompanied by high volume. High volume, liquid output will be a factor when choosing a skin barrier and perhaps the pouch capacity.

Flatus is passed from a fecal stoma and collected in the pouching system. If the amount of gas inflates the pouch to more than half its capacity, it must be released, or the inflation of the pouch will cause strain on the pouch seal. It is generally agreed that the majority of gas passed via an ileostomy is related to ingested air. Activities related to air ingestion that should be avoided in the person with an ileostomy who has a large volume of gas include drinking through a straw, chewing gum, smoking, and sucking on hard candy. Many people with ileostomies note an excessive amount of gas upon awakening after a full night's sleep. This is related to ingestion of air while sleeping. Methods to manage ingested air are avoidance of the activities already mentioned, use of a pouch with a gas filter, or the use of simethicone. Simethicone can be used with

each meal or only before sleeping, if the gas is related to swallowing air while sleeping. Although the gas from a colostomy can be related to ingested air, it is generally correlated to the bacteria in the stool and the fermentation of the bacteria. Certain foods provide bacterial overgrowth. Avoidance of notable foods (see Appendix C), and use of gas filters (see discussion later in this chapter) or enzyme preparations (see Chapter 16) can be effective.

Assessment of the output from a urinary diversion should include the characteristics of the urine, the presence of odor, the color, and the presence of substances other than fluid (e.g., the presence of mucous strands). If the person with a urostomy has an ileal or sigmoid conduit, mucus strands will be present that may give the urine a cloudy appearance. The small and large bowel secrete mucus and will continue to do so when used as a conduit. It appears that the amount of mucus decreases over time, but will always be present in a limited amount.

Peristomal Skin Integrity

The condition of the peristomal skin should be healthy and intact. Any breaks in the epidermis can result in the release of moisture, which will undermine the pouching system seal. Treatment of impaired peristomal skin is covered in Chapter 13.

Peristomal Plane Characteristics

It is extremely important to assess the area directly around the stoma. The term *peristomal plane* refers to the surface area located under the solid skin barrier and adhesive of the pouching system; it extends out from the base of the stoma in an area of approximately 4 by 4 inches around the stoma (Rolstad and Boarini, 1996). The peristomal plane evaluation provides information that helps determine the shape, size, and construction of the skin barrier. The patient's abdomen should be examined when the patient is in lying, sitting, and standing positions. The area immediately around the stoma and out to about 4 inches (i.e., the peristomal plane) is observed to determine if changes in position cause creases or folds or movement that could disrupt the pouching system seal. The stoma is visualized with the patient in sitting, supine, and standing positions to evaluate if the amount of protrusion is lessened in any position. The skin around the stoma is evaluated for firmness or excessive softness. These assessments will provide important information when choosing to use a barrier with convexity, a soft, flexible skin barrier, or perhaps a belt (see discussion in later section).

Patient Preferences and Requirements

It is important to evaluate the patient's expectations regarding stoma pouching options. A patient who has just undergone ostomy surgery may have few or no expectations. However, this is not the norm: most patients have been prepared, or have prepared themselves, regarding stoma management. They may want to use a pouching system that is not reasonable in the postoperative period; for instance, they may wish to try out a short, opaque pouch, which will not allow the visualization of the stoma or the output that is necessary during the hospitalization, and the pouch may overfill too quickly. The patient should understand that although this and other options are available, it is important to learn to work first with the postoperative pouch, and to develop basic skills before moving on to other types of products. As the stoma and abdomen heal, and as the stoma begins to function in the normal range, the person with a fecal or a urinary stoma can try out other types of pouching systems.

Wear time should be discussed with the patient. Wear time, the amount of time between pouch application and removal, should be predictable. The factors that contribute to wear time are the type of stoma, the amount and volume of stoma output, the peristomal planes, the type and shape of the solid skin barrier, and the patient's preferences. Most clinicians agree that a minimal acceptable wear time is 3 to 4 days (Gordon, Rolstad, and Bubrick, 1999; Wells and Doughty, 1994), but this may not always be achievable. Wear time can be evaluated by examination of the solid skin barrier. When the solid skin barrier is removed, the adhesive side is examined for erosion and possible undermining. If the solid skin barrier adhesive side

appears intact, with little wear and no undermining, wear time can be extended. The same examination is performed at the next change, until maximal wear time can be established.

The patient's visual acuity and manual dexterity are considered when choosing a pouching system. Patients with limited visual acuity may benefit from a precut pouching system, or a system with few pieces. A person with decreased manual dexterity may prefer a two-piece pouching system that allows the pouch to be discarded rather than emptied.

Additional considerations include the patient's activities (e.g., water sports, contact sports) and financial issues (e.g., method and amount of supply reimbursement).

When assessing a person who has had a stoma for some time, the evaluation should include average frequency of emptying the pouch (or changing it, if using a closed-ended system) to evaluate stoma output, the usual consistency of the output, the ordinary wear time, the preferred wear time, and the change procedure. The change procedure will include how the person removes the pouch, skin preparation, and the application procedure. This provides information on the patient's expectations, as well as routines that should be altered to increase wear time, or decrease potential or actual skin irritation (Table 12-1).

POUCHING PRINCIPLES

The choice of a pouching system depends on a thorough assessment of the patient, as already outlined. Once the assessment is completed the selection of a pouching system can be made. A pouching system must provide predictable wear time and protect the peristomal skin. A solid skin barrier (or in some limited instances only an adhesive interface) and the collection device are the components of a pouching system (Figure 12-3). The most important portion of the pouching system is the solid skin barrier, the interface between the patient's skin, and the pouch. If chosen appropriately, the skin barrier protects the skin from the stoma effluent and seals the pouch to the skin for a predictable wear time. The pouch, although perhaps the more obvious portion of the pouching

TABLE 12-1   Pouching System Selection: Patient Assessment

CRITERIA	CHARACTERISTICS
Stoma	Mucosa
	Texture
	Color
	Mucocutaneous junction
	Amount of protrusion
	Inches above skin
	Anatomic location
	Jejunum
	Ileum
	Ascending colon
	Transverse colon
	Descending colon
	Sigmoid colon
	Ileal or sigmoid conduit
	Ureter
	Kidney
Size and shape	Inches at widest and longest diameters
	Round, oval
Location of stoma lumen	Straight up
	Side
	Level with skin
Stoma construction	End
	Loop
	Mucous fistula
	Cutaneous pyelostomy
	Ureterostomy
	Ileal or sigmoid conduit
Stoma function	Amount of effluent
	Consistency of effluent
	Presence and amount of flatus
Peristomal skin integrity	Intact healthy skin
	Denuded areas
Peristomal plane characteristics	Presence of skin creases or folds
	Change in stoma appearance in various positions
Patient's preferences and requirements	Wear time
	Visual acuity requirements
	Manual dexterity requirements
	Activity of daily living requirements

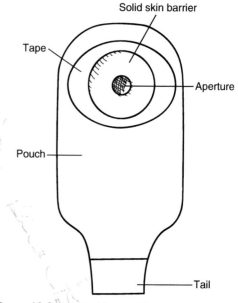

Figure 12-3 Drainable pouching system components.

system, does not contribute greatly to the pouch seal. Therefore the first and foremost decision to be made when choosing a pouching system is the choice of the solid skin barrier. One type of pouching system not widely used is a reusable pouching system. This system is covered in a separate section later in this chapter.

Pouching System Framework: Solid Skin Barrier (Figure 12-4)

A skin barrier protects the peristomal skin from the stoma output. A secondary function of the skin barrier is to create a level pouching surface (Erwin-Toth and Doughty, 1992). Skin barriers are available in several forms: solid, paste, powder, and liquid. While all skin barriers protect the skin, solid and paste skin barriers also provide an adhesive seal. Skin barrier powders contribute to the pouching system seal by providing a dry surface (typically used on denuded skin), and a skin barrier liquid can be used to protect irritated skin and to enhance the adhesive seal.

Solid skin barriers (Figure 12-5) are available in several configurations: sheet, plain, or with a flange

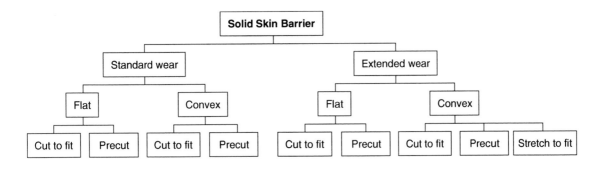

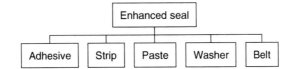

Figure 12-4 Pouching system framework: solid skin barrier.

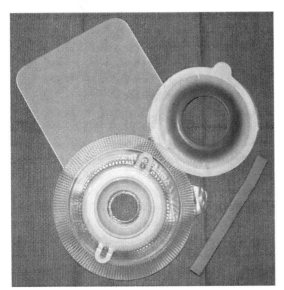

Figure 12-5 Solid skin barriers: plain sheet with flanged barrier, washer, and strip.

or coupling attached to the top side, the washer, and the strip. The sheet skin barrier has an adhesive side (applied to the skin) and a top side that carries the pouch or flange. The top side is typically covered with a film, which provides protection from moisture (i.e., stoma effluent), carries the pouch or

flange, stabilizes the adhesive for ease or removal (without the film the adhesive would break up as it was removed, making separation from the skin difficult), and influences the flexibility of the barrier (certain films make the barrier stiff or flexible).

Solid skin barriers contain several materials (e.g., polymers, tackifiers, softeners and plasticizers, hydrocolloids, fillers, and pigment). Each type of skin barrier has a unique "recipe" of these ingredients. The amount, type, and location in the skin barrier of ingredients differ among solid skin barriers, thus all skin barriers are not created equal and will perform differently. The *polymers* and *tackifiers* provide adhesiveness. *Softeners* and *plasticizers* are oils that provide softness and flow. *Hydrocolloids* are powders that absorb moisture and can consist of carboxymethylcellulose, pectin, and gelatin. Skin moisture absorption in a skin barrier is important because skin releases moisture constantly; if this moisture is allowed to sit on the skin, maceration will occur, as well as a resultant fungal overgrowth that damages the natural skin barrier. *Fillers* can influence fluid absorption, and *pigments* provide color (Table 12-2).

The majority of solid skin barriers erode slowly when in contact with stoma output. As the hydrocolloid absorbs moisture, the skin barrier swells and

TABLE 12-2   Solid Skin Barrier Components

MATERIALS	FUNCTION
Polymers	Provide various degrees of adhesion, flow, and mobility
Tackifiers	Provide adhesiveness
Softeners and plasticizers	Provide adhesive flow
Hydrocolloids	
CMC	Fluid absorption
Pectin	Fluid absorption
	Acidic (can help to decrease skin overgrowth)
Gelatin	Provides gel strength, decreases overall erosion
Fillers	Regulate water absorption
Pigment	Provides color

Each type of skin barrier has a unique "recipe" of these ingredients. The amount, type, and location of ingredients in the skin barrier differs among solid skin barriers.
CMC, Carboxymethylcellulose.

increases in size and breaks apart. This erosion depends on several factors: the amount and moisture content of the output, skin moisture (perspiration), and the type of skin barrier. The erosion of the solid skin barrier on a pouching system will cause the peristomal skin to be exposed to the stoma effluent and will negatively affect the seal of the pouching system. Thus an important factor for pouching system wear time is the type of solid skin barrier. There are two types of solid skin barriers, regular-wear and extended-wear. The difference between these two types of skin barriers depends upon the product ingredients; the extended-wear skin barrier has delayed absorption and a higher level of adhesion, generally providing longer wear time.

Both regular- and extended-wear skin barriers possess a property called *flow.* Flow is the ability of the skin barrier (and hence the adhesive) to spread over the skin, enhancing the adhesive contact. Regular-wear skin barriers have high flow, and it is important on application to use both pressure and warmth to obtain the spreading or flow of the skin barrier onto the peristomal skin. Extended-wear

skin barriers have low flow, thus when applying an extended-wear barrier it is only necessary to apply pressure to enhance the seal. A key time for adhesion is the few minutes after application when the barrier flows; thus it is important to keep strenuous movements to a minimum for the first half hour following application of the skin barrier.

A key step in determining predictable wear time of the pouching system is to ascertain at what point the skin barrier is no longer providing skin protection. This is best done by changing the solid skin barrier after a few days of wear, examining the adhesive side for erosion, and assessing the peristomal skin for signs of contact with the stoma effluent. Wear time is increased gradually, with assessment of the skin barrier at each removal. The point at which the skin barrier erodes significantly and allows stool or urine on the skin (and thus reduces the adhesive seal) is identified, and from then on the pouching system is changed before this point.

The adhesive side of the solid skin barrier is applied to the peristomal skin. A release paper coated with silicone covers the adhesive and holds the adhesive area flat. As already noted, a key concept in applying a solid skin barrier to the peristomal skin is the application of pressure. All solid skin barrier adhesives are pressure-sensitive, thus upon application of the skin barrier to the skin, pressure is applied to the entire surface to insure an adequate seal (see Table 12-3 for solid skin barrier usage tips).

The first decision when planning stoma care is to determine the type of solid skin barrier for the pouching system: standard- or extended-wear (see Figure 12-4). As previously noted there are two categories of solid skin barriers: regular-wear and extended-wear. The difference between the two skin barriers is how they interact with moisture and how high the adhesion is to the skin. Although both kinds of barriers absorb moisture, the extended-wear barrier has delayed absorption by the hydrocolloids, thus slowing down the erosion process. The life span, or length of time over which the extended-wear barrier has the ability to protect the skin and maintain the pouch seal, is generally

TABLE 12-3   **Solid Skin Barrier Application Tips**

TIP	RATIONALIZATION
Apply pressure over solid skin barrier (both types) to the skin to enhance the seal.	The adhesive in solid skin barriers is pressure-sensitive.
Apply warmth to the *standard-wear* barrier to further enhance the seal.	Standard-wear skin barriers skin have high flow and will begin the process of spreading if warmed upon application (this is not the case with extended-wear barriers).
Cut the opening in the solid skin barrier to fit around the stoma, allowing no skin between the stoma and the edge of the skin barrier to be exposed.	The skin barrier must cover all of the peristomal skin to provide protection. The skin barrier will not harm the stoma.

greater (compared to the regular-wear barrier) because of this durability. There is no definition of "longer" in connection to wear time: longer relates to the "regular" length of wear time for that specific patient. For example a standard-wear skin barrier may provide a seal for one patient for up to 4 days and for another patient for only 2 days because of a complex stoma situation. For one patient an extended-wear seal may mean 7 days, yet for another patient it can mean 4 days. Thus the terms regular- and extended-wear are relative to the specific patient's situation. It is generally agreed that the extended-wear barrier is more resistant to moisture and adheres strongly to the skin, and that in the face of moisture it will therefore maintain shape longer than the comparable standard-wear skin barrier. Therefore a person with high volume output or output with a high liquid content will benefit from the slower erosion of an extended-wear solid skin barrier. Less erosion should translate into longer wear.

The next decision in determining the type of solid skin barrier is shape. The contour of the skin barrier provides an effective seal by maintaining continuous contact of the skin barrier to the skin. The two shape options are flat and convex. A flat barrier has a level skin contact area, and a convex barrier has an outward curve that begins at the aperture of the skin barrier and extends outward (Rolstad and Boarini, 1996; Wound, Ostomy and Continence Nurses Society, 2002)

(Figure 12-6). The choice will depend upon the assessment of the stoma (height and location of the stoma lumen) and the peristomal skin planes (the presence of creases, folds, or any change in the stoma appearance when the person is in a sitting, standing, or lying position). Rolstad and Boarini (1996) recommend that the shape of the skin barrier should be a mirror image of the topography of the peristomal plane. A flat solid skin barrier is considered in the following situations: minimal shifts in the peristomal plane in the flat, lying, and standing positions; maintenance of stoma protrusion in the previously noted positions; and stoma effluent that does not undermine the skin barrier seal.

Convexity, an outward curve, is available in several options (Figure 12-7). Levels of convexity have been defined as shallow ($<\frac{1}{16}$-inch depth), moderate (depth of $>\frac{1}{16}$-inch but $<\frac{1}{4}$-inch), and deep ($>\frac{1}{4}$-inch deep) (Rolstad and Boarini, 1996). One-piece convex pouching systems are constructed with the pouch and skin barrier as one piece; the skin barrier is convex. The skin barrier of a convex one-piece pouching system can be precut, cut, or stretched to fit, or custom-constructed. Custom-constructed convex systems are created by businesses that manufacture the product from either measurements or a mold of the area on a specific patient. Two-piece convex pouching systems have a solid skin barrier with convexity precut and built in; a cut- or

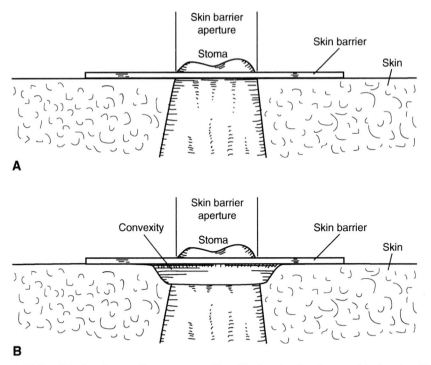

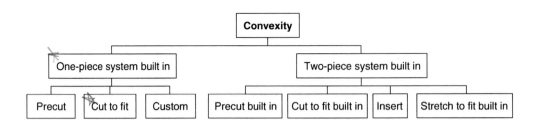

Figure 12-6   Skin barrier configurations. **A,** Flat skin barrier. **B,** Convex skin barrier. (From Rolstad BS, Boarini J: Principles and techniques in the use of convexity, *Ostomy Wound Manage* 42(1):26, 1996.)

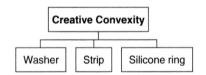

Figure 12-7   Pouching system framework: convexity.

stretched-to-fit built-in or presized insert can be placed into the skin barrier.

Convexity can be created using a skin barrier washer or strip. The washer or the strip is fitted around the stoma before the pouching system application. Another system that can add convexity to a two-piece pouching system is the use of a silicone ring that can be snapped into the skin barrier of the two-piece system.

A further option in a convex pouching system is the size of the convexity. Some convex products have a well-defined area of convexity, located at the opening of the skin barrier (Figure 12-8). The defined area of convexity provides support directly around the stoma, applying pressure to push the stoma into the pouching system opening and to flatten creases next to the stoma lumen. One

consideration in cut-to-fit or stretch-to-fit convex products is to ensure that once the skin barrier opening is made, the convexity is located where the support is required. To help carry this out, most cut-to-fit convex products are available with the convexity in various diameters. Other convex products slope the convexity in a gradual fashion from the inner opening to the outer edge of the skin barrier (Figure 12-9). The sloped or slanted section of convexity applies pressure on the peristomal plane; it keeps the uneven surface flat and is used most often to maintain a seal on a creased or folded peristomal area.

The use of a convex skin barrier should be considered in several situations. If the stoma does not protrude into the pouching system and this lack of protrusion causes the stoma effluent to drain under the solid skin barrier, convexity can provide pressure on the peristomal skin and cause the stoma to project into the pouching system opening (Wound, Ostomy and Continence Nurses Society, 2002). Other stoma situations that can cause the effluent to drain under the solid skin barrier include retraction, peristomal fistula, and location of the stoma lumen at skin level. Convexity next to the stoma opening can be used to apply pressure on the peristomal area and provide consistent, predictable wear. The degree of convexity depends upon the amount of retraction or the level of the fecal or the urinary output (i.e., lumen location).

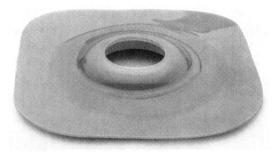

Figure 12-8   Convex cut-to-fit skin barrier, two-piece pouching system, convexity located at opening of skin barrier. (Courtesy Hollister, Inc, Libertyville, IL.)

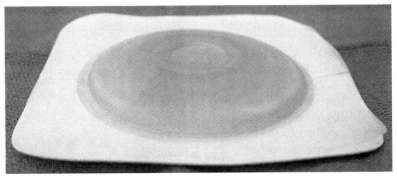

Figure 12-9   Convex precut skin barrier. Convexity slopes from inner opening to edge of skin barrier.

When there are creases and/or folds in the stoma plane with the person in sitting, standing, and lying positions, convexity may assist in flattening the area to provide an adequate skin barrier seal. The type of convexity most appropriate in many of these situations is a sloping or gradient convexity, the degree of which should reflect the degree of creasing.

The next decision in determining the type of solid skin barrier is fit. Solid skin barriers are available in *cut-to-fit* and *precut* options. *Cut-to-fit* solid skin barriers are used for stomas that are not a standard round shape. An important principle when using a solid skin barrier is that the fit should be at the mucocutaneous junction to prevent peristomal skin exposure to the stoma effluent. Exceptions to this principle can be made to manage prolapsed stomas (see Chapter 14 on stomal and peristomal complications), stoma friability, or stoma enlargement during passage of a solid large stool. If the stoma is not round, or if the desired pouching system is not available in the person's stoma size, a cut-to-fit skin barrier is indicated. A template or pattern is created. Precut solid skin barriers are used when the stoma size matches the precut size, or in selected cases when a small gap between the stoma and the solid skin barrier will not damage the skin. Examples of selected cases include a solid, dry stool or the use of additional skin barriers such as paste, skin barrier strips or washers, or a liquid skin barrier.

The function of the solid skin barrier is to protect the skin and provide a seal for the pouching system. There are several items that can be used to enhance a pouching system seal: *adhesives, strips, pastes, washers,* and *belts.*

Adhesives can be placed on the skin or the adhesive side of the skin barrier to strengthen the contact between the pouching system and the skin. Adhesives are available as brush-on contact cement (placed on both the skin and the adhesive side of the skin barrier), adhesive spray, and wipe-on liquid adhesive. Adhesives should be used with caution because in some cases they may actually reduce the adhesion of the skin barrier to the skin, for instance in the case of extended-wear barriers.

Strips are solid skin barrier material of various lengths and thicknesses; they have adhesive throughout the product (see Figure 12-5). They can be used to fill an uneven area and to provide an additional barrier around the stoma. Pressure and warmth will increase the flow of this product, making it more moldable. Some of the skin barrier strips are firm enough to be used to create convexity and are placed around the stoma, under the cut edge of the skin barrier.

Skin barrier *paste* is poorly named; it is used to fill in uneven areas and is placed as caulking around the cut edge of the solid skin barrier to prevent migration of the stoma effluent (Figure 12-10). It should be cautioned that skin barrier paste contains alcohol, which can cause a temporary burning sensation when placed upon denuded skin. Skin barrier pastes contain hydrocolloids and erode over time when exposed to moisture.

Washers, constructed of solid skin barrier material, are available in various inner and outer diameters and in various depths and convexities (see Figure 12-5). Skin barrier washers contain no top film, as is present in a solid skin barrier, and are

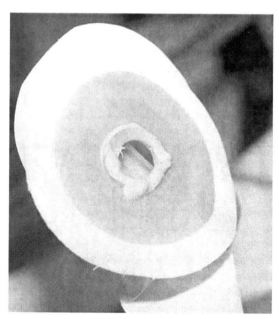

Figure 12-10   Skin barrier paste placed at edge of solid skin barrier to prevent migration of effluent.

adhesive throughout. Skin barrier washers can provide convexity (some washers are created with convexity) and may enhance a seal that is weakened by high liquid stoma output.

A pouching system *belt* can be used to strengthen a seal by applying pressure to the skin barrier against the peristomal skin, and to support the pouch. A belt is often used to magnify the pressure of the convex pouching system.

Pouches

Pouches are available in many shapes and configurations, of various fabrics, and with film that is either transparent or opaque. Pouches that are sealed to the skin barrier or adhesive seal are classified as one-piece systems (see Figure 12-3) and pouches that are separate from the skin barrier but attach to the skin barrier with a flange or adhesive seal are classified as two-piece systems (Figure 12-11).

Considerations in using a one-piece system are:
- Low profile (Erwin-Toth and Doughty, 1992)
- No risk of pouch detachment from the skin barrier flange
- Potential difficulty in application of an opaque one-piece pouch (inability to visualize placement of skin barrier opening over stoma)
- Inability to change the pouch without changing the skin barrier

Two-piece systems use a coupling mechanism to attach the pouch to the solid skin barrier. The coupling mechanism is often a flange (two pieces of plastic that snap together), and sometimes a zone that accepts an adhesive seal. One part of the flange or adhesive is on the solid skin barrier and the other part of the flange or adhesive is attached to the pouch. The coupling options include:
- A "*floating*" plastic flange that is attached to the solid skin barrier with a membrane that extends from the solid skin barrier. The pouch is attached to the flange by pinching the two pieces together.
- A flange that is *attached* to the solid skin barrier; the pouch is snapped onto the skin barrier until the connection is secured. This type of system

requires the user to place the pouch flange over the skin barrier flange and apply pressure to make the connection.
- A *locking* plastic flange *attached* to the solid skin barrier. The solid skin barrier is applied and the pouch flange snapped onto the skin barrier flange. Once in place, a locking mechanism ensures a secure connection.
- A zone on the solid skin barrier that will accept the *adhesive* portion of the pouch. Although this type of system has two pieces, it does not use a plastic flange connection.

Issues regarding the use of each two-piece flanged type of product are listed in Table 12-4. Considerations in using a two-piece system are:
- Ability to change pouch without changing skin barrier (Erwin-Toth and Doughty, 1992) (allows user to wear a short pouch for some activities and return to a longer length for other activities)
- Ease of placement of skin barrier with flange (no pouch attached so stoma easily visualized)
- Security issues of proper flange attachment
- Profile under clothing

The pouching system framework divides pouch options into two major divisions: drainable (Figure 12-12) and nondrainable (see Figure 12-15). *Drainable pouches* include open-ended pouches, indicated for fecal drainage, and pouches with a tap, indicated for drainage of urine. Drainable pouches are drained when one-third full. *Nondrainable pouches* are closed at the bottom and are removed and generally discarded when about one-third to one-half full. A common characteristic of all pouches is odor-resistant film.

Pouching System Framework: Drainable One- and Two-Piece Pouch

The first two considerations in choosing a pouch are *length* and *film*. The choice of *length* depends upon the assessment of the volume of stoma output and the person's personal preference. Current available lengths are short (5-, 6.5-, and 7.5-inch), medium (8-, 9-, and 10-inch), regular (12-inch) and long (16-inch) (Figure 12-13). There are several considerations in choosing the appropriate

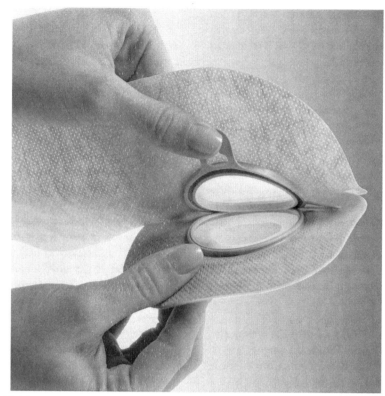

Figure 12-11   Two-piece pouching system with attached plastic flange. (Courtesy Hollister, Inc, Libertyville, IL.)

TABLE 12-4   Two-Piece Pouching Systems

FLANGE FEATURES	USAGE ISSUES
Floating	Indicated if user has a tender or painful peristomal or abdominal area
	Allows user to feel the flange connection as it is made, providing secure seal
	May allow use in an area where an attached flange would cause pouch failure
	High profile of flange on skin barrier
Attached	May cause pain if user has a tender or painful peristomal or abdominal area
	Low profile of flange on skin barrier
Locking	Provides security of pouch to skin barrier connection
	Locking mechanism may be seen as bulky
Adhesive	Low profile
	May be difficult to line up pouch to attachment zone on skin barrier
	No discomfort when applying pouch to skin barrier

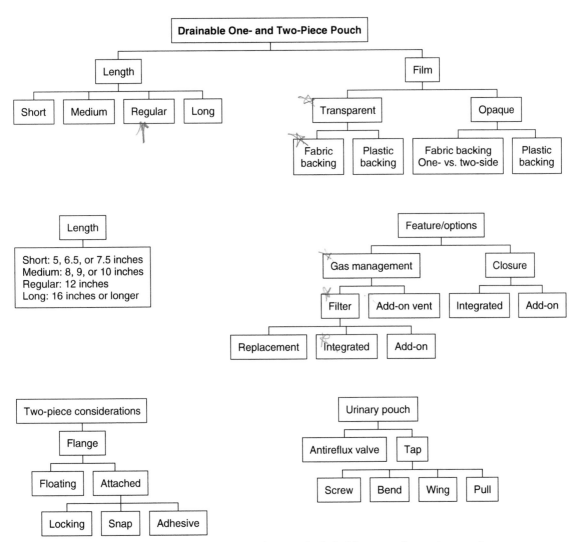

Figure 12-12 Pouching system framework: drainable one- and two-piece pouch.

length: shorter pouches contain less volume, thus frequent emptying may be necessary (compared to a longer, higher-volume pouch); shorter pouches may feel more comfortable under certain types of clothing; and although a long pouch can contain more drainage, the weight of a large volume of output may pull on the skin barrier adhesive seal.

Pouch *film* is available in transparent or opaque forms (see Figure 12-13). The considerations of a transparent film are that a clear pouch allows the wearer to assess the volume (and need for emptying) by direct visualization; the stoma can be visualized through the pouch, enhancing the ability to line the pouch opening over the stoma; and in some instances the solid skin barrier can be visualized and assessed for wear (and thus allow the wearer to change when erosion of the skin barrier is seen). Opaque film is preferred by some because it is not

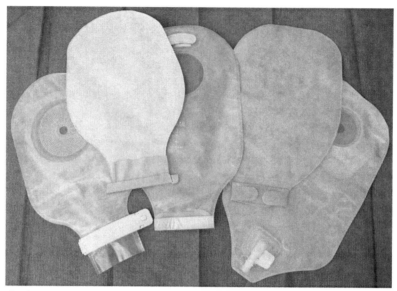

Figure 12-13   Drainable pouch options: variable lengths, pouch closures (integrated or added on), and pouch films (clear, transparent fabric).

necessary to visualize the fecal or urinary output, and this is aesthetically more acceptable. If the user positions the skin barrier opening over the stoma by looking through the pouch, the opaque film can interfere with placement. The use of a two-piece system allows the use of an opaque pouch without the placement issue: the solid skin barrier is placed over the stoma without the pouch attached, and then the opaque pouch is applied.

The next choice is between the use of a pouch with or one without *fabric.* Clear pouches have either a plastic or a fabric backing. This choice depends upon the wearer's preference. Some report that the plastic can trap moisture between the skin and the back of the pouch, and the fabric backing is reported by some to prevent moisture build-up. However, care must be taken to dry the fabric after showering or bathing.

Opaque films have several backing options: plastic on front and back, plastic on front with fabric on back, and fabric on both front and back. The placement of fabric on front and back is thought to lessen the "rustling" or crinkling of the plastic pouching material.

The final features to consider in choosing a drainable one- or two-piece pouching system are *pouch closures* and *gas filters.*

Drainable pouches have several options related to the *pouch closure.* Pouch closures that are used on pouches with tails, not attached to the pouch but *added on,* are available in several styles: of plastic or rubber, with an interlocking closure or a snap or a paper-wrapped wire (much like a bread bag closure). Another option *integrates* the closure into the bottom of the pouch, using a folding mechanism closed with a Velcrolike material (see Figure 12-13).

Urinary pouches have a tap to facilitate emptying and employ a valve or a plug to close the pouch. Tap options include screw, bend, wing, and pull. Choices in pouch closure depend on the person's personal preferences and limitations in hand mobility. Urinary pouches come with adapters that allow connection of the pouch tap to a larger drainage system (used at night). Integral to most urostomy pouches are antireflux valves to reduce backflow of the urine (Erwin Toth and Doughty, 1992). Backflow of urine can cause the skin barrier seal to erode or can undermine the seal (Wells and Doughty, 1994).

Gas filters, located on the top of some pouches, are integrated or added into the pouch film and allow flatus from the pouch to pass through a small piece of charcoal, which diminishes odor (Figure 12-14). As the gas builds in the pouch, pressure pushes the gas through the small holes under the gas filter, through the charcoal filter, and out the pouch. Some gas filters can be removed and replaced, and there are gas filters that are sold separately from the pouch and are applied with adhesive. One reason for gas filter use is excessive gas that frequently inflates the pouch; however, if the charcoal is moistened (either by liquid effluent or by bathing), it becomes saturated and does not allow gas to be vented. Manufacturers provide filter "covers," pieces of paper-coated adhesive that can be placed over the filter to keep out shower or bath moisture. Despite this intervention, gas filters lose effectiveness long before many of the pouch system adhesive seals require changing. One option to manage gas is the use of a vent, a small plastic device that can be applied to a pouch using an adhesive. The vent can be opened to release the gas,

but there is no deodorizing device. Therefore this type of system is only used in a situation where odor can be controlled.

One type of pouch that is an option on select occasions is a nonadhesive pouch. The nonadhesive pouching system uses a silicone ring placed directly around the stoma and a belt that carries the weight of the pouch and applies pressure to the silicone ring to maintain a seal. The nonadhesive pouching system must be correctly sized and the belt adjusted as the patient makes significant position changes (e.g., from supine to standing).

Pouching System Framework: Nondrainable One- and Two-Piece Pouch

Most of the options available in drainable pouches are also available in nondrainable pouches (Figure 12-15). The characteristics of one- and two-piece systems are identical for drainable and nondrainable pouches, including film options and two-piece flange considerations (see earlier discussion). Nondrainable one-piece pouches have a less aggressive skin barrier or adhesive seal compared to one-piece drainable pouches. The difference in the seal aggressiveness relates to the fact that the person using a nondrainable one-piece pouch generally removes it at least once in 24 hours. Drainable skin barrier adhesive seals are constructed with a more aggressive adhesive, since usual wear time is between 3 and 7 days. Length options for nondrainable pouches include short (5-, 6.5-, and 7.5-inch), medium (8- and 9-inch), and a cap (Figure 12-16). A cap is a small pouch with or without a gas filter that can be used if the fecal output is predictable or if the user irrigates. The cap can also be used for intimate activities, since it is small and discreet.

Nondrainable pouches may be used when the wearer prefers to remove and discard the pouch rather than empty it, when the stoma effluent is infrequent and low volume, and when a person irrigates and needs a pouch for security. Considerations for use of a drainable pouch include the cost of pouch replacements, ease in disposing the pouch, and the number of pouch changes needed on a daily basis.

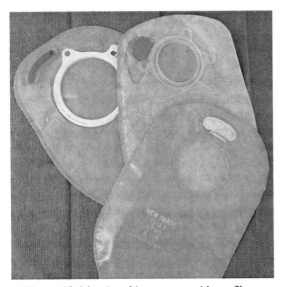

Figure 12-14   Pouching systems with gas filters.

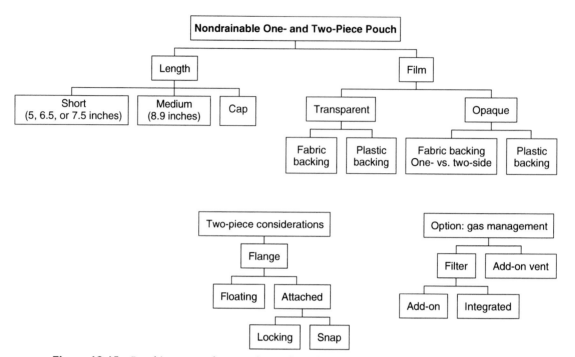

Figure 12-15   Pouching system framework: nondrainable one- and two-piece pouch.

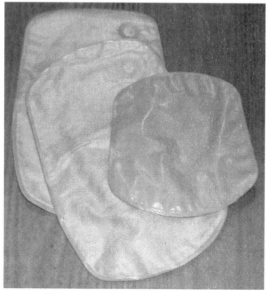

Figure 12-16   Closed-end pouches.

Accessories

Three products not mentioned in the pouching system framework are skin barrier powder, liquid skin barrier, and solvents. *Skin barrier powder* is used to decrease denuded skin moisture. A small amount is sprinkled onto the involved area, rubbed into the skin, and the excess brushed off. *Liquid skin barriers* are products that place a protective coating over the skin (Erwin-Toth, 2003). Although the use of this product is thought by some clinicians to enhance the skin barrier seal, its use may in fact prevent the hydrocolloid action of water absorption and decrease the seal. *Solvents* can be used temporarily to assist in adhesive removal. Although sealants are not generally necessary if the pouching system is worn for several days (the seal gradually loosens over the wear time, making removal easier), they may be helpful in persons with sensitive skin (Erwin-Toth and Doughty, 1992). It is important to remove any solvent residue from the skin, because residue can cause pouch seal failure and/or a reactive dermatitis.

Reusable Equipment

Reusable pouching systems are constructed of durable material such as rubber, heavy plastic, or vinyl (Erwin-Toth and Doughty, 1992). They are available as one- or two-piece systems. The components are a faceplate and a pouch (Figure 12-17). The faceplate, the interface between the skin and the pouch, has a precut opening and is available in flat and convex shapes. If the faceplate is a separate piece from the pouch, it is attached to the pouch by stretching the pouch over the inner flange; the pouch is secured with a small piece of rubber, an elastic string, or in some cases a metal device. Pouches are available in several lengths and are drainable, or for urostomy management contain a tap. The faceplate opening is cut ⅛-inch larger than the stoma, because it is an unforgiving material and can cause a stoma laceration. To protect the ⅛-inch gap between the stoma and the faceplate opening, a solid skin barrier washer is applied. The faceplate is attached to the peristomal skin with a double-faced gasket (one side to the faceplate, the other side to the peristomal skin) or with contact cement (painted on the faceplate and the skin). Wear time is variable, and when the pouching system is removed, all pieces are cleansed and reused (with the exception of the double-faced adhesive disk and skin barrier). The following should be considered when using this type of equipment:

- Initial investment can be costly; however, since most parts are reused, in the long run it may be cost-effective for the user.
- How much time will be invested in washing and reusing the equipment?
- A limited number of manufacturers make this type of equipment.

If reusable equipment is used, fitting should take place after stoma edema has subsided.

CONCLUSION

Assisting in the choice of a pouching system is one of the most important contributions the wound, ostomy and continence/enterostomal therapy nurse makes to the person with a fecal or urinary diversion. It is important to use the principles of pouching in making choices, assessing success, and supporting the person as the adjustment to living with a stoma is made.

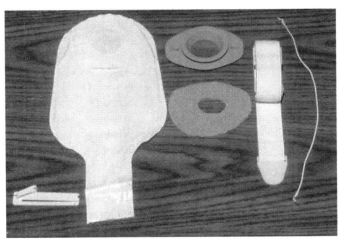

Figure 12-17   Reusable equipment: (left to right) closure, pouch, *(top)* faceplate, *(bottom)* double-faced adhesion, belt, and elastic string to secure pouch to faceplate.

SELF-ASSESSMENT EXERCISES

Questions

1. List the three principles that guide the management of a person with a fecal or urinary diversion.
2. A newly created stoma will remain edematous for up to 6 weeks. Why is this an important consideration when fitting a person with an ostomy pouching system?
3. Describe the normal output for each of the following diversions:
   a. Jejunostomy
   b. Ileostomy
   c. Colostomy
   d. Urostomy
4. The Hartmann's pouch is defined as:
   a. A continent pouch created from the small intestine and connected to the anus.
   b. A urinary diversion that uses the cecum to create an internal pouch and a continence valve.
   c. A distal segment of the intestine that is oversewn and left in the abdomen when an end stoma is created.
   d. An externally worn pouching system that is custom made with a convex skin barrier.
5. What is the purpose of the rod that is placed under a loop stoma?
6. Name two indications for the creation of a mucous fistula.
7. Compare and contrast the creation of gas in a person with an ileostomy and a person with a colostomy.
8. What is the peristomal plane?
   a. The junction of the stoma and skin
   b. The stoma-skin junction to the edge of the solid skin barrier
   c. The solid skin barrier
   d. The area in which the waterproof adhesive secures the pouching system seal
9. Define the concept of "wear time" and discuss the factors that will contribute to wear time.
10. Why is the solid skin barrier the most important portion of the pouching system?
11. Name and discuss the function of three materials found in solid skin barriers.
12. Name the two types of solid skin barriers.
13. Explain the difference between a flat and convex skin barrier.
14. List three convexity options available in a one- and two-piece pouching system.
15. In which of the following clinical situations should the use of convexity be considered?
    a. When the location of the lumen is straight up on a stoma
    b. When the person with the stoma wants the security of a belt
    c. When using reusable equipment
    d. When the stoma does not protrude into the pouching system, with the result that effluent drains under the solid skin barrier
16. When would a cut-to-fit solid skin barrier be used for stoma management?
17. The solid skin barrier should be cut to fit at the base of the stoma.
    True _____ False _____
18. After application of a pouching system that had a bead of skin barrier paste around the cut edge, the patient complained of burning in the area around the stoma that lasted for about 1 to 2 minutes. What could explain this reaction?
19. Name a clinical situation where a belt might be used to enhance the pouching system seal.
20. Differentiate a one- from a two-piece pouching system.
21. Describe the considerations relevant to choosing between a one- and a two-piece pouching system.
22. Name two options in drainable one- and two-piece pouches.
23. What is the purpose of the antireflux valve found in most urostomy pouches?
24. When might a person choose to use a nondrainable pouch?
25. Describe when and how skin barrier powder might be used in the management of a person with a fecal or a urinary diversion.
26. Explain the rationale for use of a liquid skin barrier.

27. Describe why, when fitting a person with reusable equipment, it is important to order the faceplate ⅛-inch larger than the stoma.

Answers

1. The three principles are to (a) maintain the pouching seal for a consistent, predictable wear time, (b) maintain peristomal skin integrity, and (c) support the person with a stoma.

2. A newly created stoma will gradually decrease in size as edema recedes, and the solid skin barrier of the pouching system must accommodate this shift. If the skin barrier size is not fit to the skin-stoma junction, the peristomal skin will be exposed to the stoma effluent resulting in a possible break in the skin integrity.

3. **a.** Jejunostomy: Output is watery, clear, and dark green; can be in excess of 2400 ml/24 hours

   b. Ileostomy: Immediately after creation output is liquid; amount varies between 800 and 1700 ml/24 hours and levels off to gain consistency with amounts between 500 and 1800 ml/24 hours

   c. Colostomy: Output depends on the location: the more distal to the small intestine the thicker and less frequent the output

   d. Urostomy: Normal output in 24 hours for the adult patient is approximately 1500 to 1600 ml.

4. c

5. The rod is placed to support the loop of intestine on the skin.

6. A mucous fistula is created when a primary anastomosis at the time of surgery is not indicated, if the Hartmann's closure is not done, or if there is a distal unresectable obstruction.

7. A person with an ileostomy can create gas by drinking through a straw, chewing gum, sucking on hard candy, or swallowing air while sleeping. A person with a colostomy can create gas by eating foods that support bacterial overgrowth and, in some instances, by swallowing large amounts of air.

8. b

9. Wear time is the predictable amount of time between pouch application and removal. Factors that contribute to wear time are stoma type, stoma output, peristomal planes, type and shape of the solid skin barrier, and the patient's preferences.

10. The skin barrier is the most important part of the pouching system because it protects the skin from the effluent and seals the pouch for a predictable wear time.

11. Skin barrier materials and their function:
    Polymers: provide adhesiveness
    Tackifers: provide adhesiveness
    Softeners and plasticizers: provide flow
    Hydrocolloids: absorb moisture
    Fillers: regulate absorption
    Pigment: provide color.

12. The two types of skin barriers are regular-wear and extended-wear.

13. A flat skin barrier has a level skin contact area, and a convex barrier has an outward curve that begins at the opening of the skin barrier and extends for a variable distance.

14. Convexity options for a one-piece system are (1) precut, (2) cut-to-fit, and (3) custom. For a two-piece system the options are (1) precut built-in, (2) cut- or stretch-to-fit built-in, and (3) insert.

15. d

16. A solid cut-to-fit skin barrier is used for stomas that are not round.

17. True

18. Skin barrier pastes contain alcohol, and when the alcohol contacts the denuded skin, the paste can cause a temporary burning sensation.

19. A belt might be used to enhance the pouching system seal to magnify the pressure of a convex pouching system, to support the pouch, or to apply pressure to the skin barrier against the skin.

20. One-piece pouching system: pouch that is sealed to the skin barrier. Two-piece system: pouch is separate from the skin barrier and attached to the skin barrier with a flange or adhesive seal

21. Considerations of a one-piece system: low profile, no risk of pouch detachment from skin barrier; when using a nontransparent pouch there is difficulty seeing the stoma to apply the pouch or to visualize the output; inability to change the pouch without removing the skin barrier. Considerations for a two-piece system: ability to change the pouch without skin barrier removal; ease of placement of skin barrier due to direct visualization; security issues related to the flange pouch coupling; and high profile under clothing.

22. Options in drainable one- and two-piece systems: variations in length, transparent or non transparent film, fabric covering, pouch closures, gas filters

23. The antireflux valve serves to reduce backflow of the urine that might cause the skin barrier seal to erode or might undermine the seal.

24. Nondrainable pouches might be worn when the person prefers not to empty the pouch; when the stoma output is infrequent and low-volume and the wearer prefers to discard the output rather than empty; when the person irrigates; when the pouch is used for security; or for intimate activities.

25. Skin barrier powder can be used to decrease denuded skin moisture; a small amount is sprinkled onto the involved skin, rubbed into the area, and then brushed off, leaving a light dusting. The use of the powder may improve the skin barrier-to-skin seal.

26. Liquid skin barriers provide a protective coating over skin and are thought by some clinicians to enhance the seal.

27. The faceplate should be larger than the stoma, because the material that the faceplate is constructed from is firm and can cause stoma trauma.

REFERENCES

Corman ML: Diverticular disease. In Corman ML: *Colon and rectal surgery,* ed 3, Philadelphia, 1993, JB. Lippincott

Erwin Toth P: Ostomy equipment and selection criteria. In Milne CT, Corbett LQ, Dubuc DL, editors: *Wound, ostomy and continence nursing secrets,* Philadelphia, 2003, Hanley & Belfus.

Erwin Toth P, Doughty DB. Principles and procedures of stomal management. In Hampton B, Bryant R, editors: *Ostomies and continent diversions: nursing management,* St Louis, 1992, Mosby.

Gordon PH, Rolstad BS, Bubrick MP: Intestinal stomas. In Gordon PH, Nivatvongs S, editors: *Principles and practice of surgery for the colon, rectum and anus,* ed 2, St Louis, 1999, Quality Medical.

Grotz RL, Pemberton JH: Stoma physiology. In MacKeigan JM, Cataldo PA, editors: *Intestinal stomas: principles, techniques and management,* St Louis, 1993, Quality Medical.

Keighley MRB: Stomas. In Keighley MRB et al: *Atlas of colorectal surgery,* New York, 1996, Churchill Livingstone.

Kilpatrick JA: Urinary elimination. In Potter P, Perry A, editors: *Fundamentals of nursing,* ed 5, St Louis, 2001, Mosby.

Rolstad BS, Boarini J: Principles and techniques in the use of convexity, *Ostomy Wound Manage* 42(1):24-32, 1996.

Wells JA, Doughty DB: Pouching principles and products, *Ostomy Wound Manage* 40(2):50-63, 1994.

Williams N et al: Defunctioning stomas: a prospective controlled trial comparing loop ileostomy with loop transverse colostomy, *Br J Surg* 73:566-570, 1986.

Wound, Ostomy and Continence Nurses Society: Convex pouching systems: a fact sheet for clinicians, 2003.

Pediatric Ostomies: Pathophysiology and Management

13

BETH HARRISON and JOY BOARINI

OBJECTIVES

1. Describe the presentation and etiology of these pediatric disorders: Hirschsprung's disease, imperforate anus, persistent cloaca, necrotizing enterocolitis, malrotation, intussusception, meconium ileus, exstrophy conditions, prune belly syndrome, myelomeningocele, lipoma and tethered cord, ureteropelvic junction obstruction, megaureter, and vesicoureteral reflux.

2. Explain the signs, symptoms, and diagnosis of these pediatric disorders: Hirschsprung's disease, imperforate anus, persistent cloaca, necrotizing enterocolitis, malrotation, intussusception, meconium ileus, exstrophy conditions, prune belly syndrome, myelomeningocele, lipoma and tethered cord, ureteropelvic junction obstruction, megaureter, and vesicoureteral reflux.

3. Delineate medical and surgical treatment of Hirschsprung's disease, imperforate anus, persistent cloaca, necrotizing enterocolitis, malrotation, intussusception, meconium ileus, exstrophy conditions, prune belly syndrome, myelomeningocele, lipoma and tethered cord, ureteropelvic junction obstruction, megaureter, and vesicoureteral reflux.

4. Identify four factors to consider when selecting a pouching system for a neonate.

5. Relate how ostomy management techniques for the preschool child differ from those for a teenager.

6. Discuss the main components of an ostomy teaching plan for a preschool child.

7. Relate two stoma complications in the pediatric patient and describe management solutions.

INTRODUCTION

Many of the conditions and diseases that require an ostomy in the pediatric population are similar to those of the adult population. These include trauma, cancer, and inflammatory bowel disease. The first section of this chapter reviews congenital anomalies and conditions that occur during infancy and childhood that may require an ostomy as part of treatment. The second section focuses on pediatric stoma care.

OVERVIEW

Pediatric conditions with which the child is born are called congenital. Congenital conditions are not necessarily genetically transmitted from parents. Many birth anomalies are actually disruptions in normal fetal development that occur at a particular time during the course of pregnancy, often in the first trimester, before some women are even aware that they are pregnant.

The conditions that will be described are not associated with substance abuse except for premature birth, which is a risk factor associated with necrotizing enterocolitis (NEC). NEC is a condition not limited to infants of substance abusing mothers or to lack of maternal health care. Certain conditions can be detected on amniocentesis (e.g., neural tube defects) or ultrasound (e.g., hydronephrosis and cloacal exstrophy), but there are ethical issues associated with early diagnosis of these conditions. Some parents mistrust the reliability or safety of these tests, and others have varying degrees of understanding about the results they may be given.

There are also many congenital anomalies such as imperforate anus that cannot be diagnosed before birth and result in parents' shock and grief on delivery of a less than perfect child. In some cases, parents are "informed" of findings, but feel morally compelled to proceed with the pregnancy despite limited knowledge of the specific needs their newborn will entail. Nonjudgmental care, with sensitivity to the fact that most parents are not prepared to become health care providers when they conceive a child, is essential for these families.

Table 13-1 outlines the intestinal conditions that may necessitate the creation of a stoma. Table 13-2 outlines the urinary conditions that may lead to the creation of a stoma.

Gastrointestinal System

Anorectal and Intestinal Conditions
Hirschsprung's Disease

Description. A Danish physician, Dr. Harold Hirschsprung, first described this disease in 1886. Prior to this the condition, seen in newborns, had been generically explained as aganglionic megacolon. In Hirschsprung's disease (HD) there is an absence of myenteric parasympathetic, intramural ganglion cells. During normal fetal development, the migration of nerves into the hindgut of the fetus usually occurs between the sixth and twelfth weeks of gestation. However, in HD the neuroenteric mechanism in the hindgut fails to mature and migrate. This faulty innervation results in a bowel that lacks propulsive waves and has an absent or abnormal relaxation of the internal anal sphincter.

Because the ganglion cells originate in the neural crest of the fetus and migrate downward, HD most commonly affects the rectosigmoid area. The area of aganglionosis begins at the anus and extends proximally in the bowel for varying lengths. It may involve only a few centimeters of bowel or the entire gastrointestinal system. The newborn with HD has a functional obstruction of the bowel.

HD has a continuous presentation in the bowel and skip areas are extremely rare. There may be evidence of a transition zone. This is an area where there are fewer than normal ganglion cells and

occurs between the aganglionic segment and normal, healthy bowel.

Epidemiology. This condition occurs in approximately 1 out of every 5000 live births. Usually the baby is full term. HD is more likely to be found in Caucasians than other ethnic groups. The incidence in males is greater than in females with a 4:1 ratio, although total colonic disease is almost equally common in males and females.

There is a familial tendency for HD, which can affect siblings or successive generations in about 4% to 8% of the cases. Genetic investigation into the disease is ongoing, and three genes and three chromosome locations have been identified in humans. These are the RET gene on chromosome 10 (autosomal-dominant), the endothelin receptor B (EDNRB) gene on chromosome 13 (autosomal-recessive) and endothelin 3 (EDN 3) on chromosome 20 (autosomal-recessive) (Holschneider and Ure, 2000). The patterns of inheritance are complex and are currently believed to be sex-modified (X-linked) and of variable penetrance (Teitlbaum et al, 1998).

Etiology. The cause of HD is unknown and probably multifactorial. Viral and vascular causes have been named but not proven. This condition may be associated with other anomalies such as Down's syndrome, heart defects, and deafness. The presence of other conditions makes the child's care and management more complex, but many children have no other associated medical problems.

Signs and symptoms. Failure or delay in passing meconium is usually the first observable sign. There are several reasons why a newborn does not pass meconium, and when this is seen, HD must be ruled out. During the newborn assessment, the rectal examination may stimulate the infant to pass a stool. When a rectal temperature is taken or a rectal examination performed and stool is passed, the diagnosis may be delayed. However, after rectal stimulation the infant usually has constipation and diarrhea instead of normal bowel movements.

Other symptoms are consistent with a bowel obstruction. The infant has abdominal distention, gas, discomfort, and loud, gurgling bowel sounds. Vomiting may also be present.

Text continued on p. 270.

TABLE 13-1   Pediatric Surgical Conditions: Gastrointestinal System

ANOMALY	DEFINITION	SIGNS AND SYMPTOMS	DIAGNOSIS	SURGERY/TREATMENT
Hirschsprung's disease	Absence of parasympathetic, intramural ganglion cells, commonly in rectosigmoid area The absence of cells generally begins at the anus and extends proximally in the bowel to a varying length.	Delay/failure to pass meconium Abdominal distention Gas; loud, gurgling bowel sounds Older child will have signs of: bowel obstruction, failure to thrive, poor feeding with progressive disease, no normal bowel movements, may have constipation and/or diarrhea	Rectal biopsy (gold standard) Abdominal film Barium enema (no bowel prep) Anorectal manometry	Three surgical options: (1) Swenson procedure (most common): the ganglionic segment of bowel is pulled through a 1- to 2-cm aganglionic sleeve with primary anal anastomosis. (2) Duhamel procedure: the segment of bowel with normal ganglion cells is brought behind the aganglionic rectal segment, retaining a longer segment of the aganglionic bowel as the anterior wall. (3) Soave procedure: the mucosa and submucosa of the aganglionic rectosigmoid area is removed, and the ganglionic bowel is brought down through the rectal sleeve and allowed to heal everted on the perineum. Any of these procedures may follow the creation of a temporary ostomy.
Imperforate anus (anorectal malformation)	Anus is absent or displaced from its normal anatomical location	No anal opening (or displaced opening, depending on level of malformation) No passage of gas or stool Abdominal distention Fistula (depending on level of malformation)	Physical examination	Surgery: (depending on level of the malformation) Simple: surgical opening of membrane to allow stool passage Complex: diverting colostomy (first stage), followed by an anoplasty and pull through

Continued

TABLE 13-1 Pediatric Surgical Conditions: Gastrointestinal System—cont'd

ANOMALY	DEFINITION	SIGNS AND SYMPTOMS	DIAGNOSIS	SURGERY/TREATMENT
Necrotizing enterocolitis	Acute necrosis of the bowel occurring in the premature infant	Occurs between days 3 and 10 in premature infant Vomiting Temperature instability Increased gastric residual Irritability Lethargy Occult or gross blood in stool Mild abdominal distention Sepsis	Physical examination Laboratory work Frequent x-rays to monitor for bowel perforation	Bowel rest Nasogastric decompression intravenous alimentation Antibiotics Surgery: resection, and/or diversion above the necrotic segment(s)
Malrotation	Rotation and fixation of the midgut that occurs during fetal development Abdominal wall defects: Omphalocele Gastroschisis Diaphragmatic hernia	Symptoms vary with the rotation and fixation, may include: Bilious or nonbilious emesis Diarrhea Blood in the stool Abdominal pain Anorexia, nausea Failure to thrive Irritability Duodenal obstruction and midgut volvulus	Abdominal films	Surgery: correction of malrotation and intestinal diversion if necrotic or ischemic intestine is present

Intussusception	Telescoping of the bowel into the lumen of an adjoining part	Vomiting Bloody, mucoid stools Severe, colicky, intermittent pain Palpable abdominal mass Pale and lethargic infant	Abdominal films Ultrasound Contrast enema	Nonoperative reduction with contrast enema Surgery (manual reduction) is performed when the intussusception cannot be reduced, reoccurs, or gangrene is suspected.
Meconium ileus	Obstruction of the ileum with thick, sticky meconium that forms hard pellets in the narrowed, distal bowel lumen. Earliest sign of cystic fibrosis	Uncomplicated: Distention of the ileum Vomiting in the first 24–48 hours after birth No meconium is passed Complicated: Erythema and edema of the abdominal wall Peritonitis	Abdominal films Contrast enema	Water-soluble contrast enema may emulsify the meconium and relieve the obstruction. Mucomyst via enterotomy proximal to the obstruction May need a diverting ostomy (if perforated or gangrene bowel is present)

TABLE 13-2   Pediatric Surgical Conditions: Urinary System

ANOMALY	DEFINITION	SIGNS AND SYMPTOMS	DIAGNOSIS	SURGERY/TREATMENT
Cloacal exstrophy	Bowel and bladder are exposed. Omphalocele is common. Bladder is bivalved. Genital abnormalities Types of Exstrophy: Cloacal Bladder Epispadias	Symptoms vary with the specific anomalies: Anus imperforate Inguinal hernia Renal and spinal anomalies Male: bifid or diminutive penis, undescended testicles Female: bifid clitoris, vaginal duplication, agenesis, or atresia	Physical examination X-ray films Ultrasonography	Surgery to separate intestinal and genitourinary systems Closure of the bladder and omphalocele Diverting intestinal stoma (usually permanent) Orchidectomy: gender reassignment considered Multiple surgeries and reconstruction
Bladder exstrophy	Bladder and urethra are open and exposed on the lower abdomen. Wide diastasis, wide rectum, and low umbilicus	Male: short, wide penis, urethral open on dorsal surface Female: bifid clitoris, separation of labia with short, anteriorly displaced vagina	Physical examination Renal ultrasound	First surgical stage: Primary closure of the bladder if performed in the first 48-72 hours of life without osteotomy After 72 hours: bilateral iliac osteotomies done before bladder closure Second surgical stage: Epispadias repair
Epispadias	Bladder is closed but urethra is malformed	Male: urethra is dorsal and displaced. Female: urethra opens anteriorly to normal position, characterized by bifid clitoris and separate labia.	Physical examination	Surgical correction, same as for bladder exstrophy May need more than one procedure based on congenital problems Urinary diversion created if continence not obtained after reconstruction

Condition	Pathophysiology	Symptoms	Diagnostic Tests	Management
Prune belly syndrome	Congenital absence, deficiency or hypoplasia of the abdominal musculature causing wrinkled appearance of the abdominal skin. Urinary tract anomalies; large hypotonic bladder, dilated ureters, and dilated prostatic urethra	Symptoms depend on the combination of anomalies. Frail infant. Pulmonary instability/sensitivity in newborns	Ultrasound. Voiding cysto-urethrogram. Chest x-ray. Careful examination of anus, rectum, and heart	Aggressive surgical interventions. Adequate drainage of urinary system: vesicostomy or, in some cases, ureterostomies. Surgical options: Reduction cystoplasty, urethroplasty, and abdominoplasty. In older children: intermittent catheterization or continent diversion
Myelo-meningocele	Occurs when the arches of vertebrae do not fuse together over the spinal cord "Open neural tube defect": both the meninges and cord are herniated through bony defect. Meningocele: only the meninges protrudes. Spina bifida: bony defect can be occulta form where no protrusion of neural tissue is present	Vary with the level of lesion and severity. Hydrocephalus. Detrusor sphincter dyssynergia. Bladder neck incompetence, high residual urine. Neurogenic bowel: significant constipation, altered sensation and sphincter control	Apparent at birth. Spinal magnetic resonance imaging. Voiding cystourethrogram	Surgery to close defect. Shunt placement. Vesicostomy for the infant. Clean intermittent catheterization or continent diversion for the older child. Bowel program
Ureteropelvic junction obstruction	Impairment to urinary flow at the connection between the ureter and renal pelvis	Vary with severity of disease. Frequent urinary tract infections. Abdominal mass in infant. Abdominal pain, vomiting	Ultrasonography. Intravenous pyelogram. Voiding cystourethrogram. Renal isotope scan	Percutaneous diversion (nephrostomy) until definitive corrective surgery done

As time progresses without treatment, the child exhibits poor feeding, failure to thrive, and may have anemia. In some cases, the child will show symptoms of being septic and ill from enterocolitis. This is an intestinal inflammation associated with stasis in which the stool is generally green and frothy with a foul odor and the child is extremely ill, requiring intravenous support, antibiotic therapy, and rectal irrigations. In very severe cases, children with enterocolitis have required mechanical ventilation until they have been diverted and stabilized.

These children may be perceived as more fragile by their parents and their surgeons for the rest of their lives, despite long periods of robust health later. The risk of enterocolitis is believed to persist after reconstructive surgery, as well as during the diverted phase, and may preclude a single-stage procedure.

Diagnosis. Although diagnosis of HD was often delayed in the past, as many as 90% of cases of HD are now being diagnosed in the newborn period (Teitlbaum et al, 1998).

Physical examination of the infant reveals a distended abdomen. Older infants and children may have thin limbs, pallor, and failure to thrive because retained stool in the colon impinges on the stomach and decreases appetite. A typical rectal examination reveals a snug anal sphincter with an empty rectum. In some cases, removal of the examiner's finger results in an explosion of liquid stool and gas.

Abdominal films may show levels of air and fluid on supine or erect views. Diagnostic tests may include a contrast enema that should be done without preparation; no rectal examinations or washouts should be done to avoid a false negative reading. Classic findings are a normal caliber rectum or a narrowed distal segment with a funnel-shaped dilation marking the transition zone to the more dilated colon above. Also, barium is often retained in the colon for longer than 24 hours in HD.

In total colonic disease (3% to 10% of infants) the transition zone is less easily defined, but dilated loops of intestine may be seen on x-ray films and the colon may have a question-mark shape on contrast enema (Holschneider and Ure, 2000). In the newborn a positive examination contributes to the diagnosis, but a negative examination does not rule out HD, as the classic changes in the appearance of the colon may not have yet occurred.

Anorectal manometry may be performed in some centers. If there is an intact anorectal reflex, HD can be ruled out in older infants. The anorectal reflex may not be fully developed in infants less than 12 days of age. Reported accuracy rates have varied widely (Teitlbaum et al, 1998) and operators with sufficient pediatric experience may not be available in many settings.

The gold standard test for this congenital disease is a rectal biopsy. The absence of ganglion cells in the tissue sample confirms the diagnosis. In the newborn period, this biopsy can be obtained at the bedside or on an outpatient basis by suction rectal biopsy performed two cm above the anal valves. In older infants and children, full-thickness open rectal biopsy must be performed, because suction biopsy specimens tend to be inadequate for accurate diagnosis.

Many pediatric surgeons find that pathologists must be specially trained to detect the correct quality and quantity of ganglion cells to make an adequate diagnosis of HD, and will send biopsies done at community hospitals to pathologists with this training.

Treatment. Surgical intervention is the definitive treatment, and the objective is to remove or bypass the aganglionic segment of bowel. Over the years there have been several different surgical approaches to accomplish this.

In 1948 Swenson used a pull-through procedure whereby the ganglionic segment of bowel was pulled through a 1- to 2-cm aganglionic sleeve. This procedure requires meticulous dissection close to the internal sphincter. In the 1960s Duhamel revised the procedure; he took the segment of bowel with normal ganglion cells and brought it behind the aganglionic rectal segment, retaining a longer segment of the aganglionic bowel as the anterior wall. Also in the 1960s, Soave described a procedure where the mucosa and submucosa of the aganglionic rectosigmoid area were

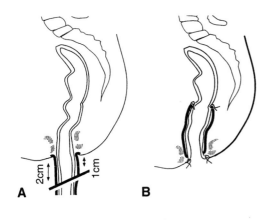

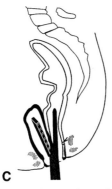

Figure 13-1 Surgical procedures for Hirschsprung's disease. **A,** Swenson procedure. **B,** Soave procedure. **C,** Duhamel procedure. (From Ashcraft KW et al: *Pediatric surgery*, ed 3, Philadelphia, 2000, WB Saunders.)

removed and the ganglionic bowel was then brought down through the rectal sleeve and allowed to heal everted on the perineum. Boley modified the procedure with a primary anal anastomosis, and this procedure, the endorectal pull-through, is the one most commonly performed as a single-stage neonatal procedure (Figure 13-1).

These procedures are considered "definitive" therapy, since they all require full or partial resection of the aganglionic bowel. Pediatric surgeons disagree on the benefits and merits of each procedure, with those surgeons trained in and adept at a particular procedure often remaining staunch advocates of that particular approach. Most experts agree that surgeons do best when they use the

operative approach with which they are most comfortable. The most important factor in the long-term success of any procedure may be the surgeon's willingness to follow the patient over the long haul of toilet training, to achieve adequate continence without the megacolon that can result from long-term constipation.

Any of the procedures just described may follow the creation of a temporary ostomy, performed at the level of normally enervated bowel. This is often called a "leveling" ostomy. The level of aganglionic bowel determines whether this will be a colostomy or ileostomy. If the diagnosis was missed or delayed, the normal bowel can be quite large when it is exteriorized, especially if this is done as a loop ostomy.

Loop ostomies in children with HD have an increased risk of prolapse. When this occurs it can be distressing for the parents. The prolapsed loop stoma may also be a challenge to pouch, since the cutting surfaces on pediatric pouching systems are limited. An adult pouching system may need to be used, which may seem to overwhelm the baby's size. If there is a loop stoma located low on the abdomen, the challenge of pouching is increased. Oval skin barriers may be useful in these children.

If the diagnosis is made early in the neonatal period and there is no enterocolitis, many surgeons can complete the repair in one stage, which avoids the creation of a temporary ostomy. With recent technical advances, all three procedures can now be done through a laparoscopic and/or transanal approach. Preoperative preparation often requires colonic lavage or irrigations via the rectum for days or weeks to ensure adequate bowel decompression and preparation. If the aganglionic segment is longer than anticipated, some surgeons will convert from a laparoscopic single-stage approach to an open procedure, often creating either a colostomy or an ileostomy.

In cases where the treatment is staged, two or three operations may be needed. First, when the diagnosis is made, a diverting stoma is done. This allows for relief of the obstructive symptoms and for normal bowel movements. When the child is older at the time the diagnosis is made, parents report a much happier child, who is less fussy about foods and who has more energy after the stoma is created.

Since the pelvis of a newborn is quite small, some surgeons delay the reparative work until the infant reaches a size of about 9 kilograms. If there are other complicating anomalies, especially cardiac anomalies, achieving adequate weight and stability may require 1 year or longer. This may also be true for longer segment disease. In the case of total colonic disease, some surgeons advocate delaying definitive repair until the child is toilet trained for urine, to decrease the severe perineal breakdown that occurs with frequent liquid stools in diapered infants.

At the second procedure, the surgeon performs one of the procedures already mentioned. In some cases, the ostomy remains in place until adequate healing at the repair site has taken place. In these cases, a third and final operation involves the takedown of the ileostomy or the colostomy. More commonly, the ostomy is closed when the pull-through is done, resulting in a two-stage procedure.

Some children continue to have persistent dysfunction of their bowel after surgery and may require irrigation and or dilation to promote evacuation. Over time, many adapt and function spontaneously. However, some will continue to suffer from constipation, as well as bouts of enterocolitis.

The exceptions are those children with very long segment disease and those with ultrashort-segment disease. Children with very long segment disease extending through the small intestine require long-term total parenteral nutrition (TPN), which is fraught with risk, particularly the risk of liver disease. In the most severe cases, with disease extending to the duodenum, diversion of the bowel may not even be possible, and the child may be managed with a gastrostomy to vent the stomach, rectal irrigations to relieve mucus plugs in the rectum and colon, and a central line for home TPN. Persons with ultrashort-segment disease can often be treated with transanal or transsacral myectomy rather than bowel resection and pull-through (Caty and Azizkhan, 2000; Holschneider and Ure, 2000; Teitlbaum et al, 1998).

Imperforate Anus

Description. Imperforate anus, a congenital anomaly in which the anus is absent or displaced from its normal anatomic location, is also known as anorectal malformation. The condition may be differentiated as high or low. A high imperforate anus occurs when the anal opening is located above the puborectalis sling. A high imperforate anus is more complicated and involves more complex surgical intervention. A low imperforate anus is located below the puborectalis sling. Females may have the more complex, persistent cloacal defect where vagina, urethra, and rectum meet and fuse into a common channel with a single perineal orifice (Kiely and Pena, 1998) (Figure 13-2).

Epidemiology. Imperforate anus occurs in approximately 1 in every 5000 live births. The incidence is more common in males than in females. There is no familial tendency for this problem.

Etiology. The cause of imperforate anus is unknown. A problem occurs in the development of the fetus, probably between the fourth and sixteenth weeks of gestation. Fistulas to other organs are common; communication may exist to the urinary bladder or posterior urethra in the male, or to the vagina in the female, or, in low anomalies, to the perineum.

Imperforate anus is frequently associated with other anomalies, especially in the urinary tract. There is a grouping of anomalies that has been identified as the VACTERL syndrome that includes imperforate anus as one of the congenital abnormalities. Each of the letters stands for another system that is affected (Box 13-1).

Signs and symptoms. If there is no outlet for meconium, the infant will fail to have a bowel movement within the first 24 to 48 hours. This will often be accompanied by abdominal distention and possibly vomiting. Should a fistula be present between the bowel and the perineum or the vagina, there may be stool in the newborn's diaper and minimal symptoms of obstruction at first. If there is a fistula between the bowel and the bladder, there may be stool or gas passed through the urethra. The anteriorly displaced ectopic anus condition may be missed altogether at first, as the anus is

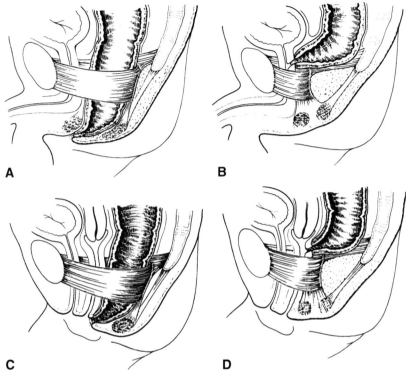

Figure 13-2 Common types of anorectal anomalies. **A,** Low lesion in male: covered anus with or without anocutaneous fistula. **B,** High lesion in male: anorectal agenesis with rectourethral fistula. **C,** Low lesion in female: ectopic anus with anovulvar or anovestibular fistula. **D,** High lesion in female: anorectal agenesis with rectovaginal fistula. (Modified from Spitz L: Hirschsprung's disease and anorectal anomalies. In Schwartz SI, Ellis H, editors: *Maingot's abdominal operations,* vol 2, ed 9, Norwalk, Conn, 1989, Appleton & Lange.)

BOX 13-1 Syndrome of Coexisting Congenital Anomalies (VACTERL)

....

V: Vertebral anomalies such as spinal curvature, tethered cord, hemivertebra, missing vertebrae

A: Anal atresia (i.e., imperforate anus)

C: Cardiac malformations such as PDA, ASD, VSD, tetralogy of Fallot, transposition of the great vessels or hypoplastic left heart

TE: Tracheo-esophageal fistula and/or esophageal atresia

R: Renal problems such as single kidney, VUR

L: Limb deformities such as extra or deformed digits, missing radius

---

PDA, Patent ductus arteriosus; ASD, atrial septal defect; VSD, ventricular septal defect; VUR, vesicoureteral reflux.

present. These children progressively develop severe constipation that generally leads to the diagnosis. There have also been cases where infants have been discharged to home with a low imperforate anus without a diagnosis being made, because there has been passage of meconium into the diaper.

Diagnosis. Careful physical examination provides a definitive diagnosis with the discovery of an absent anus or anteriorly displaced anal opening. Radiographic contrast studies can be used to confirm the location and position of fistulas that cannot be visualized.

Treatment. Treatment for imperforate anus, unless it is a very mild form, requires surgery. The simplest form of imperforate anus involves the anal opening being covered by a thin membrane that can be perforated to allow for normal bowel movements. In some cases of low anomalies in females, dilation of the existing perineal or vaginal or vestibular fistula is done to allow the child to be discharged to home to grow and develop before a two-stage surgical approach is undertaken.

Most cases of higher anomalies involve surgery at the time of diagnosis and are done as a three-stage procedure. Immediate intervention requires the creation of a colostomy to divert stool from the fistula. Although the stoma is body-altering, there may be other anomalies that are life-threatening and cause for greater concern on the parents' part.

The colostomy is usually left in place until the child reaches an adequate size for the reconstructive procedures to be done. Most surgeons prefer to perform the anoplasty and pull-through procedure when the child is young so the parents can easily perform the needed postoperative anal dilations. However, this may be delayed if there are other medical conditions or surgical repairs that are of a higher priority.

During the second operation, fistulas are closed. An anoplasty is done to create an anal opening in the correct position, usually using electromuscular stimulation to identify the appropriate muscles of the sphincter complex. Last, a pull-through procedure is done to bring bowel down through the puborectalis sling and into its correct position in the perineum. This is a major procedure, and the child's ability to be continent in the future will depend on both the success of this operation and the existing nerve and muscles structures present at the time of the repair.

The final operation involves the takedown of the colostomy once the surgeon is satisfied that there is adequate healing. Generally a series of dilations will have been performed to ensure that the anal caliber is sufficient before closing the ostomy. Following this operation, the infant usually has a period of frequent stooling.

Diaper rash is a significant issue for these children after colostomy closure. The wound, ostomy, and continence (WOC/ET) nurse should remain involved to be sure that adequate care is provided to minimize scarring of the perianal skin and to promote patient comfort, ensuring that the child will continue to eat well and thrive. Children are smart enough that if they feel pain from denuded perineal skin when they stool after eating, they will decrease the frequency of food intake. Stricture is also a concern and may require that the child undergo dilations for several more months to keep the anus patent and well calibrated.

Toilet training is often delayed in these children because of variations in sensation and ability to control the passage of stool. Constipation maybe a significant issue, especially for those with low lesions. The goal of bowel management is a daily, large, soft stool so that the rectum does not become dilated. Bowel management is highly individualized, using habit training, dietary manipulation, laxatives or bulking agents, and suppositories or enemas. In those with high lesions and a tendency to frequent, loose stools, medications to slow the transit may also be used.

The process of bowel management requires time and patience on the part of the child and the family, as well as the health care provider. WOC nurses will find ample opportunity to use their training in the long-term management of these children. Children who require enema therapy to manage their continence may be candidates for the Malone procedure, in which the appendix or a substitute is used to create a continent stoma for administering antegrade continent enemas. This procedure is also referred to as an appendicostomy or a Malone antegrade continence enema (MACE) procedure (Pope and Rink, 1999).

Persistent Cloaca

Description. Persistent cloaca is a condition in females that includes an imperforate anus but also involves a common channel genitourinary system with a single perineal opening and a rectal fistula attached to the posterior wall of the common channel. The associated anomalies are those that have already been described for imperforate anus and include a variety of uterine and ovarian configurations. Surgical repair involves perineal reconstruction with vesicourethral mobilization to bring the urethral opening to the perineum, as well as vaginal reconstruction.

Treatment. Definitive surgical repair of cloaca is more complicated than that for simple anorectal repair, and urinary decompression measures may be required in addition to colostomy creation for intestinal diversion during the newborn period. Urinary decompression may be accomplished by catheterization of the perineal orifice, although the vaginal structure is often divided by a septum that cannot be visualized, making it difficult to achieve drainage. These children may also be treated with diversion by vesicostomy, but some will require an additional vaginostomy to achieve adequate decompression of the urinary tract. Parents must cope with a daughter whose abdomen seems covered with stomas and catheters. After surgical repair, they will need to dilate the neoanus, located in an extensively reconstructed perineum. Long-term care may include the need to perform intermittent catheterization for adequate bladder decompression, as well as bowel management similar to that for imperforate anus.

Necrotizing Enterocolitis

Description. NEC is a major cause of morbidity and mortality in the low birth-weight infant. This condition was first described in 1891, but the first complete reports did not appear until the mid-1960s. It is now the most common gastrointestinal disease encountered in newborn intensive care units (NICUs). The disease occurrence is a direct result of advancements in technology that permit the survival of smaller and smaller infants, since it occurs most often in preterm neonates.

NEC involves necrosis of the bowel and frequently results in perforation. These are very sick babies, who have numerous life-threatening problems. The infection can occur in the large or small intestine or both, and often involves the ileocecal area. Skip areas of the necrosis are common, which makes surgical intervention more challenging.

Epidemiology. The incidence of NEC varies in neonatal and premature nurseries. Between 1% and 8% of all babies admitted to a NICU will have NEC. Very low birth-weight babies, of less than 1500 g, are at higher risk and have an incidence of NEC of at least 10% (Caty and Azizkhan, 2000).

This problem is seen frequently in babies who have had numerous stresses within the newborn period. Being born prematurely often results in resuscitative events, pulmonary weakness or instability, low Apgar scores, increased risk of infection because of an immature immune system, hypothermia, and a need for transfusion or even surgery. These stress factors are not additive but cumulative in their effect on newborns, increasing the chances for the newborns' developing NEC.

Etiology. The causes are somewhat controversial and still not clearly understood. However, most agree that there are three factors that are implicated in the onset of NEC: feeding, mucosal injury, and bacterial invasion (Albanese and Rowe, 1998).

Ninety-five percent of babies who develop NEC have been fed. This is an important finding. Babies who are at high risk for developing NEC must be fed very cautiously with low-volume, diluted feedings, advanced very slowly, and monitored constantly for suspected NEC. Breast milk provides antibodies such as secretory IgA, as well as lactoferrin, vitamin E, beta-carotene, and platelet-activating factor acetylhydrolase. Encouraging a new mother to pump and provide breast milk to her preterm infant gives her the ability to provide additional nutritional support that may help her newborn.

Mucosal injury can be caused directly by exposure to bacterial endotoxins or hypertonic solutions. Gastric acid and intestinal motility are also reduced in premature infants, allowing more bacterial colonization. Indirect injury results from hypoxia associated with low-flow states such as shock or vascular obstruction, or by birth asphyxia from lung or heart disease. Once bacteria are able to invade the injured mucosa, the inflammatory processes can increase edema in the bowel wall and aggravate ischemia.

Blood cultures are positive in approximately one third of NEC babies. The most common invading bacteria include *Escheria coli, Salmonella, Klebsiella pneumoniae, Proteus mirabilis, Staphylococcus aureus, Salmonella* species, *S. epidermis, Clostridium* species and enterococcus (Albanese and Rowe, 1998). NEC has been reported in epidemic clusters, and therefore infection control measures are essential in limiting spread of this condition.

Symptoms. The onset of symptoms usually occurs in the early newborn period between days 3 and 10. These symptoms include vomiting or increasing gastric residuals, temperature instability, irritability, lethargy, occult or gross blood in the stools or the gastric aspirate, and poor feeding if the infant continues to be fed. Symptoms vary widely from mild abdominal distention to sepsis.

Some NICUs use a staging system for NEC, developed by Bell, which delineates the stages of the disease process (Albanese and Rowe, 1998). Even when a formal staging system is not used, it is generally recognized that bowel rest and decompression with antibiotic therapy are essential once NEC is suspected. NEC is a progressive disease, and mortality increases if the infection is not controlled.

Diagnosis. Physical examination may reveal a distended abdomen, with edema and erythema of the abdominal wall associated with peritonitis, a later finding. Laboratory tests reveal neutropenia, thrombocytopenia, and metabolic acidosis. The C-reactive protein is often elevated but this finding is not specific to NEC. The NICU staff needs to monitor distention with abdominal girths, since changes can happen quickly.

X-rays are done as often as every 6 to 8 hours to monitor for bowel perforation, which may be asymptomatic in the very sick newborn. Common findings associated with NEC are an ileus pattern, pneumatosis intestinalis (indicative of bowel wall gas, also seen in other conditions), portal vein gas (a poor prognostic indicator), pneumoperitoneum (associated with perforation), intraperitoneal fluid, and persistently dilated loops. Contrast studies are occasionally done, with caution and using water-soluble contrast given from above, since contrast enemas are associated with an increased risk of perforation. If there is intraperitoneal fluid, a tap may be done for diagnosis of perforation.

Treatment. The key factors in the treatment regimen are early recognition and prompt treatment. Medical management of the infant is vigorous and includes bowel rest, nasogastric decompression,

intravenous alimentation, transfusions, and antibiotic therapy.

These babies are not good surgical candidates. However, surgery is indicated when there is perforation, peritonitis, intestinal infarction, or when the infant is clinically deteriorating despite aggressive supportive treatment.

Surgery involves resection of, or diversion above, any necrotic or questionable bowel segments. The surgeon's objective is to save as much intestinal length as possible, since NEC is one of the leading causes of short bowel syndrome in neonates. In selected patients with overall good health, very localized disease, and no questionable distal areas, a primary anastomosis may be possible after resecting the damaged bowel. Since these criteria are seldom met by the fragile preemies described above, many infants will require an ostomy proximal to the injured bowel and a mucous fistula distal to it. Because of technical issues at the time of surgery, most surgeons bring the stomas out through the incision to facilitate closure.

Skip areas characterize NEC; therefore surgical intervention usually involves multiple resections and anastomoses or diversions. Some surgeons make a proximal diversion and splice the distal bowel segments below the mucous fistula, which then can be used to administer contrast for evaluation before closure of the stoma. Some surgeons remove frankly necrotic bowel and leave questionable areas, then reexplore in 48 to 72 hours for more definitive diversion. This technique reduces the amount of necrotic tissue the infant's body must contend with and can often result in the salvage of bowel that appeared doomed at first-look surgery.

In cases of very extensive NEC, some surgeons elect to simply close the abdomen when resection would condemn the child to TPN support and a need for small bowel transplantation. Other surgeons perform high diversion without resection, and still others resect all necrotic bowel and leave the infant with a high ostomy.

During surgery one or more stomas may be created. This may be done in an effort to bypass an anastomosis, or as a way of monitoring questionable bowel viability or performing diagnostic testing before reanastomosis or realimentation. Because of the rampant infections often present in these infants and the local edema, the incisions between stomas are often tenuous and can dehisce. Sometimes there is subcutaneous or fascial infection that must be reduced before the wounds can heal sufficiently to provide an epithelialized surface for a pouching system to adhere to.

The stomas created in these emergency situations are often less than ideal; sloughing of residual bowel disease at the stoma level may leave a flush or retracted stoma. With sufficient retraction, skin level stenosis can result. In some cases, sutures placed in the stoma can produce fistulas at the base of the stoma. These can mature and result in a multi-lumened stoma for which pouching and seal maintenance is difficult, since the effluent often exits at skin level. Often the creativity of the WOC nurses and the NICU staff is called on to manage these sick babies.

Stoma closure is generally performed between 4 weeks and 4 months from the time of the initial surgery. Factors that determine timing of stoma closure include weight gain and stomal output. When very high stoma output precludes adequate weight gain, despite optimal parenteral support, and there is distal bowel that can aid in fluid and electrolyte balance, early closure may be the only option. Earlier closure may also be considered if the child cannot be transitioned to full enteral feeding due to the level of diversion. In the event that stomal stenosis occurs and the distal bowel is in good condition, the stoma may be closed rather than revised.

In some cases, enteral feedings can be administered via the mucous fistula or the distal lumen of a loop ostomy to the distal bowel, to aid in stabilizing weight gain and decrease the risks of prolonged parenteral nutrition. These maneuvers call for creativity on the part of the nursing staff. Strategies that are key, if the child is to be fed into the distal bowel via a stoma, are to introduce the catheter an adequate length into the stoma lumen (5 to 10 inches if possible) and to secure the catheter

carefully. Before stoma closure the distal bowel should be studied with water-soluble contrast, since strictures occur in 9% to 36% of patients recovering from NEC, whether they have had surgery or not. Surgical patients may develop strictures at one or more of their anastomotic sites.

In cases of medical management alone, scarring may result from inflammation and infection, and this is suspected when the child is symptomatic or failing to thrive. The most common site of stricture is the colon, particularly the left colon at the splenic flexure, followed by the terminal ileum (Albanese and Rowe, 1998). Strictures need repair or resection at the time of stoma closure to avoid further complications. With extensive or multiple strictures, prolonged diversion may be required.

Malabsorption, short bowel syndrome, and cholestatic liver disease are the other common complications of NEC. Infants with short bowel syndrome may eventually be weaned from TPN and onto full enteral feedings as their gut adapts, or they may become candidates for small bowel or liver and small bowel transplantation.

Abdominal Wall Defects
Malrotation, Omphalocele, and Gastroschisis

Description. Malrotation is an abnormality in the rotation and fixation of the midgut that occurs during fetal development; it is most easily understood in the context of normal rotation and fixation of the intestine (Figure 13-3). The intestinal tract elongates, develops, and rotates within the umbilical sac from around the fifth gestational week and remains there until the tenth gestational week. At that time it normally rotates and reduces back into the abdominal cavity, where it will fixate to the posterior abdominal wall during the twelfth week of fetal development.

Abdominal wall defects such as omphalocele, gastroschisis, and congenital diaphragmatic hernia are anomalies that occur during the first stage of this process. Omphalocele involves an umbilical hernia of the persistently extruded bowel, covered with a membrane that is amnion externally and peritoneum internally. The abdominal wall defect can vary in size, and the degree of normal rotation and fixation varies with the extent of intestinal

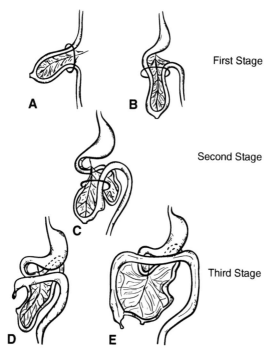

A   B   First Stage

C   Second Stage

D   E   Third Stage

Figure 13-3   Normal intestinal rotation. **A,** Six weeks' gestational age, nonrotation. **B,** Eight weeks' gestational age, incomplete rotation. **C,** Nine weeks' gestational age, incomplete rotation. **D,** Eleven weeks' gestational age. **E,** Twelve weeks' gestational age. (From Filston HC, Kirks DR: Malrotation: the ubiquitous anomaly, *J Pediatr Surg* 16:614, 1981.)

extrusion. Wound care for the larger-omphalocele patients is more likely than ostomy formation and is generally directed by the surgical team. Infection is a huge risk, since the membrane over the defect is far from normal skin (Cooney, 1998).

Gastroschisis is an extrusion of nonrotated midgut through an opening in the abdominal wall to the right of the umbilicus. There is no membrane to protect it from contact with the amniotic fluid, and the loops of bowel are often matted and thickened. Bowel atresia and ischemia can occur with this defect and may call for stoma formation.

Diaphragmatic hernias occur from inadequate diaphragm development that results in herniation of the abdominal contents into the chest cavity.

This condition requires surgical intervention for repair, but rarely leads to intestinal diversion stomas. However, it is common for gastrostomy tubes to be required for feeding. Malrotation anomalies that occur during later stages of fetal development vary in presentation but are not apparent at birth. This is because the abdominal contents are contained in their proper cavity.

Mesocolic paraduodenal hernias can result from failure of fixation. Although their occurrence is rare, they are significant as a cause of strangulating bowel injury, as is the more common and potentially lethal midgut volvulus (Figure 13-4). The severity of symptoms varies with the abnormality of rotation and/or fixation.

Epidemiology. The actual incidence of this anomaly is difficult to establish, because many cases are asymptomatic and are discovered on autopsy. The incidence of symptoms leading to clinical diagnosis is estimated at 1 in 6000 live births. Rotational abnormalities are slightly more common in males than in females (Clark and Oldham, 2000).

Etiology. No specific cause for malrotation is known at this time.

Symptoms. As noted in previous paragraphs, symptoms vary with the specifics of the rotational or fixation abnormality. The abdominal wall defects are clinically apparent at birth, and identification and stabilization of the defect is part of the surgical intervention.

About half of the children with malrotation become symptomatic in the first month of life and up to 90% in the first year of life (Clark and Oldham, 2000). Symptoms include both bilious and nonbilious emesis, diarrhea, abdominal pain, and blood in the stool. Anorexia or nausea, failure to thrive, irritability, lethargy, and fever are also reported. If the obstruction is intermittent, the symptoms may be irregular and vary with the level of obstruction. Duodenal obstruction and midgut volvulus are the most common.

Diagnosis. Plain abdominal films are generally insufficient to diagnose malrotation, and an upper gastrointestinal contrast evaluation is needed. The characteristic finding for malrotation with midgut volvulus is often described as a "bird's beak," a term

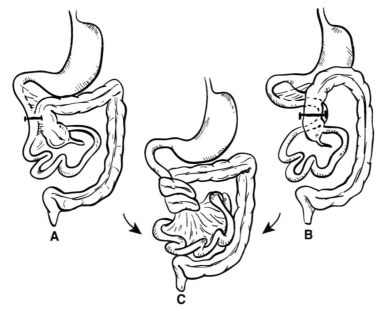

Figure 13-4   Pathophysiology of midgut volvulus with malrotation. **A,** The narrow mesenteric attachment in nonrotation, **B,** or incomplete rotation, **C,** predisposes the patient to midgut volvulus. (From Filston HC, Kirks DR: Malrotation: the ubiquitous anomaly, *J Pediatr Surg* 16:614, 1981.)

that reflects the external compression and torsion. Rotational anomalies are identified by the abnormal location of intestinal structures.

Treatment. The treatment for malrotation with or without volvulus is surgical. The presence or suspicion of volvulus makes surgery more urgent. Once the malrotation has been corrected and volvulus reversed, the presence of intestinal ischemia or necrosis determines whether intestinal diversion may be indicated. A second-look procedure similar to that described for NEC may be performed, because it is essential to preserve maximal intestinal length.

Primary anastomosis may be accomplished when there are two viable intestinal ends. If there has been necrosis of the entire midgut, the child will be left with significant short bowel syndrome. The operative correction of malrotation follows the original recommendations of Ladd, first published in the 1930s (Clark and Oldham, 2000). Corrected malrotation will always appear as an abnormality on abdominal films, with the cecum positioned on the left.

Intussusception

Description. Intussusception is the invagination of a portion of the intestine into the lumen of an adjoining part. It can also be described as a telescoping of the bowel into itself.

Epidemiology. Incidence in the United States has not been studied, but reports from Great Britain cite a range of 1.4 to 1.9 per 1000 live births, with a male/female ratio of 3:2. Intussusception occurs most commonly in infants between the ages of 4 and 12 months (Young, 1998).

Etiology. The cause of this condition is unknown, but it usually originates in the distal small bowel close to the ileocecal junction and moves into the ascending colon. Postoperative intussusception has been reported following a variety of surgeries. In other cases, there is a lead point such as a Meckel's diverticulum, a polyp, intestinal duplication, or an intestinal tumor. In the majority of cases, there is no apparent cause.

Symptoms. The classic signs of intussusception include vomiting, bloody mucoid stools that resemble red currant jelly, abdominal pain, and a palpable abdominal mass. The pain is severe, colicky, and intermittent. The abdominal mass is sausage shaped, and generally located in the right hypochondrium and along the transverse colon. The children are pale and will become lethargic.

Diagnosis. Abdominal films or ultrasound may be used to confirm the clinical diagnosis as needed. Contrast enemas have been used to diagnose and to treat intussusception.

Treatment. Nonoperative hydrostatic reduction of intussusception can be performed using barium or air, if there is no evidence of peritonitis that indicates a gangrenous intestine. Surgical intervention is required when the intussusception cannot be reduced, reoccurs, or gangrene is suspected. The intussuscepted bowel can often be manually reduced at laparotomy. Pathologic lead points or irreducible segments are resected with end-to-end anastomosis. The need for intestinal diversion is rare but can occur if the edematous bowel ends are not suitable for primary anastomosis.

Meconium Ileus

Description. Meconium ileus is the earliest sign of cystic fibrosis (CF). It is the obstruction of the ileum with thick, sticky meconium that forms hard pellets in the narrowed distal bowel lumen. The colon appears small in caliber but distends readily when the obstruction is relieved. Some of these infants will develop volvulus, gangrene, perforation, and peritonitis or bowel atresia, conditions referred to as complicated meconium ileus.

Epidemiology. The incidence of CF is approximately 1 in 3000 live births, and meconium ileus occurs in approximately 15% of CF patients (Groff, 2000).

Etiology. The tenacious meconium seen in this disease is a result of the abnormalities of exocrine mucus production seen in CF. The thick, viscous secretions of the disease will occlude air passages and pancreatic ducts, as well as the ileum. Decreased water content and pancreatic enzyme deficiency are noted in the meconium.

Symptoms. If the meconium ileus is uncomplicated, newborns will have distention and vomiting in the first 24 to 48 hours of life, and no meconium is passed per rectum. Complicated meconium ileus

may result in erythema and edema of the abdominal wall resulting from peritonitis.

Diagnosis. Abdominal films in meconium ileus reflect fewer air-fluid levels and less rectal gas than those of infants with HD or meconium plug syndrome. Contrast enemas are generally needed for definitive diagnosis and may also be therapeutic.

Treatment. As in intussusception, contrast enemas may be used in treating this condition. Water-soluble contrast is used, since the bowel could be perforated. The contrast media may cause sufficient emulsification of the thick meconium to relieve the obstruction as the enema is refluxed into the terminal ileum and distal small bowel under fluoroscopy. Additional small-volume enemas (10 to 15 ml) can be repeated in the NICU with up to 75% of uncomplicated meconium ileus responding to this treatment.

If the obstruction cannot be relieved with enema treatment, or in cases of complicated meconium ileus, surgery is indicated. Acetylcysteine (Mucomyst), a wetting agent, can be instilled into the bowel via enterotomy proximal to the obstruction. The sticky meconium and pellets can then be milked down into the colon and the enterotomy closed. For complicated meconium ileus, resection of perforated or gangrenous bowel may be required, with primary anastomosis or a diverting ostomy as needed. Minimally diverting Mickulicz loop stomas were used in the 1950s but are less common with the current methods of treatment (Groff, 2000).

Bile Diversion Stomas. This section is included to address those relatively rare stomas created for primary liver disorders. Earlier ostomy texts included a review of the partially diverting cutaneous stomas sometimes performed in the repair of biliary atresia by variations of the Kasai portoenterostomy (Bryant and Buls, 1992). Cutaneous diversion did not decrease the incidence of ascending cholangitis as originally hoped and also complicated later liver transplantation. As a result, this form of the Kasai procedure is now seldom used (Ohi and Nio, 1998).

Cutaneous stomas for the partial diversion of bile may be an option for patients suffering from intractable pruritis whose quality of life is poor because of their intense discomfort (Ng et al, 2000). This occurs as a result of cholestatic liver disease in those who are not yet eligible for liver transplantation. The surgery involves the use of jejunum or appendix as a conduit for bile from the gall bladder to the skin, where it can be collected in a pouching system. Daily volume of diverted bile was cited as 30 to 150cc (Edmond and Whitington, 1995), so a small pouch with a urinary tap can be used.

Genitourinary Anomalies

Exstrophy (Cloacal Exstrophy, Bladder Exstrophy, Epispadias)

Exstrophy (eversion of an organ) (see Table 13-2) conditions comprise a spectrum of anomalies of the lower abdominal wall and pelvis, the most complex of which is cloacal exstrophy and the least complex, epispadias. These events occur between the fourth and eighth weeks of fetal development. Bladder exstrophy is the most common, followed by epispadias and then cloacal exstrophy. All three anomalies occur in both male and female children and will be reviewed from most complex to least.

Cloacal Exstrophy

Description. With cloacal exstrophy, omphalocele is common. Below the protruding, membrane-covered umbilicus are the exposed bowel and bladder. The bladder is bivalved and surrounds the intestinal mucosa in the midline. Each hemibladder contains a ureteral orifice, and the intestinal mucosa represents the ileocecal area with one or two appendiceal orifices between lumens of proximal bowel above, and distal bowel or hindgut below (Figure 13-5).

Genital abnormalities include bifid or diminutive penis and undescended testicles, and in the female, there can be a bifid clitoris with vaginal duplication, agenesis, or atresia. Treatment includes regional practices that have varied over the years. Many centers elected to assign female gender status to males born with this anomaly because of the technical difficulties in surgically achieving satisfactory external genitalia. This practice is beginning to change, partly as a result of numerous, highly publicized cases involving litigation over gender

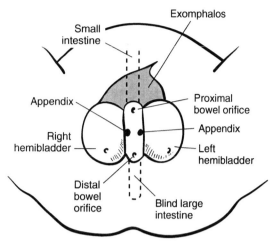

Figure 13-5 Anatomy of classic cloacal exstrophy. (From Howell C et al: Optimal management of cloacal exstrophy, *J Pediatr Surg* 18:365-369, 1983.)

assignment. If gender reassignment is to occur, it is best done in the first 24 to 48 hours of life because of the parental adjustment and apprehension that occurs (Warner and Ziegler, 2000).

In cloacal exstrophy the anus is imperforate. Inguinal hernia is common, and the midgut may be foreshortened, with a predisposition to malabsorption and failure to thrive. Spinal anomalies are frequent and include sacral and other vertebral anomalies, myelodysplasia, lipomeningocele, and tethered cord. Diverse skeletal anomalies, including dislocation of the hip and clubfoot, occur in up to 50% of patients (O'Neill, 1998). A variety of renal anomalies have been reported in up to 60% of cases, including pelvic kidney, hydronephrosis, hydroureter, ureteral atresia, unilateral renal agenesis, multicystic kidney, and crossed fused ectopia. It is important to note that despite numerous physical differences, the majority of these children have normal intelligence (Warner and Ziegler, 2000).

Epidemiology. Cloacal exstrophy is rare and occurs in only 1 in 200,000 to 400,000 live births; it accounts for only 10% of exstrophy cases. It appears to occur equally in males and females (O'Neill, 1998).

Etiology. The cause of cloacal exstrophy is unknown at this time.

Symptoms. Symptoms vary with the specific anomaly, but surgical intervention is inevitable once assessment of associated anomalies is complete. Cardiac and pulmonary anomalies are rare in these children; therefore, once preoperative screening and specialty consultation are completed, family education and consultation is done, and the first of many reconstructive surgeries is scheduled. During the assessment phase the exposed organs must be kept moist with nonadherent dressings or, on occasion, pouched to keep the organs from dehydrating.

Diagnosis. Diagnosis is facilitated by the overt visibility of the deformities, but x-ray studies and ultrasonography are used to demarcate the extent of involvement of the upper urinary tract, the central nervous system, the musculosketal system, and to assist in the assessment of gender status. Consultation of multiple specialists must be coordinated by a team leader, usually the pediatric surgeon, in order to present the family with an orderly treatment plan.

Treatment. Initial surgical intervention involves separation of the intestinal and the genitourinary systems and formation of an intestinal stoma. If possible, primary closure of the bladder, as well as the omphalocele, is done at this time. The intestinal stoma is generally located laterally, to avoid the midline incision.

Every attempt is made to preserve the hindgut and appendices for later reconstructive purposes. When possible, the hindgut and exposed intestinal plate are tubularized and incorporated into an end colostomy to maximize intestinal function. When spinal dysraphism occurs as a closed tube neural defect, neurosurgical intervention may be postponed. Open tube defects require more immediate intervention, and shunts may be needed for hydrocephalus. In cases of gender reassignment, orchiectomy is done at this initial surgery.

More extensive reconstruction of the urinary system and genital reconstruction are usually deferred until the child reaches 9 kilograms and is stable. Inguinal hernias are repaired at one of the staged surgeries. Orthopedic procedures such as osteotomy may be done at the time of bladder reconstruction. Casting for clubfeet is generally done early in infancy and orthotics used as needed. Multiple surgeries are usually needed for these children because of the number of anomalies.

Children with cloacal exstrophy will live with permanent intestinal stomas due to the continence challenges of their anatomic anomalies. Urinary continence is made possible by continent urinary diversion or reconstruction.

Changing body contours and developmental needs dictate regular assessment of ostomy care and pouching systems, with a goal of preserving skin integrity, containing effluent, encouraging self-care, and promoting self-esteem. WOC nurses who care for these children are confronted with a variety of challenges, as well as the opportunity to support the growth and development of both child and family.

Bladder Exstrophy

Description. In bladder exstrophy, the bladder and urethra are open and exposed on the lower abdomen. There is wide pubic diastasis, as well as wide rectus and a low umbilicus. Males have a wide, short penis with the urethral plate open on the dorsal surface. The testicles are usually descended with normal vas deferens and ejaculatory ducts.

Females have a bifid clitoris and separation of the labia with a short, anteriorly displaced vagina. While the uterus, ovaries, and tubes are normal, the vagina and uterus may be duplicated. Most children with this condition have vesicoureteral reflux. The anus in both males and females tends to be anteriorly displaced and may be stenotic or prone to prolapse because of pelvic floor weakness.

Epidemiology. Bladder exstrophy occurs in 1 in 10,000 to 1 in 50,000 live births. It is three to four times more common in males than in females (Brock and O'Neill, 1998).

Etiology. No cause has been found for this variation in fetal development.

Symptoms. As with cloacal exstrophy, the infant's clinical problem is readily apparent. It is uncommon for these children to have other anomalies, so the focus after birth is on preparation for the first stage of surgical intervention.

Diagnosis. Other than physical examination and routine laboratory tests, only renal ultrasound is needed to evaluate the number and the condition of kidneys and the presence of hydroureteronephrosis.

Treatment. Primary closure of bladder exstrophy can be accomplished without osteotomy if done in the first 48 to 72 hours of life, since at this point the pelvic ring is still malleable. After 72 hours, bilateral iliac osteotomies are done before bladder closure.

The goal of most first-stage surgery is to close the bladder and leave the child with epispadias to ensure decompression of the upper tracts. While some surgeons are attempting bladder closure and epispadias repair in the neonate, other practitioners are concerned about the risk of bladder outlet obstruction increasing the severity of reflux. The latter group prefers to wait a year before correcting the epispadias and allowing the bladder to enlarge (Murphy, 2000).

In either case, ureteral stents and suprapubic urinary drainage are used with Bryant's traction or external fixation, to decrease tension on the midline repair. Complications of this stage include wound dehiscence (5%), bladder prolapse (10 to 15 %), and outlet obstruction (5%) with hydronephrosis (Murphy, 2000).

The second stage of repair for most males is correction of the epispadias. This repair includes straightening and lengthening the penis and creation of a ventral urethra. The surgery is generally done between 6 and 12 months of age. Urethrocutaneus fistula is the most common complication of this stage with an incidence of 30% to 50%. Decreased penile length and residual chordee can be a problem for these boys (Brock and O'Neill, 1998). The goal of the final stage of surgery is urinary continence, accomplished with bladder neck reconstruction and reimplantation of the ureters. If adequate capacity is not achieved, augmentation may be done. If continence does not follow bladder neck reconstruction, continent urinary diversion is done, usually using a Mitrofanoff style of procedure. It is estimated that 10% to 20% of patients will require urinary diversion (Kramer, 1998).

Finally, it should be noted that there is an increased incidence of adenocarcinoma of the bladder in these children, perhaps a result of chronic inflammation and metaplasia in the exposed bladder plate. Squamous cell carcinoma and rhabdomyosarcoma have also been reported. Both males and females have been able to reproduce but have lower than normal fertility (Brock and O'Neill, 1998).

Epispadias

Description. Children with epispadias are born with the bladder closed, but the urethra is dorsal and displaced in the male, and in females the urethra opens anteriorly to the normal position and is characterized by a bifid clitoris and separation of the labia. Male epispadias is classified by the location of the urethral meatus as penopubic, penile, or glandular. Boys with glandular epispadias are continent and require less reconstruction than those with penopubic epispadias. Two thirds of those with penile epispadias need bladder neck reconstruction. Females have a urethral cleft involving the length of the urethra and sphincter and a flattened mons pubis (Kramer, 1998).

Epidemiology/etiology. Epispadias is rare and occurs 3 to 5 times more often in males. As with the other forms of exstrophy, a cause is not known.

Symptoms/diagnosis. The diagnosis of epispadias is made through physical examination. Associated anomalies have not been cited.

Treatment. Surgical correction of epispadias, as noted for bladder exstrophy, is undertaken in the older infant. Endoscopy is used to evaluate the external sphincter and bladder neck in preparation for the repair. Surgical reconstruction of male penopubic and female epispadias is complicated and may require more than one surgical procedure. Simpler reconstruction may be done as a single operation. Urinary diversion is an option, if urinary continence cannot be attained with reconstruction.

Posterior Urethral Valves

Description. Posterior urethral valves (PUV) are folds or leaflets of tissue that can obstruct the flow of urine. There are three types of valves, with type I being the most common. The condition can range from mild with nonobstructing, prominent folds, to severe with totally obstructing, diaphragm-like leaflets. Posterior urethral valves are the most common cause of urinary obstruction in newborn boys.

Epidemiology. PUV is the most common form of congenital urethral obstruction and occurs in 1 in 8,000 to 25,000 live male births. There is no comparable condition in females (Casales, 1999).

Etiology. No known causes have been noted.

Symptoms. The condition varies in severity of obstruction, so the symptoms reflect the degree of obstruction caused and also the age of the infant. About half of severe valve cases are first seen in the first year of life with abdominal mass and infection. Sepsis, metabolic acidosis, and azotemia can also occur in infants. In children over 1 year of age, a urinary tract infection (UTI) is the most common symptom. Other symptoms may include nocturnal or diurnal enuresis, frequency, dribbling, hematuria, and acute urinary retention.

Diagnosis. Voiding cystourethrogram (VCUG) is the best method of diagnosis for the valves, which are seen as filling defects as the bladder empties. Other findings might include hypertrophy of the bladder neck, trabeculation of the bladder, bladder diverticula, vesicoureteral reflux, and hydronephrosis. Although all of these findings may be secondary to the obstructing valves, it is also possible for the child to have concomitant disease such as obstructive megaureter or ureteropelvic junction obstruction.

Treatment. In very young infants, stabilizing electrolytes and renal function are the first objectives. Definitive treatment, resection or ablation of the valves, is generally performed using an endoscope and may be deferred until the infant is older and thriving. In cases where treatment is delayed, urinary tract decompression is needed. This can be accomplished by vesicostomy unless the upper tract injury requires supravesicle diversion. In these cases, ureterostomies or pyelostomies may be done.

The urinary diversion is generally closed at the time of the valve ablation. Complications of valve ablation are persistent obstruction, sphincter damage, and urethral injury with stricture formation (Retik, 1998). Surgical texts stress the use of direct visualization during valve resection and caution to avoid the external sphincter. Newer endoscopy equipment is available in smaller sizes that allows relatively early repair under direct visualization, with decreased risk of injury.

The other reported sequela of PUV is a "valve" bladder that is poorly compliant and has high pressure. This may be treated with medications or bladder augmentation.

Prune Belly Syndrome

Description. Prune belly syndrome (PBS) carries that name because of the characteristic wrinkly appearance of the abdominal skin caused by the congenital absence, deficiency, or hypoplasia of the abdominal musculature. Urinary tract anomalies include a large, hypotonic bladder with dilated ureters and a dilated prostatic urethra. The syndrome also includes bilateral cryptorchidism. Although the last two anomalies suggest that the syndrome occurs only in males, it has been reported in females, although very rarely.

Epidemiology. The incidence of PBS is about 1 in 35,000 to 50,000 live births (Keating and Rich, 2000). As noted, it occurs primarily in males although reported in a very small number of females. A variety of other anomalies also occur in children with PBS. Some of these are pulmonary hypoplasia and lobar atelectasis; cardiac anomalies such as patent ductus arteriosus, atrial septal defect, ventricular septal defect, or tetratology of Fallot; orthopedic anomalies such as pectus excavatum and carinatum, varus deformity of feet, congenital hip dislocation; and gastrointestinal anomalies such as malrotation, intestinal atresia, imperforate anus, or cloaca, HD, omphalocele, or gastroschisis.

Etiology. No genetic basis for this syndrome has been discovered. There are conflicting theories as to the specific embryologic processes that result in the physical features of the anomaly.

Symptoms. Symptoms vary according to the combination of anomalies present. Many of these children are relatively fragile as infants and require multiple surgeries, but improve significantly as they grow. Newborns may be ill and have pulmonary instability or sensitivity; however, as they grow older, renal issues tend to prevail as the leading concern. Fertility has not been documented with PBS (Keating and Rich, 2000).

Diagnosis. Workup of infants with characteristic abdominal wall and testicular findings should include x-ray studies of the chest to evaluate pulmonary status, as well as careful examination of the anus, the rectum, and the heart. Orthopedic anomalies are usually readily apparent. Urologic evaluation should include ultrasound and VCUG initially, and nuclear scintigraphy after several weeks to evaluate functional status.

Treatment. Both aggressive surgical intervention and conservative medical management have been advocated. Several caveats to early aggressive reconstruction exist:

- Renal dysplasia cannot be reversed with surgery.
- Low-pressure symptoms are the result of ureteral smooth muscle deficiency rather than obstruction.
- The technical challenges of these children's urinary tracts are not without risk (Keating and Rich, 2000).

The relatively rare occurrence of these cases makes determining best practice difficult, and gathering evidence for interventions will require a great deal of additional time and study.

The important tenets for managing these children that are clearly understood include:

- Provide adequate drainage for the urinary system.
- Prevent UTIs that can impair renal function.
- Maximize physical and social adaptation as possible.
- Use prophylactic antibiotics in untreated vesicoureteral reflux, and careful monitoring of renal growth and function.
- Use vesicostomy if drainage is needed, since it appears to be the preferred method, although some children may require higher diversion with ureterostomies or pyelostomies.

Caution with ureteral diversion is warranted, because the proximal ureters appear to be more functional than the distal and care must be taken with vascular supply. Clean intermittent catheterization (CIC) via urethra or continent abdominal stoma is another option for the cooperative older child.

Ostomies in these children can be a challenge to pouch, since the deep abdominal wrinkles preclude finding a smooth surface on which to affix the pouching system. Stomal lumens also tend to stenose more frequently than in other children because the abdominal musculature that holds the lumen stable is deficient. Routine dilation of urinary and intestinal stomas helps prevent stasis. Laxatives and active bowel management have been needed in children with both intestinal diversions and reconstructed cloaca, and imperforate anus.

Reduction cystoplasty, urethroplasty, and abdominoplasty are all potential interventions for children with PBS. Some improvement in voiding and decreased residual after voiding has been reported with abdominoplasty (Keating and Rich, 2000). Growth also results in improved voiding status, since the structures lengthen and straighten over time. As noted, with the small total number of cases and limited length of follow-up, it is difficult to determine best practices. Time and improved survival rates should increase the database and clarify future treatment regimens for PBS children.

Myelomeningocele, Lipoma, and Tethered Cord

Description. Myelomeningocele is a condition that occurs when the arches of the vertebrae do not fuse together over the spinal cord. The actual term *myelomeningocele* refers to the condition when both the meninges and the cord are herniated through the bony defect. The more modern term for this is an *open neural tube defect.*

A meningocele is when only the meninges protrude. An older term familiar to many lay people is *spina bifida,* but this actually refers only to the bony defect and can be an *occulta* form where there is no protrusion of neural tissue. Those lesions that involve the neural tissue are the *cystica* form.

Lipomas are fatty tissue growths or benign tumors that can occur around the spinal cord that can grow larger as the child lays down fatty tissue.

Tethered cord is a condition that often involves fatty tissue at the base of the spinal cord filum, which can be adherent or "tethered" to the vertebra.

This condition often requires surgery, since with growth the spinal cord is meant to rise freely upward within the spinal column. If the cord is tethered, it becomes stretched as the child's spinal column lengthens, and this can result in gait disturbance and bowel and bladder control problems.

Epidemiology. Spina bifida occulta occurs in about 5% of the population, and myelomeningocele occurs in about 0.32 of 1000 live births (Wong and Hockenberry-Eaton, 2001). Prenatal diagnosis of the condition is done with a blood test of the mother to check for serum alpha fetoprotein (AFP), which is normally found in amniotic fluid. Levels of AFP rise if the neural tube does not close, and elevation in the protein level during the first trimester of pregnancy indicates risk of neural tube defects. Tethered cord also occurs in 10% to 46% of children with imperforate anus or cloaca (Kiely and Pena, 1998).

Etiology. The cause of spina bifida and myelomeningocele is unknown, but a variety of maternal health conditions such as diabetes, folic acid deficiency, and obesity have been implicated. The increased incidence in families suggests a genetic influence (Wong and Hockenberry-Eaton, 2001).

Symptoms. Symptoms vary with the level of the lesion and severity. As many as 30% of these children have a degree of hydrocephalus, which is treated with a ventricular-peritoneal shunt to decrease the pressure on the surrounding brain tissue from the accumulated fluid. Tethered cord can occur and recur in myelomeningocele children as they grow and increase bowel and bladder problems.

The urinary tract is at risk because of detrusor-sphincter dyssynergia, in which the sphincter fails to relax when the bladder contracts. In other children, the bladder neck is incompetent, causing the bladder to empty continuously but incompletely. The child's diaper is always wet, and urine flows freely with any increase in abdominal pressure, but there is a high residual of urine in the bladder. The bladder is often high pressure and can become trabeculated over time. Most of these children are incontinent.

Bowel management is also an issue, since these children have neurogenic bowels which tend to show significant constipation and altered sensation and sphincter control. Although it is possible to toilet train children with lower lesions, high lesions require more active bowel management strategies. Even with an effective bowel management program, these children may still be subject to episodes of fecal incontinence if they have a viral illness, need to take antibiotics, or eat too much of a food to which they are sensitive.

Diagnosis. The myelomeningocele is readily apparent at birth unless it is anterior, in which case it will only be picked up on spinal magnetic resonance imaging (MRI) studies. The same is true for a tethered cord. These are generally diagnosed by MRI, as are lipomas. Other diagnostic tests include MRI of the head for hydrocephalous, ultrasounds of the kidney, VCUG, and later, urodynamics to evaluate bladder function.

Multiple orthopedic films will be taken to assess various bony anomalies that occur with growth. The variety of anomalies is too extensive to detail here but includes defects of the spine such as scoliosis, kyphosis, and lordosis, as well as anomalies of the ankle and foot such as Charcot foot. Dislocated hips are common with the higher lesions.

Treatment. Initial treatment for children with an open neural tube defect is surgery to close the defect followed by shunt placement if needed. As shunted children grow, it is not uncommon for them to require multiple shunt revisions because the tubing can get plugged or kink, or otherwise malfunction.

The urinary tract of most children with spinal lesions requires attention from birth onward. As noted, these children are at risk for upper tract deterioration and will often need assertive treatment plans.

CIC is often used to maintain regular and complete bladder decompression. For families who cannot perform CIC as needed for very young children, a vesicostomy provides continuous decompression and fits within the diaper area, thus avoiding the need to pouch. Older children can learn CIC or have a continent urinary diversion.

Continent urinary stomas (e.g., Mitrofanoff) are particularly useful for children in wheelchairs, because they can often be catheterized without get-ting out of the chair. This is convenient and a tremendous timesaver in school and later life, as well. A variety of surgical procedures can be used to provide a continent channel from the abdominal wall to the bladder.

In addition to the procedures detailed earlier, some children may need intervention on the blad-der neck and/or the use of medications to increase their continence interval, the period of time with-out urinary leakage. Anticholinergics are used both orally and intravesically to control bladder contractions and increase storage. Bladder aug-mentation with or without ureteral reimplanta-tion may be used. Artificial sphincters and injections of collagen or Teflon have been used to increase urethral resistance. A variety of sling pro-cedures have been tried, and in some cases the bladder neck can be disconnected if there is a con-tinent diversion, although this requires meticu-lous regularity of CIC to prevent distention and potential rupture of the bladder. Bowel programs range from increasing fiber in the diet and using habit training, to more active programs that use suppositories or digital evacuation. These chil-dren are often good candidates for the MACE pro-cedure described earlier, also known as an appendicostomy or neoappendicostomy. In this procedure, the appendix or a substitute is brought to the abdominal wall, often at the umbilicus, to provide a channel for catheterization and instilla-tion of enema fluid to cleanse the bowel. The goal is to prevent fecal incontinence (Pope and Rink, 1999).

A large team of specialists typically manages these children. The skills and knowledge of the WOC nurse make a valuable contribution to the health team. More of these children are reaching adulthood than ever before, and many nurses who do not practice in pediatrics may eventually have the opportunity to care for an adult with one of these spinal lesions.

Ureteropelvic Junction Obstruction

Description. Ureteropelvic junction (UPJ) obstruction is an impairment to urinary flow at the level of the connection between the ureter and the renal pelvis. This may occur unilaterally or bilater-ally. The clinical condition varies with the degree of obstruction, which may be only partial or intermit-tent, and with the extent of injury to the renal tissue from the dilation.

Epidemiology. UPJ obstruction is the most common fetal uropathy (which includes PUV). The incidence of UPJ obstruction is about 1 in 1000 and is more common in boys than in girls and more common in the left ureter. Fewer than 15% of cases are bilateral (Casales, 1999).

Etiology. The causes of the obstruction can vary. These include aberrant vessels that span the area, kinks, bands and adhesions in the area, arteri-ovenous malformations in the area, abnormal dis-tribution of muscular and collagen fibers at the level of the UPJ, valvelike processes, and benign fibroepithelial polyps.

Symptoms. As with most of the other condi-tions, symptoms vary with the severity of the dis-ease—in this case, the dilation of the renal pelvis, the presence and frequency of UTIs, and whether the disease is unilateral or bilateral. Most often the children will have an abdominal mass in infancy. They will usually have UTIs, abdominal pain, and vomiting.

Diagnosis. The diagnosis of UPJ obstruction begins with ultrasonography that demonstrates renal pelvic dilation. An intravenous pyelogram (IVP) may be needed to demonstrate the obstruc-tion at the UPJ level, as opposed to a VCUG that is used to demonstrate vesicoureteral reflux, which can also cause renal pelvic dilation. Once UPJ is demonstrated or suspected, a renal isotope scan is used to measure functional status of the kidney. These measures are repeated at intervals to ensure that there is no deterioration during periods of observation or, after an intervention, to evaluate efficacy.

Treatment. Infants who are symptomatic or have poor or deteriorating renal function or wors-ening renal dilation may require at least percuta-neous diversion to relieve dilation and stabilize function. Interestingly, unilateral drainage in the event of bilateral dilation may improve drainage from both kidneys. Percutaneous nephrostomy is usually maintained for 3 to 4 weeks so that definitive surgery can be done—pyeloplasty if dilation decreases and function improves. Nephrectomy may be required if function remains poor.

The timing of surgery during the first year of life remains controversial among surgeons. Fetal urinary diversion can be done in cases where prenatal diagnosis has been made, but its implications remain to be seen as larger numbers of cases are reported. There is some question as to whether the diversion of urine to improve amniotic fluid volume preserves pulmonary function at the expense of the lower urinary tract (Mouriquand, 1998).

Megaureter

Description. Megaureter is a descriptive term that refers to an abnormally dilated ureter that may also be elongated and tortuous. Megaureter may be due to a defect in the muscle fibers of the ureter that causes a lack of peristalsis of urine down to the bladder. This is a functional obstruction that results in dilation of the distal ureter. Megaureter may also be caused by massive vesicoureteral reflux due to a variety of conditions (Hendren et al, 1998).

Epidemiology/etiology. The occurrence of megaureter varies with its etiology, which is multifactorial.

Symptoms. Children usually have fever, abdominal pain, and hematuria. The urinary stasis can result in stones.

Diagnosis. An IVP demonstrates the dilation in the ureter. The ureters are usually tortuous, and there is less dilation of the proximal than the distal ureter and almost normal renal pelvis and calyces.

Treatment. If the megaureter is caused by vesicoureteral reflux (VUR), correction of that condition should lead to compensation of the ureter. VUR is covered in the next section. Surgical correction of primary megaureter involves tapering of the dilated ureter and reimplantation into the bladder. The children are usually followed closely for recurrence of the functional obstruction.

Vesicoureteral Reflux

Description. Reflux of urine from the bladder back into the kidney occurs when any of the normal mechanisms that maintain one-way, downward flow do not function. It is a significant and dangerous problem because it can damage the kidney.

Epidemiology. Primary VUR occurs in up to 18.5% of normal children. Of infants with UTIs, up to 70% will have reflux. Reflux is common in children with antenatal diagnosis of hydronephrosis. Primary VUR is more common in females than in males, but males with UTIs are more likely to have VUR. The highest incidence is in younger children. VUR is 10 times more common in Caucasian than in African-American girls. VUR can also occur in up to 45% of siblings of children diagnosed with VUR (Atala and Walker, 1998).

Etiology. The most common causes of VUR are a short intravesical tunnel; an anatomically abnormal ureterovesical junction as is found in bladder exstrophy, PBS, or ureteral duplication; or a high pressure bladder, which can result from functional disorders of voiding, neurogenic bladder, or posterior urethral valves (Ewalt, 1998). The ratio of tunnel length to ureteral diameter of 4:1 or 5:1 usually results in an effective one-way valve; when this ratio is altered by large ureteral diameter or short tunnel length, reflux may occur. Data suggest a dominant inheritance pattern with variable penetrance, but as can be seen with other urinary anomalies, there are multiple factors involved.

Symptoms. The earliest symptom of VUR is a UTI. Symptoms of UTI vary with age. Neonates tend to have nonspecific symptoms such as lethargy, irritability, temperature instability, anorexia, emesis, or jaundice. Older infants may have abdominal pain, emesis, diarrhea, poor weight gain, or fever, sometimes with cloudy or foul-smelling urine. Older children are apt to have dysuria with urinary frequency, urgency, and enuresis. Later symptoms are hypertension, proteinuria, voiding dysfunction, and chronic renal insufficiency (Sheldon et al, 2000).

Diagnosis. A VCUG is done to detect the presence of reflux, but it must be deferred until the UTI has cleared and the child is asymptomatic. Ultrasound of the kidney and bladder may be done even during the acute phase of a UTI. Once discovered, VUR is graded according to an international classification on a scale of one to five, based on the degree of dilation of the ureter and the renal pelvis and calyces (Figure 13-6). The diagnostic process must also determine whether the VUR is primary or secondary to another process, such as bladder outlet obstruction or neurovesical disease.

Treatment. Since the length of the submucosal tunnel increases with age, many children with VUR will be managed nonoperatively with antibiotic suppression, good hydration, perineal hygiene, and bowel management. Strict surveillance of these children includes serial urine cultures and renal imaging every 6 to12 months. Renal growth and cortical scarring are monitored as is blood pressure, and annual VCUGs are usually obtained.

Since many children with VUR are girls, it is important to note that constipation can result in incomplete bladder emptying. There is such a strong association that part of the workup of girls with constipation includes urine culture, and review of the VCUG often reveals fecal retention. Constipation has also been associated with urinary incontinence, since it is difficult to adequately constrict the urinary sphincter when the rectal ampulla is distended with a fecal bolus. The diagnosis of reflux in the presence of fecal retention may lead to referral to a WOC nurse for assistance with bowel management.

Cystoscopy is usually done for children with surgical indications such as breakthrough UTI, significant renal injury on initial evaluation, pyelonephritis, reflux of grade 4 or greater, puberty, or failure to respond to 4 years of suppressive therapy. Endoscopy may reveal a poor ureteral insertion that would benefit from reimplantation. Other surgical indications include progressive renal injury, failure of renal growth, breakthrough pyelonephritis, and intolerance of or noncompliance with antibiotic suppression (Sheldon et al, 2000).

The goal of surgical intervention is the achievement of a 5:1 ratio between ureteral diameter and tunnel length. Surgical reconstruction requires ureteral exposure and mobility, as well as meticulous preservation of blood supply to the ureter. Most children will have ureteral stents and a urethral catheter after surgery.

Complications can include de novo contralateral reflux, ureteral obstruction, and persistent reflux or diverticula formation. Ureteral obstruction may be due to ureteral kinking, problems with placement or construction of the neohiatus or anastomotic stricture, devascularization, or a tunnel that is too tight (Sheldon et al, 2000).

PEDIATRIC STOMA CARE

The focus of this section will be on the care of pediatric patients with stomas, and their unique needs. Participating in the care of the pediatric stoma patient requires knowledge regarding family issues, physical growth and development issues, preterm

GRADE OF REFLUX

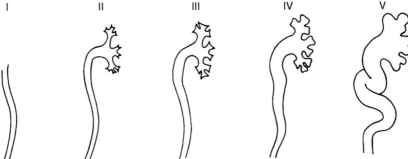

Figure 13-6 International classification of vesicoureteral reflux. (From The International Reflux Committee: Medical versus surgical treatment of primary vesicoureteral reflux, *Pediatrics* 67:396, 1981.)

infant skin development, and stoma care related to the pediatric population. Pouching principles unique to the pediatric population will be covered in this section, and the reader is referred to Chapter 12 for basic pouching principles.

Psychologic and Physical Factors

Parental Fears and Psychosocial Considerations

During the 9-month gestation, parents invest many hopes and dreams in their unborn child. Routine fetal ultrasound during prenatal visits makes their baby even more real. They can make out features and see their baby move. Therefore, when the outcome of the birth includes some type of anomaly that requires intervention, there is a period of adjustment. Parents experience many emotions, including anger, fear, anxiety, and guilt (Davies, 1992).

Parents may wonder if what they did or did not do contributed to this outcome for their newborn. When a stoma is the result of trauma or late diagnosis, parents may also feel culpable and distressed by their inability to prevent the catastrophe and protect their child. They may question their own competence and ability to care for their child. These fears need to be explored and verbalized. The WOC/ET nurse can facilitate discussion, especially when there is no clear understanding or link between cause and effect of the condition. Even if the WOC/ET nurse is not a specialist in pediatrics, helping the parents to organize and prioritize their questions is a start.

Body Image

A stoma requires an adjustment in body image, and when the person with a stoma is an infant, it is the parents who experience the body image alteration. They need to amend their dreams of the "perfect" baby. Initially fear for their child's life may be their greatest concern, especially with a preterm infant or a child born with significant, life-threatening anomalies.

During this time of stress, it is important to examine how the family has reacted to past crises. Support systems such as family, faith, and friends must be assessed and encouraged. Later stressors

may involve the care of the stoma and other surgeries that are required to correct the physical problem.

Older children need to adjust their body image to incorporate the stoma, and the parents need to adjust their vision of their child. These processes are not always simultaneous or even parallel. Children take many clues from their parents' reaction to the surgery and the stoma. Working closely with the parents is critical if the child is to develop a healthy self-concept.

Frequently the goal for older children is to demonstrate competence and independence, because they are more pragmatic about daily life issues. For most children, the primary goal is reintegration into their normal lives and daily activities, especially the things they enjoy such as school, sports, and their friends.

It may be helpful for parents to have the WOC/ET nurse list areas that will *not* be affected by the presence of a stoma, such as lying on the abdomen, bathing, swimming, turning, and crawling. Once some of the more common activities have been described, the nurse can elicit discussion of other activities parents are concerned about. In most cases, infants who happen to have stomas have more in common with other newborns than not.

In the teenage patient body image is a major concern, and this is a very vulnerable time for the child and the parent. Teenagers want to be like other teenagers, and anything that makes them feel they are different is difficult, since they may not have yet developed a strong sense of self.

In working with teens, it is often best to teach the teen directly, with the parent as an observer and possible backup, unless the teen prefers to designate an alternate caring and responsible person. This can be particularly helpful with working parents or single parents, as long as all parties agree with the role assignment.

Physical Growth

The physical growth of the infant is notably different from that of the adult. Within the first year, most infants triple their birth weight. This significant growth spurt leads to changes in the peristomal plane, body contours, and the stoma size.

It is necessary to periodically remeasure the stoma and adjust the style and size of the pouching system that was initially selected.

The growth spurt adds weight to the infant that results in the sleep pattern changing; with less sleeping during the day, the child now sleeps through the night. This may present new challenges to the pouching system in terms of capacity. For children with liquid or high output, a pouch with a urinary spout may be selected and connected to a bedside collector to increase the capacity at night.

If parents were getting up at night and changing diapers (for the child with a stoma not wearing a pouch), they may find that as their child sleeps through the night, the peristomal skin demonstrates signs of skin breakdown. Some parents choose to set an alarm clock to change their child's diaper. This may affect the parents' and the child's normal sleep patterns. A secure pouching system can allow for uninterrupted sleep and help to maintain intact skin.

Parents may also be concerned that their child is not growing at a normal rate. Physical growth is seldom delayed solely due to the presence of a stoma. The clinician needs to help the parents by examining all parameters that may impact the child's development including prematurity, concomitant health problems, and nutrition. Looking at the child's height and weight data also helps to focus on relative proportion rather than comparisons to "normal" for age only.

Since most children become more physically active as they grow, changes can be dramatic and seem to happen overnight. As infants begin to sit up, scoot, crawl, pull themselves up on furniture, and walk, significant strain is placed on the pouch seal. Any dramatic decline in wear time should be evaluated in light of these activities, which are part of a child's normal physical growth. Parents should be encouraged to report changes in wear time, and the WOC/ET nurse should reevaluate equipment on a regular basis to note any need for a stronger skin barrier adhesive, an ostomy belt, or a border of tape.

It is also important to ensure that the child's prescription and an authorization for supplies are obtained, so that adequate quantities are available. Insurance or third-party payers must be made aware that infants and children should not be limited to quantities of supplies designed for the needs of an adult or geriatric ostomate. The WOC nurse may need to write letters to third-party payers to validate the need for increased quantities of monthly ostomy supplies for the baby or child.

Skin Development: Preterm Infant

Premature infants have a less well developed epidermal barrier, leaving them ill-equipped to deal with the outside environment (Rogers, 2003). Maturation of the epidermis does occur in the neonate and usually by about one month after birth the skin is normalized to that of a full-term infant. Thus there are special considerations in the management of the low birth-weight infant's skin and stoma.

Because of the immature epidermal barrier, the preterm baby's skin has increased permeability. In addition, these babies have an increased surface area relative to their body weight. Thus they are at greater risk for toxic reactions because of greater absorption of topically applied substances. It is advisable to employ an approach of minimization and carefully evaluate any products placed on the child's skin. Preterm infant skin characteristics are outlined in Table 13-3.

The adhesive properties of skin barriers must be evaluated, and close attention should be paid to manufacturers' guidelines for use, since products may not have been tested for use with the preterm infant. In addition, products which have been tested in or developed specifically for premature infants may have specific properties the WOC nurse should be aware of, such as decreased absorption in the barrier as a tradeoff for more flexibility or easier skin release. Examples of pouching systems for premature infants are found in Figure 13-7.

Developmental Growth

Part of newborn development includes exploring the environment. Newborns play with their fingers and toes and things in their immediate environment, including their pouches. Parents may report that children have proudly displayed their pouches, pulled off when they wake up in the morning or after a nap. The WOC nurse can help by listening to the parents' concerns and by offering suggestions in managing this pouching challenge, which is usually temporary. Parents need to display their dissatisfaction to their infants through facial expression and tone of voice. This can be likened to the approach taken with their children when they teach them not to touch a hot stove or put objects into electrical sockets. Another suggestion might include providing additional toys in the children's cribs that may have more appeal than the full ostomy pouch. In addition, when their child takes a

TABLE 13-3   Preterm Infant Skin Characteristics

SKIN CHARACTERISTICS	MANAGEMENT CONSIDERATIONS
Increased skin permeability	Minimal product usage because of greater transepidermal absorption
Immature elastin fibers and diminished cohesion between the epidermis and dermis	Careful adhesive removal because of decreased ability of skin to stretch
Decreased thickness of the stratum corneum	Increased transepidermal water loss may interfere with the pouch seal. In addition, there is increased transepidermal absorption: use topical agents sparingly.
Slowly developed acid mantle	Skin more susceptible to damage with the use of alkaline products

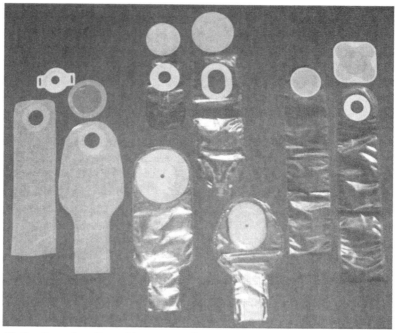

Figure 13-7 Examples of pouching systems for premature infants. (Reprinted from Rogers VE: Managing preemie stomas: more than just the pouch, *JWOCN* 30(2):105, 2003, with permission from the Wound, Ostomy and Continence Nurses Society.)

nap or goes to bed for the evening, parents should make sure the child is wearing clothes. A one-piece sleeper or a T-shirt that snaps in the crotch can help to deter curious, little fingers. An inexpensive nursery monitor may also help to alert parents when their child is awake and active, so they can arrive on the scene before problems occur.

The infant who has a temporary stoma will not remember later that he or she ever had an ostomy. However, later in life the child may be curious about a scar or ask questions about having been in the hospital, when this is discussed by their parents. For that reason, the WOC/ET nurse may advise that the parents save a pouch in the baby book and even take pictures. This is part of their child's special and unique story of growing up. There is nothing to be ashamed of, and years later it will make it easier to explain what happened.

Pouch removal by toddlers and preschool children may be an acting-out of their frustrations or angers. This can be dealt with best by employing the family's usual time-outs or other disciplinary methods, as well as by encouraging more appropriate ways to express feelings. Children this age can help parents by reporting when it is time to empty or change the pouch. Young children can be given their own responsibilities such as gathering supplies, holding tape rolls or tail clips, snapping pieces together, or whatever their manual dexterity will allow. Parents should remember that children of this age love being given responsibility and jobs.

School-age children have better manual dexterity but like their younger counterparts, they may be too busy to stop other activities to empty pouches or to take the time to properly cleanse the pouch spout when emptying. They may also have difficulty correctly coordinating all the needed steps to change their own pouches. However, children at this age are learning huge amounts of games and rules, and they can often correctly guide an adult through their stoma care if the appropriate supplies are on hand and the adult will listen to them. Children who have had their ostomy for a long time can be totally responsible for their own stoma care when provided with a supportive and non-judgmental environment. It is one of the tasks of childhood to master the intricacies of expected behaviors; part of the challenge is to be less than perfect at the beginning. Belittling the child's less-than-ideal skills and not providing enough privacy to maintain personal dignity are the most common adult errors with this age group. The use of praise and rewards and increasing privileges commensurate with increased responsibility should be encouraged with this age group, as well as with preteens.

Preteens either excel at personal hygiene from the beginning, or they slowly adopt acceptable practices; this also applies to stoma care. Acceptance of the child, and encouraging needed behaviors to ensure that social expectations for cleanliness and odor control are met, is very important at this age. Self-confidence is often lower than the outward attitude would imply; thus private time to review concerns, fears, and issues is as important for these children as it is for teens.

Teenagers usually have the manual dexterity and time management skills to handle appropriate stoma care. However, they are subject to a host of social and role stresses that may impact their coping and their stoma adaptation. It is important that they are given time and opportunity to practice skills, to role-play social situations of concern, and to express their feelings.

As a child goes through each developmental stage, parents may experience stress, and there may be especially difficult times as the child grows when they think their child is not like everyone else. Parents need help to make the presence of the stoma a normal part of life (Davies, 1992) (see Table 11-1).

Management Considerations
Stoma Site Selection
In the newborn, the creation of a stoma is often an emergency procedure, and there is no opportunity for preoperative stoma site selection. When site marking is possible, there are some general factors to take into consideration. It is difficult to predict physical growth patterns for an infant or child but in general, stomas placed above the umbilicus grow up with the body and stay in the same relative proximity to bony prominences. By the same token,

those stomas sited below the umbilicus will grow down and stay in the same relative proximity to bony prominences. The ideal location for most children would be the umbilical area, but the umbilicus is important to body image for children and parents. Possibly it can be an ideal area for a continent stoma later in life. Chapter 11 has further information on stoma siting and preoperative teaching.

Depending on the child's age, play therapy can be helpful, both in explaining the purpose for marking the stoma and for beginning the preoperative teaching. Preschool and younger, school-age children respond well to the use of dolls (see Figure 11-1).

Pouching vs. Other Containment Options

Since infants wear diapers, parents may view pouching as unnatural and may prefer to diaper the infant with a stoma. Whether or not this is an option depends upon the anatomical location of the stoma in the gastrointestinal or the urinary tract and on the stoma's bodily location. Regardless of whether there is an option to pouch or not pouch, the pros and cons of each management method should be discussed with the parents.

Urinary Stomas

When an infant has a pyelostomy, ureterostomy, or vesicostomy, diapering may be the most realistic option. These stomas are usually flush or retract over time, and are often in difficult anatomical locations. Successful pouching may be difficult and the effort and cost may not equal the return in pouch wear time.

One technique for managing a urinary stoma without a pouching system is to use a folded newborn diaper over the stoma, covering it with a larger diaper to hold it in place. Some families use sanitary pads as the absorptive layer. Staff nurses may teach the parents to use plain gauze in the mistaken belief that the area needs to be kept as sterile as possible. One way to allay parent fears when changing to a less "sterile" technique is to describe the stoma as the child's new urethral meatus. Although not strictly accurate in terms of protective mechanisms between the orifice and the kidneys, for lower diversions (i.e., vesicostomies and ureterostomies), this is a functional way of looking at this issue that can ease acceptance of more practical measures.

Pyelostomies can be difficult to manage in the described manner once the child is able to sit, because the stoma stretches up and out of the diaper area as the child bends forward. For this reason, it can be appropriate to use a pouch with the bottom tap cut off to direct the urine down into the diaper area. The use of a urostomy pouch may be problematic, since a pyelostomy is most often located on the back. This means the child will lie on the full pouch if the tap is left in place.

Most urinary ostomies in infants do not result in skin breakdown, although skin maceration can result if the diaper is not changed often. If the child is on antibiotic therapy, a fungal rash may occur. Parents should be instructed to examine the skin thoroughly for signs of fungal overgrowth, and to notify the health care provider should a reddened papular area occur. If a fungal rash occurs, it advisable to use an antifungal preparation covered with a protective barrier ointment.

Fecal Stomas

The risk for skin breakdown is higher with fecal stomas, and parents need to be taught techniques for skin protection. If the fecal stoma is not pouched, alternatives for collection should be explored. These include absorbent paper towels, cotton pads, liners, and cloth diapers cut or torn into foldable strips, which are used in conjunction with a diaper. However, the stoma mucosa should also be protected from irritation, since bleeding can result from the diaper rubbing on the stomal surface. Petrolatum gauze or petrolatum jelly applied to the absorptive material helps decrease this irritation.

Fecal stomas with high output or output that can cause peristomal skin breakdown (i.e., ileostomy) must be pouched if at all possible. The minimal acceptable goal for the child with a stoma is maintenance of the peristomal skin, and the use of a pouching system should facilitate this goal. Parents are reminded that the use of a pouching system should also control odor and may in some instances control costs.

Stomal Output

The WOC nurse must consider content and volume of the diet, the child's growth, and teething patterns when evaluating stomal output in an infant. There are many changes in the infant's diet within the first year, including a possible transition from breast milk to formula along with the addition of many new foods. These changes can significantly alter the color, volume, odor, and consistency of the stomal output.

Dietary advancements in the first year are generally managed by the pediatrician and are based on age criteria and disease state limitations. Mothers may also have preferences regarding the length of time they breastfeed. When new foods are added, it is important to evaluate how the child reacts to them, and most pediatricians recommend that only one new food be introduced at a time.

Infants suck on almost anything they can get near their mouths. They also use crying as a means of communication. These two factors lead to increased amounts of swallowed air, which can result in pouch ballooning and, potentially, premature dislodgment of the pouch seal. To manage this increased air, the WOC/ET nurse may recommend a pouching system with a filter or a two-piece system that can be "burped" when gas accumulates in the pouch. If no filter is available for a one-piece system, the WOC/ET nurse should show the family how to hold the tail of the open pouch up to release gas without soiling the tail of the pouch. Gas will normally be emptied at least twice as often as stool.

Stomal output is also influenced by the physical growth of the child. As body size and intake increase, so will the output. The pouching system used in the hospital that easily handled the output of the newborn may become too small for the 4-month-old infant. A change in pouch shape and size may improve pouch capacity.

The fecal output of a child with a stoma can be quite variable. Because many infant stomas are placed in the transverse colon, stomal output tends to be looser and greater in volume than the output of an infant with an intact gastrointestinal tract or that of a child with a sigmoid colostomy.

Children who had NEC (see earlier section) or other catastrophic, acute emergencies resulting in surgical diversion may have an ileostomy or a diversion higher in the gastrointestinal tract such as a jejunostomy or a duodenostomy. Some of these children have a functional short gut, because, although they may have additional bowel length distal to the diversion, it is not continuous and available for absorption. The output of many of these stomas is so liquid that a urinary pouch can be used, which makes emptying easier for both parent and child.

A rule of thumb to evaluate output is the formula of 1 ml/kg/hour (Boarini, 1989). A tolerable upper limit to output as feedings are being advanced is around 30ml/kg/day with an ileostomy. This can help the WOC/ET nurse to estimate what approximate output would be appropriate in an infant. When output is consistently high and enteral feeding is used, advances may need to be held temporarily. This is done in the face of significant skin breakdown or the inability to maintain a pouch seal for a reasonable period of time (generally at least 12 hours). The WOC/ET nurse needs to confer closely with medical and nursing staff in more complex situations.

It is also important to remember that a child can become dehydrated very quickly. The parents do usually not need to measure stool output, but they should have an idea of the frequency and volume of output that is normal for their baby. They can base this understanding upon the number of times they typically empty the pouch. They should also be familiar with normal urine color and weight of diapers, as well as the frequency of diaper changes.

Diarrhea can be a result of a change in diet, a medication side effect, or a flulike illness. If it is accompanied by vomiting, the infant, especially one with an ileostomy or higher stoma, can quickly get into a dangerous fluid and electrolyte imbalance.

Fluid requirements for children are determined by weight. The following are useful guidelines in calculating fluid intake for children (CHLA Pediatric Dosing Handbook and Formulary, 2001):

- If less than 10 kg of body weight: 100 ml/kg/day
- If 11-20 kg of body weight: 1000 ml plus 50 ml/kg for each kilogram over 10 kg
- If greater than 20 kg of body weight: 1500 ml plus 20 ml/kg for each kilogram over 20 kg

Parents should be educated about the signs and symptoms of dehydration and should observe for sunken eyes, lack of tears, dry lips, listlessness, and decreased urine output, as evidenced by fewer diaper changes. Parents need to know that water or juices do not replace depleted electrolytes. It is advisable to have an electrolyte solution in the home for prompt oral replacement. Infant electrolyte formulas are generally more appropriate than "sports drinks" for infants and children, especially those with small bowel stomas.

Teething also influences stomal output. As babies cut new teeth, they drool; the drool that drips can be swallowed and will produce "teething diarrhea." Children without stomas experience this, and it is often seen as diarrhea and reddened perianal skin. This liquid stool is more irritating to the skin and tends to quickly erode solid skin barriers.

This phenomenon is more familiar to mothers than to most pediatricians. The WOC/ET nurse needs to be alert to this, since the parent may report decreased wear time and skin barrier erosion. Understanding this phenomenon may mean that no specific change in equipment is necessary. If the decreased wear time is due to a teething episode, it will usually resolve when the tooth breaks the gums.

Pouching Systems

Frequent assessment of the effectiveness of the infant's or the child's pouching system should be routinely scheduled. Products used with an infant require adaptation during the first year because of growth and abdominal changes. For children with long-term ostomies, regular or at least annual contact with the WOC/ET nurse should be encouraged. Pouching systems need to accommodate physical development and the assumption of self-care (Figure 13-8).

It is often necessary for the WOC/ET nurse to promote transition of care from the parent to the child so the child achieves the normal tasks of development. If this is not done gradually and in small steps, the child may refuse to accept responsibility for self care when the parents decide they are

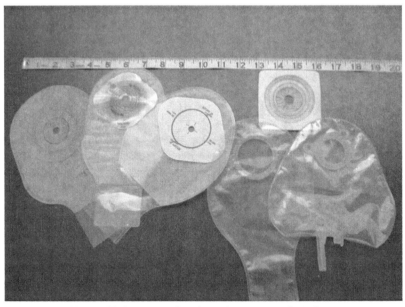

Figure 13-8   Examples of pouching systems for infants.

ready to abdicate total care. It is also easier for the child to learn things a little bit at a time rather than all at once.

Usually the pouching system needs to be flexible, since the abdomen on an infant tends to be rounded and soft. Flexibility of the pouching system is also helpful if the stoma is located near a crease or is low on the child's abdomen. Many pouching systems designed for infants have thin and less aggressive skin barriers. This improves the flexibility of the wafer, but it also means the barrier is less durable and may have to be changed after only a few days.

Parents often prefer a two-piece pouching system, for several practical reasons. With an energetic baby, it is easier to empty a fecal pouch by removing it from the barrier flange, setting it aside to empty later, and applying another pouch. This is more convenient than draining a pouch and wiping off the tail of the pouch while the baby is active.

Since infants produce a lot of gas, a two-piece pouching system can allow for easy gas release by 'burping" (i.e., releasing the pouch from the flange). Pouches with integrated or replaceable filters are an alternative to vent and deodorize gas. An add-on vent with a plastic self-cap may be easier to manage than burping a two-piece system. Eliminating the gas minimizes bulges under clothing and the risk of the pouch being dislodged prematurely.

Skin barrier paste is helpful as a caulk to fill in uneven surfaces. When working with small babies it is helpful to place the paste into a syringe for easier, more controlled dispensing (Figure 13-9). This also results in a smaller bead of paste. The plunger is removed, and the paste is squeezed into the syringe. The plunger is reinserted, and the paste is dispensed through the Luer-Lok end. No needle is used. The syringe cap should be saved and replaced after each use to prevent the skin barrier paste from drying.

Solid skin barriers can be cut and customized into small rings to protect the peristomal skin. Adhesive barrier rings or barrier strips can be cut into small pieces and formed for use in areas that require caulking.

An ostomy belt may be helpful to secure a pouching system on an active child. However, most

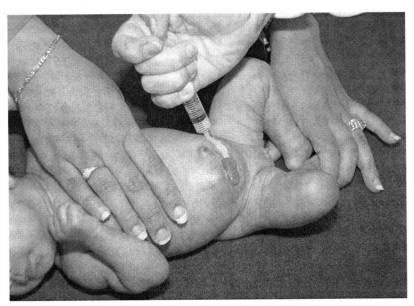

Figure 13-9   Paste in syringe. (Courtasy Hollister, Inc, Libertyville, IL.)

one-piece pediatric pouches do not contain belt tabs. Therefore if a belt is indicated, a two-piece system is usually required. Wide, elastic hernia support belts are available and can also be used to protect the stoma during active sports, or to keep the pouch out of reach of a child who keeps pulling it off.

Pouch covers are an additional accessory that can be purchased or even made by parents. The pouch cover helps to conceal the contents; in the infant, it is more for the comfort of the parents. Older children may be involved in selecting a pattern or color they like.

Fabriclike panels are integrated into some pediatric pouches at the interface of the pouch and the skin. This prevents the plastic from contacting the child's skin. If not part of the pouching system selected, fabric panels can be placed as a comfortable layer between the pouch and the skin. One simple trick is to cross-cut a hole in a washcloth or a piece of fabric and then slip the pouch through it so that the panel lies between the pouch and the skin. Another is to use a baby bib of terry cloth material, tied around the pouching system skin barrier and forming a cloth barrier between the child and the plastic pouch.

If the infant or toddler is still in a diaper, it is critical for the WOC/ET nurse to determine where the pouch is in relation to the diaper. If the stoma is high on the abdomen, the pouch is placed over the diaper. If the stoma is lower on the abdomen, the diaper may have to be rolled so the pouch can be placed on the outside.

Occasionally, because of the stoma location, the pouch may need to be placed inside the diaper. When this occurs, the pouching system seal may be compromised because of the frequent contact with urine. This can vary from boys to girls as boys tend to wet forward and girls wet more to the back of the diaper. When the pouch is inside the diaper, frequent diaper changes may help to ensure pouch wear time is reasonable. For boys, it also helps to use a bit of waterproof tape on the sides of the pouch adhesive that come in most contact with the urine—usually the medial and lower edges.

It is important to examine the skin for possible fungal overgrowth adhesive that may proliferate

under pouch film that is moist. Pouches that have clothlike backings may remain wet with urine and cause odor, skin maceration, and discomfort. Yeast overgrowth on the skin is also common following the use of antibiotics, such as those used to treat ear infections or during the early postoperative period.

Pouch Removal

To protect the peristomal skin during pouch removal, a soft cloth moistened with warm water is used to gently release the skin from the skin barrier. Adhesive removers should not be used on infants because of their potential for irritation. Adhesive and pectin can safely remain on the skin without interfering with the new skin barrier adhesion. Water is sufficient to cleanse peristomal skin in the infant; no use of soap or infant wipes is necessary (Rogers, 2003).

Pouch Emptying

It may be helpful, when emptying a newborn's pouch, to angle the pouch spout to the side rather than in a vertical orientation, since the infant is usually in a recumbent position (Figure 13-10). The angle can be adjusted toward the outer hip as the infant begins to crawl, to ensure that the weight of the effluent does not prematurely loosen the seal.

In older or more active children it is helpful to angle the pouch toward the hip until they are able to sit on the toilet or potty-chair. When they are at this point, the pouch should be angled down and inward so that the children can participate in emptying as appropriate for their age and abilities.

When an infant is still in diapers it may be easier to empty the ostomy pouch into the diaper, especially if the parents are using disposable diapers. With a fecal stoma, the parents can empty the pouch whenever they are changing their child's wet diaper. They can unfasten the diaper and insert the tail or spout of the pouch into the diaper. The diaper can then be wrapped up and disposed.

The diaper can serve as a "squeegee" to clean off the outside tail of the pouch. Baby wipes can also be useful for wiping off the tail of the ostomy pouch and are readily available to most new parents. However, these wipes are generally not recommended for cleaning the peristomal skin, since they

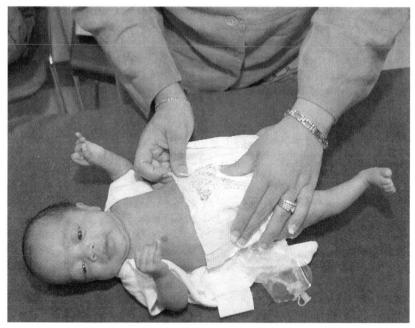

Figure 13-10   Pouch to side. (Courtesy Hollister, Inc, Libertyville, IL.)

may have ingredients that will affect the barrier seal to the skin.

Because children have a lot of gas it is important to remind parents that gas takes up space, and if the pouch is overfilled the gas can cause the pouch seal to break prematurely. It is a good practice for parents to empty the pouch of gas before naps and the child's bedtime. They should check the pouch again before they retire, in the event that more gas has accumulated.

If possible, routine pouch changes should be planned for a time of day when the infant is quiet or usually happy and satisfied. If this is not possible, pouch changes should be planned for when some assistance is available. This is especially helpful early on, when parents have doubts about their ability to handle not only a new baby but also the ostomy.

Packing extra supplies is an important survival skill. Extra supplies should include a change of clothes and everything necessary for a complete pouch change. Extra supplies can be stored in the baby's diaper bag, at a grandparent's house, and at the day care provider's. In the case of a school-age child, the school nurse or an office assistant may be entrusted with the extra supplies.

It is important to share responsibility for the child's care. Often it is the mother who learns the care, and although she may choose to do it, others do need to understand the procedures for emptying and changing. The WOC/ET nurse can encourage this by enlisting members of the family and teaching all who will be learning the care.

If the infant or child will be going to day care, the parents must discuss stoma care responsibilities with the day care providers. Although the parent may work nearby and therefore may want to be called if the pouch needs to be changed, the day care provider still needs to learn how to empty the pouch and what to do if there is a leak in the pouching system. Planning ahead is critical, and this discussion must take place before the child's first time at day care. Finding day care willing to take a child with an ostomy may take some time; therefore parents should start looking as soon as they are themselves comfortable with the child's care. It is also helpful if prospective caretakers can be offered a teaching session with a WOC nurse, to be sure that all their questions are addressed and that they feel comfortable with the added responsibilities. Concern for liability and the child's safety while in their care is a major issue for all good day care providers.

Keeping the infant or child occupied and quiet during the pouch change procedure is beneficial for the parents. Toys are helpful distractions. Other siblings can be of assistance, because they can keep the child distracted while the pouch is being changed. The older child with an ostomy can help with the procedure by holding a pouch clamp or the tape before it is applied. Children should participate as much as their age or abilities allow.

Toddlers may do well dressed in overalls, depending on where the stoma is located. It is important to have access to the pouch for easy emptying, especially if the child is involved in helping.

Potential Complications

For the pediatric patient with an ostomy, the following complications are common: dehydration, prolapse, hernia, skin irritation, and stoma color alterations.

Dehydration can happen quickly in an infant and can be life-threatening if not recognized early. Parents should learn to recognize signs and symptoms of dehydration and to be attentive to the "normal" consistency and volume of output that their child produces. Dehydration is a potential risk for any child but is more likely to happen in the infant with an ileostomy or high stoma. The parents should keep oral electrolyte solutions at home and be aware that water, juice, and sodas are not adequate electrolyte substitutes. In addition to the stomal output, the child may be losing fluids from other routes (e.g., vomiting, perspiration, teething-related drooling).

If the parents are concerned, they should contact their physician immediately or bring the infant to the emergency department for fluid replacement. If the child has an ileostomy or higher gastrointestinal stoma, the parents should mention that they were taught the importance of the need to check

electrolytes. This is especially important if the emergency department or urgent care center is not aware of the increased risk of dehydration in a child with flulike symptoms who has a stoma, compared to a child with similar symptoms but without a stoma.

Stomal prolapse and *peristomal hernia* are relatively common complications seen in infants. There are several reasons why children seem to experience these complications. First, they do not have well-developed abdominal muscles to support the stoma. Secondly, with crying there is an increase in the intraabdominal pressure that can force the bowel through the fascial opening to create a prolapse, or stretch the fascial opening to create a peristomal hernia. As in adults, it appears that the distal stoma is more likely to prolapse. With divided stomas set in an incision, a peristomal hernia may form along the entire area.

When a child has had an obstructive condition such as HD (see earlier sections of chapter), prolapse can also occur. As the bowel decompresses and the stoma shrinks in size, it may not be proportionate to the fascial opening that was created.

It is important to forewarn parents about this possibility because a prolapsed stoma can be very distressing. If the stoma color is red or pink, this condition is not an emergency. However, immediate intervention may be needed if the stoma changes color, indicating that the blood supply is compromised, and remains edematous so that it cannot self-reduce. In children, surgical intervention is not usually required. Therefore, if the stoma continues to prolapse, the WOC nurse may need to teach the parents to reduce the prolapsed bowel by placing the child on his or her back and exerting even pressure over the stoma while pushing it gently into the abdomen. A hernia belt with a prolapse addition can be considered to provide mild support. This belt comes in pediatric sizes and tends to stay in place better than other types of support products, such as an elastic wrap.

The peristomal protrusion that occurs with a hernia can be alarming to parents. This is seldom an emergency unless there is entrapped bowel, which would be signaled by a change in output, abdominal distention, and onset of acute abdominal pain. The biggest issue for children with hernias is pouching problems: at pouch change the child may be upset and cry, which increases the protrusion of the hernia. Once the pouching system is in place and the child relaxes, the hernia should self-reduce, which shifts the peristomal plane. This shift can disturb the pouching system seal. Increasing the flexibility of the pouching system seal and in some cases providing a firmer, two-piece pouching system can be a way to solve this problem.

Skin irritation is usually caused by the contact of stool with the peristomal skin. When the skin is eroded, it is painful. This can cause great distress for the parents, whose child becomes fussier and cries as a result of the discomfort. It is important to determine the cause of the skin irritation and to institute measures to correct the cause. Common causes of peristomal skin irritation include improper fit of the pouching system, erosion of the skin barrier (due to prolonged wear or high output), or skin reaction to various products or inappropriate removal. Once the cause is corrected, parents should be taught to dust the involved area with a skin barrier powder before pouch application. The powder can absorb excessive moisture and protect the peristomal skin. When applying powder to an infant's skin, care must be taken to prevent aspiration of aerosolized powder. Rogers (2003) suggests enlarging the end of the powder bottle to allow the powder to be easily sprinkled onto the skin, preventing a "puff" of powder. She further suggests applying the powder onto a gloved finger and gently rubbing the powder over the involved area.

As mentioned earlier, infants use crying as a normal form of communication at this stage of their development. When they cry, the parent may notice *a change in the stoma color*. Instead of being bright red or pink, it may briefly appear pale, gray, or even white. This can cause alarm for the parents, who have been taught that a healthy stoma is red. This change in color seems to be related to a shunting of the blood away from the bowel, and is transient and benign.

Teaching and Discharge Planning

The WOC/ET nurse has a significant role in the education of the parents. Parents are usually eager to learn the necessary procedures and to know what is best for their child. It is essential to keep in mind that this teaching is being done at a time when the family is very stressed.

It is important to schedule many opportunities for the parents to participate in their child's care when they are under the supervision of the WOC/ET nurse. Children can recover quickly and discharge may occur suddenly. Therefore the WOC/ET nurse should take advantage of every chance for a teaching experience. The staff should be encouraged to continue to work with the parents when the WOC/ET nurse is not available, to help reinforce teaching and prepare the ground for further demonstrations when the WOC/ET nurse returns.

In the initial period the parents' anxiety might be increased by the fact that the child often cries during the pouch change procedure. They should be reminded that most infants fuss over routine child care activities such as ear cleaning, bathing, and nail trimming. Children often become even more annoyed if restrained, so parents should be helped to review ideas for keeping the infant or child occupied during the pouch change procedure.

Bathing is invariably a topic for discussion before discharge. The infant or child would probably not have a tub bath in the hospital, so the parents will have questions. Children can be bathed with the pouching system on or off. It is important to help parents think through what to expect if the pouch is off and the stoma functions. If they do choose to take the pouch off during the bath, remind them that they should not use any baby oil or lotion on the skin that may interfere with good barrier adherence.

If the child has an ureterostomy or a pyelostomy, it is advisable to discuss bathing with the nephrologist. With adequate oral intake the flow of urine is usually sufficient to prevent any risk of infection. If there is concern, the parents may need to make sure the water level is below the ureterostomy when their child is in the tub.

With a toddler or a young child, play therapy can provide a very important medium for teaching skills and basic concepts of care. Most children's hospitals have a child life department. These professionals are adept and creative and base their approach upon the developmental level of the child. One creative tool they use is the Ostomy Shadow Buddy (see Figure 11-1). These special dolls are for children who have had or will have ostomy surgery. They can be used to explain what a stoma is and how it is managed. Developed by a mother (Mary Postlethwait) who had a child with special needs, dolls with a stoma can be used both to teach the person with a stoma and as a tool for the child with a stoma to explain to others how he or she is different. The Shadow Buddies are available in various styles: boy or girl, in various skin tones, and with different hair colors. Fabric or soft body dolls can also be used to fashion a "look-alike" comfort and teaching toy. For some children a stuffed animal with a stoma can serve the same purpose.

Parents may find support from other parents who have had similar experiences with their children. The WOC/ET nurse can facilitate contact with other parents as appropriate. The United Ostomy Association (UOA) began an effort to form a parent support network in 1989. Support for Parents and Ostomy Children, or SPOC, was formally recognized as a chapter of the UOA in 1990 (Davies, 1992). Its goal is peer support and education. Some local chapters have created opportunities for sharing tools they have developed, such as videos to facilitate support for families (Fort Worth, Texas, UOA Chapter Video, 2002).

For the older child the UOA sponsors the annual Youth Rally. This is usually a great learning experience for children who have ostomies or are incontinent. The Youth Rally annual summer camp is for children who are 11 to 19 years old. It is a chance for them to associate with other kids who have similar concerns, to learn from the counselors and each other, and to have fun.

Once the child is discharged from the hospital, follow-up care should be initiated. In addition to the WOC/ET nurse, there are usually many specialists the parents have seen during their child's hospitalization. It is helpful to clarify who is responsible for which specific aspects of the child's care so that if a question arises, the parents know whom to contact. Phone numbers and follow-up appointments should be given as part of the written discharge instructions.

The Role of the WOC/ET Nurse after Stoma Closure

Many of the conditions that necessitate a stoma in the pediatric patient require only a temporary stoma. The WOC/ET nurse has much to teach after takedown of the stoma, focusing on skin protection for the perineal area and, later on, bowel management or intermittent catheterization for some of the children.

Following the pull-through procedure and takedown of the colostomy, the child with imperforate anus or HD often experiences frequent, small stools. Because the child does not yet have voluntary control, there is usually some perianal skin erosion. This can be distressing for the parents, who often see the takedown of the colostomy as the end of their journey. Because of the discomfort their child experiences from the eroded perianal skin, some parents may feel that the colostomy was easier to manage.

The WOC/ET nurse can provide support to parents, who may at this point be very discouraged. In addition, knowledge of the products for skin protection and care can be invaluable to the parents. Working closely with the physician and the dietician, the WOC/ET nurse can suggest foods that may thicken the stool. This may help decrease the frequency of the bowel movements as bulk is added. However, care must be taken not to constipate the child, particularly since children with imperforate anus and HD have an increased tendency towards constipation. There is also a degree of discomfort associated with passing stools through relatively tight anal scar tissue, or with the increased anal resistance and unaccustomed sensations associated with the HD repairs.

Cleaning the child's skin after each stool is important to prevent further erosion from the stool. However, this is difficult, since the child may object and cry because of discomfort. Sometimes baths can be soothing, and using a squirt bottle to cleanse the stool instead of a washcloth or baby wipe can be less traumatic. Sitz baths used every 4 to 6 hours with a period of air-drying afterwards can be helpful. Topical creams and barriers can be applied to promote healing and provide skin protection.

Because initially stools can be frequent, a diaper liner can be helpful and cost-effective. Although this is usually a temporary problem, sometimes children with imperforate anus repair will never achieve voluntary bowel control. This may take some time to discover, since the child of this age is not yet expected to be potty trained. Later, if voluntary control is not possible because of the complexity of the congenital anomaly, the WOC nurse may work with parents who are now faced with learning bowel programs or again considering a permanent fecal diversion.

CONCLUSION

There are many conditions that may require fecal or urinary diversion in the pediatric patient. These diversions may be permanent or temporary, but all require knowledge of the disease process, the surgical procedure, and the intended outcome. The challenges of participating in the care of a child with a fecal or a urinary diversion include working with the family, identifying the developmental age of the child and tailoring interventions to meet those challenges specific to it, understanding pouching principles that pertain to the pediatric population, and providing a nurturing, supportive environment to the child and family.

SELF-ASSESSMENT EXERCISES

Questions

1. In HD there is an absence of:
   a. Myenteric parasympathetic, intramural ganglion cells.
   b. Mucosal cells that lubricate the passage of stool.
   c. Muscle bands responsible for peristalsis.
   d. An anal opening.

2. What is the most commonly affected area in HD?
   a. The terminal ileum
   b. The transverse colon
   c. The rectosigmoid area
   d. Only the anal canal

3. There is a familial tendency for HD.
   True _____ False _____

4. What is the gold standard for diagnosis of HD?

5. What is the objective of surgical management of HD?

6. Discuss the options for surgical management of HD.

7. Which of the following descriptions best describes imperforate anus?
   a. Anal area completely missing; no opening present on visual examination; on radiographic examination no sigmoid colon is present; thought to be related to maternal drug abuse
   b. Congenital anomaly in which the anus is absent or displaced from its normal anatomic location
   c. Large anal opening devoid of sphincters
   d. Condition most often found in infants with cerebral palsy

8. Imperforate anus may be differentiated as high or low. Which condition (high or low) requires a more complex surgical intervention? Describe why.

9. Persistent cloaca is a condition of females that includes an imperforate anus but also:
   a. Inability to heal the anal area.
   b. A common channel genitourinary system with a single perineal opening and a rectal fistula attached to the posterior wall of the common channel.
   c. An enlarged anal opening without the presence of sphincters.
   d. The lack of anatomic landmarks in the perineal area.

10. Describe the pathophysiology of NEC.

11. Name the three factors that are implicated in the onset of NEC.

12. List at least two options in the medical management of NEC.

13. What is the main principle of surgical treatment of NEC?

14. At the first postoperative assessment of a neonate with NEC, the WOC nurse notes three stomas. Why is this not unusual in a patient treated for NEC?

15. Malrotation is any abnormality in the rotation of the midgut and the fixation of mesentery that occurs during fetal development.
    True _____ False _____

16. Which of the following best describes intussusception?
    a. The invagination of a portion of the intestine into the lumen of an adjoining part
    b. The telescoping of the rectum through the anus
    c. The lack of ganglion cells in the transverse colon, causing folding of the colon
    d. A total bowel obstruction

17. What is meconium ileus?

18. Meconium ileus is the earliest sign of what disease?

19. What are two treatments for the patient with uncomplicated meconium ileus?

20. Which of the following exstrophy conditions is the most common?
    a. Cloacal exstrophy
    b. Bladder exstrophy
    c. Epispadias

21. Children treated for cloacal exstrophy are left with permanent intestinal stomas.
    True _____ False _____

22. Which of the following best describes bladder exstrophy?
    a. The bladder exists in a contained membrane sac.
    b. The bladder and urethra are open and exposed on the lower abdomen.
    c. The urethra exists parallel to the bladder neck.
    d. The bladder capacity is reduced to less than 75 ml.

23. Describe one clinical manifestation of a patient with posterior urethral valves.

24. Prune belly syndrome is best described as:
    a. A small abdominal cavity with externally located small and large intestine, which area is covered with wrinkly membranes
    b. A wrinkly appearance of the abdominal skin caused by the absence, deficiency, or hypoplasia of the abdominal musculature and urinary tract anomalies
    c. An inverted bladder wall located in the inguinal area
    d. Abdominal skin that is excessive in the area of the pubis, causing malformation of the urinary tract

25. Which of the following statements is true of children born with spina bifida?
    a. The infant is born with an everted bladder and fusion of the mucosa to the skin.
    b. The infant often requires gender reassignment.
    c. The infant will have some issues of bowel and bladder management.
    d. As the child ages the spina bifida abnormalities disappear.

26. UPJ obstruction impairs the urinary flow:
    a. At the level of the connection between the ureter and renal pelvis.
    b. At the level of the connection of ureter and the bladder.
    c. Between the mid- and lower ureter.
    d. Because of malformation of the ureter and the renal pelvis junction.

27. Which of the following diseases is the most common congenital abnormality of the ureter?
    a. UPJ obstruction
    b. Posterior urethral valves
    c. Megaureter
    d. Vesicoureteral reflux

28. For most children with a stoma, reintegration into their normal lives and daily activities is the goal.
    True _____ False _____

29. Discuss two considerations for the pediatric stoma patient related to physical growth issues.

30. The neonate is at a greater risk for toxic reactions when using pouching products because of:
    a. Greater absorption of topically applied substances.
    b. The numerous products used to keep the pouch seal secure.
    c. The high number of sebaceous glands that can absorb substances.
    d. The need to use high end adhesive products that are intended for adults.
31. Toddlers can be helped to participate in ostomy care by being allowed to:
    a. Use scissors to cut the skin barrier.
    b. Gather supplies, holding tape rolls.
    c. Measure the stoma.
    d. Only watch the change procedure, since they will not have skills to do much more.
32. Which type of ostomy may make diapering the most realistic option for an infant?
    a. A high-output ileostomy
    b. A pyelostomy, a ureterostomy, or a vesicostomy
    c. A left-sided, low-output colostomy
    d. All stomas should be pouched.
33. Name two techniques that can be used to manage gas in a child with a fecal stoma.
34. Discuss why parents may prefer to use a two-piece pouching system with an infant.
35. If an infant is in a disposable diaper, it may be easier to empty the ostomy pouch into the diaper.
    True _____   False _____
36. Discuss how a doll with a stoma can be used in the care of a child with a fecal or urinary diversion.

Answers

1. a
2. c
3. True
4. Rectal biopsy
5. To remove or bypass the aganglionic segment of bowel
6. (a) Pull-through procedure, whereby the ganglionic segment of bowel is pulled through the aganglionic segment, or (b) the segment of bowel with normal ganglion cells is brought behind the aganglionic rectal segment, or (c) a procedure where the mucosa and submucosa of the aganglionic rectosigmoid area is removed, the ganglionic bowel is brought down through the rectal sleeve, and allowed to heal everted on the perineum
7. b
8. Low imperforate anus usually involves an anal opening covered by a thin membrane that can be perforated to allow for normal bowel movements. Most cases of higher anomalies involve surgery at the time of diagnosis, with fecal diversion. A three-stage procedure is planned: (a) initial diversion; (b) any fistulas are closed, an anoplasty is performed, and a pull-through procedure is done; (c) the fecal diversion is closed.
9. b
10. NEC is necrosis of the variable lengths of the small or large intestine.
11. Three factors that are implicated in the onset of NEC are feeding, mucosal injury, and bacterial invasion.
12. Medical management of NEC can include bowel rest, nasogastric decompression, intravenous alimentation, transfusions, and antibiotic therapy.
13. Surgery involves resection or diversion above necrotic or questionable bowel segments.
14. NEC can skip areas, demonstrating intact, nondiseased intestine between diseased segments. Since NEC is one of the leading causes of short bowel syndrome in neonates, it may be prudent for the surgeon to resect and exteriorize the intestinal segments to preserve intestinal length. Thus the neonate with NEC may have a proximal stoma and several nonfunctioning stomas.
15. True
16. a
17. Meconium ileus is the obstruction of the ileum with thick, sticky meconium that forms hard pellets in the narrowed distal bowel lumen.

18. Cystic fibrosis

19. One treatment is contrast enema, in which the media may cause sufficient emulsification of the thick meconium to relieve the obstruction as the enema is refluxed into the terminal ileum and distal small bowel under fluoroscopy. A second treatment involves acetylcysteine (Mucomyst), a wetting agent. It can be instilled into the bowel via enterotomy proximal to the obstruction, and the sticky meconium and pellets can then be milked down into the colon and the enterotomy closed.

20. b
21. True
22. b
23. Clinical manifestations in infants include abdominal mass and infection within the first year, sepsis, metabolic acidosis, and azotemia. In children over 1 year of age, a UTI is a common symptom. Other manifestations may include nocturnal or diurnal enuresis, frequency, dribbling, hematuria, and acute urinary retention.

24. b
25. c
26. a
27. a
28. True
29. Considerations: within the first year most infants triple their birth weight, thus the pouching system must be reevaluated; as infants age they can stretch out their periods of sleep and begin to sleep through the night, placing new demands on their ostomy pouching system capacity; if diapers have been used to contain the effluent, the longer sleep patterns means less frequent diaper changes; the peristomal skin can demonstrate signs of skin breakdown

30. a
31. b
32. b
33. Two ways to manage gas are use of a pouching system with filter or use of a two-piece system that can be "burped" and an add-on vent.

34. It may be easier to empty a fecal pouch by removing it from the barrier flange, setting it aside to empty later, and applying another pouch. This is more convenient than draining a pouch and wiping off the tail of the pouch while the baby is active.

35. True
36. Dolls can be used to explain what a stoma is and how it is managed. They can be used for teaching the child, or the child can use them to explain to others how they are different.

REFERENCES

Albanese CT, Rowe MI: Necrotizing enterocolitis. In O'Neill JA et al, editors: *Pediatric surgery*, ed 5, St Louis, 1998, Mosby.

Atala A, Walker RD: Vesicoureteral reflux. In Graham SD, editor: *Glenn's urologic surgery*, ed 5, Philadelphia, 1998, Lippincott-Raven.

Boarini J: Principles of stoma care for infants, *J ET Nurs* 16(1):21-25, 1989.

Brock JW, O'Neill JA: Bladder exstrophy. In O'Neill JA et al, editors: *Pediatric surgery*, ed 5, St Louis, 1998, Mosby.

Bryant RA, Buls JG: Pathophysiology and diagnostic studies of gastrointestinal tract disorders. In Hampton BG, Bryant RA, editors: *Ostomies and continent diversions: nursing management*, St Louis, 1992, Mosby.

Casales AJ: Posterior urethral valves and other obstructions of the urethra. In Gonzales ET, Bauer SB, editors: *Pediatric urology practice*, Philadelphia, 1999, Lippincott, Williams & Wilkins.

Caty MG, Azizkhan RG: Necrotizing enterocolitis. In Ashcraft KW, editor: *Pediatric surgery*, ed 3, Philadelphia, 2000, WB Saunders.

CHLA pediatric dosing handbook and formulary, ed 14, Hudson Oh, 2001, Lexi-comp.

Clark LA, Oldham KT: Malrotation. In Ashcraft KW, editor: *Pediatric surgery*, ed 3, Philadelphia, 2000, WB Saunders.

Cooney DR: Defects of the abdominal wall. In O'Neill JA et al, editors: *Pediatric surgery*, ed 5, St Louis, 1998, Mosby.

Davies A: Children with ostomies: parent helping parents, *J ET Nurs* 19(6):207-212, 1992.

Edmond JC, Whitington PF: Selective surgical management of progressive familial intrahepatic cholestasis (Byler's disease), *J Pediatr Surg* 30(12):1635-1641, 1995.

Ewalt DH: Renal infection, abscess, vesicoureteral reflux, urinary lithiasis, and renal vein thrombosis. In O'Neill JA et al, editors: *Pediatric surgery*, ed 5, St Louis, 1998, Mosby.

Fort Worth, Texas UOA Chapter video: Social interaction for young people with ostomy and related surgeries, 2002.

Groff DB: Meconium disease. In Ashcraft KW, editor: *Pediatric surgery*, ed 3, Philadelphia, 2000, WB Saunders.

Hendren WH et al: Megaureter and prune-belly syndrome. In O'Neill JA et al, editors: *Pediatric surgery*, ed 5, St Louis, 1998, Mosby.

Holschneider A, Ure BM: Hirschsprung's disease. In Ashcraft KW, editor: *Pediatric surgery*, Philadelphia, 2000, WB Saunders.

Keating MA, Rich MA: Prune-belly syndrome. In Ashcraft KW, editor: *Pediatric surgery*, ed 3, Philadelphia, 2000, WB Saunders.

Kiely EM, Pena A: Anorectal malformations. In O'Neill JA et al, editors: *Pediatric surgery*, ed 5, St Louis, 1998, Mosby.

Kramer SA: Exstrophy and epispadias. In Graham SD, editor: *Glenn's urologic surgery*, ed 5, Philadelphia, 1998, Lippincott-Raven.

Mouriquand P: Congenital anomalies of the pyeloureteral junction and the ureter. In O'Neill JA et al, editors: *Pediatric surgery*, ed 5, St Louis, 1998, Mosby.

Murphy JP: Exstrophy of the bladder. In Ashcraft KW, editor: *Pediatric surgery*, ed 3, Philadelphia, 2000, WB Saunders.

Ng VL et al: Long-term outcomes after partial external biliary diversion for intractable pruritis in patients with intrahepatic cholestasis, *J Pediatr Gastroenterol Nutr* 30:152-156, 2000.

Ohi R, Nio M: The jaundiced infant: biliary atresia and other obstructions. In O'Neill JA et al, editors: *Pediatric surgery*, ed 5, St. Louis, 1998, Mosby.

O'Neill JA: Cloacal exstrophy. In O'Neill JA et al, editors: *Pediatric surgery*, ed 5, St Louis, 1998, Mosby.

Pope JC, Rink RC: Surgical options in the management of the neurogenic bladder. In Gonzales ET, Bauer SB, editors: *Pediatric urology practice*, Philadelphia, 1999, Lippincott Williams & Wilkins.

Retik AB: Posterior urethral valves. In Graham SD, editor: *Glenn's urologic surgery*, ed 5, Philadelphia, 1998, Lippincott-Raven.

Rogers VE: Managing preemie stomas: more than just the pouch, *JWOCN* 30:100-110, 2003.

Sheldon CA et al: Urinary tract infection and vesicoureteral reflux. In Ashcraft KW, editor: *Pediatric surgery*, ed 3, Philadelphia, 2000, WB Saunders.

Teitlbaum et al: Hirschsprung's disease and related neuromuscular disorders of the intestine. In O'Neill JA et al, editors: *Pediatric surgery*, ed 5, St Louis, 1998, Mosby.

Warner BW, Ziegler MM: Exstrophy of the cloaca. In Ashcraft KW, editor: *Pediatric surgery*, ed 3, Philadelphia, 2000, WB Saunders.

Wong DL, Hockenberry-Eaton M: The child with neuromuscular or muscular dysfunction. In Wong DL et al, editors: *Wong's essentials of pediatric nursing*, ed 6, St Louis, 2001, Mosby.

Young DG: Intussusception. In O'Neill JA et al, editors: *Pediatric surgery*, ed 5, St Louis, 1998, Mosby.

RESOURCES

Katy Hirsch: *Making friends*. A book to be used for 5-10 year old children who are recovering from ostomy surgery. 5987 E. 71st Street, Suite 101, Indianapolis, Indiana, 46220, http://hirschinc.com, Hirsch & Associates.

Mary Postlethwait and Kathleen Patton: *Shadow buddies: know your buddy book*. A resource guide to educate children about disabilities, illnesses, and medical challenges. The buddies covered include orthopedic, diabetic, oncology, respiratory, burn, heart, cerebral palsy/pump, dialysis, Down syndrome, HIV/AIDS, liver transplant, lung transplant, ostomy, seizure, and vision, 401 Clairborne Rd., Suite 103A, Olathe, KS 66062, www.shadowbuddies.com, 2000, Shadow Buddies Foundation.

Suzanne LeVert: *When your child has a chronic illness* New York 1995, Dell.

Michael Bérubé: Life as we know it, a father, a family, and an exceptional child, 1996, Random House.

Thomas H. Powell and Peggy Ahrenhold Gallager: *Brothers & sisters—a special part of exceptional families*, 1985, Paul Brodes.

Sandy Tovray and Maria Wilson-Portunondo: *Helping your special needs child: a practical and reassuring resource guide*, Rocklin, Calif, 1995, Prima.

Christine Williams, MD and John J. Connolly EdD, editors: The parent's helper: who to call on health and family issues, 1996, Fairview Press.

Paul E. Hyman, editor, Carlo Di Lorenzo, associate editor: *Gastrointestinal motility disorders*.

The Assoc. for Bladder Exstrophy Children: *Living with bladder exstrophy* www.bladderexstrophy.com

Mark L. Batshaw, MD: *Your child has a disability, a complete sourcebook of daily and medical care*, 2002, Paul H Brookes Publishing.

T. Berry Brazelton, MD: *Going to the doctor*. Reading, Mass, 1996, Addison-Wesley.

Robert E. Cole and David Reiss, editors: *How do families cope with chronic illness?* 1982, Laurene Erbaum Associates.

Pat Baird, MA, RD: *Be good to your gut, recipes and tips for people with digestive problems*, 1996, Blackwell Scientific.

American Pseudo-Obstruction & Hirschsprung's Disease Society, Inc, P.O. Box 772, Medford, Mass, 617-395-4255.

TEF/VATER support network, 15301 Grey Fox Road, Upper Mariboro, Md 20772, 301-627-2131.

Pull-thru Network, Bonnie McElroy, 316 Thomas Street, Bessemer, Ala 35020, 205-428-5953.

United Ostomy Association, Coloring book in Spanish: Ale has an ostomy; Coloring book in English: Chris has an ostomy.

Stomal and Peristomal Complications

JANICE C. COLWELL

OBJECTIVES

1. Describe the presentation, incidence, etiology, diagnostic assessment workup/assessment and management of the following *stomal* complications: hernia, prolapse, necrosis, mucocutaneous separation, retraction, stenosis, fistula, and trauma.
2. Describe the presentation, incidence, etiology, assessment, diagnostic workup/assessment and management of the following *peristomal* complications: peristomal varices, peristomal candidiasis, folliculitis, mucosal transplantation, pseudoverrucous lesions, peristomal pyoderma gangrenosum, suture granulomas, peristomal irritant contact dermatitis, peristomal allergic contact dermatitis, and peristomal trauma.
3. Discuss the presentation of the following uncommon stomal and peristomal conditions: malignancy, herpes, pemphigus, and psoriasis.

INTRODUCTION

The incidence of stoma-related complications is difficult to determine. A review of the literature finds incidence reported as varying from 6% to 66.8% (Shellito, 1998; Makela, Turku, and Laitinen, 1997; Pearl et al, 1985; Park et al, 1999; Cheung, 1995; Leenen, 1989; DelPino et al, 1997; Arumugam et al, 2003; Ratliff and Donovan, 2001) depending on the type of stoma, the time frame of the complication (early postoperative to late postoperative), the type and definition of the complication, and the type of diversion (fecal versus urinary, end versus loop). It appears that a large percentage

of persons who undergo ostomy surgery will experience some type of complication while they live with a stoma.

Several studies have looked at risk factors associated with stomal and peristomal complications (Duchesne et al, 2002; Arumugam et al, 2003), and although findings vary, obesity, inflammatory bowel disease, and stomas created in an emergency setting have all been implicated.

STOMAL COMPLICATIONS
Hernia

A parastomal hernia occurs as a defect in the fascia that allows loops of intestine to protrude into the area of weakness. During stoma creation an opening is made into the fascia to allow the intestine to be advanced. In some patients this defect can enlarge, allowing the intestine to bulge into the area.

Presentation

The hernia is visualized when abdominal pressure is increased with the patient in a sitting or standing position (Color Plate 6). An unsightly bulge appears (size is variable depending upon the size of the defect) in one area around the stoma. The patient may encounter difficulty maintaining the seal of the ostomy pouching system, because the abdominal skin of the area alternates between stretching and relaxing, thus shifting the pouch seal. The difficulty in maintaining the pouching system seal can cause leakage and irritated peristomal skin. The patient may report insecurity related to the variability of the pouch seal, as well as psychologic stress resulting from the unsightly bulge that may be quite noticeable under clothing.

Some patients note occasional pain or discomfort in the area of the hernia, probably related to the stretching of the hernia ring at the level of the abdominal wall. In extreme cases the patient reports intense pain at the site of the parastomal hernia that is due to obstruction or ischemia of an intestinal loop.

Incidence

The reports of the incidence of parastomal hernias are difficult to compare, because some describe patients with asymptomatic hernias and others relate percentages of patients requiring surgical interventions. The reported rates of hernia formation (nonsurgical as well as surgical candidates) ranges from 6.5% for persons with urostomies (Franks and Hrebinko, 2001), and 16% to as high as 62.5% in patients with fecal diversions. (Shellito, 1998; Makela, Turku, and Laitinen, 1997; Williams et al, 1990; Cheung, 1995; Pearl, 1989; Rubin, Schoetz, and Matthews 1984).) Pearl notes that "the cumulative risk of a hernia developing seems to increase with time, although most occur within the first 2 years after stoma formation."

Etiology

Although there is no clear identified etiology of parastomal hernias, siting of the stoma to outside of the rectus muscle has been strongly implicated (Londono; Pearl; Corman, 1993). Others cite poor surgical technique (Cheung, 1995; Gordon, Rolstad, and Bubrick, 1998), a large fascial opening (Edward, 2001; Corman, 1993; Gordon, Rolstad, and Bubrick, 1998), the placement of the stoma through the incision (Pearl, 1989), or even weak abdominal musculature (Cheung, 1995; Shellito, 1998; Londono-Schimmer, Loeng, and Phillips, 1994).

Diagnostic Workup/Assessment

On visual examination, with the patient in a sitting or standing position an asymmetric bulge is present in one area, beginning next to the stoma and reaching out a variable distance. In an infrequent presentation the bulge is noted in the entire parastomal area. A digital examination of the stoma allows the fascial defect to be felt when the patient coughs or bears down to increase the abdominal pressure. An incomplete ring is felt in the area of the herniation. To confirm the presence of a hernia, an upper gastrointestinal x-ray film with a small bowel or a retrograde contrast study, both through the stoma, can be obtained to visualize bowel loops around the stoma and above the abdominal wall; alternatively a computed tomography (CT) scan with oral contrast can be requested to diagnose the fascial defect.

Management

If the patient is asymptomatic (i.e., maintains a consistent ostomy pouching system seal, has minimal or no discomfort, and can conceal the bulge under clothing), no surgical intervention is recommended. Several nonsurgical management techniques can be considered, depending upon the size and location of the hernia. Hernia support belts, binders constructed of elastic material with an opening for the pouch, can be worn over the hernia and are manufactured by NuHope Laboratories (Pacoima, CA). These belts are thought to provide support to the parastomal hernia, decreasing the protrusion and stabilizing the parastomal plane and thus assisting in maintaining the pouching system seal. The belts are custom-fit according to the size and location of the hernia and the type of ostomy pouching system used. The belt must be placed around the abdomen, and the pouch brought through the opening in a flat position, while the hernia is reduced. The success of a hernia belt is variable; it might be considered for a patient who is not a surgical candidate. A flexible pouching system is recommended; options include a one-piece appliance with a flexible skin barrier or a two-piece system with a floating flange. The stoma size should be evaluated with the patient in both the sitting and flat positions, since the stoma can enlarge when the patient is in the upright position and the hernia protrudes. Colostomy patients who use irrigation as a management system should be advised to suspend irrigation if difficulty is encountered when introducing water, or if they begin to note prolonged or incomplete evacuations following irrigation. Because the intestine can tunnel into the hernia, the irrigant or cone tip of the irrigation kit may not be easily introduced into the stoma. Patient education points include:

- Regulation of diet and fluid intake to ensure pasty stool and prevent constipation

- The necessity of seeking immediate medical attention should the stoma darken in color together with severe onset of unremitting pain
- The importance of scheduled follow-up visits with the health care provider to monitor the hernia condition

Three surgical options for hernia repair are:

1. Primary fascial repair: an incision is made over the herniated area, and the peristomal fascia is reapproximated. This method has a high incidence of recurrence.
2. Local repair with prosthetic material such as Gortex or Marlex mesh. There is a high incidence of erosion of the prosthetic material into the intestinal stoma.
3. Relocation of the stoma to the opposite side of abdomen. The stoma is taken down, a new one is brought out through the presited stoma site, and the fascial repair is done at the old site. This is the preferred method of repair.

The results of hernia repair are not encouraging. In a series of 94 parastomal hernia repairs (Rubin, Schoetz, and Matthews, 1994), 43% of the patients had a recurrence. The authors reported a fascial repair recurrence rate of 76%, a stoma relocation recurrence rate of 33%, and 50% recurrence with local repair using prosthetic material. Other studies report similar results (Shellito, 1998). If surgical repair is necessary, relocation of the stoma is apparently superior to fascial repair.

Prolapse

A prolapse is the telescoping of the bowel through the stoma.

Presentation

A stoma prolapse varies in length and will protrude at least 5 to 13 inches into the pouching system (Color Plate 7). The mucosa becomes edematous and a deep red color. The enlarged stoma is susceptible to trauma. The bulk of the prolapse can make fitting a pouching system difficult and be impossible to conceal under clothing, causing the patient psychologic distress. In extreme cases the blood supply to the stoma may become compromised, causing stoma necrosis.

Incidence

Reports on the incidence of colostomy prolapse vary. A study by Cheung (1995) reported the rate of prolapse development to be 6.8% in patients with colostomies, 38.5% in transverse colostomies, and about 4% in end sigmoid colostomies or ileal conduits. Chandler and Evans (1978) noted that prolapse was seen more frequently in stomas created for obstruction and that 40% of loop stomas using the right colon prolapsed. Other reports concur that the highest prevalence of stoma prolapse is seen in loop transverse colostomies, and that the distal limb is predominantly involved (Shellito, 1998; Gordon, Rolstad, and Bubrick, 1998).

Etiology

Suspected etiologies include:

1. The use of a large fascial opening in the abdominal wall (Gordon, Rolstad, and Bubrick, 1998)
2. Colostomy brought out through an abdominal incision (Corman, 1993)
3. The presence of an obstruction at the time of colostomy formation (Chandler and Evans, 1978)

Diagnostic Workup/Assessment

The stomal mucosa is examined for color and the presence of edema. Occasionally, on a very long, dependent prolapse, the prolapsed section can become edematous.

Management

Conservative management is suggested, since most loop stomas are temporary. A pouching system should be selected that can accommodate the length of the stoma. The pouching system should be flexible; a two-piece pouching system with a rigid ring should be avoided to prevent stoma trauma. The pouch opening should accommodate the stoma at its largest size (notably when patient is standing). For most patients it is easiest to apply the pouch when the stoma is reduced. The patient is instructed to lie flat and reduce the stoma by applying gentle pressure (WOCN Society, 2003). The reduction of the stoma can best be accomplished by the application of cold to the stoma for several minutes; this can be achieved by placing an ice pack on the pouch over the stoma. The pouching system is applied with the stoma reduced while the patient is supine. This position will be difficult for many patients, and assistance may be required. The patient is advised to observe the stoma for color changes and to seek immediate attention should the stoma become ischemic. Support belts are available that contain a prolapse flap or strap, but they do not apply enough pressure to contain the stoma prolapse in most patients.

Patients should be made aware that a stoma that becomes dark in color and becomes painful is a medical emergency that requires immediate medical intervention. An ischemic stoma caused by strangulation can be treated on an emergency basis with table sugar (sprinkled directly on the exposed stoma) to shrink an incarcerated prolapse and allow bowel reduction until surgical repair is undertaken (Shellito, 1998).

Surgical repair is indicated in the presence of ischemia, congestion, or inability of the stoma to be reduced. Surgery involves resection of the prolapse and fashioning of a new stoma. Generally this can be done after incising the mucocutaneous junction circumferentially and taking down the colostomy. Since a loop transverse colostomy is usually temporary, the best treatment is closure (Corman, 1993).

Necrosis

Stoma necrosis results from impairment of blood flow through the stoma tissue, resulting in tissue death.

Presentation

The stoma appears dark in color, varying from maroon to black, and feels flaccid (see Color Plate 4). Necrosis can be seen immediately after stoma creation, generally occurring within 24 hours of the surgical procedure. The degree of necrosis can vary from a small area on the stoma to more than half of the stoma above the skin level and/or down to below the fascia.

Incidence

Reports of necrosis include 1% to 10% of colostomies, 1% to 5% of the patients with ileostomies (Shellito, 1998), and 12% to 22% of fecal stomas (DelPino et al, 1997; Duchesne et al,

2002). Leenen and Kuypers (1989) report a high rate of necrosis in obese patients as a result of the traction that is placed on both the mesentery and bowel wall. This same study reported a higher percentage of necrosis occurring, more often, in acutely ill patients. DelPino et al (1997) in a review of 1758 patients with stomas, noted that necrosis was the most frequent complication (13%) in end stomas and end loop stomas had the lowest rate of necrosis. They suggest that this may be due to the relative ease of exteriorizing a loop configuration than an end stoma, resulting in less tension and better blood supply.

Etiology

Ischemia is generally caused by mesenteric tension, by trauma to the stoma during its creation, or by excessive trimming of the mesentery from the bowel end.

Diagnostic Workup/Assessment

The degree of necrosis is variable and can be assessed by passing a small, lubricated, glass tube into the stoma and inspecting the mucosa with a pen light. If the necrosis extends to the fascial level, urgent reoperation is warranted. If the necrosis only involves a few millimeters, it may be observed; no surgical intervention is immediately indicated. The presence of bright red bleeding is also noted (as may occur with vigorous rubbing of the stoma), which could indicate viable tissue below the necrosis.

Management

The necrotic tissue will slough and may need debridement. If the dead tissue is allowed to remain in place, there may be a significant odor from the area. Once the necrotic tissue is removed or falls away, there is a mucocutaneous separation (see following paragraphs). As the necrotic area and the mucocutaneous separation heal, stenosis in the area of healing will be noted. Loose necrotic tissue can cause the patient distress; the patient should be instructed that the tissue loosens and falls away as part of the healing process. The stoma should be monitored at periodic intervals to watch for healing and to assess the degree of stoma stenosis.

The use of a transparent pouching system during hospitalization is recommended to allow for visualization. A two-piece appliance allows direct visualization on a daily basis without the need for removal of the skin barrier.

Mucocutaneous Separation

A mucocutaneous separation is the detachment of the stoma from the skin.

Presentation

On examination a variable degree of separation between the skin and stoma is noted (see Color Plate 5).

Incidence

There are few reports of the incidence of mucocutaneous separation. Lefort et al (1995) report five patients with a mucocutaneous separation in a series of 23 patients with colostomies; Park et al (1999) reported an incidence of 4% in their review of 1616 stoma patients.

Etiology

Separation may be the result of poor healing, tension, or superficial infection (Gordon, Rolstad, and Bubrick, 1998). The risk factors include prior administration of corticosteroids, diabetes, malnutrition, infection, stoma necrosis, and recurrence of disease. Stoma necrosis causes a mucocutaneous separation as the dead tissue detaches from the skin.

Diagnostic Workup/Assessment

The area of separation is gently probed to determine depth. The degree of separation is noted and the amount of circumference involved are noted and used to determine progress toward healing. If the defect is large, the base should be assessed to determine the type of tissue present (i.e., necrotic, granular). Any stool draining from this area should be noted, since this may indicate a fistula.

Management

Mucocutaneous separations are managed conservatively. The etiology is determined and corrected or reduced if possible. The separation is filled with an absorbent material that absorbs drainage and prevents excessive soiling from stool or urine. Absorbent materials include skin barrier powder, hydrofiber, and calcium alginate. The skin barrier of the pouching system is fitted over the area to provide protection from the effluent. The pouching system is changed at frequent intervals to

assess healing and change the filler material. If necrotic tissue is present in the mucocutaneous separation, changing the pouch frequently may be necessary because of excessive drainage.

As the mucocutaneous separation heals, the stoma should be assessed for stenosis and retraction.

Retraction

Stoma retraction is the disappearing of the normal protrusion of the stoma to or below skin level.

Presentation

The stoma is level with or below the skin level (Color Plate 8). Patients may report that the stoma disappears when they are sitting. They may also report inability to maintain a seal on the pouching system and note effluent undermining the pouch seal.

Incidence

Retraction has been reported to occur in as many as 10% to 24% of all stoma patients (Gordon, Rolstad, and Bubrick, 1998; Makela, Turku, and Laitinen, 1997). Shellito (1998) reports 1% to 6% of colostomies and 3% to 17% of ileostomies become retracted. Arumugam et al (2003) analyzed risk factors and found that a high body mass index (i.e., obesity) was associated with an increased rate of stoma retraction.

Etiology

Retraction results from tension on the stoma caused by one or more of the following factors: short mesentery, thickened abdominal wall, excessive scar or adhesion formation, obesity, inadequate initial stoma length, improper skin excision (Corman, 1993), necrotic stoma, and mucocutaneous separation (WOCN Society, 2003; Shellito, 1998; Pearl et al, 1985).

Diagnostic Workup/Assessment

The stoma should be viewed without the pouching system, with the patient in sitting and supine positions. The level of the stoma to the skin and the shape of the peristomal skin are noted.

Management

For many cases of retraction a convex pouching system and the use of a belt can provide a predictable seal (see Chapter 12). Surgical revision may be considered should the patient not be able to achieve a predictable seal that protects the peristomal skin. Local revision is possible in cases where there is adequate intestine to mobilize above the skin level. In this instance an incision is made around the stoma, the intestine mobilized, and a new stoma fashioned. In some cases a laparotomy is necessary to create a new stoma.

Stenosis

Stenosis is a narrowing or contracting of the stoma occurring at the skin or fascia that impairs the drainage of effluent (WOCN Society, 2003; Hampton, 1992).

Presentation

The patient with a fecal stoma may complain of constipation followed by a large volume of output; explosive, loud, and excessive gas; pain at the time of stoma emptying; and narrowing of the caliber of the stool. The stoma opening appears small (Color Plate 9). The patient with a urinary diversion may note recurring urinary tract infections, projectile emptying of the urine, and/or flank pain (WOCN Society, 2003).

Incidence

Stoma stenosis has been reported to occur in 2% to 10% of ileostomies and end colostomies (Shellito, 1998) but almost never in transverse colostomies. Cheung (1995) noted an overall stenosis rate of 10% in 322 stomas, with 11.5% in end sigmoid colostomies and 7.3% rate in ileal conduits. DelPino, Cintron, and Onsay (1997) reported a 4% incidence rate in 1758 patients with stomas of all types.

Etiology

Stenosis occurs as a result of ischemia (Gordon, Rolstad, and Bubrick, 1998; Pearl et al, 1985). Contributing factors include necrosis, excessive tension, retraction, recurrent Crohn's disease, mucocutaneous separation, and recurrence of cancer. Chronic peristomal dermatitis with stoma and peristomal skin encrustation in ileal conduit patients has been noted to create a "late" stenosis, appearing in one study at median of 128 months (Cheung, 1995).

Diagnostic Workup/Assessment

A digital examination using a gloved, lubricated finger is performed to assess the size and the mobility of the skin and fascial rings. When a digital examination is not possible because of severe stenosis, a retrograde contrast study through a small rubber catheter may be performed.

Management

For mild stenosis of fecal diversions, a low-residue diet, stool softeners, or high liquid intake may be all that is necessary to allow for easy passage of the stool through the stoma.

Stoma dilation has been reported (Potter, 2000) but there is a lack of evidence-based literature to support this practice. The use of Hager dilators has been suggested, starting by introducing a small one into the stoma and increasing the size as tolerated. When performed over a prolonged period of time, this may provide relief. Others report that chronic dilations can cause stoma stenosis (Hampton, 1992).

For more severe cases, surgical treatment is necessary and is based on the cause of the stenosis. If the stenosis is located only at the skin level, it can be managed by surgical detachment of the skin from the mucosa and the fashioning of a new stoma after excising a small amount of skin to increase the skin opening (Gordon, Rolstad, and Bubrick, 1998). If the stenosis is the consequence of excessive tension, retraction, or full-thickness necrosis, the stoma will need to be refashioned after advancement of the intestinal loop. The procedure often requires a laparotomy. In the presence of recurrent Crohn's disease or cancer, the stoma needs to be resected and refashioned through a laparotomy.

For the patient with a stenotic ileal conduit related to hyperplasia of the peristomal skin, treatment to decrease the hyperplasia should be instituted (see p. 317). The stenosis may be relieved once the stomal tissue and the peristomal tissue have been cleared of the hyperplastic tissue.

Fistula

A fistula is an abnormal communication between the stoma and the surrounding area.

Presentation

It appears as an opening in the peristomal skin with communication from the intestinal lumen (Color Plate 10). The fistula can be complete, allowing 100% of the effluent to drain, or partial, in which a percentage of the effluent drains from the fistula and the remainder from the stoma lumen. The patient may first note difficulty maintaining the pouching system seal and be unaware of the presence of a fistula; alternatively, the patient may have noted stool exiting from a location other than the stoma lumen. A fistula from the intestine to the peristomal skin can cause the patient burning and pain, whereas a fistula on the stoma will generally be painless. The patient may experience discomfort, because the pouch seal is inadequate and the peristomal skin becomes irritated and denuded.

Incidence

It is reported that 15% of all ileostomy revisions are related to fistula formation (Corman, 1993). In a review of 126 patients with colostomies, one patient developed a peristomal fistula (Porter et al, 1989); and a second study of 49 patients with inflammatory bowel disease (IBD) had four patients with fistulas (Weaver, Alexander-Williams, and Keighley, 1988).

Etiology

Fistulas are reported to be nearly unique to ileostomies (Shellito, 1998), and most are related to recurrence of disease. Although the fistula may occasionally occur from a suture placed full-thickness through the side of the stoma at the time of creation, more common causes include recurrences of Crohn's disease, poor healing, and mechanical trauma from the pouching system.

Diagnostic Workup/Assessment

Stoma effluent drains from an area other than the stoma lumen. Conventional contrast studies (i.e., upper gastrointestinal films with small bowel follow-through or retrograde studies through the fistula) or a CT scan with oral contrast can be used to visualize the fistula.

Management

Although some superficial fistulas can heal spontaneously, most fistulas require formal stoma reconstruction and in some cases stoma relocation (Gordon, Rolstad, and Bubrick, 1998). If surgical intervention must be delayed, a pouching system that can accommodate both the skin fistula and the stoma should be considered; in the case of a fistula

on the side of the stoma, the use of a convex pouching system may provide an adequate seal.

Stoma Trauma

The stoma presents with mucosal injury.

Presentation

A laceration is present on the stomal mucosa, usually a small, white line with minimal depth (Color Plate 11). In other cases the stoma will appear denuded, with a deep red area that may bleed easily.

Incidence

No reports exist pertaining to incidence.

Etiology

Stoma injuries generally occur from pouch injury, a hard surface applying pressure to the stoma (i.e., seat or pant belt), or being hit with a ball.

Diagnostic Workup/Assessment

The stoma injury appears at the area of trauma and is characterized by a shallow, white mark or a deep red area. There may be small pinpoint bleeding in the area. The patient does not feel any pain in the area.

Management

The etiology of the stoma trauma must be determined and corrected. There are no topical therapies for a stoma injury; the area is observed at pouch change for a decrease in the size as an indication of healing. Stoma injuries usually heal spontaneously.

PERISTOMAL COMPLICATIONS
Peristomal Varices

Varices are large, portosystemic venous collaterals and occur at the site of a stoma in patients with portal hypertension.

Presentation

A purple hue caused by the dilation of mucocutaneous vessels is noted around the stoma (Color Plate 12). Intermittent, spontaneous, profuse bleeding can be seen by the patient, either in the pouch or during pouch change at the stoma-skin junction. As a result of the portal hypertension, the volume of blood loss can be large and can occur quickly.

Incidence

Ectopic (abnormally dilated veins associated with gastrointestinal mucosa) varices account for between 1% and 5% of all variceal bleeding (Norton,

Andrews, and Kamath, 1998). In a review of 169 cases of bleeding ectopic varices, 27% bled from peristomal varices (Norton, Andrews, and Kamath, 1998).

Etiology

As mentioned, peristomal varices (referred to by some as caput medusae) are large, portosystemic venous collaterals. Collaterals develop where the portal venous system communicates with the systemic circulation. The placement of bowel through the abdominal wall creates such a situation and may result in the formation of collaterals. With the development of portal hypertension, intrahepatic vascular resistance increases, allowing the portosystemic collaterals to open and varices to develop at the mucocutaneous junction. The most common scenario for stomal varices occurs in the patient with an ileostomy after proctocolectomy for inflammatory bowel disease with associated primary sclerosing cholangitis (i.e., fibrosing inflammatory destruction of intrahepatic and/or extrahepatic biliary ducts) (Norton, Andrews, and Kamath, 1998). Varices can also be seen in those patients with malignancies involving the liver and patients with cirrhosis.

Diagnostic Workup/Assessment

A thorough examination of the stoma site is performed, looking for a stomal site of bleeding. Upper and lower endoscopy are used to identify varices. Hemoglobin and hematocrit levels are monitored to assess blood loss and initiate resuscitation of the patient.

Management

The first priority is to stop bleeding and then to identify and manage the underlying disease. Once that is addressed, a conservative management approach is advocated. Initial interventions to stop peristomal bleeding include direct pressure, cauterization with silver nitrate, gel foam, epinephrine-soaked gauze, and suture ligation (Norton, Andrews, and Kamath, 1998; Johnson and Laurin, 1997). The patient should be advised to use a pouching system that will not apply direct firm pressure to the peristomal area. Two-piece systems should not be used because of the need to apply pressure to attach the pouch, and because the flange can rub on the engorged vessels. Patients

should be cautioned against wearing snug clothing that could constrict or rub the stoma, precipitating a bleed. While the patient is at risk for a variceal bleed, silver nitrate, pressure bandages, and gel foam are kept at the bedside for quick access. Other interventions include injection sclerotherapy and mucocutaneous disconnection of the stoma with ligation of the portosystemic channels. A transjugular intrahepatic portosystemic shunt (TIPS) or a surgical portosystemic shunt may be indicated to lower portal pressure. In patients with end stage liver disease, liver transplantation is considered.

Bleeding from the stoma can be a frightening and, in some cases, life-threatening event. The patient should be educated regarding how vulnerable the peristomal area is to pressure and injury and how to protect the area. If bleeding starts, he or she should be advised to apply firm, direct pressure; if this does not stop the bleeding after several minutes, the patient should seek immediate medical attention.

Peristomal Candidiasis

Peristomal candidiasis is an overgrowth of a *Candida* organism of sufficient magnitude to cause an inflammation, infection, or disease on the skin surrounding a fecal or a urinary diversion (Evans and Gray, 2003). The most common cutaneous *Candida* species is *C. albicans*.

Presentation

The primary lesion with candidiasis is a pustule. The pustule is abraded during the removal of pouching system adhesive, and the chief findings include papules, erythema, and maceration (Color Plate 13). The patient may complain of burning and/or itching. Satellite lesions can be found at the edge of the advancing candidiasis, an important diagnostic finding (Habif, 1996). The involved area can be encountered anywhere on the peristomal skin, but it is generally limited to under the adhesive seal of the pouching system, since the spread of lesions is inhibited when it reaches dry skin (Evans and Gray, 2003).

Incidence

Ratliff and Donovan (2001) report a 1% incidence in a study looking at 161 patients with stomas. No other reports were noted.

Etiology

As mentioned, candidiasis is an overgrowth of a *Candida* organism (generally *C. albicans* or *C. tropicalis*) on the skin around the stoma. It has been suggested that prolonged exposure of the peristomal skin to either fecal or urinary effluent provides a moist medium that allows *Candida* colonization and proliferation (Evans and Gray, 2003). Risk factors include long-term antibiotic administration, diabetes mellitus, use of immunosuppressive drugs, surgery, hospitalization, and a moist environment. The moist environment may be caused by an inadequate pouching system seal that resulted from cutting the skin barrier seal larger than the stoma, or by prolonged wear time that allowed effluent to contact the peristomal skin.

Diagnostic Workup/Assessment

Peristomal candidiasis is generally diagnosed based upon the clinical findings of pustules, papules, inflammation, and pruritis, and on the presence of risk factors. A potassium hydroxide, or KOH, preparation using skin scrapings from an intact pustule can confirm the diagnosis (Evans and Gray, 2003).

Management

The first line of treatment is to identify and correct whatever caused the moist environment. Pouch fit is checked to be sure that the stoma effluent is not making skin contact. The peristomal skin should be thoroughly dried before application of the skin barrier (a hair dryer on a low setting can be effective in drying the peristomal skin). A topical antifungal preparation that will not interfere with the pouch adhesion is recommended, generally a powder. Two types of antifungal powders are available: polyene antibiotics such as nystatin (e.g., Mycostatin), available by prescription, and topical azole agents such as miconazole, available as an over-the-counter product. The peristomal area is cleansed and dried, and a modest amount of powder is applied to the affected area. The powder is rubbed into the peristomal skin, and any excess is brushed off. The powder is applied at pouch change until the area appears dry and intact.

Anecdotal reports of the use of an antibacterial, antifungal skin cleanser (Technicare) have indicated it to be a successful antifungal treatment.

Folliculitis

Folliculitis is an inflammation of hair follicles usually caused by *Staphylococcus aureus* (Lyon and Smith, 2001).

Presentation

Pustules are present around a hair follicle. They progress from pustules to papules to crusted areas (Color Plate 14).

Incidence

No reports are available on incidence.

Etiology

Peristomal folliculitis generally results from shaving of the peristomal skin, friction, and in some cases occlusion. Risk factors include diabetes mellitus, obesity, malnutrition, immunodeficiency, and chronic staphylococcal infections (Bryant, 2000).

Diagnostic Workup/Assessment

This bacterial infection can generally be diagnosed by clinical findings of a pustule pierced by a hair and the secondary lesions with crusts and erythema (Bryant, 2000).

Management

The cause should be identified and addressed. Reducing the frequency of shaving, lightly shaving the area to prevent skin damage, clipping of hair, and gentle adhesive removal using an adhesive removal product are recommended. Use of an antibacterial soap at pouch change has been advocated, as well as the use of antibacterial wash.

Mucosal Transplantation

Mucosal transplantation is the seeding of viable intestinal mucosa along the suture line onto the peristomal skin.

Presentation

Intestinal mucosa are present in and around the peristomal area, flush to the epidermis (Color Plate 15). The mucosal tissue remains moist and in many cases interferes with the pouching system seal.

Incidence

No reports on incidence are available.

Etiology

Mucosal transplantation occurs at the time of stoma formation if the sutures used to mature the stoma are placed through the peristomal skin rather than through the dermis.

Diagnostic Workup/Assessment

Areas of moist, red mucosal tissue are scattered in the peristomal area. Attempts to "heal" the tissue by use of skin barrier powders or to cauterize the tissue prove worthless.

Management

The only effective treatment is excision, which generally necessitates a stoma revision and infrequently necessitates stoma resiting (Corman, 1993).

Pseudoverrucous Lesions

Pseudoverrucous lesions are wartlike lesions in the peristomal area. Several terms are used to refer to this condition: hyperplasia, chronic papillomatous dermatitis (Lyon and Smith, 2001), and pseudoepitheliomatous hyperplasia.

Presentation

Pseudoverrucous lesions are found around the stoma in the area of chronic irritation from moisture (Color Plate 16). The amount and size of lesions is related to the chronicity of the skin moisture, the type of moisture, and the seal of the pouching system. The raised areas are thickened epidermal projections, and the size and color vary (white to light gray, deep red, or brown). The epidermis in the involved area is moist. The lesions may be painful, and bleeding is common. First reported in the literature as occurring around urinary diversions (Borglund, Nordstrom, and Nyman, 1998), pseudoverrucous lesions have also been described around fecal diversions (Hampton, 1992).

Incidence

Because of the use of unspecific terms to describe pseudoverrucous lesions, there are no consistent reports of incidence.

Etiology

The cause is chronic irritation from moisture that leads to reactive thickening of the epidermis. This can result from the chronic use of an opening in the skin barrier larger than the stoma that allows effluent to contact skin, or from habitual use of an improperly fitted pouching system that traps the effluent between the skin barrier and the skin. The tendency in a person with a urostomy to develop pseudoverrucous lesions is greater if the urine is alkaline (Lyon and Smith, 2001).

Diagnostic Workup/Assessment

Pseudoverrucous lesions are diagnosed by clinical findings; see the earlier section under presentation.

Management

The cause of the peristomal moisture must be determined and corrected. As previously noted, the opening in the skin barrier should be checked to be sure that it fits up to the stoma-skin junction. The wear time should be determined and shortened, if erosion of the skin barrier is noted at removal. The skin barrier should be assessed for overhydration, which could increase skin moisture levels. In select cases the judicious use of silver nitrate on large lesions may hasten healing and provide a flat surface for the pouching system. In severe cases, surgical resection may be necessary.

Although alkaline urine alone is not thought to cause the development of pseudoverrucous lesions (Lyon and Smith, 2001), a high urine pH can cause moist encrustations in addition to the pseudoverrucous lesions. Correcting the pH (the average urine pH should be 6.0) of the urine can be accomplished by adequate fluid intake (1800 to 2400 ml/24 hours) and intake of cranberry juice and vitamin C. Cranberry juice has been noted to contain active ingredients that lead to a transient acidification of urine (Gray, 2002); however, the reports of the volume of cranberry juice that must be taken vary between 10 and 16 ounces in 24 hours. Cranberry capsules (a dietary supplement) are recommended for a variety of conditions, including prevention and treatment of urinary tract infection (recommended dosage is from 1 to 2 tablets per day to 1 to 2 tablets with each meal) (Gray, 2002). See Chapter 16 on medications with contraindications of urine acidification.

Stoma and peristomal encrustations can be treated with vinegar soaks applied to the area at pouch change. A pad soaked in vinegar is placed over the involved area for 5 minutes, rinsed, soaked again in the vinegar, and replaced. At the end of the soaks the area should be lightly rubbed to loosen the encrustations. The use of an acidic skin barrier such as karaya or CollySeals (Torbot,

Cranston, RI) can be used under the pouching system to maintain an acidic environment that will dissolve the encrustations.

Peristomal Pyoderma Gangrenosum

Peristomal pyoderma gangrenosum (PPG) is a rare, ulcerative skin condition of unknown etiology that occurs in the area surrounding the stoma.

Presentation

PPG is thought to start as one or more pustules that break open and form full-thickness ulcers with irregular, ragged, overhanging margins. A necrotizing inflammatory process extends peripherally from the primary lesion, resulting in a necrotic ulcer with undermined edges (Habif, 1996). The surrounding skin becomes red and purple, and the entire area is very painful (Color Plate 17). PPG is thought to be a variant of pyoderma gangrenosum, 70% of which occurs on the lower legs. PPG generally does not extend beyond the adhesive edge of the pouching system. Healing typically results in a cribriform scar.

Incidence

It is difficult to determine the true incidence, since PPG is seldom recognized and not reported (Sheldon et al, 2000). The majority of patients with PPG have been diagnosed with IBD. It occurs in approximately 2% of patients with IBD (Callen, 1998), and more often with Crohn's disease than ulcerative colitis (Hughes, Jackson, and Callen, 2000; Cairns et al, 1994). There are reports in the literature of a small number of patients with PPG and malignancies (Hughes, Jackson, and Callen, 2000; Lyon and Smith, 2001). The onset of PPG has been reported to occur from 2 weeks to 25 years following stoma construction (Hughes, Jackson, and Callen, 2000; Cairns et al, 1994). At least 50 cases have been reported in the literature (Mancini, Floyd, and Solla, 2002).

Etiology

There is no clear understanding of the pathogenesis. It is reported that women are more likely to develop PPG than men (Sheldon et al, 2000; Cairns et al, 1994). Pathergy (a process whereby in susceptible persons, trauma to the skin results in pustules and/or ulcers) has been suggested to play a role, since the skin can be irritated from the pouch adhesive or leakage of effluent (Hughes, Jackson, and Callen, 2000).

Diagnostic Workup/Assessment

Diagnosis is a clinical one based upon history and ulcer assessment. There are no diagnostic tests. Biopsy only serves to exclude disorders such as malignancy or vasculitis.

Management

No single therapy has been demonstrated to be effective in the treatment of PPG (Sheldon et al, 2000). The principles of management include decreasing the inflammatory process and maintaining the seal on the pouching system for a predictable time period. Patients should be screened for the presence of active inflammatory bowel disease. Topical treatment may include antiinflammatory agents such as steroid preparations in a paste (e.g., Orabase with Kenalog) or topical immunomodulators such as tacrolimus (e.g., Protopic) (Lyon and Smith, 2001) and pimecrolimus (e.g., Elidel) (Lyon and Smith, 2001; Hughes, Jackson, and Callen, 2000; Sheldon et al, 2000). In cases of small areas of involvement, topical therapy is instituted to determine response. Systemic medical therapy is considered if there is no response or worsening of the area with the use of topical treatments. Systemic medical therapy may include administration of metronidazole, prednisone, cyclosporine, dapsone, or infliximab. Surgical removal and resiting of the stoma may be necessary in extensive cases of PPG, especially if the underlying bowel is affected by active IBD.

The principles of PPG wound care include moisture control, maintenance of a clean wound base, protection of the wound base, delivery of topical antiinflammatory/immunosuppressive preparations, and achieving a predictable pouching system seal of at least 24 hours. Products that may be employed to meet these goals and that are applied over the topical therapy include hydrofiber and/or calcium alginate dressings to control wound drainage, hydrocolloid dressings placed directly over the ulcers or as a secondary dressing (to provide a dry surface for the pouching system), skin barrier powder in shallow, minimally draining ulcers (for absorption), and foam dressings (with a nonstrike-through outer covering to provide a dry pouching surface). The use of a topical anesthetic may be needed because of the discomfort or pain associated with dressing and pouch changes. The frequency of changing the dressings and the pouching system depends upon the amount of wound exudate. A new presentation of PPG may have excessive wound drainage that requires daily pouching system and dressing changes until therapeutic levels of the anti-inflammatory or immunosuppressive drugs are reached. Healing rates are variable, and the patient requires ongoing support during the treatment and healing phases. Because of the full-thickness destruction, the healed areas are frequently uneven and may cause pouch seal problems that will necessitate refitting of the pouching system once the PPG heals.

Suture Granulomas

Suture granulomas are granulation tissue that occurs at the skin-stoma base in areas of retained or reactive suture material.

Presentation

Red, friable tissue, usually in a small, round shape, is scattered around the mucocutaneous junction (Color Plate 18).

Incidence

No reports are available on incidence.

Etiology

The cause is cutaneous reaction to retained or reactive suture material.

Diagnostic Workup/Assessment

The area should be probed to determine if the red bumps are firm or fluid-filled. Granulomas are friable granulation tissue that bleeds easily. Some patients complain of pain on examination.

Management

Each granuloma should be examined to determine if suture material can be visualized and removed. Silver nitrate can be used to decrease the amount of tissue. In severe cases, cauterization can be used.

Peristomal Irritant Contact Dermatitis

Peristomal irritant contact dermatitis (PICD) is skin damage resulting from contact with fecal or urinary drainage or chemical preparations.

Presentation

Skin damage is located in the areas that have been exposed to stool, urine, or chemicals (e.g., solvents, cleansers, liquid skin barriers, soaps, or adhesives). The effluent or chemical destroys or erodes the epidermis, and the patient complains of pain and burning in the involved area. The area initially shows erythema or an erythematous macular rash and can quickly progress to denudement if exposure continues (Bryant, 2000). The area is moist because of the loss of epidermis (Color Plate 19).

Incidence

In the literature the incidence of patients with PICD varies from 2.5% to 55% (Ratliff and Donovan, 2001; Lyon and Smith, 2001; Porter et al, 1989; Duchesne et al, 2002; Arumugam et al, 2003; Cheung, 1995; Park et al, 1999; DelPino, Cintron, and Orsay, 1997; Lefort et al, 1995).

Etiology

The skin damage can result from an inadequate pouch-to-skin seal, that allows the stool or urine to remain in prolonged contact with the skin, or the use of chemicals in direct contact with the peristomal skin. The cause of the inadequate seal is variable and may include incorrect pouch sizing, poor pouch application technique, excessive wear time, inappropriate pouching system, stoma dysfunction, poor stomal location, or poor stomal or peristomal skin conditions (Table 14-1). The use of substances such as solvents, cleansers, soaps, and liquid skin barriers can cause irritation.

Diagnostic Workup/Assessment

The following should be assessed: location of the area of skin damage, the skin barrier on the removed pouching system to check the barrier's integrity (i.e., size and erosion), the peristomal area with the patient in a supine and a sitting position (noting creases, folds, and skin integrity), and the stoma when patient is in the supine and the sitting positions (noting amount of protrusion, the location of the lumen, and the size). The patient should be questioned about the usual wear time and any changes in the normal wear or the amount and consistency of the effluent, a recent shift in weight, pouch application and removal technique, and product usage.

TABLE 14-1   Determining the Cause: Inadequate Pouching System Seal

CAUSE	ASSESSMENT	INTERVENTIONS
Poor pouch application technique	Discuss with patient the steps involved in pouch application; note the products used.	Correct technique; determine if all products are necessary
Excessive wear time	Examine the skin barrier on the pouching system for erosion.	Decrease wear time to the point at which the skin barrier is not showing erosion. Cut back on the wear time by one day at a time until the skin barrier is not eroded to the point where the stoma effluent is in contact with the skin. Consider the use of an extended-wear barrier for longer wear and less erosion.
Inappropriate pouching system	Examine the stoma and the peristomal skin with patient in a sitting and a flat position. Note skin creases and folds and the location of the stoma lumen.	Match the shape and size of the skin barrier to the peristomal skin and stoma. Consider use of convexity for creased or folded peristomal areas. Consider flexible systems for a flat peristomal area. Consider use of convexity if stoma lumen is close to skin.
Stoma dysfunction	Determine the amount and consistency of the effluent. Perform digital examination to note skin and fascial rings: r/o hernia, stenosis. Watch stoma as effluent discharges to see if stoma changes in shape or size or there is a shift in the peristomal plane.	Consider dietary or medication manipulation of fecal output to thicken stool. Consider use of extended-wear barriers.
Poor stoma location	Examine patient in sitting and flat positions. Note skin creases and folds, presence of open incisions, bony prominences.	Match the shape and size of the skin barrier to the peristomal skin and stoma. Consider use of convexity for creased or folded peristomal areas. Consider use of belt.
Poor stoma	Examine stoma, note lumen location and position on abdomen, note amount of protrusion above skin. Perform digital examination to note skin and fascial rings: r/o hernia, stenosis.	Consider use of convexity for a flush stoma, lumen at skin level, etc. Consider referral to surgeon for site relocation.
Peristomal skin condition	Note skin integrity next to stoma and out to the end of the adhesive. Review with patient the products that are used in stoma management.	Determine irritant (i.e., effluent, chemical, or mechanical) and eliminate skin contact. Denuded skin treatment: skin barrier powder for superficial, small areas, steroid preparations for involved areas.

Management

Correction of the etiology of the skin-effluent-chemical contact is the first objective. The appropriate pouching system provides a secure, predictable wear time and protects the peristomal skin from the effluent. Identifying and eliminating the offending substance will allow the skin to heal. If possible it is best to reduce the amount of products used next to the skin and add new products slowly to note possible reactions.

The denuded skin must be treated to decrease the inflammatory process. A steroid preparation that contains no oily substances can be used. Triamcinolone acetonide (e.g., Kenalog) is available in a spray form and will not leave a greasy film on the skin. Corticosteroid scalp lotions (e.g., betamethasone valerate, brand name Luxiq) to treat PCID have been reported to be useful; however, although they appear to be efficacious, they contain 40% to 50% isopropyl alcohol, which can cause an initial burning sensation (Lyon and Smith, 2001). Occlusion (such as occurs under the skin barrier) enhances penetration of the steroid preparation. Long-term use (for months) may result in thinning of the epidermis (Habif, 1996). The use of the topical steroid preparation should be limited, since once the offending agent is removed the area should begin to show signs of recovery.

Skin barrier powder can be sprinkled and rubbed gently onto the denuded area, and the excess brushed off. The powder will absorb excessive moisture, enhancing the pouching system seal.

Peristomal Allergic Contact Dermatitis

Peristomal allergic contact dermatitis (PACD) refers to hypersensitivity to chemical elements resulting in an inflammatory reaction.

Presentation

Erythema is noted in the involved area followed by pruritis. Primary lesions are vesicles, bullae, papules, plaques, and wheals. Secondary lesions include moist desquamation, edema, fissure, excoriation, and crust (Bryant, 2000). The location of the reaction is confined to the skin where the product is applied (Color Plate 20). For example, the shape of the erythema will be the same round size as the skin barrier.

Incidence

No reports are available regarding incidence.

Etiology

PACD is an immunologic response to an allergen.

Diagnostic Workup/Assessment

The peristomal skin should be examined for the presence of redness, warmth, moisture, and pruritis. The configuration of the reaction is the clue to the root of the reaction.

Management

Management consists of determining and discontinuing the offending product (usually by noting any of the products in contact with the skin in the affected area). Patch testing can verify the offending product. Antiinflammatory agents (see previous paragraphs) should be used.

Peristomal Trauma

Peristomal skin trauma presents with loss of epidermis.

Presentation

Denuded epidermis and, in some cases, dermis are seen in the area of injury. The size varies depending on cause (Color Plate 21). The patient notes pain and moisture in the area.

Incidence

No reports are available on peristomal trauma.

Etiology

Peristomal skin injury is generally related to friction from tape removal. Injudicious tape removal will strip the epidermis, leaving a moist, painful surface. Other types of peristomal skin injury can include ulcer formation from convex faceplates, belts, and belt tabs.

Diagnostic Workup/Assessment

Peristomal skin injury appears as a full- or partial-thickness skin loss located in the area of the trauma.

Management

The cause of the trauma must be determined and corrected. The peristomal skin injury can be sprinkled with a skin barrier powder and covered with a thin hydrocolloid dressing until healed.

UNCOMMON STOMA AND PERISTOMAL COMPLICATIONS

Malignancy

Recurrent malignancy at the stoma site is rare and potentially a fatal complication (Corman, 1993, Ramanujam and Venkatesh, 2002). Causes are thought to be implantation at the time of tumor resection or inadequate resection margins. Resection of the area with stoma relocation is the suggested therapy. Carcinoma on the peristomal skin is also rare. The patient is seen with discolored skin, bleeding, and a mass (Color Plate 22). Ramanuman and Venkatesh (2002), reported a case of carcinoma at the ileocutaneous junction of a person with an ileostomy. They suggest that the "old-fashioned, ill-fitting" pouching system used by the patient caused chronic peristomal skin irritation and a squamous cell carcinoma. Following biopsy, treatment consists of a wide excision of the abdominal wall and resiting of the stoma.

Herpes

Herpes zoster and herpes simplex are viral illnesses triggered by illness, stress, and fatigue. Herpes zoster (shingles) occurs along dermatone distributions and forms vesicles, causing pain. Herpes simplex manifests itself with grouped vesicles on an erythemic base and can occur on any cutaneous site (Color Plate 23). Treatment of herpes consists of antiviral therapy and pain relief. Herpetic lesions in the peristomal area are quickly unroofed because of the pouch adhesive. If the area is contained, a hydrocolloid dressing can be used to contain the wound fluid, provide protection, and enhance the pouching system seal.

Pemphigus

Pemphigus is a rare, blistering, autoimmune skin disease that has been described as involving the peristomal skin (Lyon and Smith, 2001). Several forms of pemphigus have been classified that depend on the level of intraepidermal split formation. In pemphigus vulgaris (PV), the blisters are located just above the basal level, whereas in pemphigus foliaceus (PF) the blisters occur within the upper layers of the epidermis (Hertl and Veldman, 2001) (Color Plate 24). In PV the blisters most commonly present in the oral cavity but may occur on the skin as well. Skin lesions are flaccid bullae without surrounding erythema. In PF there is no mucosal involvement. Skin lesions present as erythematous, scaling plaques; intact bullae are rarely seen (Blauvelt, Hwant, and Udely, 2003). Immediate dermatologic referral is necessary. Treatment options include administration of corticosteroids, dapsone, or mycophenolate mofetil. The moist bullae may be present in the peristomal area, complicating the pouch seal. The temporary use of a nonadhesive pouching system may be necessary. In select cases the use of a hydrocolloid or a foam dressing as the primary dressing may provide a dry surface for pouch adherence.

Psoriasis

Psoriasis is a chronic disease characterized by proliferation of the epidermis. The plaque type is the most common form of the disease, occurring in more than 80% of cases (Lebwohl, 2003). Psoriasis presents with sharply demarcated, erythematous, thick, silvery-white, scaling plaques (Color Plate 25). IBD occurs more commonly in patients with psoriasis (Blauvelt Hwant, and Udely, 2003). The areas generally affected are palms, scalp, elbows, knees, and soles. Plaques occur in sites of repeated trauma. It appears that the immune system plays a prominent role in the development of this disease (Lebwohl, 2003). Topical steroids are commonly used for treatment of psoriasis. Psoriasis can occur on the peristomal skin, and the plaques can become denuded from adhesive removal and cause pouch failure. Referral to the dermatology staff is recommended for evaluation and treatment. The role of tumor necrosis factor in this disease has recently been documented, and new therapies targeting the pathogenesis include infliximab and etanercept (Lebwohl, 2003).

CONCLUSION

It is likely that the majority of patients with a fecal or a urinary diversion will develop a peristomal or stomal complication. For this reason it is suggested that a person with a stoma should be periodically assessed for the appropriate use of the ostomy pouching system, for the integrity of the peristomal skin, and for the function of the stoma. Prevention and early intervention are key principles in the management and prevention of stomal and peristomal complications. A team approach (wound, ostomy, and continence nurse, surgeon, gastroenterologist, and dermatologist) is key to identifying and managing stomal and peristomal problems.

SELF-ASSESSMENT EXERCISES

Questions

1. What surgical intervention has the best outcome for a patient with a peristomal hernia?
2. Eighteen hours after the creation of an end stoma, the nurse notes that the stoma mucosa is black and flaccid. What would be the appropriate assessments and interventions?
   a. Check the hydration level of the patient and provide hydration, because the flaccid stoma may be the result of dehydration.
   b. Remove the stoma pouch, and gently rub the stoma to note any surface bleeding. Notify the surgical service and prepare to examine the stoma using a small, lubricated, glass tube and a flashlight.
   c. Encourage the patient to ambulate, since this activity may precipitate bowel function.
   d. Remove the stoma pouch and cut a larger opening in a new pouch, and place a gauze pad in the pouch to prevent that plastic from contacting the stoma.
3. Name two interventions to decrease the edema in a prolapsed stoma.
4. Discuss the etiology of mucocutaneous separation.
5. What type of pouching system should be considered for the patient with a retracted stoma?
6. Why does stomal stenosis occur?
7. Following stoma trauma a patient will complain of pain at the area of trauma.
   True _____ False _____
8. After a proctocolectomy a patient with sclerosing cholangitis comes to the stoma outpatient clinic noting that she had two bleeding episodes in the last 7 days. During each episode she reports the pouch filled up to one-third full with bright red blood. Upon examination of the stoma, no bleeding areas are noted; however, the peristomal skin has a purple hue. What would be a differential diagnosis for this patient?
9. Discuss the clinical presentation of peristomal candidiasis.
10. What is folliculitis?
11. Mucosal transplantation is caused by a large skin barrier opening on the pouching system.
    True _____ False _____
12. What is the cause of pseudoverrucous lesions?
13. Name the diagnostic test commonly done when ruling out the presence of peristomal pyoderma gangrenosum.
14. What is peristomal irritant contact dermatitis?
15. Name two uncommon stomal or peristomal complications.

Answers

1. The best surgical intervention would be stoma relocation.
2. b
3. Interventions to reduce edema in a prolapsed stoma are patient should be supine, applying cold packs to the stoma, and applying sugar to the stoma mucosa.
4. Possible etiologies of mucocutaneous separation are poor healing, tension or superficial infection, and risk factors that can include prior administration of corticosteroids, diabetes, malnutrition, infection, stoma necrosis, and recurrence of disease.
5. A convex pouching system
6. Stoma stenosis occurs because of ischemia.
7. False; a stomal injury will not cause the patient pain but will only be noted on examination.
8. Portal hypertension
9. Clinical presentation of peristomal candidiasis consists of papules, erythema, maceration, and patient complaints of burning and itching.

10. Folliculitis is the inflammation of a hair follicle caused by *S. aureus*.
11. False; mucosal transplantation is caused by the suturing of the intestinal mucosa to the epidermis.
12. Excessive moisture is the cause of pseudoverrucous lesions.
13. There is no diagnostic test to rule out peristomal pyoderma gangrenosum.
14. PICD is skin damage resulting from the contact of fecal or urinary drainage or chemical preparations.
15. Uncommon stomal or peristomal complications are malignancy, herpes, pemphigus, and psoriasis.

REFERENCES

Arumugam PJ et al: A prospective audit of stomas: analysis of risk factors and complications and their management, *Colorectal Dis* 5:49-52, 2003.

Blauvelt A, Hwant ST, Udely MC: Allergic and immunologic disease of the skin, *J Allergy Clin Immunolo* 111:S560-570, 2003.

Borglund E, Nordstrom, G, Nyman CR: Classification of peristomal skin changes in patients with urostomy, *J Am Acad Dermatol* 19(4):623-628, 1998.

Byrant RA: Skin pathology and types of damage. In Bryant RA, editor: *Acute and chronic wounds: nursing management*, ed 2, St. Louis, 2000, Mosby.

Cairns BA et al: Peristomal pyoderma gangrenosum and inflammatory bowel disease, *Arch Surg* 129(7):769-772, 1994.

Callen JP: Pyoderma gangrenosum, *Lancet* 351:581-585, 1998.

Chandler JG, Evans PG: Colostomy prolapse, *Surgery* 84:577-582, 1978.

Cheung MT: Complications of an abdominal stoma: an analysis of 322 stomas, *Aust N Z J Surg* 65:808-811, 1995.

Corman M: Intestinal Stomas. In, *Colon and rectal surgery*, ed 3, Philadelphia, 1993, Lippincott.

DelPino A et al: Enterostomal complications: are emergently created enterostomas at greater risk? *Am Surg* 63(7):653-656, 1997.

Duchesne JC et al: Stoma complications: a multivariate analysis, *Am Surg* 68(11):961-986, 2002.

Edwards DP et al: Stoma-related complications are more frequent after transverse colostomy rather than loop-ileostomy: a prospective randomized clinical trial, *Br J Surg* 88(3): 360-363, 2001.

Evans EC, Gray M: What interventions are effective for the prevention and treatment of cutaneous candidiasis? *JWOCN* 30:11-16, 2003.

Franks ME, Hrebinko RL: Technique of parastomal hernia repair using synthetic mesh, *Urology* 57:551-553, 2001.

Gordon PH, Rolstad BS, Bubrick MP: Intestinal stomas. In Gordon PH, Nivatvongs S, editors: *Principles and practice of surgery for the colon, rectum and anus*, ed 2, St. Louis, 1998, Quality Medical.

Gray M: Are cranberry juice or cranberry products effective in the prevention or management of urinary tract infection? *JWOCN* 29:122-126, 2002.

Habif TP: *Clinical dermatology: a color guide to diagnosis and therapy*, ed 3, St Louis, 1996, Mosby.

Hampton BG: Peristomal and stomal complications. In Hampton BG, Bryant RA, editors: *Ostomies and continent diversions: nursing management*, St Louis, 1992, Mosby.

Hertl M, Veldman C: Pemphigus: paradigm of autoantibody-mediated autoimmunity. *Skin Pharmacol Appl Skin Physiol* 12:408-418, 2001.

Hughes AP, Jackson JM, Callen JP: Clinical features and treatment of peristomal pyoderma gangrenosum, *JAMA* 284:1546-1548, 2000.

Johnson PA, Laurin J: Transjugular portosystemic shunt for bleeding of stomal varices, *Dig Dis Sci* 42:440-442, 1997.

Lebwohl M: Psoriasis, *Lancet* 361:1197-1204, 2003.

Leenen LH, Kupyers JHC: Some factors influencing the outcome of stoma surgery, *Dis Colon Rectum* 32:500-504, 1989.

Lefort MM et al: The definitive stoma: complications and treatment in 50 patients, *Acta Chir Belg* 95:63-66, 1995.

Londono-Schimmer EE, Loeng AP, Phillips RK: Life table analysis of stomal complications following colostomy, *Dis Colon Rectum* 37(9): 916-970, 1994.

Lyon CC, Smith AJ: Infections. In Lyon CC, Smith AJ: *Abdominal stomas and their skin disorders: an atlas of diagnosis and management*, Malden, Mass, 2001, Blackwell Science.

Makela JT, Turku PH, Laitinen ST: Analysis of late stomal complications following ostomy surgery, *Ann Chir Gynaecol* 86(4):305-310, 1997.

Mancini GJ, Floyd L, Solla JA: Parastomal pyoderma gangrenosum: a case report and literature review, *Am Surg* 68(9):824-826, 2002.

Norton ID, Andrews JC, Kamath PS: Management of ectopic varices, *Hepatology* 28(4):1154-1158, 1998.

Park JJ et al: Stoma complications: the Cook County Hospital experience, *Dis Colon Rectum* 42:1575-1580, 1999.

Pearl RK: Parastomal hernias, *World J Surg* 13:569-572, 1989.

Pearl RK et al: Early local complications from intestinal stomas, *Arch Surg* 120:1145-1147, 1985.

Porter JA et al: Complications of colostomies, *Dis Colon Rectum* 32(4):299-303, 1989.

Potter KL: Surgical oncology of the pelvis: ostomy planning and management, *J Surg Oncol* 73:237-242, 2000.

Ramanujan P, Venkatesh KS: An unusual case of squamous cell carcinoma arising at the stoma site: case report and review of the literature, *J Gastrointest Surg* 6:630-631, 2002.

Ratliff CR, Donovan AM: Frequency of peristomal complications, *OWM* 47(9):26-29, 2001.

Rubin MS, Schoetz, DV, Matthews, JB: Parastomal hernia: is stomal relocation superior to fascial repair? *Arch Surg* 129:413-419, 1994.

Sheldon DG et al: Twenty cases of peristomal pyoderma gangrenosum: diagnostic implications and clinical management, *Arch Surg* 135:564-569, 2000.

Shellito PC: Complications of abdominal stoma surgery, *Dis Colon Rectum* 41:1562-1572, 1998.

Weaver RM, Alexander-Williams J, Keighley MR: Indications and outcomes of reoperation for ileostomy complications in inflammatory bowel disease, *Int J Colorectal Dis* 3(1):38-42, 1998.

Williams JG et al: Paraileostomy hernia: a clinical and radiological study, *Br J Surg* 77(12):1455-1457, 1990.

Wound, Ostomy and Continence Nurses Society: Stoma complications: a best practice document for clinicians, 2003, In press.

CHAPTER

15 *Ostomy Adjustment*

CRAIG A. WHITE*

OBJECTIVES

1. Describe areas that are of psychologic concern to the new ostomy patient.
2. List risk factors for psychologic problems following ostomy surgery.
3. Relate the most common psychologic disorders that present after ostomy surgery.
4. Define the term *body image*.
5. Illustrate the types of aims and goals that may appear in a psychologically sensitive care plan.
6. Explain the main psychosocial concerns of ostomy patients.
7. Name the area that is key to planning ostomy patient care.
8. List the guidelines to be used in the providing of information during the preoperative visit.
9. Describe the teaching technique in the postoperative period that will promote the patient's confidence.
10. Explain how negative thinking affects the adjustment of the person with a new ostomy.

*The author is supported by a Cancer Research UK Fellowship in Psychosocial Oncology (CP1047/ 0101). Grateful thanks are extended to Alison Carnegie and Melanie Mackie for assistance with the preparation of this manuscript.

This chapter is largely based on that which appeared in Taylor P, editor: *Stoma care in the community: a clinical resource for practitioners*, London, 1999, Nursing Times Books, Emap Healthcare. Reproduced here by kind permission of NT Books/ Emap Healthcare.

INTRODUCTION

It is not possible to provide care to people who have had ostomy surgery without considering the psychologic impact of the surgery on their lives. This surgery involves significant changes in body form and functioning that are associated with increased self care demands and involve adaptation in almost every life domain (Bekkers et al, 1996). These changes can have a profound and lasting psychosocial impact. Patients often report concerns about appearance, smell, odor, relationships, and sexual and social functioning. This chapter outlines the main psychologic issues that are relevant to people who undergo stoma surgery with particular emphasis on psychologic assessment and management. The importance of understanding psychologic processes that underpin adjustment to this form of surgery will be highlighted throughout the chapter.

THE PROCESS OF PSYCHOLOGIC ADJUSTMENT

The process of psychologic adjustment to ostomy surgery differs among individual patients. However, there are common themes occurring in the psychologic concerns of patients (White and Hunt, 1997). To varying degrees, all patients will be concerned with their appearance and the day-to-day impact of the changes in their bowel or bladder functioning. For a very few people these concerns and issues will precipitate the signs and symptoms of a mental disorder requiring treatment. For some the surgery will cause other problems that may compromise their overall quality of life. However, there are also a sizeable proportion of patients for whom the surgery results in an improvement in their mental health (Thomas, Madden, and Jehu, 1984), which may have been previously significantly compromised by the effects of a chronic medical problem such as ulcerative colitis. A further group of patients may have psychologic problems relating to events that are separate from their illness and surgical treatment. Examples might include a preexisting relationship problem, social anxiety, or an eating disorder. Significant psychologic symptomatology following stoma surgery (irrespective of origins or preoperative psychologic status) is experienced by approximately 18% to 26% of patients (Thomas, Madden, and Jehu, 1984; Wade, 1990; White and Unwin, 1998). These figures are of a similar magnitude for patients who have undergone other forms of major surgery and/or following the diagnosis of diseases such as cancer.

The factors associated with postoperative psychologic problems can be thought of in terms of preoperative and postoperative factors. Patients with a past psychiatric history are at a greater risk of psychologic problems following surgery (Thomas, Madden, and Jehu, 1987; Wade, 1990; White and Unwin, 1998), as are those patients who report lower levels of satisfaction with preoperative preparation (Follick, Smith, and Turk, 1984; Thomas, Madden, and Jehu, 1987). Patients experiencing stoma-related physical symptoms such as leakage, peristomal skin problems, or prolapse are more likely to experience psychologic symptoms (Thomas, Madden, and Jehu, 1987; Oberst and Scott, 1988; Wade, 1990; White and Unwin, 1998).

Cognitive factors have also been shown to be associated with poorer psychologic adjustment. White and Unwin (1998) found that patient beliefs about physical integrity and the impact the stoma will have on their lives, and whether they felt in control of their bodies, were significantly related to levels of psychologic distress. Bekkers et al (1997) reported patients with higher levels of self stoma care efficacy (confidence in their abilities to provide self stoma care) had higher levels of psychosocial adjustment in the first four postoperative months.

Data suggest that a proportion of patients not satisfied with their stoma pouch change and disposal routines have a level of dissatisfaction that is positively correlated with levels of psychologic distress (White, unpublished). McVey, Madill, and Fielding (2001) identified lowered personal control as the most important concept to emerge from their analysis of transcribed interviews of patients who underwent ostomy surgery for cancer. They also investigated social self-efficacy (confidence with regard to social functioning with a stoma) and found that higher levels of social self-efficacy were associated with better psychosocial adjustment at both 4 months and at 12 months after surgery. Factors such as age, marital status, severity of illness, preoperative diagnosis, gender, and type of stoma have not been shown to be related to psychosocial adjustment following stoma creation (see White and Hunt [1997] for review).

ASSESSMENT OF PSYCHOSOCIAL VARIABLES

Psychologic concerns, problems, and symptoms can present before, during, and after surgical treatment. The most common psychologic disorders that present following stoma surgery are adjustment disorders, anxiety disorders such as panic disorder, generalized anxiety disorder, agoraphobia, major depressive disorder, and/or sexual dysfunction. There is an increasing amount of evidence indicating that a significant degree of posttraumatic stress disorder is prevalent among people who have had a life-threatening illness such as cancer (Baider and de Nour, 1997). It is possible that some people will experience these symptoms after surgery. There are also many persons who will have symptoms that, although not present with sufficient frequency and intensity to warrant a formal diagnosis, will significantly compromise their overall psychologic well-being, and the quality of social and sexual aspects of their lives (Bekkers et al, 1996). Care should integrate psychosocial support and symptom screening with vigilance for the occurrence of psychologic problems (Borwell, 1997). Screening questions that can be used to assess for psychologic problems are listed in Table 15-1.

TABLE 15-1 **Main Symptoms of Common Psychologic Disorders (with Screening Questions)**

PSYCHOLOGIC DISORDER	MAIN SYMPTOMS	SCREENING QUESTIONS
Panic disorder	Recurrent panic attacks Concern about more attacks Worry about losing control Changed behavior related to attacks	Do you ever get a sudden rush of fear or discomfort? Is that accompanied by physical sensations? What is the worst thing that could happen when this is going on? Do you do anything differently to cope with these attacks?
Major depressive disorder	Depressed mood Diminished interest in activities Weight loss or appetite change Sleep problems Agitation Loss of energy Feeling worthless or guilty Recurrent thoughts of death or suicide	How have you been feeling in your spirits? Do you get the same amount of enjoyment from what you do? How do you feel about yourself compared to other people? Do you ever feel that life is not worth living?
Generalized anxiety disorder	Excessive worry and anxiety most days for at least 6 months Difficult to control the worry Associated with restlessness, fatigue, irritability, muscle tension, sleep problems, or concentration problems	Are you ever troubled by worrying thoughts that go round and round in your head? Are you able to control these worrying thoughts?
Social phobia	Persistent fear of one or more social or performance situations Anxious about acting in humiliating or embarrassing way Exposure to situation almost always results in anxiety Recognizes fear is excessive Avoids situations or endures with distress	How do you feel about being in social situations? Do you ever worry about being embarrassed or making a fool of yourself? When you are not in the situation, how do you think and feel?
Posttraumatic stress disorder	Experience of event involving actual or threatened death or injury Person intensely fearful, helpless, or terrified Recurrent distressing thoughts, images, or nightmares of event	Does the event ever come back to your mind when you don't want it to? How do you feel when you are reminded of the event? Is there anything you do to avoid thinking about the event? Are you bothered by being on edge or very jumpy?

TABLE 15-1 **Main Symptoms of Common Psychologic Disorders (with Screening Questions)—cont'd**

PSYCHOLOGIC DISORDER	MAIN SYMPTOMS	SCREENING QUESTIONS
Posttraumatic stress disorder—cont'd	Intense physical and psychologic distress when reminded of event	
	Makes an effort to avoid being reminded of event	
	Diminished interest in activities	
	Hypervigilance or exaggerated startle response	
	Irritability or outbursts of anger	

Many of the concerns that people with a stoma have are often discussed in terms of body image problems. Fisher (1990) has argued that ". . . .one also needs to recognize that there are indeed quite different and perhaps largely independent dimensions represented under the rough rubric of body image." There is no such single entity as *body image*. The term is often used to refer to different components of the same construct by different researchers and clinicians. A detailed review of the main psychologic dimensions of body image is outside the scope of this chapter (see White [2002]). Recent evidence suggests that body image should be regarded as a cognitive structure that represents the sum of previous appearance-related experiences and that serves as a template to direct attention, influence encoding and interpretation, and facilitate recall of information regarding self-evaluative information about one's appearance.

Psychologic signs, symptoms, problems, and concerns are often not identified by the health care team (Bridges and Goldberg, 1984; Feldman et al, 1987; Mayou and Hawton, 1986). There are many potential reasons for this, including concern that it will be difficult to manage problems once they are elicited, that this will be emotionally overwhelming, and/or that there is not enough time to

BOX 15-1 **Main Psychosocial Concerns of Ostomy Patients**

- Not being complete as a person
- General impact of stoma on life (e.g., rules my life)
- Feeling in control of body
- Whether other people will hear or smell stoma
- Influence on intimacy and sexual function
- Being able to deal with stoma care

assess psychologic aspects of personal experiences (Faulkener and Maguire, 1994). Patients undergoing stoma surgery should be routinely screened for the most commonly occurring psychosocial concerns (Box 15-1). It is often assumed that if a concern is important it will be mentioned by the patient. This is not always the case: patients may actively avoid mentioning certain concerns for fear that they are inappropriate or that it will result in wasting a busy staff member's time. It has also been suggested that the manner in which outpatient consultations are organized, and their settings, may not always be conducive to the disclosure of concerns (Rubin and Devlin, 1987).

Self-report questionnaires can be used as part of the process of determining a patient's precise psychologic needs, to monitor changes in symptoms over time, and in some situations to evaluate responses to an intervention. The Stoma Cognitions Questionnaire (White and Unwin, 1998) measures the degree to which patients agree or disagree with statements regarding their stomas. This measure can complement clinical interviewing and be a useful way of eliciting concerns about life with a stoma.

The Stoma Self Efficacy Scale (Bekkers et al, 1996) is particularly useful for the assessment of confidence in ability to manage the demands of the stoma care routine (stoma care self-efficacy) and the ability to manage the social impact of living with a stoma (social self-efficacy). The Hospital Anxiety and Depression (HAD) Scale (Zigmond and Snaith, 1983), a well-known tool, is used as a screening measure for symptoms and has been included in psychosocial research to measure outcomes. The usefulness of the HAD has recently come under question, and it has been suggested that the 12-item version of the General Health Questionnaire (Goldberg, 1992) is a better measure to use for screening for psychologic symptoms (Hall, Hern, and Fallowfield, 1999).

MANAGEMENT OF PSYCHOLOGIC HEALTH

The aim of psychosocially sensitive assessments is primarily to identify psychologic concerns, issues, and problems. There are many strategies that can be implemented in the management of psychosocial aspects of patient care. These include psychosocial support by means of listening and counseling, interventions to address physical problems compromising psychologic health (e.g., leakage, odor), monitoring of psychologic symptoms, referral to a specialist in mental health, or the implementation of strategies to address concerns and promote optimal well-being. Staff concerns about not knowing what to do when issues are identified can significantly contribute to problems with their identification.

Prevention

Assessment of factors that may contribute to problems following ostomy surgery is key to planning ostomy patient care. In a substantial proportion of cases, patients will know in advance that they are to have stoma surgery. A preoperative assessment of psychologic status can determine if the patient has ongoing psychologic problems and should be screened for the presence of risk factors that may place the patient at increased risk after surgery. The preparation of a psychologically sensitive care plan should always be a priority. This is not always easy, since there are few models to assist with identifying optimal models of psychologic care delivery. However, Box 15-2 contains examples of some of the types of aims and goals that may appear in a psychologically sensitive care plan.

Preparation for Surgery

Psychologic preparation for surgical procedures has been shown to result in numerous psychologic and physical health benefits (Johnston and Vogele, 1993) and should be an integral part of the preoperative patient preparation (Borwell, 1997; Black, 1998). It is generally accepted that such preparatory work should cover what is going to happen before, during, and after surgery (procedural information) and how the patient will feel throughout the process (sensory information).

BOX 15-2   Examples of Psychologically Oriented Components of Nursing Care Plans

· ·

- Prepare patient for surgery by providing information on procedural and sensory aspects.
- Determine if any risk factors for psychologic problems are present.
- Promote stoma care self-efficacy.
- Assess patient satisfaction with information.
- Enhance satisfaction with information.
- Monitor psychologic symptoms at outpatient appointment.
- Inform colleagues in hospital and community of risk factors for psychologic problems.

Efforts should be made to enhance an individual patient's satisfaction with the information he or she has been given, since this may confer a prophylactic effect psychologically. The most sensible first steps are to establish what is already known and to ensure that patients are provided with the information that they want. They should be encouraged to consider the potential impact of receiving information (they may not have thought about how they will feel if the information they get differs from hopes or expectations). Information needs should always be assessed individually. Patients can be asked to list questions and, when practical, to take these to a subsequent appointment. Given the established links that exist between preoperative providing of information and patient level of satisfaction, it is imperative that people are asked first to report how satisfied they are with the information that they have been provided and second, what would need to happen for them to be more satisfied. Information provision aimed at enhancing satisfaction can then take place. Subsequent satisfaction checks can be done to determine whether the information has had the desired enhancing effects.

There are guidelines that can be followed when providing information for patients. These guidelines are based upon work by psychologists regarding what information provision strategies promote enhanced recall, compliance, satisfaction, and quicker recovery from illness (Ley and Llewelyn, 1995). It is recommended to start by providing the most important information first. This is more likely to be recalled because of the *primacy effect.* Stressing the importance of information, explicitly categorizing the information, and repeating the categories as information giving progresses will increase recall. Repetition of material increases recall and has beneficial effects on satisfaction. This is an example of how explicit categorization can be used:

Knowing three things might help you to live with a pouching system. First, a description of what pouching systems look like and how they work; second, how you will learn to deal with your pouching system; and third, what arrangements there will be for providing you assistance. First, what the pouching system looks like and its purpose. It is a method of collecting the waste material

that will be discharged from the newly created opening located on your abdomen. . . .

INCREASING SELF-EFFICACY

Some patients will have difficulty mastering the skills involved in managing their stoma. These skill acquisition difficulties may relate to a global lack of confidence in their ability to manage anything in their lives, may be confined to the tasks involved or specific situations, or may be attributable to a lack of information. Factors associated with problems such as depression (i.e., lack of motivation) and dementia (i.e., impaired memory and praxis) can make assimilation of the skills difficult.

The choice of interventions in these cases depends on the main factor contributing to the problem. Most psychosocial problems in ostomy care can be conceptualized as related in some way to a lack of self-efficacy in the component parts of the stoma care routine. As a result, in most cases, enhancing stoma care self-efficacy leads to an improvement in psychosocial functioning. An example of this would be social anxiety mediated by a lack of confidence that the appliance has been securely attached. Addressing patient confidence in this aspect of their self care should address the patient's social anxiety.

The promotion of self-efficacy can be achieved if patients are supported as they learn each component part of their stoma care routine—in isolation, repeatedly, and until they notice changes in their confidence levels. These changes can be monitored using a confidence diary. This will provide patients with information on their progress and/or the health care provider with information on areas of difficulty. It can be reinforcing for patients to monitor the changes in their confidence levels. White (1997) has suggested how the components of changing a pouching system can be broken down and data collected on confidence ratings as postoperative recovery progresses (Box 15-3). Patients may also find it easier to learn skills if they are first demonstrated by someone else (for example, by using a video or live demonstration), and if they learn them in a similar setting to that in which they will carry them out.

BOX 15-3   Confidence Diary

Date:
Location:
Postoperative day:
Confidence scale:

                          0 10 20 30 40 50 60 70 80 90 100
                      Not at all   Very
                      confident   confident

Activity   **Confidence Rating (0-100)**
Removing appliance from skin
Emptying the appliance
Washing and drying the stoma site
Measuring stoma size
Putting appliance on
Disposal of used appliance

Note: Component activities differ according to stoma care routine.

Many patients become concerned about their first encounters with situations that previously would not have caused problems. Much of the rehabilitation process following surgery is characterized by enabling people to tackle problems in manageable steps, at a pace that suits the overall context of their postoperative recovery. Clinical psychologists often use a treatment technique called graded exposure to tackle avoidance mediated by anxiety. This can be a useful way to think of helping people tackle the small steps they will need to take to make a full recovery in separate life domains. This technique consists of two components. First, breaking a larger goal or task into as many smaller steps as possible, and then ranking these steps according to degree of difficulty, anxiety, pain, and so on. Each small step can be tackled in increasing order of difficulty until the patient has mastered the final step. Problems and setbacks can be dealt with by suggesting that the patient may be stuck at an earlier stage, or that they insert a smaller leap from one step to the next.

Reviewing and Responding to Negative Thinking

Many psychologic problems are characterized by negative thinking patterns. These thoughts are often key factors for serious and more clinically significant problems with depression and anxiety. In such circumstances it is unlikely that simple advice on how to review and respond to thinking will have lasting effects (indeed, to provide only advice would be inappropriate). However, patients with less serious problems relating to anxiety and low mood may find it helpful to consider the way in which their thinking is influencing their psychosocial adjustment to surgery. Patients can be helped to identify their thoughts and evaluate them to see if there are more constructive alternatives. They should be advised to pay attention to what is going through their minds when they notice a change in their feelings (e.g., a dip in their mood or a surge in anxiety). When they have identified some of the thoughts they are encountering, they can look for thinking biases, or come up with alternatives by asking themselves a series of questions designed to shift their perspective or promote more helpful alternatives. Thoughts can be identified by asking a series of simple questions when there is a mood change. The evaluation of thoughts can be facilitated by reviewing common thinking biases and by asking another series of simple questions to facilitate a shift in perspective (Box 15-4). Further details on the basic elements of this strategy can be found in White (2002) and in Leahy (1997).

BOX 15-4   Reviewing and Responding to Negative Thinking

. . . .

A. Questions for Identifying Problem-Thoughts

1. What was going through my mind just as I started to have this problem-mood?
2. What does this situation mean to me? What does this situation say about me?
3. What is the worst thing that could happen in this situation?
4. What have I just been thinking about?
5. What do I guess that I was thinking about just then?

B. Common Thinking Biases

Problem-thoughts are often the result of biases or distortions in thinking. These biases or distortions have special names. When you are trying to change problem-thoughts it can be helpful to look for these biases. Some of the common biases are described below.

All-or-Nothing Thinking
Seeing things in black-and-white categories: either everything is going completely well, or it is a complete disaster
Over-Generalization
Seeing a single event as part of a never-ending pattern of events or generalizing from one isolated event to the rest of our lives
Mental Filter
Picking out a single negative detail and focusing on it exclusively
Discounting the Positive
Saying that positive experiences don't count
Jumping to Conclusions
Drawing conclusions when there are no facts to support your conclusion. "Mind-reading" is an example of this: you make predictions about what other people think as if you had mind-reading abilities. "Fortune-telling" is another bias that involves jumping to conclusions. This involves predicting that something won't work out as if you can really see into the future.
Magnification
Exaggerating the importance of your difficulties and problems, and minimizing your abilities to cope and your positive qualities
Emotional Reasoning
Assuming that your negative feelings are a reflection of the way that things really are
Personalization
Holding yourself personally responsible for an event that is not entirely under your control

C. Questions for Changing Problem-Thoughts

1. What experiences have I had that show me that this thought is not completely true all of the time?
2. If I were trying to help someone I cared about to feel better when this person had this thought, what would I tell the person?
3. What advice might someone I cared about give to me if he or she knew that I was thinking about things in this way? Would the person agree with me? If not, why not?
4. When I am not experiencing this problem-mood, how would I think about things?
5. What have I learned from previous events or experiences in my life that might help me to cope with this problem-thought?
6. Is my problem-thought an example of a thinking bias? If so, which one is it?
7. What is the evidence to support this thought? What is the evidence against this thought?
8. What is the worst thing that could happen? Could I live through and cope with this?
9. What is the best thing that could happen? What is the most realistic outcome?
10. What would be the effect of changing this problem-thought? What can I do now?

Case Management Role

To manage psychosocial aspects of ostomy surgery the health care team must be confident about the processes of case management and know which specialist colleagues they can refer patients to and the nature of some of the interventions that may be recommended.

There are times when it may be necessary to make a referral to a clinical psychologist or psychiatrist for a specialist opinion on the patient's psychologic problems. Patients will often be concerned about issues such as mental illness and/or their physical problems not being taken seriously when such referral is suggested. The health care team should be confident in the ways to explain such a referral as a positive step in a patient's care. Retaining involvement with a patient after such a referral has been made is often helpful in terms of addressing concerns about referral and monitoring fluctuations in symptoms. The types of questions that could be used at this stage are outlined in Box 15-5.

Troubleshooting

Undertaking assessment and management of psychosocial aspects following ostomy surgery can mean that the health care team will encounter difficult situations (e.g., when a patient refuses to talk about how he or she feels, or when a patient relates that everything is fine but behavior does not

support this statement). Sometimes patients make unreasonable demands on the staff. Although these situations are difficult to manage, there are some general guidelines that can help staff respond.

When patients refuse to talk about how they are feeling, this should be acknowledged, and they should be told that someone will be available to listen when they feel able to talk. It is helpful to offer the patient an explanation about why they might be finding it difficult to talk (e.g., because of fear of powerful emotions) and to make the suggestion that not talking can make things worse. In some circumstances, patient refusal to speak about issues troubling them could be part of a serious mental illness needing urgent intervention. In such circumstances the person is likely to demonstrate other signs and symptoms such as crying or unusual behaviors. When problems are suspected that the patient denies, one way to handle this is to summarize what has been heard from the patient and to follow this with a summary of concerns. Patients can be given information on how to access assistance if they become aware of problems and/or find they want someone to talk to at a future time. Attempts to persuade the patient that things are not fine do not usually work and can alienate the patient. Gentle questioning about the discrepancies between health care provider and patient perspectives can sometimes be attempted by those who have confidence in their use of counseling skills (e.g., "You were saying that you have had no problems since I last saw you. One of the nurses has been worried about some of the things you have said about your feelings. Do you know what she has been concerned about?").

CONCLUSION

The providing of care for those with a stoma is an inherently psychologic process. Many of the concerns that people have are psychologic in nature and a substantial number of people will struggle with problems related to anxiety and depression. Psychologic well-being can be enhanced by preparing people for surgery, providing information that is sensitive to their needs, promoting confidence in the stoma care routine and the gradual steps

---

BOX 15-5   Questions to ask Mental Health Professionals

· ·

- Are there things that I could be doing to help this patient with these problems until he or she is seen?
- What would be signs that the patient is getting worse?
- Is there any information that you could give me that you think would help this patient?
- Are there any treatments or strategies that might help while the patient is waiting to see you?
- Under what circumstances should I contact you again for further advice?

involved in recovery, providing advice on how to tackle negative thinking patterns, and ensuring appropriate and timely speciality referral as necessary. Assessment and management of psychosocial issues can be challenging, and all members of the health care team must work together to achieve a successful outcome.

SELF-ASSESSMENT EXERCISES

Questions

1. A person with an ostomy that complains of difficulty sleeping, poor appetite, and decreased energy might have the following psychologic disorder?
   a. Anxiety disorder
   b. Posttraumatic stress
   c. Major depressive disorder
   d. Social phobia
2. List three psychosocial concerns of an ostomy patient.
3. Assessment of factors that may contribute to problems following ostomy surgery is key to planning ostomy patient care.
   True _____ False _____
4. Describe the term *body image.*
5. Which of the following teaching techniques would be the most effective to promote the patient's confidence in ostomy care?
   a. Provide a teaching video on pouching system
   b. Provide simple, small steps in emptying and changing the pouching system
   c. Provide a teaching booklet on ostomy care
   d. Provide a pouch and tail clip to practice with
6. Discuss suggested guidelines for providing ostomy-related information to patients.
7. Depression and anxiety can be attributed to a negative thinking pattern of the person with an ostomy.
   True _____ False _____
8. Psychologic symptoms following stoma surgery can be experienced in 40% of patients.
   True _____ False _____

9. Severity of illness, age, and type of stoma are significant factors in poor psychosocial adjustment.
   True _____ False _____
10. List three risk factors that can be related to postoperative psychologic problems.

Answers

1. c
2. (a) The ability to feel they have control of their body; (b) the ability to deal with stoma care; (c) the impact of living with the stoma and its effect on intimacy and sexual function; (d) the issue of odor and noise control
3. True
4. Body image can be defined as a cognitive structure that represents previous appearance-related experience and serves as a template to recall information regarding self-evaluation about one's appearance.
5. b
6. Start by providing the most important information first. Stressing the importance of information, categorizing the information, and repeating the categories as information giving progresses will increase recall. Repetition of material increases recall and has beneficial effects on satisfaction.
7. True
8. False; 18% to 26%
9. False
10. Cognitive factors, past psychiatric history, problems with leakage of pouch and prolapse, and peristomal skin problems

REFERENCES

Baider L, de Nour A: Psychological distress and intrusive thoughts in cancer patients, *J Nervous Ment Dis* 185(5):346-348, 1997.

Bekkers NJTM et al: Prospect of evaluation of psychosocial adaptation to stoma surgery: the role of self-efficacy; *Psychosom Med* 58:183-191, 1996.

Black PK: Colostomy, *Professional Nurse* 13:851-857, 1998.

Borwell B: Psychological considerations of stoma care nursing, *Nurs Standard* 11(48):49-53, 1997.

Bridges KW, Goldberg DP: Psychiatric illness in in-patients with neurological disorders: patients' views on discussion of emotional problems with neurologists, *Br Med J* 286:656-658, 1984.

Faulkener A, Maguire P: *Talking to cancer patients and their relatives,* Oxford, 1994, Oxford Medical.

Feldman E et al: Psychiatric disorder in medical inpatients, *QJ Med* 63:405-412, 1987.

Fisher S: The evolution of psychological concepts about the body. In Cash TF, Pruzinsky T, editors: *Body images: development deviance and change,* New York, 1990, Guildford Press.

Follick MJ, Smith TW, Turk DC: Psychosocial adjustment following ostomy, *Health Psychol* 3:505-517, 1984.

Goldberg D: *General health questionnaire (GHQ-12),* Windsor, 1992, NFER-NELSON.

Hall A, Hern RA, Fallowfield L: Are we using appropriate self report questionnaires for detecting anxiety and depression in women with early breast cancer? *Eur J Cancer* 15:79-85, 1999.

Johnston M, Vogele C: Benefits of psychological preparation for surgery: a meta-analysis, *Ann Behav Med* 15:245-256, 1993.

Leahy R: *Cognitive therapy: basic principles and applications,* Northvale, NJ, 1997, Jason Aronson.

Ley P, Llewelyn S: Improving patients' understanding, recall, satisfaction and compliance. In Broome A, Llewelyn S, editors: *Health psychology: processes and applications,* ed 2, London, 1995, Chapman & Hall.

Mayou RA, Hawton KE: Psychiatric disorders in the general hospital, *Br J Psychiatry* 149:172-190, 1986.

McVey J, Madill A, Fielding D: The relevance of lowered personal control for patients who have stoma surgery to treat cancer, *Br J Clin Psychol* 40:337-360, 2001.

Oberst MT, Scott DW: Postdischarge distress in surgically treated cancer patients and their spouses, *Res Nurs Health* 11:223-233, 1988.

Rubin GP, Devlin HB: The quality of life with a stoma, *Brit J Hosp Med* 38:300-306, 1987.

Thomas C, Madden F, Jehu D: Psychosocial morbidity in the first three months following stoma surgery, *J Psychosom Res* 28:251-257, 1984.

Thomas C, Madden F, Jehu D: Psychological effects of stomas – II: Factors influencing outcome, *J Psychosom Res* 31:317-323, 1987.

Wade BE: Colostomy patients: psychological adjustment at 10 weeks and 1 year after surgery in districts which employed stoma-care nurses and districts which did not, *J Adv Nurs* 15:1297-1304, 1990.

White CA, Hunt JC: Psychological factors in postoperative adjustment to stoma surgery, *Ann R Coll Surg Engl* 79(1):3-7, 1997.

White CA, Unwin JC: Postoperative adjustment to surgery resulting in the formation of a stoma: the importance of stoma-related cognitions, *Br J Health for Psychol* 3:85-93, 1998.

White CA: *Living with a stoma. A practical guide to coping with colostomy, ileostomy or urostomy,* London, 1997, Sheldon Press.

White CA: Body image in oncology. In Cash T, Pruzinsky T, editors: *Body image: a handbook of theory, research, and clinical practice,* New York, 2002, Guildford Press.

White CA (unpublished): *Pouch change and disposal study:* Final Report.

Zigmond AS, Snaith RP: The Hospital Anxiety and Depression Scale, *Acta Psychiatr Scand* 67:361-370, 1983.

RESOURCES

Maguire P, and Haddad: Psychological reactions to physical illness. In Creed F, Guthrie E, editors: *Seminars in liaison psychiatry,* London, 1996, Gaskell Press.

(Although originally written for trainee psychiatrists and medical students, this chapter provides a general introduction to the many issues that are relevant to the assessment and management of psychosocial aspects of medicine and surgery.)

White CA: *Positive options in living with your ostomy,* Alameda, 2002, Hunter House Publications.

Leahy R: *Cognitive therapy. Basic principles and applications,* Northvale, NJ, 1997, Jason Aronson.

PART

V

RELATED ISSUES

16 *Medications Affecting Ostomy Function*

·····························

GILBERT J. CUSSON

OBJECTIVES

1. List three oral preparations that are thought to control fecal and, in some instances, urinary odor.
2. Discuss factors that the person with an ileostomy should take into account when considering enteric or coated medications.
3. Define the action of antidiarrheal agents.
4. List two commonly used antidiarrheal medications and their recommended dosages.
5. Describe the potentially detrimental effect of broad-spectrum antibiotics in the person with an ostomy.
6. Explain the interaction of urinary acidifiers and antibiotics in the person with a urostomy.
7. Identify the potential side effects to the person with an ostomy of sodium bicarbonate antacids, calcium carbonate-containing antacids, and magnesium-containing antacids.
8. Discuss the types of drugs that can cause constipation in the person with a colostomy.
9. Name one bulk-forming laxative agent and one osmotic laxative.
10. Differentiate between the following antiflatulents: simethicone and alpha-galactosidase (e.g., Beano).

INTRODUCTION

This chapter discusses ingested substances that can affect the appearance and odor of the stoma output, the effects of medications on stoma functioning, medications that can alter the consistency of stool and/or urine, and classes of medications, including antidiarrheals, laxatives, and antiflatulents and other medications or substances as they relate to stoma functioning.

INTERNAL DEODORIZERS

Most ostomy pouching systems are odor-resistant. Deodorizing options can be considered to decrease the amount of odor that is released upon emptying the pouch, rather than for "covering" odor while the pouch is in place. If the person with a fecal or a urinary pouch detects an odor when the pouch is sealed, this indicates pouch adhesion failure or failure to thoroughly clean the drainage area of the pouching system. Internal agents that have been used to deodorize the fecal or the urinary output include bismuth subgallate 200 mg (e.g., Devrom), charcoal 260 mg (e.g., Charco Caps), and chlorophyllin copper complex 100 mg (e.g., Derifil) (Beart and Curlee, 1978; PDR, 1998).

Bismuth subgallate is a heavy metal, and the mechanism of deodorizing action is unknown. It is usually used in doses of 200 mg before each meal and at bedtime. Bismuth subgallate decreases peristaltic activity and causes a dark coloration of the stool. Long-term use has been associated with general malaise, lack of energy, and peculiar sensations in the fingers and toes; however, these side effects disappear when the drug is discontinued. It is thought that charcoal reduces fecal odor by reducing the malodor of intestinal gas. Suarez et al (1999) studied the efficacy of ingested activated charcoal to reduce the release of gas by colonic flora. They reported that activated charcoal produced no significant reduction in fecal gas and suggested that this is explained by the saturation of the charcoal during passage through the gut. A study examining the effect of fecal odor reduction in patients with colostomies found no evidence of decreased odor (Christiansen et al, 1989). Charcoal will turn the stool dark and can cause constipation. Chlorophyllin may have a laxative effect and can turn the stool green (Selekof, 2002). Chlorophyllin has been reported to control body and fecal odor (Young and Beregi, 1980). The U.S. Food and Drug Administration Advisory Review Panel on over-the-counter drugs has suggested that chlorophyllin is safe in oral doses up to 100 mg tid (Egner et al, 2001).

DRUG ABSORPTION IN THE PERSON WITH AN OSTOMY

Many factors can influence how well a medication is absorbed within the normal gastrointestinal tract, and these factors can be significantly altered in the person with a fecal diversion. The most important consideration for the person with an ostomy is the length of small bowel available for drug absorption. Persons with ileostomies and those with transverse colostomies associated with excessive gastrointestinal motility and high output should avoid enteric-coated and sustained-release products because of their slow dissolution properties (Schwartz, 1986). In this population, the amount of drug absorption may be inadequate. In general, persons with distal colostomies probably absorb drugs as well as persons without stomas. Prompt-acting dosage forms such as solutions, suspensions, gelatin capsules, and uncoated tablets are usually well absorbed and well tolerated in people with ileostomies. Crushing tablets into a powder is an effective way of improving dissolution and absorption. The person with an ostomy should be counseled to monitor for signs of drug malabsorption by checking the pouch for remnants of the drug whenever new drugs are prescribed. Table 16-1 lists selected prescription drugs and their potential to cause adverse effects in persons with an ostomy.

Some newer drugs on the market are packaged in acid-stable microspheres (e.g., pancreatic enzymes,

lansoprazole [e.g., Prevacid], and omeprazole [e.g., Prilosec]), which will not break up in the acidic pH of the stomach but will disintegrate only in the alkaline milieu of the small intestine. This form of drug may be erratically absorbed in some people with short bowel syndrome or pancreatic insufficiency with loss of bicarbonate secretion.

THE INS AND OUTS OF DRUG THERAPY IN THE PERSON WITH AN OSTOMY

The pharmacologic effects of certain drug classes are of major importance for persons with a colostomy, ileostomy, and/or urostomy. Drug categories to be addressed include antidiarrheal agents, antibiotics, antacids, laxative agents, and antiflatulents.

Antidiarrheal Agents

Antidiarrheals have the pharmacological effect of slowing intestinal peristalsis and may be effective in providing relief from loose stools and decreasing ostomy output. The most frequently used antidiarrheal agents are diphenoxylate and atropine (e.g., Lomotil) which is only available by prescription, and loperamide (e.g., Imodium) which is an over-the-counter medication. Diphenoxylate is a synthetic opioid agonist that inhibits intestinal peristalsis by acting on mucosal receptors responsible for peristalsis. The usual dosage of Lomotil is 2.5 to 5 mg qid titrated to patient response, not exceeding 20 mg per day (8 tablets). Lomotil is available in 2.5-mg tablets and liquid form (2.5 mg/5 ml). Loperamide is a synthetic opioid agonist that exerts its antidiarrheal effects by stimulating mu opioid receptors located on the intestinal circular muscles. Other pharmacologic actions of loperamide include disruption of cholingeric and noncholinergic mechanisms involved in peristaltic regulation, inhibition of calmodulin function, and inhibition of voltage-dependent calcium channels (Daly and Harper, 2000). In its gastrointestinal motility effects, loperamide is approximately fiftyfold more potent than morphine and 2 to 3 times more potent than diphenoxylate. The usual dosage of loperamide is 4 mg initially, then

TABLE 16-1 Potential Effects of Selected Prescription Drugs in Patients with Ostomies

AGENT	POTENTIAL PROBLEMS	TYPE OF OSTOMY	COMMENTS
Histamine₁-Receptor Antagonists			
Cetirizine (Zyrtec) Loratidine (Claritin) Fexofenadine (Allegra)	No known problems for these agents	Ileostomy, colostomy, urostomy	
Analgesics			
Celecoxib (Celebrex)	No known problems	Ileostomy, colostomy	NSAIDs are associated with GI irritation and bleeding. COX-2 inhibitors may have a lower-risk profile. Use caution in patients with history of GI ulceration or bleeding.
Tramadol (Ultram)	Constipation		Tramadol has opiate agonist activity and, similar to oxycodone, can cause constipation.
Oxycodone (Oxycontin)	Constipation; ER formulations may exhibit erratic absorption		ER products have been associated with erratic absorption in the ostomate. Oxycontin is an ER tablet form of oxycodone. General recommendations are to avoid these formulations and use liquids or immediate-release products.
Selective Serotonin-Reuptake Inhibitors			
Sertraline (Zoloft)	No known problems	Ileostomy	
Paroxetine (Paxil)	Hyponatremia; diarrhea/loose stools		Monitor fluid and electrolyte status closely while on Paxil.
Citalopram (Celexa)	No known problems		
Fluoxetine (Prozac)	No known problems		
Antipsychotics			
Olanzapine (Zyprexa)	Constipation	Colostomy	Anticholinergic activity of olanzapine is associated with constipation.
Risperidone (Risperdal)	No known problems		
Antidiabetics			
Metformin (Glucophage)	Diarrhea	Ileostomy	Metformin can cause dose-related GI effects. As a weak base, metformin is primarily absorbed in the small intestine, which may have variable absorption in ileostomates.
Rosiglitazone (Avandia)	No known problems		
Pioglitazone (Actos)	No known problems		

ACE, angiotensin converting enzyme; *CSA*, cyclosporine; *ER*, extended-release; *GI*, gastrointestinal; *NSAIDS*, nonsteroidal antiinflammatory drugs; *SR*, sustained-release; *Vd*, volume of distribution.

Continued

TABLE 16-1   **Potential Effects of Selected Prescription Drugs in Patients with Ostomies—cont'd**

AGENT	POTENTIAL PROBLEMS	TYPE OF OSTOMY	COMMENTS
Anticonvulsants			
Divalproex Na (Depakote)	Erratic absorption of enteric-coated and SR formulations	Ileostomy	Enteric-coated and SR products have resulted in erratic absorption in ileostomates. General recommendations are to avoid these formulations and use liquids or immediate-release preparations.
Antilipidemics			
Atorvastatin (Lipitor)	No known problems for these agents	Ileostomy, colostomy, urostomy	
Simvastatin (Zocor) Pravastatin (Pravachol)			
Cardiac/Hypertensive Medications			
Amlodipine (Norvasc)	No known problems	Ileostomy	Fluid and electrolyte abnormalities are common in ileostomates. Careful monitoring is recommended while on ACE inhibitors.
Lisinopril (Zestril, Prinivil)	Hyperkalemia		
Quinapril (Accupril)	Hyperkalemia		
GI Medications			
Omeprazole (Prilosec)	No known problems	Ileostomy, colostomy	
Lansoprazole (Prevacid)	Diarrhea		Diarrhea may occur more often with use of Prevacid. Monitor fluid and electrolyte status in ileostomy patients.
Famotidine (Pepcid)	No known problems		
Antimicrobial Agents			
Amoxicillin/ clavulanate (Augmentin)	Diarrhea (Augmentin, Cipro, Zithromax, Combivir)	Ileostomy, urostomy, colostomy	Broad-spectrum antibiotics have the propensity to alter normal bowel flora and cause diarrhea, which can be a significant problem for patients with ileostomies.
Ciprofloxacin (Cipro)	Crystalluria (Cipro)		Crystalluria with Cipro is associated with an alkaline urine and high doses. Urinary acidification, a process used to avoid bacterial overgrowth in urostomy patients, should be monitored carefully.
Azithromycin (Zithromax)			
Fluconazole (Diflucan)	No known problems with Diflucan		

TABLE 16-1   Potential Effects of Selected Prescription Drugs in Patients with Ostomies—cont'd

AGENT	POTENTIAL PROBLEMS	TYPE OF OSTOMY	COMMENTS
Lamivudine/ zidovudine (Combivir)			
Selected Agents for Therapeutic Drug Monitoring			
Warfarin (Coumadin)	Hypoprothrom- binemia	End jejunostomy, ileostomy	Some reports of drug failure associated with malabsorption of warfarin in patients with short-bowel syndrome
Cyclosporine (CSA, Sandimmune)	Possible delayed absorption of capsules		Length of functionally intact proximal small bowel is important in dosing of CSA. Liquid formulation or IV may be required. More frequent monitoring is recommended.
Gentamicin (various)	Increase clearance; variable Vd		Variable Vd and increased clearance of gentamicin has been reported in patients with ileostomies. More frequent monitoring may be required.
Digoxin (Lanozin, others)	Variable absorption		Bioavailability of digoxin is highly variable, depending on length of remaining bowel. Monitor for drug failure.

From Selekov JL: Ostomy care and suppliers. In Berardi RR, editor: *Handbook of nonprescription drugs*, ed 13, Washington, DC, 2002, American Psychiatric Association.
ACE, Angiotensin converting enzyme; *CSA*, cyclosporine; *ER*, extended-release; *GI*, gastrointestinal; *NSAIDs*, nonsteroidal antiinflammatory drugs; *SR*, sustained-release; *Vd*, volume of distribution.

2 mg after each loose stool, not to exceed 16 mg/day. A person with an ileostomy (with concomitant high output) will generally take 4 mg with each meal and, if necessary, 4 mg at bedtime.

Other antidiarrheals include opium preparations, which decrease intestinal motility by stimulating mu opioid receptors. Camphorated tincture of opium (e.g., Paregoric) and deodorized tincture of opium (DTO) both require prescriptions, but DTO is a class II narcotic and requires close regulation by the U.S. Drug Enforcement Administration. The usual dosage of Paregoric is 5 to 10 ml qid. DTO is dosed at 0.6 ml qid and can be diluted in water and taken with food: 1 ml DTO = 10 mg morphine. It is essential to be extremely vigilant when using the opium tinctures of these two products, which have been mistaken for each other: DTO is 25 times more potent than Paregoric.

Lomotil and Imodium have not been associated with physical dependence. However, chronic use of opium derivatives (e.g., Paregoric and DTO) may result in physical dependence, and long-term use should be avoided. Patients with extensive short-bowel syndrome and high output may require DTO therapy long-term. Octreotide acetate (i.e., Sandostatin) has been used to control excessive ostomy output not controlled adequately with the aforementioned antidiarrheal agents (American Hospital Formulary Service, 2003). The major disadvantages of Sandostatin are that it requires parenteral administrations (subcutaneously, intravenous push, or continuous infusion), is very expensive, and has a short duration of action. The correct dosage depends on the cause of the high output (e.g., an adult with a gastrointestinal fistula may receive 50 to 200 µg every 8 hours. An initial subcutaneous dose of 50 µg is given qd or bid, and the dose is titrated based on patient tolerance and response. The initial intravenous dose is 50 to 100 µg every 8 hours, increased by 100 µg/dose at 48-hour intervals to achieve a maximum dose of 500 µg every 8 hours.

Other agents used to treat high output from the small intestine are methylcellulose and psyllium (e.g., Metamucil), which work by adding bulk to the stool (American Hospital Formulary Service, 2003). The water content of the stool is decreased; the methylcellulose dosage for adults is 60 to 120 ml, according to the consistency and volume of the fecal output. Psyllium forms fecal bulk; the dose is administered by mixing the powder in liquid, in chewable pieces, or in wafer form, and is generally given up to three times per day. Drugs that have been associated with causing diarrhea are listed in Table 16-2.

Antibiotics

Diarrhea caused by broad-spectrum antibiotics is a major concern to the person with an ostomy. Broad-spectrum antibiotics may significantly alter the normal bacterial flora of the intestinal tract, and this can result in diarrhea, which can rapidly cause dehydration. Antibiotic-associated diarrhea (AAD) may be caused by an overgrowth of antibiotic-resistant bacteria, fungi, or toxin-producing

Clostridium difficile. All antibiotics, including metronidazole and vancomycin, have been associated with *C. difficile* overgrowth and diarrhea; however, clindamycin, ampicillin, amoxicillin, and the cephalosporins are most frequently associated with this disorder. *C. difficile* produces enterotoxins A and B. Enterotoxin A is the primary cause of the secretory diarrhea associated with *C. difficile,* and it is also cytotoxic to enterocytes. Toxin B is not enterotoxic, but it is a potent cytotoxin that causes the release of proinflammatory mediators and cytokines. Both toxins are necessary to cause the full tissue damage that characterizes AAD (Mylonakis, Ryan, and Calderwood, 2001). The secretory diarrhea usually starts during antibiotic treatment, but it can begin up to 4 weeks after the antibiotic has been discontinued. Treatment necessitates discontinuing the offending antibiotic and prescribing an appropriate alternative antibiotic. Metronidazole is the preferred initial antibiotic because it costs less than vancomycin; also, there is a lower propensity of the person to develop vancomycin-resistant enterococcus infection. In adults, metronidazole is given orally at a dosage of 500 mg tid for 10 to 14 days.

Antibiotic therapy in the person with a urostomy has different implications. Sulfa-containing antibiotics including sulfisoxazole (i.e., Ganstrisin),

TABLE 16-2   Medications that cause Diarrhea

MEDICATION/ACTION	BRAND NAMES
Antibiotics	Numerous
Metoclopramide/prokinetic	Reglan
Lactulose	Cephulac
Digitalis	Digitoxin
	Digoxin
Guanethidine/antihypertensive	Ismelin
Lithium carbonate/antipsychotic	Eskalith, Lithane
Magnesium salts/laxative	Milk of Magnesia
Phosphate salts	Neutraphos, Fleet Phospho-soda
Methyldopa/antihypertensive	Aldomet
	Amodopar
Reserpine/antihypertensive	Serpasil
Sulfasalazine/antiinflammatory	Azulfidine

sulfamethoxazole (e.g., Gantenol), and trimethoprim/sulfamethoxozole (e.g., Septra, Bactrim), can cause crystallization in the urine if high concentrations are reached, or in the presence of an acidic urine (Schwartz, 1986). Since urostomy patients may be using urinary acidifiers to prevent encrustations and urinary tract infection, they are at increased risk for developing sulfa crystals in the kidneys and ureters. Increasing fluid intake by 2 to 3 L per day can minimize the risk of crystallization. Patients taking urinary acidifiers should discontinue them during treatment with sulfa-containing antibiotics (Karlstrand, 1977). Vitamin C (ascorbic acid) has been used for urinary acidification in urostomy patients at dosages of 1 to 2 g 4 to 6 times a day around the clock to achieve an ideal urinary pH of <6.5. Ascorbic acid should be discontinued in the presence of sulfa antibiotics, as mentioned. Isolated cases of impaired warfarin (e.g., Coumadin) response associated with large doses of ascorbic acid (≥10g/day) have been reported, but this effect has not been confirmed. Box 16-1 lists medications that can discolor feces and urine.

Antacids

The antacid of choice for the person with an ostomy depends largely on the type of ostomy and the person's individual gastrointestinal response to the particular antacid. Sodium bicarbonate antacids (e.g., Alka-Seltzer, Bromo Seltzer, baking soda) may result in alkalinization of the urine, which is undesirable in the person with a urostomy because it increases the risk of urinary tract infection and encrustation (Karlstrand, 1977). Calcium carbonate-containing antacids (e.g., Tums, Titralac) should be used with caution in the urostomy patient (because of the risk of calcium stone formation) and colostomy patient (because of the risk of constipation) (Karlstrand, 1977). Magnesium-containing antacids such as Milk of Magnesia

BOX 16-1 Selected Drugs That Discolor Feces and Urine

Drugs That Discolor Feces	
Black	Hydralazine
Acetazolamide	Iodide-containing drugs
Aluminum hydroxide	Iron
Aminophylline	Levodopa
Amphetamine	Melphalan
Amphotericin B[*]	Methotrexate
Anticoagulants[*]	Nitrates
Aspirin[*]	Nonsteroidal antiinflammatory
Barium	drugs[*]
Bismuth	Phenylephrine
Charcoal	Potassium salts[*]
Chloramphenicol	Procarbazine
Chlorpropamide	Sulfonamides
Cholestyramine	Tetracycline
Clindamycin	Thallium
Corticosteroids	Theophylline
Cyclophosphamide	Thiotepa[*]
Cytarabine	**Blue**
Digitalis	Chloramphenicol
Ethacrynic acid	Methylene blue
Fluorouracil	**Gray**
	Colchicine

From Selekof JL: Ostomy care and suppliers. In Berardi RR, editor: *Handbook of nonprescription drugs*, ed 13, Washington, DC, 2002, American Pharmaceutical Association.
[*]Discoloration may be caused by bleeding.
[†]Discoloration caused by nonabsorbable complex between cefdinir or metabolites and iron in the gastrointestinal tract.

Continued

BOX 16-1   Selected Drugs That Discolor Feces and Urine—cont'd

Green
Chlorophyllin copper complex
Indomethacin
Iron
Medroxyprogesterone
Pancrelipase

Drugs That Discolor Feces
Green-Gray
Oral antibiotics
Orange-Red
Phenazopyridine
Rifampin
Rifapentine
Orange-Brown
Rifabutin
Pink-Red
Anticoagulants[*]
Aspirin[*]
Barium
Cefdinir[†]
Nonsteroidal antiinflammatory drugs[*]
Tetracycline syrup
Red to Brown-Black
Clofazimine
White or speckled
Aluminum hydroxide
Barium
Oral antibiotics
Yellow or Yellow-Green
Senna

Drugs That Discolor Urine
Black
Cascara
Ferrous salts
Phenacetin
Blue or Green
Amitriptyline
Cimetidine (injection)
Flutamide
Methocarbamol
Mitoxantrone
Promethazine (injection)
Propofol (injection)

Triamterene
Dark
Metronidazole
Phenacetin
Orange
Chlorzoxazone
Phenazopyridine
Warfarin[*]
Orange-Red
Phenazopyridine
Rifampin
Pink-Red
Phenothiazine
Phenytoin
Purplish-Red
Chlorzoxazone
Red
Daunorubicin
Dimethylsulfoxide
Doxorubicin
Idarubicin
Red-Brown
Aloe
Levodopa
Methyldopa
Phenothiazines
Phenytoin
Warfarin[*]
Violet
Senna
Yellow
Aloe
Riboflavin
Vitamin B_{12}
Yellow-Brown
Cascara
Nitrofurantoin
Senna
Sulfonamides
Yellow-Orange
Vitamin A
Yellow-Pink
Casara

---

[*]Discoloration may be caused by bleeding.
[†]Discoloration caused by nonabsorbable complex between cefdinir or metabolites and iron in the gastrointestinal tract.

(magnesium hyrdoxide) may cause diarrhea in the person with an ileostomy, whereas aluminum hydroxide-containing antacids (e.g., Amphogel, Alternagel) may cause constipation. Altering the type of antacid based on side effects may be necessary for persons with ostomies to help tailor specific therapeutic manipulations to the person's needs.

Laxative Agents

Laxatives can be either beneficial or extremely harmful, depending on the types of ostomy and laxative. Laxatives are classified by their mechanism of action on the colon (Table 16-3).

Laxatives should never be used by a person with an ileostomy because of the potential for severe dehydration and electrolyte imbalance (American Hospital Formulary Service, 2003). A person with a colostomy and constipation should undergo an assessment to identify the causative factors (i.e., insufficient fluid and/or fiber intake, slow transit, and whether neurologic, metabolic, or medication-induced) (Table 16-4). Narcotic analgesics can cause constipation in the colostomy population because of their pharmacologic property of slowing intestinal peristalsis. Narcotic analgesics include natural and synthetic opioid derivatives such as meperidine (e.g., Demerol), morphine (e.g., MS Contin,

TABLE 16-3   Laxative Agents

MECHANISM OF ACTION	AGENTS/BRAND NAMES
Osmotic Laxatives	
Hypertonic solutions of nonabsorbable salts that attract or retain water in the lumen of the colon, distending the bowel and promoting contractions	Magnesium Citrate
	Magnesium Hydroxide (Milk of Magnesia)
	Sodium phosphate (Fleet Phospho-soda)
Rapid onset of action (30 minutes to 3 hours)	Polyethylene glycol lavage solution (GoLytely, Colyte)
The osmotic laxatives containing magnesium or phosphate are contraindicated in renal failure patients.	Unabsorbed carbohydrate (lactulose and sorbitol)
Stimulant Laxatives	
Solutions that increase the motor activity of the colon by direct irritation of the mucosa or by selective action in the intramural nerve plexus of the intestinal wall	Cascara Sagrada
	Senna (Fletcher's Castoria, Senokot)
	Phenolphthalein (Correctol, Ex-Lax)
Increase propulsion of the stool	Diphenylmethanes (Dulcolax)
Suggested not to be used long term	
Fiber Therapy	
Solutions that are natural or semisynthetic polysaccharides and cellulose derivatives that dissolve or swell in the intestinal fluids	Methylcellulose (Citrucel)
	Psyllium (Metamucil, Fibercon)
The bulkier stool produces distention, which should initiate peristalsis	Bran (bran cereals, wheat bran)
20 to 40 g of fiber is recommended for patients with constipation	
Stool Softeners	
Products that are surfactants, which promote water retention in the stool by increasing the wetting efficiency of intestinal water	Docusate Sodium (Colace)
	Pericolace (combination stool softener and stimulant laxative)

Oramorph), hydromorphine (e.g., Dilaudid), pentazocine (i.e., Talwin), oxycodone (e.g., Percodan), codeine, and propoxyphene (i.e., Darvon). Persons with a colostomy can safely use the bulk-forming agents (e.g., psyllium, methylcellulose, bran), whereas the fast-acting, harsher stimulant laxatives (e.g., bisacodyl, senna) should be used with caution or not al all (Karlstrand, 1977). The osmotic agents magnesium hydroxide (e.g., Milk of Magnesia), magnesium citrate (e.g., Crystal), and sodium phosphate (e.g., Fleet Phospho-soda) can be used as a second-line therapy, if poor results are noted with the bulk-forming laxatives (Doughty, 2002).

Antiflatulents

Antiflatulents work by dispersing mucus-surrounded gas pockets in the gastrointestinal tract, as well as preventing their formation. Simethicone acts in the stomach and intestine to change the sur-

face tension of gas bubbles, enabling them to coalesce and thus making the gas easier to pass by means of belching. The usual dosage of simethicone (e.g., Mylanta Gas, Phazyme) is 80 mg tid to qid. There is no systemic absorption of simethicone.

The food enzyme called alpha-galactosidase is available as a dietary supplement (e.g., Beano) that helps to prevent gas by digesting the indigestible carbohydrate (raffinose) contained in beans and some vegetables. Beano breaks down the complex sugars in gassy foods, making them more digestible. Beano thus prevents gas related to complex sugars but has no effect on gas associated with other carbohydrates, such as sorbitol, lactose, wheat, and fiber. It cannot be added to food while it is being cooked, since heat degrades the enzyme. Beano is added to food before eating by putting 5 or more drops directly into the serving.

TABLE 16-4   Medications That Can Cause Constipation

MEDICATION CLASS	GENERIC/BRAND NAMES (EXAMPLES)
β-adrenergic blockers	Atenolol/Tenormin
	Propranol/Inderal
Aluminum hydroxide antacids	Aluminum hydroxide/AlternaGEL
	Aluminum hydroxide/Amphojel
Antidepressants: tricyclic	Amitriptyline/Amitril
	Amitriptyline/Elavil
	Imipramine/Trofranil
	Nortriptyline/Pamelor
Anticholinergics	Atropine
	Dicyclomine/Bentyl
Antiparkinsonism preparations	Levodopa/Dopar
	Carbidopa/Sinemet
Benztropine	Cogentin
Calcium carbonate/antacid, calcium supplement	Tums E-X Strength
	Titralac
	Caltrate 600
Iron	$FeSO_4$/Feosol
	FeGluconate/Fergon
Opiates	Codeine, Morphine/MS Contin,
	Oramorph
	Meperidine/Demerol
	Hydromorphone/Dilaudid,
Oxycodone	Percodan
Phenothiazines	Chlorpromazine/Thorazine

CONCLUSION

The wound, ostomy, and continence/enterostomal therapy nurse and the pharmacist must be aware of the potential problems and pitfalls of drug therapy in the person with an ostomy and should take great care to educate the person in self-monitoring and drug therapy awareness. If possible the person with an ostomy should choose a pharmacy whose staff is knowledgeable in the use of drugs in patients with fecal and urinary diversions, and should ensure that the pharmacist is made aware of his or her surgical history. In addition, anyone with an ostomy should monitor the effects of any and all medications and should be encouraged to relate this information to the physician, the wound, ostomy, and continence/enterostomal therapy nurse and the pharmacist.

SELF-ASSESSMENT EXERCISES

Questions

1. Chlorophyllin used as a deodorizing agent has the following side effect:
   a. After 10 days of use, can cause dizziness
   b. Can turn the stool green
   c. Will cause the stool to become loose
   d. May cause excessive flatus
2. Persons with ileostomies and those with transverse colostomies associated with excessive gastrointestinal motility and high output should avoid:
   a. Enteric-coated and sustained-release products because of their slow dissolution properties.
   b. The use of powdered medications.
   c. Drinking orange juice and taking enteric-coated medications because of the high acidity.
   d. All of the above.
3. Name one form of drug that may be erratically absorbed in some people with short bowel syndrome.
4. The mechanism of action of antidiarrheals is:
   a. Adding bulk to the small intestine.
   b. Slowing peristalsis.

   c. Providing an absorptive surface that decreases fluid in the stool.
   d. Causing a craving for salty foods.
5. Which of the following antidiarrheals is available by prescription only?
   a. Imodium
   b. Lomotil
6. Deodorized tincture of opium is 25% more potent than Paregoric.
   True _____ False _____
7. Name two disadvantages of using octreotide acetate (i.e., Sandostatin).
8. Define the mechanism of action of methylcellulose and psyllium.
9. What is the preferred initial antibiotic in the treatment of *C. difficile*?
10. What is the recommended dosage of vitamin C (ascorbic acid) when used for urinary acidification in urostomy patients?
    a. 1 to 2 g four to six times per day around the clock
    b. 1 to 2 g bid
    c. 4 to 6 g one to two times per day around the clock
    d. 2 g taken at mealtime
11. Which of the following antacids can cause constipation in the person with a colostomy?
    a. Sodium bicarbonate antacids
    b. Calcium carbonate-containing antacids
    c. Magnesium-containing antacids
12. What is the mechanism of action of osmotic laxatives?
    a. They attract or retain water in the lumen of the colon, distending the bowel and promoting contractions.
    b. They increase the motor activity of the colon by direct irritation of the mucosa.
    c. They are natural or semisynthetic polysaccharides and cellulose derivatives that dissolve or swell in the intestinal fluids.
    d. They are surfactants, which promote water retention in the stool by increasing the wetting efficiency of intestinal water.
13. Describe how the antiflatulent simethicone works.

14. What is the mechanism of action of alpha-galactosidase (Beano)?

Answers

1. b

2. a

3. Drugs that are packaged in acid-stable microspheres may be erratically absorbed in some people with short bowel syndrome.

4. b

5. b

6. True

7. Sandostatin requires parenteral administrations (subcutaneously, intravenous push, or continuous infusion), is very expensive, and has a short duration of action.

8. Methylcellulose and psyllium work by adding bulk to the stool.

9. Metronidazole

10. a

11. b

12. a

13. Simethicone acts in the stomach and intestine to change the surface tension of gas bubbles, enabling them to coalesce, thus making the gas easier to pass by means of belching.

14. Beano breaks down the complex sugars in gassy foods, making them more digestible.

REFERENCES

American Hospital Formulary Service, Bethesda, 2003, American Society of Health System Pharmacist.

Beart RW, Curlee F: Intestinal stomas: managing the unmentionable, *Geriatrics* 33:45, 1978.

Christiansen S et al: Can chlorophyll reduce fecal odor in colostomy patients? *Ugeskr Laeger* 151:175-333, 1989.

Daly JW, Harper J: Loperamide novel effects on capacitative calcium influx, *Cell Mol Life Sci* 57:149-157, 2000.

Doughty D: When fiber is not enough: current thinking on constipation management, *OWM* 48:30, 2002.

Egner P et al: Chlorophyllin intervention reduces aflatoxin-DNA adducts in individuals at high risk for liver cancer, *Proceedings of the National Academy of Science* 98:14601, 2001.

Karlstrand J: The pharmacist and the ostomate, *J Am Pharm Assoc* 17:735, 1977.

Mylonakis E, Ryan ET, Calderwood SB: *Clostridium difficile* associated diarrhea, *Arch Intern Med* 161:525-533, 2001.

PDR: *Physician's Desk Reference for Nonprescription Drugs*, ed 19, Montoale, NJ, 1998, Blackwell.

Selekof JL: Ostomy care products and supplies. In Berardi RR, editor: *Handbook of Nonprescription Drugs*, ed 13, Washington, DC, 2002, APhA.

Suarez F et al: Failure of activated charcoal to reduce the release of gases produced by the colonic flora, *Am J Gastroenterol* 94:208, 1999.

Schwartz NJ: Drug therapy with the ostomy patient, *J Enterostom Ther* 13:157, 1986.

Young RW, Beregi JS: Use of chlorophyllin in the care of geriatric patients, *J Am Geriatr Soc* 28:46, 1980.

17 *Tube Management*

••••••••••••••••••••••••••••••

JANE E. CARMEL and JODY SCARDILLO

OBJECTIVES

1. Explain the main indications for placement of gastrointestinal tubes.
2. Describe three types of procedures for placement of an enteral feeding tube.
3. Describe the advantages of a percutaneous versus a surgical gastrostomy tube placement.
4. Identify indications for placement of a percutaneous jejunostomy tube.
5. List four complications of enteral feeding tubes.
6. Describe appropriate management of each complication.
7. List disadvantages of the use of a Foley catheter for gastrostomy feedings.
8. Discuss strategies to prevent leakage around tubes.
9. Describe commonly used drains and tubes.
10. Relate management strategies for drainage tubes.
11. Describe skin complications associated with tracheostomy tubes.
12. Discuss a discharge plan for the patient on continuous enteral feedings.

INTRODUCTION

Over the past 10 years, nutritional management has been gradually recognized as playing an important role in patients' recovery. Poor nutrition has a profound effect on wound healing, development of pressure ulcers, infection, and longer length of stay in the hospital (Bowers, 2000). Nurses have long recognized the importance of good nutrition in the process of healing. As Florence Nightingale (1859) noted, "Every careful observer of the sick will agree in this that thousands of patients are annually starved in the midst of plenty from want of attention to the ways which alone make it possible for them to take food."

Maintenance of the gut's integrity in the critically ill patient has become an important aspect in the treatment plan. The gut is one of the largest immune organs in the body, and the degree to which the gut is used affects patient outcomes. Enteral feeding is superior to parenteral feeding. Aggressive enteral nutritional support plays an important role in successful patient recovery. In 1980, Alexander et al (1980) reported that high-protein enteral feeding improved survival and lowered the rate of sepsis in severely burned children. Kudsk (2001) found that 50% of the body's immunity that protects moist mucosal surfaces depends on enteral stimulation, as evidenced by the improved clinical outcome in enterally fed patients. Advantages of enteral nutrition are the physiologic promotion of mucosal growth and function, improvement of nutrient use, and a decrease in bacterial translocation. The contraindications for enteral nutrition are peritonitis, obstruction, ileus, vomiting, and enteral fistulas. Optimal care of critically ill patients requires achievement of early enteral access, as well as adequate infusion of enteral feedings for patients prone to ileus, aspiration, and intolerance.

This chapter includes a discussion of the indications for tube placement, the different types of enteral feeding tubes, the placement procedures, tube characteristics, nursing management, and common complications. Other types of tubes and drains that the nurse may encounter in the clinical settings are also discussed.

GASTROINTESTINAL FEEDING TUBES

Indications

The major indications for tube feedings are the inability to ingest sufficient nutrients by mouth, prolonged "nothing per mouth" status, and poor nutritional absorption (Martyn-Nemeth and Fitzgerald, 1992). Enteral access devices are placed after comprehensive assessment of the gastrointestinal tract's functional status, the risk for aspiration, and the estimated duration of enteral nutritional support. Enteral routes can be established by placement of a tube through the nose, the stomach, or the small intestine. Gastrostomy and jejunostomy devices are placed when enteral nutrition support is required long-term, generally more than 6 to 8 weeks (Lord, 1997). Between 1988 and 1995, Abukis et al (2000) reported that the number of gastrostomy procedures doubled for hospitalized patients, with most of these patients being elderly, debilitated, and chronically ill.

Enteral Access Options

The three methods that can be used to achieve enteral access include surgical placement, endoscopic placement, and radiologic placement. The location of the enterostomy may be at either the gastric or the jejunal level. The tube placed into the stomach is called a gastrostomy tube, and the tube placed into the jejunum is called a jejunostomy tube. The feeding tube may be temporary or permanent. Choosing the most appropriate type of feeding tube requires assessment of a number of factors, including the specific pathologic condition, the duration of the enteral feedings, the patient's level of consciousness, and the patient's ability to become independent in enteral tube feeding management.

Surgical Placement

Gastrostomy. There are several surgical techniques for placing the tube into the stomach. Common techniques are named Stamm, Witzel,

and Janeway. Surgical gastrostomy tubes are placed through the abdominal wall into the stomach.

The Stamm gastrostomy procedure was first performed in 1894 and is still widely used today. With the Stamm technique the wall of the stomach is affixed to the fascia of the anterior abdominal wall. This ensures that the stomach will remain in that position if the tube is inadvertently removed. An opening is made to allow the tube to be placed directly into the stomach, exiting through the abdominal wall. The Stamm technique helps greatly with replacement of the tube (Figure17-1, *A*).

The Witzel method involves involuting the wall of the stomach over a length of the tube. This procedure provides an additional 4 to 6 cm of seromuscular tunnel of the stomach wall through which to place the tube (Bryant, 2000). This technique helps to secure the tube in place. A tract is formed that makes tube replacement easy (Figure 17-1, *B*).

The Janeway method is rarely used today. This is a more difficult placement that includes suturing the gastric mucosa to the abdominal surface, creating a mucocutaneous stoma. During each feeding a tube is placed; it is removed once feeding is completed. This surgical gastrostomy requires longer operative time than the previous mentioned techniques. The Janeway procedure is indicated for long-term or permanent use.

Jejunostomy. There are some situations in which a jejunal feed is superior to a gastric feed. It is most commonly indicated when patients have a high aspiration risk, esophageal or gastric cancer, previous gastric, duodenal, or pancreatic surgery, or severe gastric paresis (Allen and Spain, 2001). The anatomic location of the jejunal tube is very important. It should be inserted approximately 40 cm from the ligament of Treitz. The Stamm and Witzel procedures just outlined can be used to surgically create a jejunostomy. The Stamm procedure is advocated by some surgeons to secure the jejunum to the abdominal wall. The Witzel tunnel may be created by involuting the wall of the jejunum over the tube.

Endoscopic Placement

Percutaneous Gastrostomy. The introduction of the percutaneous endoscopic gastrostomy (PEG)

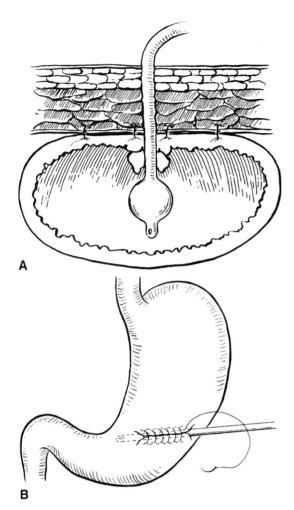

A

B

Figure 17-1 Gastrostomy site creation. **A**, Stamm technique. **B**, Witzel tunnel technique. (From Allen J, Spain D: Open and laparoscopic surgical techniques for obtaining enteral access, *Tech Gastrointest Endoscop* 3(1):51, 2001.)

in 1980 by Gauderer became widely accepted because of the advantage offered by its placement procedure. The advantage of placing the tube under local anesthesia and outside of the operating room, as compared to surgical placement, is that it does not necessitate general anesthesia, operating room time, or an abdominal incision. The procedure is faster, less invasive, less expensive, and requires less recovery time. The placement of a PEG depends on successful intubation of the esophagus

and stomach with an endoscope and safe passage of a needle and wire into the lumen of the stomach. The majority of review articles have validated the safety and cost-effectiveness of the PEG procedure (Baskin, 2001).

Contraindications for this procedure are esophageal stricture, head and neck malignancies, previous history of upper abdominal surgery that can distort the normal anatomy, significant gastroesophageal reflux, and inability to illuminate the abdominal wall (Cullen, 2001; Ganga, Ryan, and Schafer, 1994).

The patient receives conscious sedation and a topical pharyngeal anesthetic, and the endoscope is passed through the mouth into the stomach. The scope light transilluminates the abdominal wall at the level of the stoma site after the stomach is distended with air. A small (1-cm) incision is made into the abdomen after the site has been selected. A cannula needle is inserted through the abdominal incision into the stomach, and a guidewire is placed within the cannula after the needle is removed and then advanced into the stomach. The snare from the endoscope is closed over the guidewire, and the guidewire is grasped with the snare and retracted into the endoscope tip (Figure 17-2). The endoscope is withdrawn through the mouth, pulling the wire loop with it. Both the snare and the endoscope are removed. The loop end of the PEG tube is placed through the wire loop protruding from the mouth. The guidewire is pulled from the end that protrudes from the abdominal wall, facilitating passage of the feeding tube along with it through the mouth, esophagus, and stomach, until resistance is felt. The endoscope is passed again to check for proper position of the PEG. Once placement is confirmed, the endoscope is removed and the PEG external bumper is secured to the skin (Cullen, 2001). This is known as the *Ponsky pull technique.* The PEG tube does not have a fluid-filled balloon; the stomach end has an internal bumper to prevent outward migration. A similar *Sachs-Vine push endoscopic technique* can also be used. A scope is passed into the stomach, and a small incision is made externally at the selected site for the feeding tube. An angiocatheter is placed through the

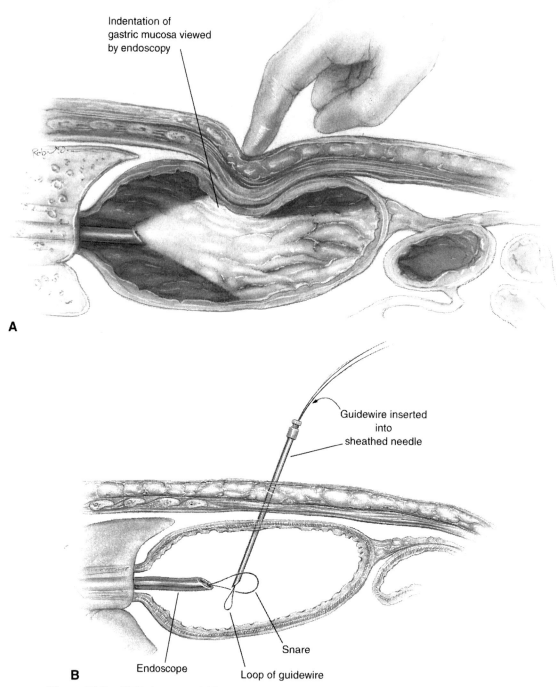

A

Indentation of
gastric mucosa viewed
by endoscopy

Guidewire inserted
into
sheathed needle

Snare

Endoscope

Loop of guidewire

B

Figure 17-2   PEG placement. **A**, To ensure proper gastrostomy tube placement, the abdominal wall site is palpated with a sterile finger to identify the entry site for the sheath and needle. **B**, A plastic cannula over a needle is placed through the abdominal wall incision into the stomach. The needle enters the stomach through the snare, which is positioned under the entry site. The cannula is held in place during needle removal to prevent dislodgement. The needle is removed and a guidewire is placed within the cannula and advanced through the cannula directly into the stomach. The snare from the endoscope is closed over the guidewire.

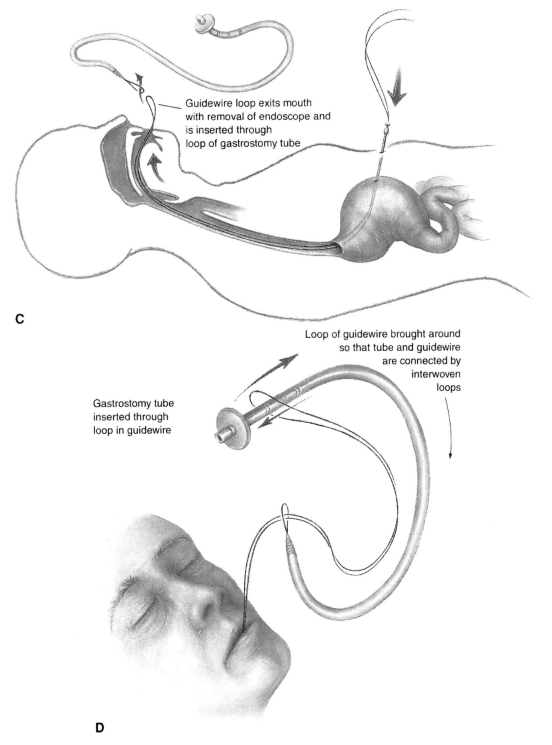

C, Guidewire loop exits mouth with removal of endoscope and is inserted through loop of gastrostomy tube

C

Loop of guidewire brought around so that tube and guidewire are connected by interwoven loops

Gastrostomy tube inserted through loop in guidewire

D

Figure 17-2 cont'd C, The guidewire is grasped with a snare through the endoscope. The snare is retracted into the endoscope tip, and the endoscope is withdrawn through the mouth, pulling the wire loop with it. **D**, The loop on the end of the PEG tube is placed through the wire loop protruding from the mouth, and the end of the PEG tube is threaded into the loop, thus securing the PEG tube.

Continued

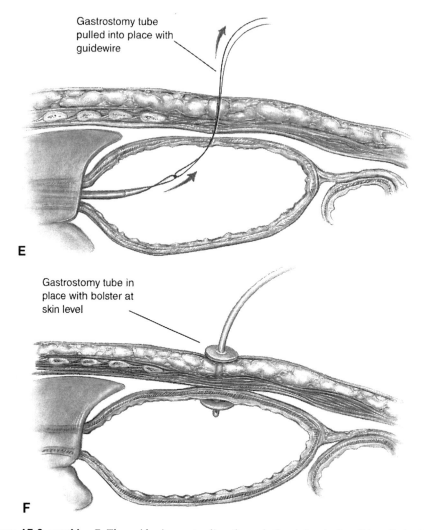

Gastrostomy tube
pulled into place with
guidewire

E

Gastrostomy tube in
place with bolster at
skin level

F

Figure 17-2 cont'd   E, The guidewire protruding through the abdominal wall is pulled with the passage of the tube through the mouth, esophagus, and stomach until resistance is felt. The gastrostomy tube is pulled until resistance is felt. The endoscope is reintroduced to check the position of the tube in the stomach. **F**, The gastrostomy tube is secured with an external bolster to keep the gastric and anterior abdominal walls in close apposition. (From Cullen JJ: Percutaneous endoscopic gastrostomy, *Operative Tech Gen Surg* 3(4):264-267, 2001.)

incision, and a long guidewire is inserted through the angiocatheter into the stomach. The wire is pulled with a biopsy snare through the esophagus and out through the patient's mouth. The PEG tube is pushed over the guidewire and advanced from the esophagus to the stomach and positioned against the anterior abdominal wall. Once the

placement is confirmed with the endoscope, the scope is removed and the tube secured (Bryant, 2000). There are many modifications of these techniques that have been developed over the years.

Percutaneous Endoscopic Jejunostomy. The percutaneous endoscopic jejunostomy (PEJ) placement is a minimally invasive procedure similar to the PEG placement. There are two techniques that will be described, the transpyloric PEJ and the direct PEJ.

The *transpyloric PEJ* procedure involves insertion of the tube through a previously placed PEG tube. A scope is passed into the stomach to the level of the gastrostomy tube, and a small, weighted-tip tube with an attached heavy suture tie is passed through the PEG tube. Under endoscopic visualization, the jejunostomy tube tip with the suture is dragged through the pylorus and positioned in the jejunum. This device, also known as the jejunal extension tube, can result in functional problems because of retrograde migration of the tube back into the stomach. A technique to secure the tube in place is to fasten the tube to the intestinal mucosa with endoscope clips. The small diameter of the tube (8 to 12 Fr.) can cause kinking and occlusion of the tube. A modification of this technique is the *direct percutaneous endoscopic jejunosotmy* (DPEJ).

The DPEJ procedure involves passing the endoscope past the pylorus into the jejunum, where the abdominal wall is transilluminated. The anesthesia needle is inserted at the site of transillumination and advanced until it enters the jejunal lumen under endoscopic visualization. The cannula is inserted alongside the needle, and the insertion wire is advanced through the cannula once the needle is removed. The snare at the tip of the scope grasps the insertion wire, and the scope is removed. The insertion wire is withdrawn so that one end of the insertion wire extends from the mouth and the other end extends from the abdominal wall. The attached loop of the pull type of feeding tube is tethered to the mouth end of the insertion wire, and the assembly is pulled internally until the tube has traversed the jejunal and abdominal walls and is pulled up snugly (Ginsberg, 2001). The DPEJ technique is technically challenging, and patient selection and attention to detail by the gastrointestinal endoscopists will enhance success. Shikem (1998) reports that there has been an 85% success rate in direct placement of the DPEJ and a minimal complication rate as compared to the PEG placement complication rate.

Radiologic Placement

Percutaneous Gastrostomy. Patients who are poor candidates for percutaneous endoscopic gastrostomy (PEG) or have unsuccessful PEG placements attempts may undergo radiologic percutaneous gastrostomy (PG) placement. The procedure may be successfully completed despite an obstructing pharyngeal or esophageal cancer that might prevent insertion of a scope. The basic imaging modality for PG is fluoroscopy. By a combination of fluoroscopy, ultrasound, and computed tomography, a PG can be placed for most patients. The procedure is similar to PEG placement except that once fluoroscopic identification of the stomach is obtained, a gastrostomy tube is pushed through the epigastrum, usually over a guidewire, and then secured internally with a balloon and externally with a bumper or disk. The rate of success with PG placement is very high, with complication rates reported as low as 3.2% (Stoner and Cantwell, 2001).

This technique has developed into other procedures that include percutaneous gastrojejunostomy, percutaneous jejunostomy, and percutaneous cecostomy. Radiologic placement of a gastrostomy tube has become increasingly common.

Percutaneous Jejunostomy. This procedure requires radiologic access to the stomach as previously described in the procedure for PG via radiologic technique. Under fluoroscopic guidance a guidewire is threaded through the duodenum into the jejunum. A balloon occluder catheter is inserted over the guidewire and placed in the jejunum. The position of the balloon is checked by inflating it with a water-soluble contrast. The balloon is then punctured by an 18-gauge needle under fluoroscopic guidance. The tract is slowly dilated with a guidewire (approximately 10 Fr.) until it can accommodate a feeding catheter. The balloon occluder catheter is removed, and the feeding catheter is secured to the skin with a suture or a stabilizing device (Bryant, 2000).

Image-Guided Percutaneous Gastrojejunostomy. Feeding into the stomach is preferable to using the jejunum because of the ability it offers to give bolus feedings, lower tube maintenance problems, and maintain gastric and duodenal activity. A gastrojejunostomy tube (GJ) is indicated for patients with gastric outlet obstruction, gastroesophageal reflux, and gastroparesis. The combined GJ will meet the needs of these patients. This double-lumen tube has a gastric drainage port and a jejunal feeding port that can accomplish both gastric decompression and simultaneous postpyloric enteral nutrition. The GJ tubes that have a balloon have triple-lumen ports. GJ tube placement by the use of imaging (fluoroscopy and ultrasonography) with guidewire techniques usually results in fewer complications and high success rates (Mayhew and Guidos, 1988).

When a combined GJ tube is needed, the gastrostomy tube is first removed, and a guidewire and angiocatheter are inserted and advanced through the pylorus via the scope. The angiocatheter is removed once the guidewire is positioned distal to the ligament of Treitz. The GJ tube is then inserted over the guidewire into the jejunum, and the guidewire is then removed. The internal bumper or balloon is secured snugly against the stomach wall. The tube is secured against the skin with a bumper or a commercial stabilizing device.

Contraindications for a GJ tube are total gastrectomy, gastric carcinomas, and portal hypertension with gastric varices. The most common postprocedural complications are clogged tubes and dislodgement. Recent modifications in the design of these tubes have decreased their tendency to migrate back into the stomach.

Image-guided GJ tube placement procedure is now well established, and placement has a 95% success rate (Mauro, 2001). The timeliness and cost-effectiveness of this technique compares favorably with traditional surgical and endoscopic enteral tube placement.

Enteral Feeding Tube Characteristics

Through the years, manufacturers have made improvements and produced tubes to meet the unique challenges and requirements of both pediatric and adult patients. Foley catheters have traditionally been used for gastrostomy tubes. Most Foley catheters are balloon-tipped and are available in different materials. Latex is the most common, but there are several silicon-coated varieties. The size of the lumen is generally based upon the patient's needs, although 20 Fr is most commonly used. The Foley catheter was originally designed for urologic use and not for gastrostomy placement and thus has limitations such as the lack of a flush or medication port or a cap, as well as having no interlocking features. Latex catheters are known to cause skin irritation and allergic reactions in latex-sensitive patients. And finally, Foley catheters have a smaller internal diameter than that of a comparably sized silicone tube.

Gastrostomy Tubes

Types. Today there is a selection of many different gastrostomy tubes, the use of which has largely replaced Foley catheters in practice. Commercial gastrostomy tubes have balloon tips that are inflated to prevent dislodgement of the tube, graduated markings to help assess tube position, and an external bumper to stabilize the tube. They are available in sizes ranging from 10 to 30 Fr. have built-in plugs, and can contain several feeding or medication ports.

Management Issues. Before insertion of the tube it is a good practice to inflate the balloon to check for leaks or defects. The balloon should be inflated with a solution that will not congeal with time. Sterile water is most commonly recommended. Many of the balloons have a 3- to 6-month life, necessitating periodic tube change. Bolus feedings can be administered using a large volume of formula (>250 ml) and a large syringe that is attached to the tube. The feeding can be administered by gravity (i.e., pouring the formula into the syringe) or by pushing it in with the syringe plunger. Bolus feedings are only recommended for gastrostomy tubes, since large volumes of formula may cause osmotic diarrhea if given into the jejunum. Continuous pump infusion into the stomach has shown a decreased incidence of gastric distention and aspiration as compared to bolus feedings.

Jejunostomy Tubes

Types. Jejunostomy tubes are usually red rubber catheters, Silastic tubes, or T-tubes. They are smaller in lumen size (i.e., 10 to 16 Fr.) than the gastrostomy tube and do not have a balloon tip. A 30-ml inflated balloon in the small bowel could cause a partial or complete bowel obstruction. Commercially manufactured jejunostomy tubes have built-in plugs.

Management Issues. Complications that can occur with a jejunostomy tube are migration of the tube, occlusion of the lumen, and pneumatosis. Misplacement of the tube can lead to diarrhea, "short-gut" syndrome, and malabsorption. Continuous pump infusion is better tolerated by the small intestine than are bolus feedings, and there is a lower risk of aspiration and abdominal discomfort.

Percutaneous Endoscopic Gastrostomy Tubes

Types. PEG tubes are manufactured in numerous sizes ranging from 18 to 22 Fr. The tubes have an internal bumper to provide proper placement and prevent migration from the stomach, and an external bumper or disk to stabilize the tube and help prevent its migrating in either direction.

Management Issues. Complications associated with the PEG tube are intraperitoneal leakage, puncture of the colon, intestinal obstruction, gastrocolic fistula, and tube site infection. These tubes have an internal bumper that is neither air- nor fluid-filled, thus this type of tube does not have a great risk of falling out of the stoma.

Low-Profile Gastrostomy Devices

Types. The low-profile gastrostomy device (LPGD) (Figure 17-3) was originally developed to deal with the problem of inadvertent tube removal that occurred among pediatric patients. Since their advent the low-profile devices have become popular in the adult population for the confused patient or the patient concerned with body image. Because they are almost flush with the abdomen, there is no tube end to be pulled, and there is no bulk under clothing. The LPGD device is kept in place by either an inflatable balloon or a mushroom tip. An antireflux valve keeps gastric content from leaking onto the skin. These devices are durable and difficult to dislodge, and they prevent skin irritation. The manufacturer provides a special adaptor for administering the enteral feeding or to check gastric content (Bowers, 2000). They are distributed with an insertion kit and a stoma measuring device kit.

Management Issues. Advantages of the LPGD include simplified care, decreased skin irritation, low risk of migration and dislodgement, comfortable wear, minimal leakage, and cosmetically pleasing. Disadvantages are limited sizes, the requirement of a mature stoma tract, expense greater as compared to traditional tubes, the potential dislodgement of tubes during feeding, and possible pressure necrosis as a result of inappropriate sizing.

These devices can be placed initially; however, common practice is placement once the gastrostomy tract is established. It is important to measure the length of the stoma tract to select the appropriate size tube. It is recommended that the stoma tract be measured every time the tube is changed, since patients may gain or lose weight, and since children are continuing to grow. The measuring device consists of a small-lumen catheter with a balloon. The lubricated tip of the device is carefully inserted into the tract once the gastrostomy tube has been removed. The balloon is inflated with 3 cc of air and gently pulled against the gastric mucosa. The skin disk is moved down until it touches the skin, and the markings (in centimeters) above the skin disk are read to determine the length of the LPGT most appropriate for the patient. The balloon is deflated and the device removed and discarded. Correct measurement will ensure obtaining the correct length. A tube that is too long allows leakage, and a short tube causes pressure necrosis (Box 17-1).

Nursing Management of Enteral Feeding Tubes

When caring for a patient with an enteral feeding tube, it is the nurse's responsibility to know the type of tube, its location, and the reason for the tube's placement. A gastrostomy or a jejunostomy tube adds little to a patient's quality of life if the patient has to endure leakage and painful, eroded skin.

Basic daily skin care should be done around the tube site. Mild soap and warm water is recommended

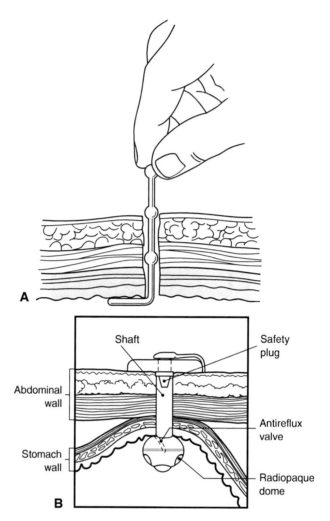

Figure 17-3 Gastrostomy button. **A,** Correct gastrostomy button size is determined by using a device to measure the width of the abdominal wall. **B,** Gastrostomy feeding button in place. (From Bryant RA: *Acute and chronic wounds: nursing management,* ed 2, St Louis, 2000, Mosby.)

for cleaning the site and rinsing the area. A cotton swab, gauze, or a washcloth can be used. Cleaning should be done in a circular pattern starting from the site and working outward, and the skin should be allowed to air-dry. It is not recommended to use hydrogen peroxide or any antiseptic creams. If there is a build-up of crusted, dry drainage around the tube, a diluted hydrogen peroxide solution may be used, followed by a thorough rinsing. The exter-

nal bumper or disks should be rotated daily to prevent pressure. The use of dressings should be avoided with this type of tube. The external bumper should be close, but not snug, against the skin; otherwise, ulceration of the peristomal skin could occur. The patient and the caregiver should be taught to assess daily for signs of redness, pain, swelling, or unusual drainage, and report any of these symptoms to the health care provider. By per-

BOX 17-1 Procedure for Changing a Low-Profile Tube

Equipment
Gloves
4- by 4-inch gauze
10-ml Luer-Lok syringe
Sterile water
Lubricant (e.g., K-Y jelly)
Low-profile tube (LPT)
Stoma-Measuring Device
Stoma-measuring devices are available to accurately measure for the correct size LPT. This determines the shaft length. If the patient has lost or gained weight and has encountered leakage or soreness around the stoma, consider remeasuring. As the abdominal fat changes in size, the shaft length size of the tube may need to be changed by remeasuring with the proper device. Children need to be measured more frequently due to their continued growth.

Procedure
1. Explain the procedure to the patient. (It is best to discontinue enteral feeding 1 to 2 hours before the procedure.)
2. Position the patient no higher than 30 degrees.
3. Wash hands with soap and water and apply gloves.
4. Assemble equipment.
5. Draw up 4 to 6 ml of water.
6. Inject the water into the balloon port of the new LPT. Inspect the balloon for any leakage; if the balloon inflates properly, withdraw the water, and set the syringe aside.
7. Withdraw the water from the balloon port of the tube that is being removed, and gently remove and discard the tube.
8. If resistance is met at the halfway mark (check the length of the tube against the new one), attach a syringe and try to withdraw any water left in the balloon. There may be some blood when the tube is withdrawn. There may also be a sound (i.e., "swooshing") once it is released.
9. Place gauze around the area to collect drainage. Advise the patient to remain flat and to not raise his or her head, since this will cause tensing of the abdomen and make tube removal difficult.
10. Clean around the site with a damp gauze and dry well.
11. Lubricate the end of the tube and gently insert; when done, the external hub is flat against the abdomen.
12. While holding the tube in place, attach the syringe to the balloon port and SLOWLY push the water in. Remove the syringe.
13. Allow the tube to have slight in-and-out movement. No dressing is required.
14. Document the procedure, patient's tolerance, size of the tube, amount of water in the balloon, and verification of placement.

---

forming these skills on a daily basis, complications can be prevented.

Complications of Enteral Feeding Tubes

Three types of complications associated with enteral feeding tubes are mechanical, gastrointestinal, and metabolic ones (Guenter, 2001) (Table 17-1).

This section will discuss prevention and treatment interventions for mechanical complications, which include tube displacement, tube occlusion, skin breakdown, aspiration, hypergranulation tissue (i.e., peristomal hyperplasia), *Candida* infection, buried bumper syndrome, and poor tube placement.

TABLE 17-1 **Tube Complications**

COMPLICATION	CAUSE	INTERVENTIONS
Skin breakdown of the peristomal area	Leakage around tube	Stabilize the tube by taping or use a commercial stabilizing device.
		If a balloon-inflated tube, be sure that the balloon is snug against the abdominal wall by gently tugging on the tube and securing the outer disk against the skin to hold the balloon in place.
		If a balloon-inflated tube, check the amount of fluid in the balloon and be sure it is the amount the manufacturer recommends.
		If a balloon-inflated tube, check to be sure that the balloon is inflated (intact) by trying to withdraw the fluid from the balloon port.
		Replace the tube if the balloon is defective.
		If the balloon is in the stomach, check for large residual.
		Treat the skin with a barrier cream or skin sealant.
		Pouch the tube if excessive drainage is present.
	External bumper too snug against the skin causing pressure-induced skin breakdown	Release the bumper by stabilizing the tube with one hand and gently pulling the bumper away from the tube site.
		Treat ulcerated areas per skin protocol.
		Reposition the bumper to avoid pressure.
		Avoid dressings under the bumper.
Tube displacement	Improperly secured tube or deflated balloon	Secure the tube; if no external bumper, apply commercial tube stabilizer device.
		If a balloon-inflated tube, check the amount of fluid in the balloon and be sure it is the amount that the manufacturer recommends.
		If balloon-inflated tube, check to be sure the balloon is intact (try to withdraw fluid from the balloon port).
		If the tube has come out of the stoma, replace it immediately to prevent stoma closure.
Tube occlusion	Inadequate flushing	Institute a routine flush schedule.
		If unable to flush, instill warm water into the tube with gentle pressure.
		Gently milk tubing: lubricate the outside of the tube with water-soluble lubricant and pull from the stoma to the end of the tube.
		Instill pancreatic enzyme and sodium bicarbonate solution.
Peristomal hyperplasia	Chronic irritation from the movement of the tube (or) The type of tube material causes irritation (or) Excessive moisture	Determine the etiology and correct.
		Cauterize the tissue with silver nitrate by rolling the silver nitrate stick across only the affected tissue; may require several treatments.
		Debridement of the tissue by use of electric cautery or use of scalpel; refer to surgeon.
		Change the tube, using another type of material.
		Use foam dressing to absorb excessive moisture.
Fungal infection	Excessive moisture trapped at the insertion site	Treat the skin with an antifungal barrier cream or powder.
		Use a foam dressing.

Mechanical Complications

Tube Displacement. Tube displacement is a common problem with enteral feeding tubes and can easily be avoided by stabilizing the tube when it is placed. It is essential that the tube stay in its original place, and thus it is very important to secure it to prevent migration or dislodgement. There are several ways to secure a tube, depending on its type. When a Foley catheter is used for gastrostomy feedings, it is a good practice to mark the tube where it exits the stoma site to help monitor for tube migration. By measuring and documenting the length of the tube that emerges from the opening, a baseline will be provided for observing the tube for potential problems. One way of marking the tube is by applying a "flag" with a piece of tape at the exit site of the tube. The tube can also be marked with a waterproof marker. Some tubes are marked with measurement increments.

A device called a *drain tube attachment device* can be used to secure the gastrostomy tube (Figure 17-4). This device can both secure the tube and protect the peristomal skin from drainage. The retention device has a skin barrier surrounded by a microporous, adhesive border and a plastic holding device to keep the tube in proper position. The device can accommodate a 5 to 40 Fr. tube or drain. The manufacturer (Hollister, Inc, Libertyville, IL) recommends that the device be changed every 7 days. Other manufacturers of external stabilizing devices include Kells and Cook; these devices are also easy to apply and accommodate a wide variety of tube sizes.

Another method to secure a tube is to use a piece of ½-inch tape, twisted around the tube and adhered to the abdomen. Some people prefer to secure the tube further by using Montgomery straps or a binder. Dale Medical Products manufactures a binder that serves to secure the tube.

A surgically placed jejunostomy tube has no inflated balloon to secure it internally, therefore an external anchoring device is necessary to prevent dislodgement. Some surgeons secure the tube with one or more sutures, but this does not always prevent the tube from pulling; in fact, any

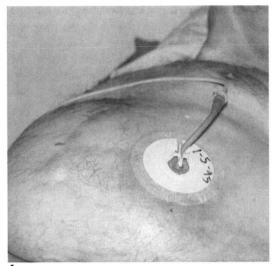

A

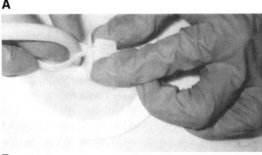

B

Figure 17-4 **A,** Stabilizing device in place. **B,** Tube stabilized with a holding device.

pulling can cause stoma enlargement that will lead to leakage around the tube. Sutures also can cause skin tearing, ulceration, and pain for the patient.

An older method for tube stabilization that has been used is the baby-bottle nipple method. This technique uses a solid skin barrier and a baby-bottle nipple to prevent lateral movement of the tube. A slit is made in the middle of the solid skin barrier wafer, and an opening made at the end so the slit is shaped like a keyhole. This opening is placed around the tube. The opening is based on the size of the tube, and it is frequently necessary to cut this opening slightly larger than the tube diameter to allow for drainage around the tube. The nipple is slit along one side, placed around the tube, and secured to the solid skin barrier with tape.

Faller and Lawrence (1992) developed a cost-effective technique for tube stabilization using foam dressing, a Molnar disk (VPI/Cook), and stretch cloth tape. This dressing is changed every 7 days and was reported to be less expensive compared to 10 other dressing procedures.

Some gastrostomy tubes come with an external disk or bumper to stabilize the tube. The purpose of the disk is to hold the balloon or internal stabilizer against the abdominal wall, thus preventing tube migration and providing stabilization. It is important to monitor disk placement: if too tight against the abdomen it can cause pressure-related skin breakdown. The external stabilizer is flush with the skin and should not have a dressing under it. If the disk is too loose, it will not adequately stabilize the tube.

Tubes with an inflatable balloon should be checked for volume on a regular schedule, generally once a week. The balloon should be refilled with the correct amount of solution, and this amount is documented. Occasionally balloons can develop a slow leak. If the balloon ruptures, the tube must be replaced.

Most radiologically placed gastrostomy and jejunostomy tubes have an outer disk or bumper that will provide external stabilization, and a mushroom tip or balloon for tube stabilization internally. These tubes should be checked daily to be sure that the internal stabilizer (mushroom tip or balloon) is firmly against the abdominal wall. This is done by gently pulling the tube outward until resistance (the internal stabilizer) is felt. After the internal stabilizer is snug to the abdominal wall, the outer disk can be gently pressed against the patient's skin.

If a gastrostomy tube falls out, the tube must be replaced quickly. If the stoma is mature (over 3 weeks old in a person with no delayed wound-healing problems), a new tube should be placed into the stoma tract. Delay in replacing the tube can cause the stoma to close, making replacement difficult or impossible (Boxes 17-2 and 17-3).

Tube Occlusion. The most common reason for tubes to clog is improper administration of medication through the tube. Another cause for occlusion is when a strict flushing protocol is not followed. Over the years there have been many "home remedies" for de-clogging a tube. Some of these solutions have used carbonated soda, cran-

---

BOX 17-2   **Procedure for Removal of Balloon Replacement Gastrostomy Tube**

Equipment
Gloves (nonsterile)
20-ml Luer-Lok syringe
4- by 4-inch gauze

Procedure
1. Explain the procedure to the patient.
2. Position the patient's head no higher than 30 degrees.
3. Plan to remove the tube before a bolus feeding or after the continuous feeding has been stopped for 1 to 2 hours. This will avoid the residual feeding draining onto the skin once the tube is removed.
4. Wash hands with soap and water and apply gloves.
5. Attach the syringe to the balloon port and slowly withdraw the water from the balloon.
6. Once assured all the water has been removed from the balloon, gently withdraw the GT.
7. Cover the opening with 4- by 4-inch gauze until ready to insert replacement tube. The tube should be inserted immediately to prevent closure of the tract.

Adapted from Bryant R: *Acute and chronic wounds: nursing management*, ed 2, St Louis, 2000, Mosby.
GT, Gastrostomy tube.

berry juice, and meat tenderizer. Due to the acidic content of cranberry juice, the solution may precipitate with protein and obstruct the tube (Stoner and Cantwell, 2001). Tubes of any diameter can clog in the absence of a routine flushing schedule. The most effective solution for flushing a tube is water. Patients on continuous tube feedings should flush their tubes every 4 hours with at least 30 ml of warm water, as well as before and after medication administration. Patients on bolus feedings should flush before and after feeds with a minimum of 30 ml of water, and before and after medication

---

BOX 17-3   Procedure for Insertion of a Balloon Replacement Gastrostomy Tube

Equipment
Replacement tube (do not change tube size)
Gloves (nonsterile)
Normal saline
4- by 4-inch gauze
Lubricant (e.g., K-Y jelly)
20-ml Luer-Lok syringe
20 ml sterile water
60-ml syringe with a male tip

Procedure
1. Explain procedure to the patient.
2. Position the patient's head no higher than 30 degrees.
3. Wash hands with soap and water.
4. Draw 20 ml of sterile water into the syringe. DO NOT use saline.
5. Insert syringe into the balloon port of new tube and fill the balloon. Check the balloon for any defects. Withdraw the water from the balloon and set syringe aside.
6. Apply gloves, move the outer disk up and down the tube to facilitate movement once the tube is in place, and place the disk higher up on the tube to be out of the way when inserting. Lubricate the tip of the tube. Do *not* use petroleum-based lubricant.
7. Cleanse the tube insertion site and 5 cm beyond the site with normal saline; cleanse in a spiral movement starting from the stoma site and moving outward. Dry the skin well.
8. Insert the tube gently into the established tract. If resistance is met, rotate the tube; do not use force but withdraw the tube and try another angle for insertion. If resistance is still met, do not try to reinsert. Call the physician; it may be necessary to downsize to a smaller tube to allow passage into the stomach.
9. Instill water into the balloon port. Be sure to check the balloon port for exact amount of water needed, and remove the syringe.
10. Gently pull back on the tube until resistance is felt; then slide the external bumper or disk down until it rests lightly on the skin.
11. Rotate the tube 360 degrees to confirm the tube has free rotation.
12. To verify proper placement, attach 30- to 60-ml syringe to the GT and withdraw; gastric content should be freely aspirated. The tube can also be flushed with water to be sure of patency and no leakage.
13. Cleanse the skin around the tube with soap and water, rinse, and dry well. No dressing is required.
14. Note (or mark) the tube's exit measurement. If the tube has no markings on it, then mark with a waterproof pen, or apply a flag (made from tape).
15. Document procedure, patient's tolerance, amount of water in the balloon, size of the tube, and measurement of the tube extension from exit site.

Adapted from Bryant R: *Acute and chronic wounds: nursing management*, ed 2, St Louis, 2000, Mosby.
GT, Gastrostomy tube.

administration. It is also recommended to give 5 ml of water between each medication if more than one is given.

Only liquid forms of medication should be administered because this decreases the risk of tube clogging and ensures better absorption of the medication. The nurse should consult with a pharmacist when enteric-coated or sustained-release medications are prescribed and determine if the form of medication can be changed. Medications that can be administered via enteral tubes are immediate-release oral tablets, soft gelatin capsules, and liquid medications. Soft gelatin capsules filled with liquid can be given by squeezing out the liquid from a pin hole punctured in the capsule.

Medication that has to be crushed should be pulverized to a fine powder. There are devices available to crush medication, such as the HandiCrush Irrigation Syringe. This device crushes, dissolves, and administers crushable tablets and water and makes it unnecessary to transfer the medication to another container.

Once occlusion of the tube has been identified, it is important to assess the tube and institute treatment. First the tube should be checked to see if it is kinked. The tube can be milked with the fingers from the insertion site outward. If a blockage is found, an attempt should be made to irrigate with warm water. A successful technique described by Mancuard and Segall (1990) for declogging a tube uses a solution of a pancreatic enzyme and sodium bicarbonate (Box 17-4).

Clog-Zapper is a kit available from CORPAK MedSystems (Wheeling, IL) that provides a "multienzyme cocktail," a formulation of acids, buffers, and antibacterial agents. This formula is a food-grade powder designed to break up clogs in most enteral feeding devices. It will not negatively affect silicone or urethane tubes.

There are mechanical instruments available to unclog tubes. Bard Endoscopic Technologics has a PEG cleaning brush for use with 20 Fr. silicone PEG tubes. Only experienced clinicians should use these devices because of the risk of tube rupture.

BOX 17-4   Procedure for Obstructed Feeding Tube
. . . .

Equipment
30- to 60-ml irrigation syringe
Warm water
Viokase tablet or powder and sodium bicarbonate tablet
Gloves (nonsterile)

Procedure
1. Check the tube for kinks. Attach a 30- to 60-ml syringe to the end of the tube and aspirate as much fluid as possible. Discard the fluid.
2. Instill 5 to 10 ml of warm water with a 30- to 60-ml irrigation syringe under manual pressure for 1 minute, using a back-and-forth motion with the plunger to loosen the clog.
3. Clamp the tube for 5 to 15 minutes.
4. Try to aspirate or flush the tube with warm water after unclamping the tube.
5. If the tube remains clogged, repeat the procedure using a pancrease and sodium bicarbonate solution.*
6. Repeat procedures 2 to 4 with the prepared solution until the tube is patent.
7. If still unsuccessful in declogging the tube, notify the physician.
8. Document the interventions used to attempt to declog the tube.

From Lord L: Enteral access devices, *Nurs Clin North Am* 32(4):685-704, 1997; and Mancuard S, Segall K: Unclogging feeding tubes with pancreatic enzyme, *J Parenter Enteral Nutr* 14:198-200, 1990.
* Prepare the solution by crushing 1 Viokase tablet or 1 teaspoon of Viokase powder mixed with 1 sodium bicarbonate tablet (nonenteric) in 5 ml warm water. (In acute care setting this may be prepared by the pharmacist.)

Skin Breakdown. Skin breakdown around the tube site is often caused by leakage of gastric drainage and enteral feeding formula. Once this occurs, meticulous skin care must be given. Interventions to stop leakage or contain the drainage must also be provided.

The peristomal skin is at high risk for damage because of the acidic pH of the gastric content. The insertion site should be monitored for erythema, induration, or pain. If soft tissue infection is suspected, a swab culture should be taken so a culture-based antibiotic can be prescribed.

Management of a measurable volume of gastric content leakage around the tube can be addressed with an ostomy pouching system (Boxes 17-5 and 17-6). The tube can be left in the pouch or brought out of the pouch with an access port (commercially manufactured access ports are available). Another

common method is to use waterproof tape to secure the tube where it exits the front of the pouch (Figure 17-5).

Some clinicians think that increasing the size of the tube or the amount of fluid in the balloon will solve the leakage problem. Increasing the size of the tube and not stabilizing the tube begins a vicious cycle of increasing the size of the tract and thus increasing leakage around the tube, and it is not recommended. One intervention that has been reported is the replacement of the larger tube with a smaller tube to promote shrinkage of the enterostomy around the smaller device (Bodnar and Fraher, 1989). Anecdotal reports suggest that taking the gastrostomy tube out for several hours will shrink the stoma, allowing the regular-sized tube to be replaced, since it now fits snugly into the stoma. Whatever approach is used, containing drainage

---

BOX 17-5   One-Piece Pouch Application Procedure for Leaking Tube or Drain

Equipment
One-piece ostomy pouching system (drainable or urostomy pouch)
Skin barrier wipes
Waterproof tape or commercial access port
Normal saline or tap water
Scissors
Gloves (nonsterile)

Procedure
1. Gather all supplies.
2. Remove dressing, if present, from around tube. Cleanse skin around wound with saline, and pat dry gently.
3. Apply skin barrier wipes to skin around the tube. If skin is irritated, treat with skin barrier powder before applying the barrier wipe. Apply an antifungal powder if indicated. Alcohol-free barrier wipes are indicated if the peritube skin is denuded.
4. Cut barrier on pouching system to the size to fit around tube or drain.
5. Remove paper backing from skin barrier and apply. Guide the tube or drain into the pouch. Seal the skin barrier by gently pressing to the skin.
6. Depending on volume of output and the purpose of the tube, the tube can be left in the pouch (to drain into the pouch) or guided through a small opening in the front, top end of the pouch (to allow the drain to be connected to a drainage system or a suction source). If the tube is to be brought out of the ostomy pouching system, make a very small slit to accommodate the drain and pull through the slit.
7. Use waterproof tape around the tube and over the pouch slit to prevent leakage around the tube where it exits the ostomy pouch.
8. The drain can exit the ostomy pouch through a commercially available access port that is cut to the size of the tube diameter per manufacturer's instructions.
9. Document procedure and patient's tolerance.

BOX 17-6   Two-Piece Pouch Application Procedure for Leaking Tube or Drain

Equipment

Two-piece ostomy pouching system (drainable or urostomy pouch)
Skin barrier wipes
Skin barrier powder
Waterproof tape or commercial access port
Normal saline or tap water
Scissors
Gloves (nonsterile)

Procedure

1. Gather all supplies.
2. Remove dressing, if present, from around tube. Cleanse skin around wound with saline and pat dry.
3. Apply barrier wipes to skin around the tube. If skin is irritated, treat with skin barrier powder before applying the barrier wipe. Apply an antifungal powder if indicated. Alcohol-free barrier wipes can be used if the peritube skin is denuded.
4. Cut skin barrier on pouching system to the size to fit around the tube or drain.
5. Remove paper backing from the skin barrier and apply to skin. Seal the skin barrier by gently pressing to the skin.
6. Guide the tube or drain into the pouch.
7. Depending on volume of output and the purpose of the tube, the tube can be left in the pouch (to drain into the pouch) or guided through a small opening in the front of the pouch (to allow the drain to be connected to a drainage system or a suction source). If the tube is to be brought out of the ostomy pouching system, make a very small slit near the top of the pouch to accommodate the drain site and pull the drain through the slit.
8. Use waterproof tape around the tube and over the pouch slit to prevent leakage where the tube exits the ostomy pouch.
9. The drain can exit the ostomy pouch through a commercially available access port cut to the size of the tube diameter per manufacturer's instructions.
10. Secure the pouch to the barrier carefully, ensuring that there is no leakage.
11. Document the procedure and the patient's tolerance.

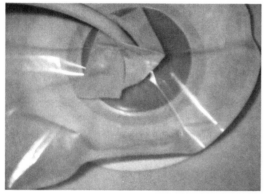

Figure 17-5   Pouching a gastrostomy tube with a one-piece ostomy pouch and waterproof tape.

while the enterostomy shrinks will prevent and even heal skin irritation. The desired outcome is to achieve a tighter cutaneous closure around the tube and thus stop leakage around it.

Denuded peristomal skin should be treated with a barrier cream such as a zinc oxide ointment (unless a hydrocolloid dressing is being used). Skin barrier powder can be used for weepy, denuded skin. Alcohol-based barrier wipes should not be used, since they will cause more patient discomfort. There are alcohol-free skin barrier wipes available. The skin should be cleaned and barrier cream applied after each episode of leakage; aggressive scrubbing of the skin to remove the previous cream should be avoided.

Aspiration. The risk of aspiration is not significantly different in patients fed by gastric or post-pyloric infusion (Levy, 1998). McClave (2001) states that the greater the number of medical risk factors that the person has, the greater the risk of aspiration. Associated risk factors are large-bore tube, dislodgement, diminished gag and cough reflex, decreased level of consciousness, previous history of pneumonia, ileus, or gastroparesis, use of a mechanical ventilator, and greater age of the patient (Rabeneck, Wray, and Petersen, 1996). The literature varies on the incidence of aspiration pneumonia, reporting ranges from 4% to 44%. The patient that is identified at high risk should have the tube placed below the ligament of Treitz.

In the placement of the PEG tube, aspiration can be related to oversedation, overinflation of the stomach, and placement while the patient is supine. However, aspiration related to the PEG procedure has been reported to be less than 1%. If there is a continual aspiration problem after placement of a PEG, a jejunal extension tube should be considered.

Nursing interventions to prevent aspiration include elevating the head of the bed 30 to 45 degrees, checking the residual every 4 to 6 hours and holding feedings if the residual is greater than 100 to 150 ml, using a small-bore feeding tube, continuous feeds as opposed to bolus feeds, and feeding beyond the stomach into the small intestine if possible.

Hypergranulation Tissue (Peristomal Hyperplasia). Hypergranulation tissue (i.e., overgrowth of friable granulation tissue also known as "proud flesh") may form around the stoma site as a result of moisture, tube migration, or rapid epithelization. Bryant (2000) reports that tubes made of certain materials, especially latex, can cause chronic irritation. This tissue can bleed easily if left untreated and is often painful. It is important to determine and correct the etiology of the tissue build-up before treatment is started. There is some controversy in the literature on treatment of hypergranulation tissue. Traditionally, cautery has been performed with silver nitrate sticks.

Sharp debridement or diathermy to the site may be required (Blakley, 1998). Once the etiology is identified and corrected, the hypergranulation tissue should resolve. Another method reported in the literature and in expert opinion is the use of steroid creams (e.g., triamcinalone 0.5%). Foam dressings applied snugly around the tube to help compress the overgrowth tissue have been noted to be of benefit.

Candida **Infection.** Fungal infections can occur when moisture is trapped at the insertion site in a susceptible host. The peristomal skin demonstrates a rashlike appearance starting with small, red papules, and coalescing into a red, moist, patchy area. This may cause burning or itching at the site. Use of an antifungal powder or cream is indicated to treat the infection. If the rash does not resolve within 7 days or becomes more extensive, systemic treatment should be considered. Tubes placed within a skin fold or below pendulous breasts may be prone to fungal infection because of the increased moist, dark area, which provides an excellent medium for yeast growth. For patients who cannot view the tube site, the nurse should teach them to use a mirror to inspect the skin daily.

Patients should be instructed to perform diligent skin care around the tube, especially in hot weather or with increased perspiration from exercise. The skin should always be kept dry. If moisture is a problem, skin sealant or a barrier cream can be used.

Buried Bumper Syndrome. This major complication of percutaneous endoscopic gastrostomy placement has been reported to occur in 1.3% to 3% of cases (Grant, 2000). The buried bumper syndrome (BBS) is defined as a partial or a complete growth of the gastric mucosa over the internal bumper. This syndrome is characterized by leakage around the tube, immobilization of the tube, or pain with feedings. Risk factors for this complication include excessive tension on the tube with the external device, smaller surface bumpers, an internal bumper made of stiffer material, malnutrition, and rapid weight gains (McClave, 2001).

This complication is not always easily identified. BBS is confirmed by endoscopy to determine where the internal bumper has migrated into the gastric wall.

Several techniques have been developed to manage this complication. Ideal treatment of BBS consists in endoscopic removal of the embedded tube and its replacement with a new one.

Endoscopic removal of a translocated PEG tube is useful only when the internal bumper has partially migrated. In the case of deeper migration into the gastric wall, the treatment of choice is minimal surgical technique.

The "push-pull T technique" consists of pulling the tube back into the stomach and removing it through the mouth. The tube is cut close to the skin and a snare is placed via endoscope through the PEG and looped around the cut piece of tube. This method requires the combined movement of endoscopic traction, after the snare has looped around a rigid tube and created a T mechanism out of the PEG, and external manual pushing that results in the oral removal of the embedded tube.

Another technique is the procedure that uses a needle knife through the endoscope to make short, radical incisions in the gastric mucosa overlying the dome of the bumper. This is done until the bumper can be exposed and removed. There is a risk of bleeding with this technique.

The incidence of BBS has decreased, since tube manufacturers have changed the shape and width of the internal bumper of PEG tubes to prevent this complication.

Poor Tube Placement. Poor tube placement can lead to problems that will impact the patient's quality of life. Site selection should be done before surgery, similar to ostomy site selection, to provide better patient outcomes. The site selection should be done by a certified wound, ostomy, and continence/enterostomal therapy nurse or a physician. Gastrostomy tube placement is most easily accomplished in the left upper quadrant, since this is the usual location of the stomach. Skin folds, creases, and dimples should be avoided. The patient should be able to see the site when in a sitting position, for better self care. There are some guidelines, such as keeping 3 to 5 cm below the costal margin and avoiding the costal margin (Hanlon, 1998). Special consideration must be given to site selection for persons confined to a wheelchair or those who wear a brace, are obese, or have other special needs.

Psychologic Implications

Many cultures recognize eating as a social and family tradition. Eating is a time for social gathering. The person who is maintained nutritionally by tube feedings may feel isolated and no longer part of family events such as the Thanksgiving dinner. It is important to have the person join the family at mealtime. With the infant or child who is receiving tube feedings, the parent should be encouraged to hold the child during the feedings (bolus method). This provides the child with a sense of security and closeness to the parent. It is important to try to focus on non–food-related traditions so the person, regardless of age, does not feel isolated and left out of family events.

COMMONLY USED TUBES AND DRAINS

Although there have been few recent changes in tube design, the modality and number of them in use in patient care has changed dramatically. Many more patients require multiple drains, especially those who undergo complex abdominal surgeries. With the use of advanced technologies, the interventional radiologist can now place some tubes that previously required a surgical placement. Frequently, patients are discharged home with tubes or drains in place that require thorough patient and caregiver education to facilitate a smooth transition to the home setting. Several of these tubes or drains are covered in the following paragraphs.

Tubes

Nephrostomy Tubes

The use of nephrostomy tubes was first described in 1941 (Primus, 1977). They provide urinary drainage through a tube inserted into the renal pelvis, which exits from the flank and is attached to extension tubing that drains into a standard urinary leg bag or a bedside drainage bag. The nephrostomy tube is designed to divert the drainage away from a partial or complete obstruction of the urinary tract. The nephrostomy tube is used for stone removal, biopsy of lesions, stricture dilatation, and stent placement, or to allow healing of leaks or fistulas in the urethra (Bartolomei and Refsnyder, 1997).

Acute obstructions caused by an enlarged prostate or nephrolithiasis (Palmieri, 2002) can also be managed with a nephrostomy tube. These tubes can be used as temporary or permanent devices. In cases of stricture or calculus, the nephrostomy tube is used temporarily. With an obstructing tumor, nephrostomy tube placement will be indefinite (Cofield, 1995). Untreated obstruction may cause hydronephrosis, pyelonephritis, pain, sepsis, or impairment in renal function (Primus, 1997).

Management. Nephrostomy tube irrigation may be prescribed to clear the tube of sediment, debris, or blood clots. The recommended amount for irrigation is 5 to 10 ml of sterile normal saline, inserted gently or according to the preference of health care provider. The fluid should not be forced in and should not be withdrawn after irrigation.

The tube must be secured adequately to prevent kinking that can cause blockage. The method of tube stabilization depends on the person who places it. These tubes can be sutured in place or secured to an attachment device. The tube should be secured so it is reasonably comfortable when the patient is lying on the affected side. Securing the tube at a perpendicular angle to the body is to be avoided, so it is not occluded when the patient turns on the side (Guidos, 1988).

The skin around the nephrostomy tube must be kept dry. The dressing should be changed at least once a week, or more often if needed. A transparent, occlusive dressing may be used to keep the area clean and dry. The skin around the tube site should be assessed for any signs of irritation, drainage, or infection. If the tube is covered to keep water away from the tube and site, the patient may shower.

The physician should be notified if the person with a nephrostomy tube experiences fever, chills, flank pain, sweats, leakage around the tube, bloody drainage from or around tube, tube dislodgement, inability or difficulty irrigating the catheter, or absence of drainage from the tube. The nephrostomy tube should be changed every 2 to 3 months. The patient is instructed in the importance of follow-up for tube replacement and ongoing monitoring. This will decrease the risk of tube blockage or dislodgement. Other patient education topics related to the nephrostomy tube include the importance of not allowing tension on the tube, which could lead to dislodgement, and of cleansing of skin around the tube, the significance of adequate fluid intake to promote drainage and prevent urinary tract infections, and the procedure for changing the dressing around the tube.

Some patients choose to wear a leg bag during the day and change to a night drainage bag, which holds a larger volume, for ease of management. Daily cleansing of the drainage bag and tubing is recommended; they should be submerged in warm, soapy water and the entire system well rinsed to remove all soap. The bag can be disinfected using a solution of 1 tablespoon of bleach and 2 cups of water and rinsing well. The bag can be hung to air-dry between uses (Smeltzer and Bare, 2000). The literature varies on the recommended time to replace a drainage bag; weekly replacement was cited as the most frequent recommended time (Cofield, 1995; Mayhew and Guidos, 1988).

Biliary Tubes

Biliary or T-tubes are soft, thin, rubber tubes that pass through skin and liver into the bile ducts to facilitate bile drainage. These tubes are placed surgically or by the interventional radiologist. Biliary drainage tubes can be used to temporarily drain bile before or after surgical procedures, to relieve blockage of the bile ducts, or to bypass a hole in the duct. They are attached to dependent drainage, using a small bag that can be periodically emptied.

Management. The biliary drainage tube must be anchored to prevent dislodgement, and secured to prevent kinking. The drainage bag should be placed below the level of the insertion site to promote gravity drainage. Overly tight securing should be avoided, since it will cause excess tension at the insertion site. Accurate output from the tube is essential to ensure drainage of the bile. When removal of the tube is considered, the tube is clamped intermittently to make sure the patient does not develop obstructive symptoms.

Backflow of bile in the tube must be prevented. This can be achieved by means of free drainage of the bile, by avoiding tubing kinks, and by proper positioning below the insertion site. The tube should be flushed daily if it was placed to prevent blockage (McConnell, 1993). The skin around the insertion site should be kept clean and dry to prevent infection and skin irritation. The tube site can be cleansed with normal saline and gauze using aseptic technique, and dried well (McConnell, 1993). The tube must be secured to prevent accidental dislodgement and covered with a dry sterile dressing.

The patient should be instructed to notify the health care provider of signs of fever or chills, leakage of bile around the tube, bleeding in or around the tube, or a dislodged or broken tube. If the patient has been instructed to irrigate the catheter and develops difficulty with irrigation, the health care provider should be notified (Society of Cardiovascular and Interventional Radiology, 1992).

Nasogastric Tubes

Nasogastric (NG) tubes are indicated for treatment of gastric distention or gastric outlet obstruction, assessment and treatment of upper gastrointestinal bleeding, gastric and esophageal diagnostic tests, gastric lavage, aspiration of gastric secretions, feedings, medication administration, gastric decompression, small bowel obstruction, or emptying the stomach before emergency surgery (Core Curriculum Committee, Society of Gastroenterology Nurses and Associates, 1998).

Contraindications for use of nasogastric tubes include nasopharyngeal or esophageal obstruction, maxillofacial trauma, or uncontrolled coagulopathy. The NG tube must be used with caution in persons who are pregnant or those with an aortic aneurysm, a recent myocardial infarction, esophageal varices, or gastric hemorrhage (Core Curriculum Committee, Society of Gastroenterology Nurses and Associates, 1998).

Management. The NG tube must be securely taped at a downward angle from the nostril to prevent pressure on the edges of the nares. The tube is secured to the patient's clothing to prevent excess tension on the tube. Pain from the presence of the tube can be managed with topical anesthetic sprays. All patients with NG or nasointestinal tubes require frequent mouth care.

The usual adult size is 14 to 16 Fr. The length of tubing needed to reach the stomach is determined by placing the end of the tube at the patient's earlobe and extending it to the nose and down to the xiphoid process.

Sump Tubes

The Salem sump NG tube is commonly used for gastric suction. It is radiopaque with a drainage lumen and a smaller vent lumen. Airflow through the vent prevents a vacuum from forming or the plugging of the tube's drainage holes by gastric mucosa. The tube is connected to suction using the larger drainage lumen. Continuous low suction or intermittent high suction can be used.

Management. The tube should be assessed every 2 hours for adequate function. The vent lumen should be placed above the patient's midline. Many tubes have an antireflux valve. A low, whistling sound may be heard, denoting that the air vent is sumping air.

Levin Tube

The Levin tube is a single-lumen NG device. The gastric mucosa can be injured if a vacuum forms and the tube adheres to the stomach lining. Suction should be maintained at the intermittent low setting to prevent this. The tube is approximately 3 feet long with a number of openings along its side. It is used to remove secretions and bloody drainage, obtain specimens, or give feedings.

Extended-Use Nasogastric Tubes

Extended-use NG tubes, also known as small-bore feeding tubes, are soft and flexible with a weighted tip. These tubes often require the use of a guidewire to facilitate proper placement. An x-ray film is needed to confirm placement before administration of feedings or medications. These tubes are commonly placed in the person who requires short-term feedings and does not need a permanent gastrostomy or jejunostomy tube. Adequate flushing is particularly important because of the decreased size of the tube lumen.

Management. After insertion, the tube should be taped securely or held in place with a commercially available tube device, to prevent injury or pressure areas to the nostril or the nasal mucous membrane. The tubing should be angled below the nares, rather than upward, to prevent damage to the nose from pressure.

Complications of all NG tubes include respiratory distress, aspiration, nosebleed, sinusitis, esophagitis, esophagotracheal fistula, gastric ulceration, hemorrhage, perforation, and pulmonary or oral infection (Core Curriculum Committee, Society of Gastroenterology Nurses and Associates, 1998).

Long Intestinal Tubes

Long intestinal tubes are used to reach the bowel beyond the duodenum. These tubes are used to treat bowel obstruction by attempting to remove secretions and gas and decompress the bowel. They are as long as 10 feet and have a weighted balloon on the end. The weighted balloon is filled with mercury or tungsten to help the tube move through the intestine. A long intestinal tube with a tungsten tip can be used to avoid the risk of tube rupture and mercury leakage. The physician passes the tube initially, and the nurse is responsible for advancing the tube. The patient changes position so that the tube advances 1 to 2 inches per hour until it reaches the desired location. It is then secured in place.

Additional Tube Types

Other tube types include the Cantor tube and the Miller-Abbott tube. The Cantor tube is a single-lumen tube, 10 feet long and used for intestinal decompression. The Miller-Abbott tube is a double-lumen tube, 10 feet long. It has a rubber balloon that is inflated after the tube is in the stomach. Fluid or gas can be aspirated from the other lumen.

Drains

Simple drains provide an exit for drainage. Commonly this is an accumulation of fluids, pus, blood, or necrotic debris that interferes with wound healing and provides a source for proliferation of bacteria. The simple drain is usually placed in a stab wound near the involved area.

A *Penrose drain*, of a soft, flat, flexible latex material, allows fluid to escape by gravity and capillary action. Gauze dressing is used around and over the drain to absorb drainage. A pouching system can be used to contain high-volume output that exceeds the capacity of dressings. A suture and a safety pin is used to hold the drain in place to prevent migration of the drain into the wound. The cigarette drain is similar to the Penrose drain except that it has a piece of gauze placed in the lumen to increase its absorptive ability (Meehan and Fraher, 1995).

Closed drainage systems are low-pressure suction devices that continuously remove fluids against gravity. The drain is attached to a collapsible reservoir that exerts a negative pressure to pull accumulated fluids from the wound bed. The collection reservoir expands as it collects drainage. Advantages that these systems provide include minimal tissue trauma, accurate drainage quantification, and the decrease in infection risk of a closed system. Most Jackson-Pratt-style reservoirs hold 100 ml, whereas the Hemovac style of reservoir can hold 500 ml.

Management of these drains includes ensuring that tubing is in a dependent position and free of kinks. The reservoir should be maintained in an empty and collapsed status to maintain negative pressure and suction. The amount and color of drainage should be monitored. The tubing is milked or stripped as needed to remove clogs of blood or tissue shreds and keep the system functioning (Meehan and Fraher, 1995).

Sump drains are double-lumen tubes with a large outflow lumen and smaller inflow lumen. The venting mechanism is activated when air enters the draining area through the small inflow lumen. Air breaks the vacuum and displaces air or fluid into the larger lumen of the tube. Certain types of sump drains have a third lumen that can be used for infusing an irrigation solution without interrupting suction from the other lumen. Management of the sump drain includes making sure the tubing is maintained free of kinks, debris, or small clots, so it drains properly. If the air vent lumen is patent, a sucking sound will be heard.

Percutaneous Drainage Catheter

Advanced techniques in radiology permit nonoperative diagnosis and drainage of fluid collections at many body sites. Percutaneous drainage is indicated if there is concern that fluid is infected, if characterization of fluid is necessary, or if the collection is producing symptoms to justify drainage.

Percutaneous drainage is avoided if there is a coagulopathy or necrotic tissue present that requires debridement. Complications of percutaneous fluid drainage can include sepsis, bacteremia, hemorrhage, or bowel or pleural transgression (Standards of Practice Committee, 1995). Length of time for drainage is determined by patient's response, volume of drainage, and complexity of the condition being treated.

Principles of management are similar to those for other drainage tubes. Sometimes tube irrigation is performed to maintain patency. When irrigating, aseptic technique must be used, as well as the prescribed type, frequency, and volume of irrigation solution. The practitioner should not use force or aspirate to return the fluid inserted. The return of fluid, color, and consistency should be documented.

The risk to the skin depends on the type of drainage. Abscess or bloody drainage may cause maceration, depending on the volume of exudate (Faller, 1997). Skin barriers should be used to prevent and treat skin irritation around drain sites. Pouching can be used if there is significant leakage around the tube exit site (see Boxes 17-5 and 17-6).

Nursing Management of Tubes and Drains

Tubes and drains can have many purposes (Box 17-7). Goals of management include maintenance of skin and tissue integrity around the tube or drain site, accurate monitoring of output, maintenance of patient comfort, including odor management, cost containment, and prevention of complications or dislodgement. The nurse must know the type of tube inserted, the exact location of the tube, the intended purpose, the nursing management, the potential complications associated with the tube or drain, and the corrective action for problems associated with drain function or surrounding skin (Meehan and Fraher, 1995). See Box 17-8 for patient education related to feeding tubes and drains.

When the patient has more than one drain, the practitioner should label each drain by location or number and record the output separately. Labeling should be consistent from caregiver to caregiver to

---

BOX 17-7   Purposes of Tubes and Drains

••
• Remove fluid for decompression, diagnosis, or analysis
• Remove fluid (serosanguinous or purulent) from wound, chest, or peritoneal cavities
• Prevent infection and promote wound healing
• Administer antibiotic solutions
• Administration of medications, fluids, feedings

From Meehan P, Fraher J: Gastrointestinal tubes and drains: nursing management, *Progressions* 17(3):3-18, 1995.

---

avoid confusion about volume and character of output. Instillation of irrigation solution should be noted separately on the intake form.

TRACHEOSTOMY TUBE

A tracheostomy tube is used to intubate an airway tract stoma. It can be used temporarily or permanently. There are many varieties, including cuffed or uncuffed, fenestrated or nonfenestrated, plastic or metal. Tracheostomies are used for prolonged airway maintenance with or without mechanical ventilation, for pulmonary toilet and secretion management, to treat upper airway obstruction (e.g., trauma, tumor), or for prevention of aspiration pneumonia.

Potential complications include local infection, local skin breakdown, tracheal stenosis, tracheal malacia, tracheoesophageal fistula, accidental dislodgement, aspiration, and altered ability for verbal communication.

Tracheostomy tubes are frequently sutured in place for the first 4 to 5 days after placement. Cotton twill tapes or commercially available securing devices are used to stabilize the tube. The stoma site should be monitored for bleeding in the immediate postoperative period. Secretions around or through the tracheostomy tube can cause local skin irritation or breakdown. Sutures should be removed as soon as possible to prevent irritation.

Management. The tracheostomy flange should be cleansed with half-strength hydrogen peroxide and normal saline at each dressing change. Cotton-

BOX 17-8   Patient Education Related To feeding Tubes and Drains

General Instructions
- Name, manufacturer, and size of the tube in place and date it was last changed
- Type of tube or drain (include name)
- Name of the procedure and purpose of tubes and drains
- How often the tube or drain will need to be drained
- The type and frequency of dressing and irrigation (if indicated)
- If a feeding tube, the amount, frequency and procedure for feeds
- Written instructions that include problem solving and contact names and numbers
- When and whom to call for help should problems arise

Instruct the patient to:
1. Inspect the skin around the tube daily.
2. Clean around the skin daily with mild soap and water. Allow to air dry.
3. If the tube has a bumper or disk, clean under it with a cotton swab.
4. Clean in a circular motion from the site outward.
5. Check the amount of water in the balloon weekly, if indicated.
6. Gently rotate percutaneous tube 360 degrees daily.
7. Do not have the bumper or disk snug against the skin.
8. Use liquid medication when possible and avoid using crushed tablets.
9. Do not force food or water if resistance is met.
10. Report any signs of redness, swelling, pain, and inability to unclog the tube or drainage and leakage around the tube to your physician.
11. Irrigate and follow drain-emptying procedure and document the amount, if indicated.
12. Know what to do if the tube or drain falls out. The opening should be covered with gauze and either call your physician or go the emergency room.
13. Notify the physician or the home care agency, or go to the emergency room, if the tube is cracked or slips in or out.
14. Keep a back-up replacement tube and adaptor available.
15. Be sure to irrigate with water on a regular basis. Bolus feedings flush with 30- to 60-ml of water before and after feedings and medication. Continuous feedings flush every 4 hours with 30 ml warm water.
16. Stabilize the tube if it does not have an external bumper or disk. This prevents lateral movement of the tube in the tract.
17. Observe the feeding tube for any changes in color, such as dark discoloration that can be related to yeast in the tube.

Adapted from Bryant R: *Acute and chronic wounds: nursing management,* ed 2, St. Louis, 2000, Mosby.

tip applicators permit thorough cleansing under the flange. Application of a small amount of antibiotic ointment around the stoma is sometimes used to prevent infection in the early postoperative period. Split 4- by 4-inch gauze or fenestrated foam dressings should be used around the tube to absorb excess secretions. Dressings are changed as often as needed to prevent excess moisture accumulation on the skin around the tracheostomy.

The tracheostomy tube should be held securely while ties are being removed and replaced. The ties are placed tight enough to secure the tube, and loose enough to prevent skin breakdown. The frequency of tie changes varies significantly from patient to patient, depending on volume of secretions (American Thoracic Society, 2000). The health care provider should observe the ties for proper fit as postoperative edema in the neck resolves. The tracheostomy tube and potential pressure areas under the tube flanges should be monitored.

The skin around the stoma and under the ties (circumscribing the neck) should be assessed for redness, irritation, and drainage. The area must be kept clean, dry, and free of secretions. The practitioner should monitor the back of the neck of the bedridden patient for signs of redness or irritation from secretions that drain down toward the back of the neck. Adequate suctioning and secretion management will minimize the presence of drainage around the tracheostomy or on the skin surrounding the tracheostomy tube.

Particular care is needed in the obese patient with a tracheostomy to prevent wounds in deep creases of the neck. These areas should be cleansed and dried well. The wider commercially available tracheostomy holders are helpful in this population because they do not slide into the crease of the neck. Skin breakdown under the ties or the tube holder is most commonly caused by friction or shear (Burke-Davis and Polowczyk, 1995). An extra tube and obturator should be kept at the bedside in case of emergency. If a disposable inner cannula is used, it should be replaced daily (Harkin and Russell, 2001).

Anecdotal reports in the literature describe success with barrier creams, hydrocolloids, and absorptive dressings for the management of skin issues in and around the tracheostomy area (Burke-Davis and Polowczyk, 1995; Harkin and Russell, 2001). General principles of wound care related to moist wound-healing, exudate management, and ease of a product's use, its availability, and its costs are considered when selecting a dressing. Since most skin breakdown around tracheostomies is related to moisture, products that absorb and manage drainage are appropriate. It is essential to evaluate the fit and condition of the tracheostomy ties. Ties that are too snug and are saturated with drainage predispose the patient to skin breakdown under the ties.

Skin barriers can be applied as needed to protect the skin around the tracheostomy. When applying barrier creams, a small amount should be used, rubbed into the skin, and well covered with a gauze dressing. A thin hydrocolloid can be used on superficial skin breakdown. The hydrocolloid will absorb moisture, provide a healing environment, and act as a protective barrier. A piece of thin hydrocolloid that extends at least 1 cm beyond the involved area should be used. The edge of the hydrocolloid must not be allowed to be in close contact with the edge of the tracheostomy, because absorption of moisture can cause the softened hydrocolloid to ooze into the trachea. Placement of the hydrocolloid too close to the stoma allows drainage to seep under the hydrocolloid, resulting in poor adherence and skin maceration.

The use of absorptive dressings such as foams, hydrofibers, and calcium alginates assists with management of drainage and filling of dead space when a wound is located near the tracheostomy site. Appropriate dressing size needs to be considered according to the wound, the patient's body habitus, and the volume of drainage that is expected. Many foam dressings are fenestrated with a precut slit for ease of use for nurse or caregiver. These dressings are usually changed 3 times per week and as needed when saturation occurs. Calcium alginates or hydrofibers that break apart when saturated should not be used near the tracheostomy stoma to prevent migration of small particles of the dressing material into the trachea.

PEDIATRIC PATIENT

Adequate nutrition during infancy and early childhood is critical for growth and development, and may even affect long-term health. The selection of the access device for the enteral tube feedings should be carefully considered while taking into consideration safety, efficacy, cost-effectiveness, and the parent's ability to manage the care.

When teaching parents, there are different issues to be considered with different age groups. It is important to monitor the toddler, who is curious and may try to disconnect the tube or change settings on the infusion pump. The older, school-age child may tamper with the pump settings and may require supervision.

The child who requires continuous feedings should have a designed pediatric pump that comes with a backpack so the child will not be restricted from activities. Tubing must be long enough for the child at the crawling stage to allow for this activity. A concern that the tubing may become wrapped around the child's neck during nocturnal infusion should be discussed during the education session. The tubing can be placed within the night clothing and tucked under the mattress to ensure the child's safety (Harrington and Lyman, 2001).

Another important consideration is the need to reassess children for the correct size tube as they gain weight. If the child has a low-profile device, the manufacturers will provide stoma-measuring devices.

It is important when teaching to stress the importance of oral stimulation by the use of a pacifier so the infant can identify the sensation of a full stomach with the acts of sucking and swallowing. Parents need to be taught how to change a tube in case of dislodgement or obstruction. It is important that they have a back-up enteral feeding tube kit in the home to prevent any stress when the situation occurs. The nurse's role would be to teach and supervise the parent performing this procedure.

Children are sent home from the hospital with drainage tubes less commonly than adults. The school-age child can be taught self care of these drains if interested, and if it is developmentally appropriate. The caregiver of the child with a tracheostomy needs instruction on preventive skin care, as well as suctioning technique, tracheostomy care, tube change, and safety measures (American Thoracic Society, 2000). Preprinted teaching sheets with illustrations are helpful for the parent to follow and provide to others who will be caring for the child (Young and White, 1992).

CONCLUSION

Enteral feeding has become the preferred form of nutritional support for patients who can no longer consume adequate nutrition. With earlier discharges and same-day procedures, the clinician is challenged to provide appropriate care and education for successful management of tubes and drains after the patient is discharged. Care for these patients should be provided by a multidisciplinary health care team consisting of the surgeon, the gastroenterologist, nutritionists, the case manager, and the nurse. In addition to increased numbers of patients receiving enteral feeding, many patients are discharged with tubes and drains. The challenge

in tube and drain management is to identify the type and purpose of the tube or drain, prevent complications, plan the appropriate interventions, and assist the family and the patient in learning to become independent in the care.

SELF-ASSESSMENT EXERCISES

Questions

1. An important point to teach nurses who care for a patient with a gastrostomy tube is to:
   a. Stabilize the tube.
   b. Change the tube every month.
   c. Flush the tube daily with saline.
   d. Flush the tube with water after every feeding.
2. Which of the following interventions would prevent a gastrostomy tube from clogging?
   a. Irrigate the tube daily with 10 ml of saline.
   b. Irrigate before medication administration.
   c. Only give liquid form of medications.
   d. Crush pills and mix with 10 ml of warm water.
3. When changing a low-profile gastrostomy tube on a 3-year-old child, what should be an important part of the procedure?
   a. Use sterile gloves.
   b. Measure the length of the stoma tract.
   c. Cleanse the skin with Betadine solution.
   d. Medicate the child for pain.
4. One of the important features of an endoscopy gastrostomy procedure, compared to a surgically placed gastrostomy, is that enteral feedings can be started right away.
   True _____ False _____
5. The low-profile feeding tubes are only for children under 5 years of age.
   True _____ False _____
6. How frequently should the balloon volume be checked on a gastrostomy tube?
   a. Daily
   b. Once a week
   c. Every month
   d. Does not need to be checked
7. It is 5 days after Mrs. Smith's total proctocolectomy. She asks the nurse why the bulb on

her Jackson-Pratt drain is collapsed. The best response by the nurse is:

a. To connect the drain to low wall suction.

b. To instruct the patient that the negative pressure of the system is working.

c. To empty the drain and record the output.

d. To tell the patient that the drain should be removed.

8. A patient is having large amounts of leakage around a Penrose drain. The best action by the nurse is to:

a. Irrigate the drain.

b. Apply an ostomy pouch around the drain.

c. Discontinue the drain.

d. Notify the physician.

9. What statement by Mr. Jones demonstrates that the teaching plan for home care of his permanent nephrostomy tube has been effective?

a. I need to follow-up with my physician for regular tube changes.

b. I don't have to worry about bladder infections.

c. I am glad I can take a tub bath.

d. I am not going to flush the tube.

10. What would be the best choice of a wound drain when an irrigation solution needs to be infused?

a. Penrose drain

b. Jackson-Pratt drain

c. Sump drain

d. Levin tube

Answers

1. a; One of the leading causes of tubes migrating and leaking the tube's not being stabilized. There are many ways to stabilize a tube to prevent complications.

2. c; The most common reason tubes clog is inappropriate administration of medication.

3. b; It is important to use a measuring device issued by the low-profile tube company to ensure that the correct size tube will be inserted. This is especially important with growing children and patients that undergo a significant weight gain.

4. True; The surgical placement of a gastrostomy tube requires a recovery period before feeding can be introduced. The noninvasive endoscopy procedure does not require a delay period before feedings can start.

5. False; The low-profile tube is not only for the pediatric patient but can be used for other ages, especially in the confused elderly person to decrease the risk of having the tube pulled out.

6. b; It is good practice to check the fluid in the balloon weekly to ensure that the correct amount of fluid is present. If the amount is less than indicated, fluid should be instilled to the correct amount and documented. Sometimes the fluid can evaporate, or the balloon can develop a slow leak over time.

7. b; The collapsible reservoir of a Jackson-Pratt drain provides a negative pressure system to collect the drainage.

8. b; The ostomy pouch will contain and quantify the amount of drainage while protecting the skin around the site. The ostomy system can stay on 5 to 7 days, providing improved quality of care and comfort for the patient.

9. a; Regular nephrostomy tube changes prevent dislodgement or blockage of the tube.

10. c; A sump drain is a triple-lumen drain that can apply suction and instill an irrigation solution.

REFERENCES

Abuksis G et al: Percutaneous endoscopic gastrostomy: high mortality rates in hospitalized patients, *Am J Gastroenternol* 95:128-132, 2000.

Alexander J et al: Beneficial effects of aggressive protein feeding in severely burned children, *Ann Surg* 192:505-517, 1980.

American Thoracic Society: Care of the child with a chronic tracheostomy, *Am J Respir Crit Care Med* 161:297-308, 2000, website: www.atsjournals.org.

Bartolomei SA, Refsnyder C: *Patient care in interventional radiology,* Gaithersburg, Md, 1997, Aspen.

Baskin W: Percutaneous endoscopic gastrostomy and placement of jejunostomy extension tube, *Tech GI Endoscop* 3(1):30-41, 2001.

Blakley P: *Practical stoma wound and continence management,* Vermont Vic, Australia, 1998, Research Publications.

Bodnar B, Fraher J: Tube feeding enterostomies: indications, techniques and management strategies, *Progressions* vol 1, no 2, 1989.

Bowers S: All about tubes, *Nursing 2000* 30(12):41-47, 2000.

Bryant R: *Acute and chronic wounds: nursing management,* ed 2, St Louis, 2000, Mosby.

Burke-Davis M, Polowczyk B: Tracheostomy skin care: managing the forgotten stoma, *Progressions* 7(3):19-23, 1995.

Cofield V: Percutaneous nephrostomy tubes: nursing care, *Urol Nurs* 15(4):128-130, 1995.

Core Curriculum Committee, Society of Gastroenterology Nurses and Associates: *Gastroenterology: a core curriculum,* St Louis, 1998, Mosby.

Faller N, Lawrence K: Hold that tube.... cost effectively, *OWM* 38(9):37-40, 1992.

Faller N: When a wound is not a wound: tubes, obvious fistulae, and draining wounds. In Krasner D Kane D: *Chronic wound care: a clinical source book for healthcare professionals,* ed 2, Wayne, Pa, 1997, Health Management Publications.

Ganga U, Ryan J, Schafer: Indications, complications and long-term results of percutaneous endoscopic gastrostomy: a retrospective study, *South Dakota J Med* 5(5):49-52, 1994.

Gauderer M: Gastrostomy techniques and devices, *Surg Clin North Am* 76(6):1285-1298, 1992.

Ginsberg G: Direct percutaneous endoscopic jejunostomy, *Tech GI Endoscop* 3(1):42-49, 2001.

Grant J: Mortality with percutaneous endoscopic gastrostomy, *Am J Gastroenterol* 95(1):3, 2000.

Guenter P: Enteral nutrition complications. In Guenter P, Silkroski M, editors: *Tube feeding, practical guidelines and nursing protocols,* Gaithersburg, Md, 2001, Aspen.

Guidos B: Preparing the patient for home care of the percutaneous nephrostomy tube, *J Enterostom Ther* 15(5): 187-190, 1988.

Hanlon M: Preplanned marking for the optimal gastrointestinal and jejunostomy tube site location to decrease complications and promote self-care, *Nutr Clin Pract* 13:167, 1998.

Harkin H, Russell C: Tracheostomy patient care, *Nurs Times* 97(25):34-36, 2001.

Harrington M, Lyman B: Special considerations for the pediatric patient. In Guenter P, Silkroski M editors: *Tube feeding, practical guidelines and nursing protocols,* Gaithersburg, Md, 2001, Aspen.

Kudsk K: Importance of enteral feeding in maintaining gut integrity, *Tech GI Endoscop* 3(1):2-7, 2001.

Levy N: Nasogastric and nasoenteric feeding tubes, *Gastrointest Endosc Clin North Am* 8(3):329-350, 1998.

Lord L: Enteral access devices. In Evans-Stoner N, Lysen, L: *Nurs Clin North Am* 32(4): 685-704, 1997.

Mancuard S, Segall K: Unclogging feeding tubes with pancreatic enzyme, *JPEN J Parenter Enteral Nutr* 14:198-200, 1990.

Martyn-Nemeth P, Fitzgerald K: Clinical considerations: tube feeding in the elderly, *J Gerontol Nurs* 18(2):30-36, 1992.

Mauro, M: Image-guided percutaneous gastrostomy and gastrojejunosotmy, *Operative Tech Gen Surg* 3(4):269-282, 2001.

Mayhew P, Guidos B: Development and evaluation of a protocol for percutaneous nephrostomy tubes, *J Enterostom Ther* 15(5):183-186, 1988.

McClave S: Managing complications of percutaneous and nasoenteric feeding tubes, *Tech GI Endoscop* 3(1):62-68, 2001.

McConnell EA: Caring for a biliary drainage tube, *Nursing* 23:6, 1993.

Meehan P, Fraher J: Gastrointestinal tubes and drains: nursing management, *Progressions* 17(3):3-18, 1995.

Palmieri P: Obstructive nephropathy: pathophysiology, diagnosis, and collaborative management, *Nephrol Nurs J* 29(1):15-23, 2002.

Primus P: Evolution and care of the percutaneous nephrostomy tube, *IMAGES* 16(3):4-9, 1997.

Rabeneck L, Wray N, Petersen N: Long-term outcomes of patients receiving percutaneous gastrostomy tube feedings, *J Gen Intern Med* 11:267-293, 1996.

Shikem LS: Direct percutaneous endoscopic jejunostomy, *Gastointest Endosc Clin North Am* (3):568-80, 1998.

Smeltzer S, Bare B: *Brunner & Suddarth's medical-surgical nursing,* ed 9, Philadelphia, 2000 Lippincott.

Society of Cardiovascular and Interventional Radiology: *Biliary catheter care,* Fairfax, Va, 1992,

Standards of Practice Committee, Society of Cardiovascular & Interventional Radiology: *Quality improvement guidelines for adult percutaneous abscess and fluid drainage;* website: www.sirweb.org/clinical/T25.htm 1995.

Stoner N, Cantwell C: Management of clients with malnutrition. In Black J, Hawks S, Kerne A editors: *Medical-surgical nursing,* ed 6, Philadelphia, 2001, WB Saunders.

Young C, White S: Preparing patients for tube feeding at home, *Am J Nurs* 4:46-53, 1992.

RESOURCES

Enteral Feeding Tubes

American Society for Parenteral and Enteral Nutrition
8630 Fenton Street, Suite 412
Silver Spring, MD 20910
1-800-727-4567
E-mail: aspen@nutri.org

Bard Interventional Products
129 Concorde Road
Billerica, MA 01821
1-800-225-1332
Website: www.bardinterventional.com

Bard Medical Division
8195 Industrial Boulevard
Covington, GA 30014
1-800-526-4455
Website: www.bardmedical.com

CORPAK MedSystems, Inc.
100 Chaddick Drive
Wheeling, IL 60090
1-800-323-6305
Website: www.corpakmedsystems.com

Medical Innovations Corporation
1600 Wyatt Drive
Santa Clara, CA 95654
Website: www.aedi.com

Oley Foundation
Albany Medical Center
214 Hun Memorial
Albany, NY 12208-3478
1-800-776-OLEY (6539)
Website: www.wizvax.net/oleyfdn

Ross Laboratories
Division of Abbott Laboratories
625 Cleveland, OH 43215
1-800-544-7495
Website: www.ross.com

Tube Attachment/Securing Devices
ConvaTec
Bristol-Myers Squibb Company
PO Box 5254
Princeton, NJ 08543-5254
1-800-422-8811
Website: www.convatec.com

Cook Wound Ostomy Continence (VPI)
1100 West Morgan Street
Spencer, IN 47460
1-800-843-4851
Website: www.cookwoc.com

Dale Medical Products, Inc.
PO Box 1556
Plainville, MA 02762
1-800-343-3980

Genetic Laboratories Wound Care, Inc.
2726 Patton Rd.
Roseville, MN 55113
1-800-328-2634
Website: www.geneticlabs.com

Hollister, Inc.
2000 Hollister Drive
Libertyville, IL 60048
1-800-323-4060
Website: www.hollister.com

MC Johnson Co., Inc.
2037 J & C Blvd.
Naples, FL 34019
1-800-553-8483
Website: www.mcjohnson.com

Sterion, Inc. (formerly Oxboro Medical)
13828 Lincoln St. NE
Ham Lake, MN 55304
1-800-328-7958
Website: www.sterion.com

NOTE: This list can be used for reference. It is not all-inclusive.

18 *Fistula Management*

PAULA ERWIN TOTH, BARBARA J. HOCEVAR, and JUDITH LANDIS-ERDMAN

OBJECTIVES

1. Define an enterocutaneous fistula.
2. List the predisposing factors leading to the formation of an enterocutaneous fistula.
3. Discuss the clinical presentation of a patient with an enterocutaneous fistula.
4. Describe the workup for a patient who presents with symptoms of an enterocutaneous fistula.
5. Identify the medical management of a person with an enterocutaneous fistula.
6. Discuss when the person with an enterocutaneous fistula may be a candidate for surgical interventions.
7. List the nursing goals for a patient with an enterocutaneous fistula.
8. Describe the types of pouching systems available in enterocutaneous fistula management.
9. Differentiate among the types of skin barriers available to manage an enterocutaneous fistula.
10. Discuss how an enterocutaneous fistula can be managed with a closed suction setup.

INTRODUCTION

Enterocutaneous fistulas (ECFs) present a myriad of challenges for patients and clinicians alike. An ECF is an abnormal connection between the intestine and the skin. Common predisposing factors to the formation of an ECF include Crohn's disease, an anastomotic leak, cancer, small bowel obstruc-tion, and abdominal sepsis, to name a few. ECFs range from the simple to the complex; medical, sur-gical, and nursing management depends on specific patient factors. Although there is no universal clas-sification system for ECFs, most clinicians describe external fistulas based on complexity, anatomic location (Table 18-1), and volume of output. Wong and Buie (1993) classify a fistula that demonstrates a short, direct tract without an abscess as a simple fistula. Complex fistulas are described as either type 1 or type 2. A type 1 complex fistula is associated with an abscess and multiple organ involvement. A type 2 fistula opens into the base of a disrupted wound (Box 18-1).

ETIOLOGY

The etiology of ECFs is varied and can be related to postoperative or spontaneous occurrences. Postoperative development of an ECF can be due to a breakdown of the intestinal anastomosis from technical errors during surgery, problems with the intestine itself, or systemic factors. Excessive ten-sion on the anastomosis and compromised vascular supply can predispose the surgical patient to fistula formation. Systemic factors such as the presence of malignant disease, infection, poor nutritional sta-tus, steroid therapy, and metabolic and endocrine disorders can all predispose to the development of an ECF. Persons with Crohn's disease are especially vulnerable to fistula formation because of the transmural nature of their disease (Wong and Buie, 1993; Rolstad and Bryant, 2000; Milsom and Ky, 2001). When an ECF is forming, it follows the path of least resistance. Common locations for fistula

TABLE 18-1   Fistula Terminology

FROM	TO	NAME
Bladder	Skin	Vesicocutaneous
Bladder	Vagina	Vesicovaginal
Colon	Skin	Colocutaneous
Colon	Bladder	Colovesical
Intestine	Colon	Enterocolonic
Intestine	Skin	Enterocutaneous
Intestine	Bladder	Enterovesical
Intestine	Vagina	Enterovaginal
Rectum	Vagina	Rectovaginal

BOX 18-1   Fistula Classification

Simple Fistulas
Short, direct tract
No associated abscess
No other organ involvement

Complex
Type 1
Associated with abscess
Multiple organ involvement

Complex
Type 2
Opens into base of disrupted wound

development and exit sites include a wound dehiscence, an abscess site, an incision, a drain site, the site of active disease, or any devascularized tissue.

PRESENTATION

Clinically, patients commonly develop fever, localized erythema, induration, and progressive local discomfort. Electrolyte imbalance, especially low potassium, and alterations in mental status are frequently present. Sepsis, malnutrition, dehydration, anemia, tissue destruction, and severe acid/base imbalances can occur. Mortality in patients with ECF is linked to fluid and electrolyte imbalances, malnutrition, and especially uncontrolled sepsis (Wong and Buie, 1993). Timely and vigorous med-

ical management of patients with an ECF is essential. Efforts are undertaken to stabilize the patient by controlling sepsis, restoring fluid and electrolyte balances, and providing nutritional support.

WORKUP

Once the patient has been stabilized, a thorough investigation to determine the exact location of the fistula's origin is undertaken. Although the type of output can indicate the origin, it is important to accurately identify the source, as well as any associated problems such as a persistent abscess or a distal obstruction. Radiographic studies generally commence with a fistulogram. A small, soft catheter is gently inserted into the fistula tract, and a water-soluble contrast is introduced. Limited inflation of the balloon may be performed to permit the flow of the contrast into the tract. Care is taken to avoid undue trauma to the tract. Based on associated symptoms and conditions, an upper gastrointestinal x-ray series with small bowel follow-through, barium enema, a computerized tomography scan, cystoscopy, or an intravenous pyelogram may be conducted (Wong and Buie, 1993; Rolstad and Bryant, 2000).

MEDICAL MANAGEMENT

The goal of medical management of the patient with an enterocutaneous fistula is spontaneous closure.

Spontaneous closure of an enterocutaneous fistula allows the fistula to heal over time. Conservative treatment can facilitate spontaneous closure in approximately 60% to 70% of all enteric fistulas, and the time to spontaneous closure is reported in a range from 4 to 7 weeks (Rolstad and Bryant, 2000). Decreasing the secretions of the gut and nutritional support are the goals in the conservative treatment regimen for the patient with a fistula. Decreasing the gut secretions can be accomplished by restricting oral intake and the use of somatostatin analogues. The patient is restricted to nothing by mouth (NPO). NPO status will decrease intestinal contents, gastrointestinal stimulation, and pancreatic and biliary secretions. Somatostatin (i.e., Octreotide) has been demonstrated to be especially effective in decreasing small bowel secretions (Elson and Iqbal, 2001).

Nutritional supports dependent on the type of fistula and the patient's overall condition. For instance, a patient with a colocutaneous fistula may be able to tolerate enteral support. Enteral nutrition is preferred because it provides maintenance of the normal intestinal function. However, the patient with small bowel fistulas will most likely require total parenteral support. Once the patient has been stabilized, a strategy to manage the fistula is determined. The etiology will, in large part, determine the overall goal and the specific interventions that will be designed to close the fistula.

Surgical closure of fistulas may be considered if the following impediments to spontaneous closure are present: complete disruption of bowel continuity, distal obstruction, foreign body in the fistula tract, epithelium-lined tract contiguous with the skin, cancer in the site, previous irradiation to the site, Crohn's disease, or presence of a large abscess (Rolstad and Bryant, 2000).

Complex fistulas and those in which the tract has epithelialized require a long-term, staged approach to closure. Despite the appeal of a quick fix and the desire to "make it better," the best approach is to wait. It is generally advisable to delay surgery for a minimum of 6 to 8 weeks after the sepsis has been controlled and the patient stabilized. This will reduce the risk of peritonitis and the creation of more fistulas. Exceptions to this recommendation may be made if reoperation can be safely undertaken within 10 days of surgery and there is no evident sepsis. Surgical intervention that is undertaken too early places the patient at a higher risk of morbidity and mortality than if surgery is delayed (Wong and Buie, 1993). In select cases where the pathway of a low-output fistula can be well visualized, endoscopic injection of a compound such as fibrin glue may be used to seal up the fistula tract (Hwang and Chen, 1996). When surgery is undertaken, options include resection with primary anastomosis with or without proximal diversion, proximal diversion or intestinal bypass of the fistula, or, as in the case of a rectovaginal fistula, an endorectal advancement flap may be performed.

NURSING MANAGEMENT

Nursing management focuses on providing comprehensive nursing care to the patient. Control of sepsis, restoration of fluid and electrolyte balance, and nutritional support are all critical parameters that must be addressed. The actual nursing management of the fistula itself is one of the most significant and frustrating aspects of care for the nurse, the physician, and especially the patient. Nursing goals for the patient with a fistula can be seen in Box 18-2.

Knowledge of the anatomic location and origin of the fistula, condition of the perifistular skin, and color, consistency, and volume of the effluent will assist the nurse in selecting the best management options. A wound, ostomy, and continence (WOC/ET) nurse can be of invaluable assistance in determining the best plan of care for the patient with a fistula and in educating the staff, the patient, and the caregivers in application of the system. The psychologic implications of fistula development on patients and caregivers should not be underestimated. The WOC/ET nurse can offer supportive care and information to persons experiencing those significant alterations in elimination and body image that a fistula creates.

Decisions for fistula management include: (1) what will be used for skin protection—solid skin barriers, sealants, skin barrier powders, and/or pastes, and (2) what containment devices will be chosen—pouches, suction catheters, and/or drains.

BOX 18-2 **Nursing Goals for the Patient With a Fistula**

- Protection of the perifistular skin
- Containment of the fistula output
- Quantification of the output
- Implementation of a cost-effective system
- Promote patient comfort, optimize physical function
- Control odor

Generally a creative combination of a variety of products is selected to tailor the plan to the needs of the patient. Changes over time in output, external diameter, abdominal contour, and patient activity may necessitate modification of the management system. Application of the system may be complicated and time-consuming. The frequency of changing will vary greatly, depending on the patient's activity level and the characteristics, size, and location of the fistula (O'Brien, Landis-Erdman, and Erwin Toth, 1998).

SKIN PROTECTION

Low-output fistulas (less than 150 ml/24 hours) may best be managed with skin protection and dressings. Skin protection can be provided by using a *solid skin barrier,* a *liquid skin sealant, skin barrier powders,* or *pastes.* The principle in using these products is to construct a barrier over the perifistular skin to prevent skin contact with the fistula output. The perifistular skin is covered with the barrier, and an absorbent dressing is applied over the fistula opening. The dressing can be changed as needed, and the skin barrier is left in place until it no longer provides protection. *Solid skin barriers* generally are resistant to fistula output and can remain in place as long as the barrier function is intact. The degradation of solid skin barriers depends upon the volume and consistency of the fistula output. Most *liquid skin barriers* provide protection for up to 24 hours in the presence of a low-output fistula, and *skin powders* and *skin pastes* (usually zinc-based) require reapplication at least once a day, depending on the amount and consistency of the output.

CONTAINMENT DEVICES

A small- to medium-size fistula that drains more than 500 ml/24 hours, or any volume of output that is extremely irritating to the skin, can be managed similarly to conventional ostomies. Pouching options include solid skin barriers of various sizes, shapes, and materials, and drainable pouches, pouches with adapters to connect to bedside drainage collectors, and pouches with access windows to allow direct visualization of the pouched area and application of a dressing, if indicated.

The *skin barrier* provides skin protection and an adhesive seal. Skin barriers can be integrated into the pouch, or they can be applied to the skin and a pouch attached over the skin barrier. Skin barrier options include regular-wear or extended-wear. The choice between regular- and extended-wear depends on the volume and consistency of the fistula output. An extended-wear barrier is best suited for high-volume, liquid output.

The size of the skin barrier depends on the size of the fistula. A general rule of thumb is to extend the solid skin barrier 1½ inches beyond the fistula edge. In select cases a convex skin barrier may be appropriate to obtain a seal on a small fistula that is located below the skin surface. Unlike fitting an ostomy pouch, in which the aperture of the skin barrier or pouch will be within one-eighth of an inch of the base of the stoma, sizing the opening for the fistula may vary. It is important to cut the skin barrier opening large enough for it to rest on relatively even skin. Most fistulas tend to have scarring and depressions in the area around the opening, so skin barrier pastes, washers, and powders can be used to protect any exposed skin and fill in uneven surfaces. The shape of the skin barrier and pouch depends on the size and shape of the fistula and the surrounding area. Skin barriers integrated into pouches are available in round, oval, and rectangular shapes. Frequently the shape of the fistula will not fit a standard skin barrier and pouch, and customization will be necessary (see following paragraphs and the case studies later in this chapter).

The *pouch* will contain the fistula effluent or direct the effluent to a bedside drainage collector. Pouches are available in various capacities, and the size will depend upon the amount of fistula output. Although most pouches are sized by length, there are also a limited variety of widths available. All fistula pouches should be drainable; the emptying port may be the standard drainable end, or the pouch may contain an adapter that facilitates attachment to a larger bedside container. Most pouches used for fistula management are made of transparent film, and at least one manufacturer provides an opaque pouch film, should this be preferred.

Small and midsize fistulas located on the mid-abdomen may benefit from a wound pouch that has an *access port* on the pouch that can be opened between pouch changes. Advantages of an access port include the potential for direct visualization of the involved area, placing dressings, instilling contrast materials, performing assessment of the skin barrier seal, and adding skin protection to the perifistular area as needed.

A very large fistula (with a width or length greater than 4 inches) can present a challenge to secure a collection device. A large wound pouch may be appropriate for an incisional fistula, but a fistula located in a skin fold or the groin, or covering a large portion of the abdomen, will require a more creative approach. Since most commercial pouches are not large enough to accommodate fistulas of this size, the WOC nurse may make a collection device from a food storage bag, a bowel isolation bag, or even a trash bag. First, skin folds, creases, and depressions are filled with skin barrier paste, skin barrier wafers, and/or skin barrier powder. Then a solid skin barrier is applied around the skin edges of the fistula. The "pouch" is secured to the skin barrier using skin cement or medical grade adhesive. Once the pouch is applied over the fistula and attached to the skin barrier, the opening is cut to allow the fistula drainage to be collected (it must be remembered that the type of pouch used in this application does not have an "opening" that is placed around the fistula opening—such an opening must be created). The outer edges of the pouch are secured to the patient's abdomen with a transparent film dressing or tape. The inner aspect of the pouch is sealed with skin barrier paste applied with a gloved finger along the entire rim of the fistula, and dusted with skin barrier powder. The skin barrier powder can be sprinkled along the entire base of the wound, and a skin barrier ointment may in some cases be applied directly to unprotected skin. Depending on the amount of fistula drainage, the "pouch" may be connected to constant drainage, or absorbent gauze dressings applied directly in the wound. Unlike with larger conventional wounds, use of modern wound care products such as calcium alginates is not recommended, since the rapid output of the stool will erode the dressing too quickly to make it a cost-effective option. Between pouch changes the nurses can change the gauze dressings without disturbing the seal. Some of these complex systems can take up to 2 hours to apply, but in the long run the system is cost-effective because it prevents frequent, costly dressing changes; it is also a plus that the patient does not need to endure frequent dressing changes along with the resultant skin stripping. There are no standard intervals for changing a fistula pouch. Some systems will require changing every 24 hours, and others will remain secure for up to 7 days. The changing schedule will depend on individual patient factors (O'Brien, Landis-Erdman, and Erwin-Toth, 1998; Rolstad and Bryant, 2000).

SUCTION CATHETERS AND DRAINS

A pouching system can be connected to suction to facilitate pouch drainage. This might be indicated if the volume of the drainage overwhelms and loosens the seal. The pouch end can be connected to low constant suction, or an opening can be made into the pouch, the suction catheter placed into the pouch (caution should be taken not to place the suction catheter directly on the fistula), and the pouch opening around the catheter sealed using waterproof tape. Commercial access ports can also be placed on the pouch, and the catheter threaded through the access port into the pouch.

Another option to manage a fistula using suction is to create a closed suction system over the fistula site. Solid skin barrier is used to line the skin edges of the fistula. A layer of moistened and wrung out/damp saline gauze dressings is placed over the wound/fistula base to provide protection to the tissue and prevent the tissue from desiccation. A suction catheter or suction drain is placed over the gauze and attached to low continuous suction. The entire area is covered with a transparent dressing; the solid skin barrier accepts the transparent dressing and helps to secure the seal. The concept behind this dressing is to have an airtight seal, therefore the transparent dressing seal must be without wrinkles or folds. To secure the transparent dressing around the suction catheter or drain, a bead of skin barrier paste may be used. The length of wear time of this type of system depends upon the seal, the amount and consistency of the fistula drainage, and the activity of the patient. If the system is without suction for a prolonged period of time, the seal will not be maintained.

CASE STUDIES

The following four case studies illustrate the concepts that were outlined above.

Case Study I

A high-output small bowel fistula developed in a midline wound following small bowel surgery. The patient had a loop ileostomy proximal to the wound, which had a moderate amount of mucoid drainage. Both the ileostomy and fistula output required containment for quantification, as well as for skin protection. The patient was maintained on NPO status and was receiving total parenteral nutrition. Abdominal retention sutures within red rubber catheters were used to support the abdominal musculature and maintain incisional closure. When the incision opened because of the fistula, three retention sutures were left in place to keep the wound from enlarging and prevent further displacement of the rectus muscles. Uneven contours created by the retention sutures took form as creases and depressions. The tension on the sutures resulting from abdominal swelling caused the sutures to lacerate or erode through tissue from the original insertion sites. A skin barrier powder was applied to the eroded areas. The powder was also used to fill the mucocutaneous separation where the rod exit sites of the ileostomy were healing. The powder protected healing tissue and absorbed excess moisture, enhancing the pouch skin barrier seal. The ileostomy pouch was applied first, using a drainable pouch with a compact outer diameter (Figure 18-1, *A*). The compact outer diameter avoided contact with the fistula pouch barrier. A synthetic-based washer was applied over the karaya washer on the pouch to extend wear time.

Next the fistula was pouched. Depressions and creases were filled using solid skin barrier wedges and paste strips. The skin barrier wedges were used

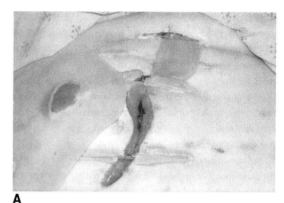

A

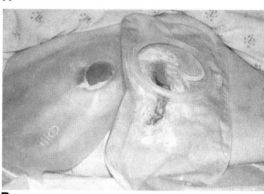

B

Figure 18-1 **A,** Ileostomy pouch with compact outer adhesive diameter placed over stoma; skin depressions and creases filled with solid, paste, and strip skin barriers to provide a flat pouching surface. **B,** Wound pouch cut off-center to avoid ileostomy pouch, inner opening cut slightly larger than wound, and exposed skin protected with skin barrier paste and powder.

to fill larger and deeper depressions. The strip paste was molded around the retention sutures, filling narrower creases (strip paste is thicker than tube paste and does not require time to set) (see Figure 18-1, *A*). A commercial wound pouch with a solid skin barrier and outer paper collar was used, because the solid skin barrier dimensions accommodated the wound size and had adequate barrier around the margins to provide skin protection and an effective seal. The pouch opening was cut off-center to prevent overlapping barriers with the ileostomy pouch (which tends to make both pouch seals less stable). The opening was cut ½-inch larger than the wound size to prevent the effluent from undermining the seal. The wound pouch was applied by centering the opening, so that a small margin of skin was exposed circumferentially (Figure 18-1, *B*). The pouch barrier was sealed by pressing at the inferior edge (closest to the fistula opening) of the barrier opening first, and then securing the remainder of the barrier seal. This prevented leakage in case the fistula started to function. The paper collar was then sealed to the skin, and the collar area that overlapped the ileostomy pouch was trimmed to avoid the ileostomy pouch barrier. The exposed skin inside the pouch opening was protected by skin barrier paste and covered with skin barrier powder. The window on the pouch facilitated access to the wound and the inner skin barrier. The powder was gently patted over the paste to increase resistance to the effluent and prevented the paste from sticking to the front of the pouch. The window of the pouch was closed by pressing the plastic rings together all the way around the rim. The pouch was connected to a leg bag or gravity drainage bag as needed.

Case Study 2

Following a bowel resection, a 65-year-old woman developed an ECF through the midline wound. The patient's abdomen was round, and the wound extended from below the umbilicus to the suprapubic crease. The wound dimensions were 3 inches by 1½ inches. Fistula drainage was small bowel effluent of a moderate amount that could be managed without the additional capacity supplied by a leg bag or a gravity drainage collector. A one-piece cut-to-fit pouch with a flexible barrier and a 3-inch cutting surface was chosen. The barrier on this pouch was not considered resistant enough to the effluent to achieve a 4- to 5-day wearing time. An additional extended-wear skin barrier was added as a washer to the pouch to lengthen the pouch's wear time. Wedges were also cut from that barrier to fill the suprapubic creases. The pouch opening was cut ½-inch larger than the washer size to prevent leakage between the two pieces. Six skin barrier wedges were cut in varying widths and lengths.

With the patient lying flat to stretch out the suprapubic creases, a thin layer of skin barrier paste

was applied to the creases. After exposing the paste to air to allow the alcohol to evaporate (about 1 minute), the skin barrier wedges were layered into the creases. This was done by layering the narrowest wedge into the deepest area of the crease first and adding successively wider wedges on top to fill the V-shaped contour of the crease. When all creases were filled, all edges of the wedges were sealed with a thin layer of skin barrier paste to prevent its lifting away when the patient changed position (Figure 18-2, *A*). Next, the washer was applied by centering the opening over the wound so that a margin of skin was visible all around the wound.

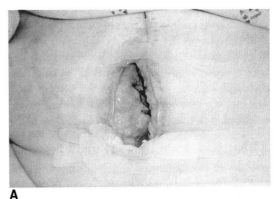

A

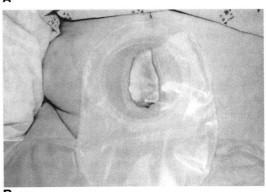

B

Figure 18-2 **A,** Skin barrier paste applied to creases followed by layering of solid skin barrier wedges; edges of wedges sealed with skin barrier paste. **B,** One-piece cut-to-fit pouch with flexible barrier cut slightly larger than wound was placed over wound (a washer was in place around the wound edges), exposed skin protected with skin barrier paste.

The exposed skin was protected with a layer of paste. The pouch was applied with the same centering technique, with a margin of the washer visible all around the opening (Figure 18-2, *B*). A bottle of skin barrier powder was introduced through the drainable end of the pouch, and powder was applied to cover the paste. This made the paste more resistant to the effluent and prevented the paste from sticking to the front plastic of the pouch. The pouch end was closed with a hinge style of clip.

Case Study 3

A 47-year-old man underwent a subtotal colectomy for a lower gastrointestinal bleed. Complications resulted, including fascial dehiscence, avascularized bowel, and necrotic fascitis. He developed small fistulae following abdominal debridement and skin grafting. As a result, much of the skin graft was lost from the contact with the enzymatic effluent. The wound bed was red and moist with granulation tissue, and shallow in depth. Three fistulas were present near the wound perimeter. The wound extended from the tip of the xyphoid process to the pubis and measured approximately 11 inches long and 7 inches wide. No commercially made pouch was known to accommodate these dimensions. An extended-wear skin barrier was chosen because it would resist the small bowel effluent and allow the patient to bend with comfort. The 8- by 8-inch skin barrier was cut into strips approximately 2 inches wide and placed petal-fashion around the wound and skin margin. The barrier strips were placed onto the skin with a ¼-inch clearance from the wound to prevent the effluent from undermining the barrier (Figure 18-3, *A*). A surgical isolation bag was selected for its size, offering as it did an ample cutting surface, and for its heavy-gauge plastic, which would not tear. The bag was not a pouch and did have a drainable end; it was closed with a drawstring tie. The opening was traced onto the bag by overlaying it on the wound bed. The opening was cut a ½-inch larger than the skin barrier size to prevent leakage between the bag and the barrier. Skin adhesive liquid was painted onto the skin barrier strips. The liquid adhesive was aired for 1 to

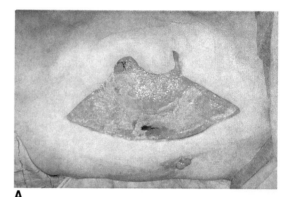

A

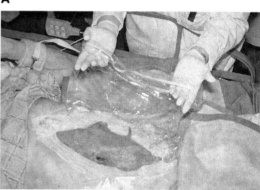

B

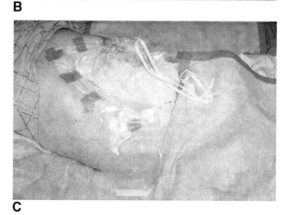

C

Figure 18-3 **A,** An extended-wear skin barrier was cut into 2-inch strips and placed petal-fashion around the wound and skin margin. **B,** An opening in a surgical isolation bag was cut ½ - inch larger than the skin barrier, and an adhesive painted onto the skin barrier strips. The bowel isolation bag was applied to the adhesive-coated skin barrier by attaching one side at a time. **C,** The edges of the isolation bag were taped to the skin, gauze packed into the wound, and the drawstring pulled closed.

2 minutes to achieve strength. The bowel isolation bag was applied to the adhesive-coated skin barrier by attaching one side at a time (Figure 18-3, *B*). The most intricately cut side was pressed into place first. The superior and inferior ends (with the bag seam) were sealed. Finally, the other side was attached, a task which involved the practitioner walking around to the other side of the bed to obtain good manual control of the bag. No creases in the plastic could be permitted, since the effluent would track through to the outside. (During the application, such a plastic bowel bag can be readjusted to smooth out wrinkles or creases and reattached to the barrier without adding more adhesive.) A skin barrier paste was applied to the exposed skin between the wound bed and the solid skin barrier and was covered with skin barrier powder. The powder was patted into the paste to enhance resistance to the effluent. The wound bed was protected with skin barrier powder and then covered with fluffed gauze. The drawstring at the top of the bag was closed and taped onto the bag (Figure 18-3, *C*). The gauze was changed when saturated, about every 4 to 6 hours depending on the amount of effluent. An abdominal binder held the gauze in the bag in place and was used when the patient was out of bed.

Case Study 4

A 55-year-old woman was seen with a small bowel fistula. Since she was not a surgical candidate, the plan included keeping her on NPO status, home total parenteral nutrition (TPN), and fistula containment. The husband of the patient received training for TPN and fistula care. The patient's contours varied with fluid retention; sometimes creases were deeper and other times more shallow. The husband was taught the principles of the pouching system and learned to vary the number of wedges according to the need to even out the surface for pouch adhesion.

All creases that were moist were dusted with skin barrier powder. A thin layer of skin barrier paste was applied before the skin barrier wedges were layered (Figure 18-4, *A*). When the wedges were level with the adjacent skin, a solid skin barrier was

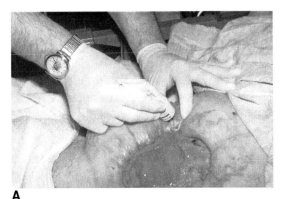

A

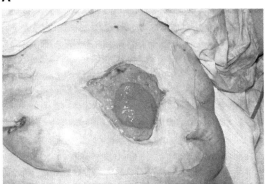

B

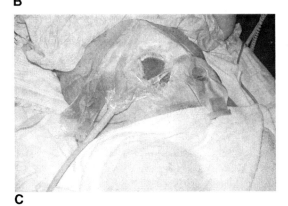

C

Figure 18-4 **A,** Moist creases were dusted with skin barrier powder and filled with a thin layer of skin barrier paste. **B,** Solid skin barrier was placed petal-fashion around the wound margins and the skin barrier inner edge was caulked with skin barrier paste. **C,** The pouch was placed over the skin barrier; exposed skin was covered with skin barrier paste followed by skin barrier powder. A waterproof tape framed the outer pouch, and an extension tube was secured to the bottom of the pouch and attached to a gravity drainage collector.

placed petal-fashion around the wound margins to accommodate its irregular shape. The skin barrier inner edge was caulked with skin barrier paste (Figure 18-4, *B)*. The postoperative pouch (with no skin barrier attached) was applied to the petaled skin barrier. (The pouch was cut approximately ½-inch larger than the wound size.) After the pouch was pressed into place, skin barrier powder was applied to the exposed skin barrier paste and the wound bed around the fistula. Waterproof tape was applied as a frame around the pouch to add stability. The drainable end of the pouch was gathered around an extension tube and taped securely to prevent leakage. The extension tubing was connected to either a leg bag or a gravity drainage collector (Figure 18-4, *C)*. After lessons with the husband, he was successful in achieving a 5- to 7-day seal at home.

CONCLUSION

An ECF presents clinicians with a complex set of problems. The physical and psychologic challenges to the patient can be enormous (Erwin Toth, 2001). Nursing interventions, designed to stabilize the patient's condition and address his or her physical and psychologic needs, assist the patient in coping with the numerous complications a fistula presents.

SELF-ASSESSMENT EXERCISES

Questions

1. Define an ECF.
2. List two causes of postoperative development of an ECF.
3. Describe the clinical presentation of a person with an ECF.
4. What will be the first radiographic study done when investigating the origin of the ECF?
   a. CBC
   b. Colonoscopy
   c. Fistulogram
   d. Barium enema
5. Name the two goals in conservative treatment of the patient with a fistula.

6. List the two methods that are used to decrease gut secretions in the person with an ECF.
7. Which of the following are impediments to spontaneous fistula closure?
   a. High small bowel output and dehydration
   b. Distal obstruction and the presence of a foreign body in the fistula tract
   c. Inability to pouch the fistula and loss of the periwound skin
   d. Patient intolerance
8. List five goals for nursing management of a patient with an enterocutaneous fistula.
9. Discuss the product options that can be used to manage an enterocutaneous fistula.
10. Which of the following can be used directly on the skin around ECFs to provide protection? (Select all that apply.)
    a. Skin barrier powder
    b. A thick layer of cornstarch
    c. Solid skin barrier
    d. Transparent dressing
11. Describe the difference between regular- and extended-wear solid skin barriers.
12. Discuss how suction can be used to manage an enterocutaneous fistula.

Answers

1. An enterocutaneous fistula is an abnormal communication between the intestine and the skin.
2. Postoperative development of an ECF may be the consequence of excessive tension on the anastomosis, compromised vascular supply, malignant disease, infection, poor nutritional status, steroid therapy, metabolic/endocrine disorders, and patients with Crohn's disease.
3. Patients may present with some of the following findings: fever, localized erythema, induration and local discomfort, electrolyte imbalance, alterations in mental status, sepsis, malnutrition, dehydration, anemia, tissue destruction, and severe acid/base imbalance.
4. c
5. Conservative treatment involves decreasing the secretions of the gut and nutritional support.

6. To decrease gut secretions, two methods are restricting the patient to NPO status and the use of somatostatin analogs.

7. b

8. Nursing management aims to provide protection of the perifistular skin, containment of the fistula output, and quantification of the output, as well as implement a cost-effective system, promote patient comfort, and optimize physical function and control odor.

9. Products include solid skin barriers, sealants, skin barrier powders and/or pastes, containment devices (pouches), suction catheters, and/or drains.

10. a, c

11. An extended-wear barrier is better suited for high-volume liquid output.

12. Suction can be applied to a pouching system to aid in removal of the fistula drainage and thus improve the pouch seal. A closed suction system can be created by lining the skin edges around the fistula with pieces of solid skin barrier. The base of the wound or fistula is covered with gauze saturated with saline and wrung out. A suction catheter or drain is placed over the gauze and the entire area is covered with a transparent dressing. The suction catheter or drain is connected to low, continuous suction. The entire setup is changed as needed when the dressing no longer provides an airtight seal.

REFERENCES

Elson C, Iqbal N: Options in managing enteral fistulas in inflammatory bowel disease. In Bayless T, Hanauer S, editors: *Advanced therapy of inflammatory bowel disease*, Hamilton, 2001, BC Decker.

Erwin Toth P: Sexual adjustments and body image. In Bayless T, Hanauer S, editors: *Advanced therapy of inflammatory bowel disease*, Hamilton, 2001, BC Decker.

Hwang T, Chen M: Randomized trial of fibrin tissue glue, *Br J Surg* 83:112, 1996.

Milsom J, Ky A: Therapeutic expectations: surgical management of Crohn's disease. In Bayless T, Hanauer S, editors: *Advanced therapy of inflammatory disease*, Hamilton, 2001, BC Decker.

O'Brien B, Landis-Erdman J, Erwin Toth P: Nursing management of multiple enterocutaneous fistulas located in the center of a large abdominal wound: a case study, *OWM* 44(1):20, 1998.

Rolstad B, Bryant R: Management of drain sites and fistulas. In Bryant R, editor: *Nursing management of acute and chronic wounds*, St Louis, 2000, Mosby.

Wong W, Buie W: Management of intestinal fistulas. In Mackeigan J, Cataldo P, editors: *Intestinal stomas: principles, techniques and management*, St Louis, 1993, Quality Medical.

19 *Outcomes Measurement*

·······························

BONNIE SUE ROLSTAD and DEBRA NETSCH[*]

OBJECTIVES

1. Discuss the historical and theoretic basis of health care outcomes studies and their relevance to WOC/ET nursing.
2. Distinguish between medical and WOC/ET nursing outcomes in ostomy and continent diversion care.
3. Identify outcomes in WOC/ET nursing practice relevant to the patient with an ostomy or continent diversion.
4. Describe a model used in an Outcomes Management Program.
5. Discuss the design and implementation of outcomes studies.
6. Explain the importance of standardized nursing language in clinical information systems.
7. Compare and contrast measurement instruments relevant to ostomy and continent diversion patients.
8. Identify potential research questions related to ostomy care.

INTRODUCTION

We create the future by what we do or fail to do today. *Fecal and Urinary Diversions: Management*

Principles is a text dedicated to the articulation of principles and techniques of this discipline-specific practice. Policies, pathophysiology, procedures, and standards of care are presented. Within this context, a chapter on outcomes management (OM) is obliged to inquire, "As wound, ostomy, and continence (WOC/ET) nurses, does what we do make a difference?"

Patients and physicians alike acknowledge the essential role of the WOC/ET nurse in providing quality care for people with ostomies and continent diversions (CDs), yet there exists little empirical evidence to support these claims. Ostomy and CD patients have benefited from the specialist role since its origin in 1958. At that time, practice was dedicated to ostomy and fistula management. Subsequently, wounds and continence have been included in the scope of practice (Alterescu, 1991). However, unlike wound care and continence care, which are often shared to some extent with other health care professionals, ostomy and fistula care remain the exclusive purview of the WOC/ET nurse. Thus the responsibility for documenting and reporting the WOC/ET nurse's contributions to improved patient care and care delivery lies within this professional role and those closely related medical specialties.

Changes in health care reimbursement and management have led to practice changes for the WOC/ET nurse. Resources are limited, and resource allocations are under scrutiny. "It will be through OM that the data will emerge to support the value of WOC/ET nurses in the care of the patients with ostomy, wound, and continence needs" (Cullen, 2001).

[*]The authors thank Kathryn Hoyman, PhD, RN, ET, Knowledge Engineer, Fairview Health Services, Minneapolis, Minn, and Ruth A. Bryant, RN, MS, CWOCN, Program Director, webWOC Nursing Education Program, Minneapolis, Minn, for their contributions to this chapter.

This chapter explores the definitions and processes of OM as they apply directly to the ostomy and CD patient population. Previously published resources on WOC nursing practice standardization are woven into the context of an OM program. A discussion is presented of the history of OM, types of OM, and the role of standardized nursing language and research methodology in an OM program, along with a call for further development by the specialty. Nursing informatics and the role of technology are explored as well as the role of teams that collaborate on quality improvement activities. Internet sites were extensively reviewed in the preparation of this chapter and appear in the references for the reader's further inquiry.

OVERVIEW

Today's consumer-driven health care system expects high quality and the best care for the most competitive price. Whether the customer is a patient, health care organization, or regulatory body, performance measurement and benchmarking, which provide outcomes information, is a means of improving quality of care (American Nursing Association, Quality Indicators: Outcomes measurement using the ANA Safety and Quality Indicators, 1999).

Quality as defined by Webster is a desired characteristic and a degree of excellence. Medicare defines quality as "doing the right thing at the right time, in the right way, for the right person, and getting the best possible results" (Centers for Medicare and Medicaid Services, 2002). Quality patient care should produce optimal health outcomes in the most cost-effective manner and result in high patient satisfaction.

Dimensions of quality encompass characteristics such as safety, morbidity/mortality, accessibility, timeliness, patient satisfaction, prevention of disease, and comprehensiveness, in addition to effectiveness of care provided. Quality is measured by studying indicators or characteristics of care (Box 19-1). Although most of these characteristics have been related to the practice of medicine rather than nursing, nursing-sensitive outcomes have also been identified and will be reviewed later in this chapter.

BOX 19-1   Components of Quality in Health Care

Equity	Services are provided to all, without discrimination.
Accessibility	Services are readily available.
Acceptability	Care meets the expectations of those using them.
Appropriateness	Care provided meets practice standards and avoids harm, as is possible.
Comprehensiveness	Care includes all aspects of disease management including prevention, treatment, and psychosocial aspects.
Effectiveness	Care provides positive change in health status or quality of life.
Efficiency	Quality care is provided at the lowest cost.

Adapted from Woodward CA (2000): Strategies for assisting health workers to modify and improve skills: developing quality health care—a process change. In *Issues in health services delivery, improving provider skills* (pp 1-60), Geneva, World Health Organization. Retrieved December 0202, from website: www.who.int /health-services-delivery/disc_papers/Process_Change.pdf.

Outcomes are the results of actions. This broad perspective includes outcomes of performance improvement studies as well as patient care. *Patient care outcomes are the results of care and represent what happened to the patient as a result of the care delivered.* The key to understanding the effectiveness of cost-sensitive, quality patient care is in part the measurement and management of outcomes (Wojner, 2001). Outcomes- and evidence-based practice are closely linked. Evidence-based practice is when findings from outcomes research are integrated into practice to improve patient outcomes and care delivery (Oermann and Floyd, 2002).

Within this evidence-based practice, decisions are predicated on the integration of research evidence, the health care provider's experience, and patient preferences; this is referred to as *best practice*. Best practice sets new standards and creates new innovations (Hickey, Ouimette, and Venegoni, 2000). Care plans, pathways, and algorithms for care are developed based on best practice.

Why Measure Outcomes?

The relevance of outcomes initiatives in WOC nursing practice is multifaceted. Outcomes research examines critical issues that impact on clinical care or the delivery of care to reduce risk, increase benefits, and improve treatment. Results are used by customers (i.e., patients, payers, and other providers) to make more informed decisions. For example, a patient may choose a surgical procedure based on outcomes studies.

In WOC/ET nursing practice, OM provides feedback that helps evaluate the care provided. This allows the WOC/ET nurse to understand the effects of interventions on the patient and the patient's overall functioning. This statement may seem to attribute undue importance to interventions practiced by the WOC/ET nurse. However, the patient who continues to experience leakage and odor with the pouching system following an intervention recommended by the WOC/ET nurse will most certainly experience changes in overall functioning— changes related to daily living activities, concepts of self-esteem, financial expenses, and health-seeking behavior.

In addition, and on a larger scale, the measurement of patient care outcomes leads to evidence-based interventions and contributes to the identification of patient-based benchmarks that will guide and improve patient care (Flarey, 1997). It also assists in the development of standardized approaches to practice that are consistent with existing corporation-wide quality improvement activities.

Finally, resources within a corporation are typically allocated based on evidence of their value. Outcomes data is used to demonstrate that the WOC/ET nursing role contributes to effective, cost-sensitive care. Furthermore, the data may be incorporated into the health care system's marketing campaigns. In the absence of adequate substantia-

tion of the WOC nurse's value, administrative support wanes and position cuts become common.

HISTORY OF THE QUALITY MOVEMENT IN HEALTH CARE

The origin of outcomes reporting is attributed to Florence Nightingale during the Crimean War (1853-1856) (Lang and Clinton, 1990; Salive, Mayfield and Weissman, 1990). Ms. Nightingale performed the first systematic analysis and reporting of patient outcomes as a means of evaluating the results of care provided.

In 1917, E. Codman, a physician, presented the "end-result idea," wherein he proposed that physiologic and psychosocial outcomes of care be tracked and publicized by physicians and hospitals to improve patient care and help patients choose physicians and hospitals. He was labeled an eccentric and his ideas were quite unpopular with physicians, who thought them detrimental to medical practice (Codman, 1917). During that same year, the American College of Surgeons published a set of minimum standards for hospitals in the United States to identify and eliminate poor health care (Brooks, 1995). These standards were the origin of today's review and accreditations process of the Joint Commission on Accreditation of Healthcare Organizations and demonstrate the intent to improve patient care by monitoring and regulating quality.

Integration of Business Practices with Health Care

The unsustainable, soaring health care costs of the 1980s and geographic inconsistencies in medical practice resulted in the restructuring of the U.S. health care system. Every care setting would be affected over the following 20 years, as prospective payment replaced fee for service reimbursement (Agency for Healthcare Research and Quality, 1998; President's Advisory Commission on Consumer Protection and Quality in the Health Care Industry, 1998). The evolving health care industry was required to provide efficient, quality health care; therefore, practices from industry and business were applied to health care (Agency for Healthcare Research and Quality, 2000).

Deming, a statistician and industrial quality control expert, brought Total Quality Management (TQM) and Continuous Quality Improvement (CQI) to the forefront as a means of providing greater efficiency and increased productivity in health care (Deming, 1982). He championed teamwork, employee empowerment, and customer satisfaction as the essential components of an effectively functioning system.

Donabedian's quality improvement framework, which separated structure, process, and outcomes components to evaluate quality, became the basis of quality improvement efforts. Structure, as Donabedian described it, encompasses features of the health care setting: staffing, types of equipment, technology, and how the health care organization functions (e.g., committees). Process was defined as the "how" of providing care (e.g., timeliness, continuity), and outcomes were defined as the results achieved (i.e., patient care) (Donabedian, 1992; Donabedian, 1985). This efficiency culture emphasized standardization of health care practices to control cost and ensure consistent patient care.

The current era in health care began in 1988, when Ellwood challenged health care to join the era of "outcomes management": the measurement and global sharing of health care outcomes amongst providers to determine what works. This approach emphasized outcomes, assessment, and accountability (Relman, 1988). It recognized that practice variation and suboptimal care are expensive, and that "linking the care people get to the outcomes they experience" makes outcomes research pivotal to monitoring and improving patient care (Agency for Healthcare Research and Quality, 2000).

Federal Involvement in Quality of Care

The U.S. federal government established the Agency for Health Care Research and Quality as part of its "Effectiveness Initiative" (Agency for Health Care Policy and Research, 1999). Regulatory bodies, such as the Joint Commission on Accreditation of Healthcare Organizations (JCAHO), now mandate process improvement and clinical outcomes as measurements of quality. Ironically, JCAHO has established the Ernest A. Codman Award to recognize organization performance and quality of care that has been improved through process and OM (Joint Commission on Accreditation of Healthcare Organizations, 2002). Consumers can use outcomes from a variety of health care settings, now widely available on the Medicare website, as decision-making tools. For example, a comparison of outcomes in long-term care facilities is currently posted on the Medicare website.

Strategies to Improve Quality

Strategies to improve quality still use Donabedian's framework of structure, process, and outcomes. Methodologies may encompass formal research or quality improvement frameworks. In either instance, the goal is to obtain useful data to improve patient care and care delivery.

Quality Assurance is one of the oldest quality strategies. This approach, establishing a minimum standard of performance to monitor effectiveness, is still useful to licensing and accrediting bodies (Woodward, 2000). CQI and TQM are ongoing, proactive processes whereby customer needs and customer-defined outcomes are emphasized (Newell, 1996; Creech, 1994). These processes operate under the assumption that all providers are committed to high-quality care. When a problem occurs the process is evaluated rather than blame assigned.

Today a merging of these approaches to quality is commonly seen, dependent in part on the culture and tolerance for change within the health care setting. Six Sigma is a more recent entrant in the field of strategies to improve quality. It is a disciplined, data-driven system for achieving, sustaining, and maximizing business success based on close understanding of customer needs and eliminating variations (i.e., defects) (Pande, Neuman, and Cavanagh, 2000).

Quality Initiatives in WOC/ET Nursing Practice

WOC/ET nurses have been reporting results of care in peer-reviewed journals for decades as a means of providing evaluative feedback about the effectiveness of ostomy and CD patient care and improving their care. All levels of evidence have been used, from randomized, controlled studies to case studies and expert opinion; the majority of the published reports are case studies or anecdotal. For example, the earliest recorded history of the WOC/ET nurse's practice is chronicled in the Fall 1972 issue of ET Quarterly, the official publication of the International Association for Enterostomal Therapy (IAET) and the precursor to the Journal of Wound, Ostomy and Continence Nursing. In this issue alone, there are six ostomy or fistula case studies that discuss problem solving and results of care (ET Quarterly, 1972). However, the standards for writing case studies were not as comprehensive as those used today.

In 1986, the IAET (now Wound, Ostomy and Continence Nurses [WOCN] Society,) sponsored a major initiative to justify the role of the enterostomal therapy (ET) nurse by documenting outcomes. The competition yielded case studies, discussion of financial strategies for WOC/ET nursing practice, and a longitudinal study of organizational improvement in a Visiting Nurses Association (Etris et al, 1987; Rolstad and Scheel, 1987). The IAET then published a White Paper on ET Nursing and its cost benefits (Kynes et al, 1987). Since that time, WOCN Society initiatives have encompassed practice standards, a database project, and reimbursement for services. However, justifying the role of the WOC/ET nurse and measuring its contribution to care with outcomes is research waiting for a champion.

PROGRAMS FOR OUTCOMES MANAGEMENT

The implication of the term *outcomes management* may lead one to conclude erroneously that the management of outcomes occurs as a final step in evaluating care. Actually, OM should be considered a program that contains a sequence of steps fundamental to any and all WOC/ET nurse practices.

Definition of Terms

Specifically, OM is a research-based, interdisciplinary endeavor to "enhance physiologic and psychosocial patient outcomes through development and implementation of exemplary health practices and services" (Wojner, 1997). This process researches

the effectiveness and value of health care products and services as well as the quality with which they are delivered. The measurement of outcomes provides objective evidence for decision making about treatment options and care delivery and enables patients, providers, and payers to make more informed decisions.

OM is distinguished from other quality initiatives in that it is more globally focused in a health care system and is customer focused, population based, and outcomes centered. It represents a mindset and attitude that uses techniques of CQI.

OM addresses principles previously established by Ellwood: (1) use of standards for clinical interventions, (2) inclusion of functional status and well-being as well as disease-specific clinical outcomes, (3) pooling of data into large databases, and (4) analysis and dissemination of data to decision-makers (Ellwood, 1988). These principles provide a roadmap for WOC/ET nurses when planning an OM program.

Obstacles to OM

Today the quality movement and outcomes management are "a tide in which we are all swimming" (Pierce, 2002). WOC/ET nurses practice in health care environments that value efficient, quality care. Thus effective WOC/ET nurses, having recognized the relationship of quality, evidence-based practice, OM, and role viability, are immersed in outcomes initiatives. However, the paucity of outcomes data in ostomy patients hints at underlying problems. If OM were easy to do, why hasn't it been done and its results made available in the published literature?

There are numerous obstacles to OM, from the incidence and prevalence of the ostomy and CD patient population to deficiencies in the supply of nurses, educational preparedness, technologic support, structured care methodologies (SCMs), and uniform nursing terminology. The typical WOC/ET nursing practice is very busy addressing immediate patient care issues and systems projects. This service is frequently understaffed. The WOC/ET nurse works with a general nursing staff that is characterized by shortages, turnover, and lack of knowledge regarding ostomy care. Immediate issues of patient care and nursing education take priority in these situations and leave little time for the details of nursing research.

The demographics of the WOC/ET nursing profession reveal another obstacle: the lack of formal education in research. A minority of WOC/ET nurses have master's degrees (24%) and a formal academic background in nursing research (WOCN Society, 2002). This group is likely to be employed in positions that require some level of research ability. In contrast, the majority of WOC nurses have B.A. degrees and have taken only introductory courses in research; thus their position descriptions are less likely to include a research component. However, in spite of this educational gap, it is important to point out that a significant amount of reporting of outcomes has been observed from each educational background. It is anticipated that the presence of quality improvement teams will benefit the WOC/ET nurse by providing additional resources for research initiatives.

Technology and Information Services support services provide the infrastructure required to organize and analyze large groups of data. These resources are generally focused on systems activities and high-volume, high-cost services (e.g., admissions, operating room scheduling, staffing). While ICD-9 codes identify the incidence of ostomy surgery, other useful information regarding nursing outcomes is not currently available. Rather, outcomes of WOC/ET nursing care are generally identified with focused chart reviews. Data collection tools include paper-based instruments, customized computed-based spreadsheets or the WOCN Society software PIDS (Patient Information Data System) (WOCN Society, 1999). Unfortunately, the data tracked do not reflect outcomes; rather they focus on productivity and patient demographics.

Unlike the high incidence of wounds or incontinence, ostomy patients are a low-volume population. With decreased lengths of stay, this group requires well-organized OM efforts designed within the phases of care (i.e., preoperative, immediate postoperative, and long-term). Large, randomized, controlled studies of WOC/ET nursing outcomes are impractical with this patient population. However, unique study designs and small, focused studies are available and meritorious.

SCMs and standardization of practice are needed to perform research that may be shared and compared with that from other facilities. These methodologies include critical pathways, algorithms, protocols, and guidelines for practice. When these tools are available (i.e., WOCN Society Ostomy/CD critical pathway), they should be used in research.

One of the most common methods used to measure outcomes is to manually review charts and tabulate the number of times a specific event is recorded. Unfortunately this is both laborious and fraught with potential errors. In addition, when events are recorded in the chart, the language used to label the event can vary widely, within the health care setting as well as nationally. This situation is the result of an absence of a standardized language for nursing, or the lack of a uniform terminology.

The American Nursing Association (ANA) Committee on Databases to Support Clinical Practice was created to review and critique nursing languages and to establish the Uniform Nursing Language System. Currently this system recognizes five standardized languages: The North American Nursing Diagnosis Association, or NANDA, Classification; the Nursing Interventions Classification, or NIC; the Nursing Outcomes Classification, or NOC; the Omaha System; and the Home Health Care Classification. The first three languages are broad and comprehensive throughout different health care settings and specialties, whereas the last two nursing languages are primarily for home health care specialties (Maas and Johnson, 1998).

Although the creation of standardized nursing language systems was intended to standardize the terms used within nursing, having five languages also creates an obstacle in the tracking of nursing diagnosis and activities. The nursing minimum data set (NMDS) was created in an attempt to reduce this obstacle and identify the common nursing core elements involved in patient care in long-term care and skilled nursing facilities. The three types of elements identified include nursing care, patient/client demographics, and service elements. The aforementioned nursing languages are used as the nursing care elements of the NMDS, which demonstrates that no single language is universally used (Hickey, Ouimette, and Venegoni, 2000). With the use of such a minimum data set, nursing language can be computerized so that retrieval of data can be achieved with a keystroke rather than a manual chart review. These new databases present an area of considerable interest to potential nursing researchers (Maas and Johnson, 1998). Data sets already established that aid in the standardization of information for further research use include Outcome and Assessment Information Set (OASIS), Minimum Data Set (MDS), and the United Ostomy Association registry.

Outcomes Management Models

The concept of creating an OM program can feel quite overwhelming for the already busy WOC nurse, particularly if there is any trepidation about

using components of the research process. However, many models for an OM program exist. A basic OM model will guide and direct the phases of the project (Figure 19-1).

During Phase I the population for the study is identified, the project questions are formed and instruments selected, intermediate outcomes are identified along with significant variables and variance, and the population database is developed. In Phase II the literature review and practice review are performed. Changes to practice are determined with new SCMs, which are pivotal to this phase. In Phase III the new practices developed and standardized in the previous phase are now implemented (i.e., tested). Data are collected regarding the new practices. During Phase IV analysis of data occurs, and potential revisions are identified. New questions can be generated, and Phase II begins again, demonstrating continuous practice improvement (Wojner, 2001).

Two specific models for OM include the Stetler Model and the Iowa Model of Research. While both

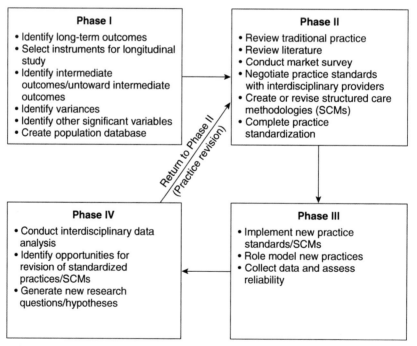

Figure 19-1   A model for outcomes management. (From Wojner AW, editor: *Outcomes management: applications to clinical practice*, St Louis, 2001, Mosby.)

models have unique features, each is based on the premise of the researcher needing to use or implement the findings.

The Stetler model focuses on the individual clinician implementing the research findings and is divided into six phases: (1) preparation, (2) validation, (3) comparative evaluation, (4) decision making, (5) translation and application, and (6) evaluation. The Stetler model is based upon the premise of the individual clinician using decision making and critical thinking at each phase (Hickey, Ouimette and Venegoni, 2000).

The Iowa Model of Research in Practice is based on the assumption that a change in evidence-based practice is triggered by a problem or a change in knowledge. Examples of problem-focused triggers include data obtained from risk management and quality improvement activities (such as a survey revealing that a large number of nurses do not know how to change an ostomy pouch), total quality management programs, and the identification of a clinical problem. In contrast, knowledge-focused triggers are stimulated by new information, new research findings, new or changed standards of care, and recent changes in expert opinion. The findings of the research are then evaluated for implementation with innovation or change of practice (Hickey, Ouimette, and Venegoni, 2000).

Once a problem or knowledge trigger is identified, the literature is reviewed to determine if there is an adequate research base for a practice change. If adequate research exists the steps to follow are:

1. Clarify the expected outcomes and document the baseline or current status of these outcomes.
2. Design nursing and multidisciplinary practice innovations.
3. Implement the research-based practice changes on a pilot unit.
4. Evaluate practice change from a process and outcomes perspective.
5. Modify practice intervention and implementation methods as needed for implementation on other units.

The OM project must be adapted into a research project if there is not an adequate research base;

this creates a base for further studies (Hickey, Ouimette, and Venegoni, 2000).

DELINEATING OUTCOMES OF WOC NURSING PRACTICE

Historically the focus of outcomes in the scope of the WOC/ET practice has been clinically based. However, Gallagher identifies three domains of nursing practice: microsocial (relationships between two or more professionals or between the WOC/ET nurse and the patient), intermediate (i.e., organizational or institutional), and macrosocial (i.e., related to policy making in large populations) (Gallagher, 2002). Each of these domains is a point of focus in WOC/ET nursing OM. When discussing the clinical nurse specialist role, Dayhoff and Lyon recognize changes in disease state, nurse-sensitive outcomes, nursing personnel outcomes, organization/ network sphere, and economic domains (Dayhoff, Lyon, 2001). Both models recognize the contribution of nurse specialist roles beyond patient care.

A distinction between outcomes of medical practice, general nursing, and WOC/ET specialty nursing practice is key. To show a contribution, outcomes affected by the WOC/ET nursing role must be isolated (e.g., mortality, morbidity, and length of stay are typically influenced by medical practice patterns rather than WOC/ET nursing practice). Although the WOC/ET nurse contributes to these outcomes, they are not primary results of WOC/ET nursing actions. However, there are discipline-specific outcomes related to morbidity that lend themselves to outcomes assessment in WOC/ET nursing.

Outcomes targeted for assessment in the WOC/ET nursing role depend on the nurse's care setting and role within the health care system as defined in a position description. However, the WOC/ET nurse's role generally encompasses three spheres: (1) clinical, (2) nursing staff support, and (3) organizational improvement. Each of these areas should be addressed in an OM program.

Clinical Outcomes

The "Clinical Value Compass" was published by the Joint Commission on Quality Improvement and provides a useful framework for the selection and reporting of outcomes to demonstrate the WOC/ET nurse's value (Nelson et al, 1996). Four types of outcomes are identified: (1) clinical (physiologic), (2) functional status, risk status, and well-being, (3) satisfaction with care provided and perceived benefit, and (4) cost (Gray, 2000).

Research in these areas asks questions about what has been achieved by an action and whether that outcome makes a difference. Benefits of an intervention, associated risks, and results of treatment are addressed as components of clinical outcomes. Box 19-2 provides ideas for OM for WOC/ET nurses. These areas closely follow the role responsibilities that are common to the WOC/ET nurse position description. For example, the WOC/ET nurse may be interested in stoma site

selection and how it affects postoperative management. A comparative study could be done to look at differences in postoperative care between those receiving elective stoma site marking versus those who had emergency procedures without a stoma site marking. The results from this study might validate the value of preoperative marking and identify potential areas for cost reduction.

Most WOC/ET nurses are familiar with economic outcomes. Productivity and time studies are typical examples. Additional examples include cost savings with more efficient product usage, reduction in complications, and preventive teaching. The information gleaned from these types of studies not only affects the quality of patient care, but also can be used to justify new positions, reinforce the need for current staffing, and document the need for program expansion.

Nursing Staff Support Outcomes

Activities related to education and support of nursing staff include orientation, ongoing education, and general emotional support. Ostomy patients are recognized as consuming significant nursing time and expertise on the unit. These two factors cause nursing staff frustration and represent a good area for the WOC/ET nurse to demonstrate the value of the role.

Opportunities for significant teaching occur 24 hours a day, each day the patient is in the hospital. For example, the nurse is giving a medication and the patient asks a question about the stoma. The nurse must be prepared to provide teaching at any time during the course of the patient's stay in the hospital. Nurses working on units where ostomy patients reside need extensive knowledge and training to be able to provide correct information and education. Even when the WOC/ET nurse is providing primary teaching, the staff nurse must know what to do whenever a situation can arise. Patients learn skills, attitudes, and information both formally and incidentally. The value of the staff nurse's knowledge in these informal teaching moments cannot be minimized.

A well-educated nursing staff is the result of ongoing educational efforts and access to supportive

---

BOX 19-2   **Topics for Outcomes Measurement (Partial Listing)**

···

Preoperative Phase

Stoma site selection and marking

Patient education

Emotional support

Family education and support

Postoperative Phase

Assessments: Stoma, peristomal skin, mucocutaneous juncture, function/complications/treatment

Technical skills acquisition (e.g., pouch emptying, assembly, and change; basic peristomal skin care)

Discharge teaching (e.g., fluid and electrolytes, diet, complication recognition, emergency contacts)

Patient's sense of well-being

Patient's satisfaction with WOC/ET nursing care

Patient's satisfaction with nursing staff's ability to provide basic ostomy care

Cause and effect relationship of preoperative activities to postoperative or long-term management

Long-Term

Assessments: Stoma, peristomal skin, mucocutaneous juncture, complications/treatment

Patient's sense of well-being

Return to school/life work/social/sexual activities

Patient's satisfaction with WOC nursing care

Quality of life

information such as procedure sheets, assessment forms, teaching documentation forms, standardized care plans, and discharge planning forms. Educational activities with nursing staff result in several important areas. Outcomes of the WOC/ET nursing role can be measured by increased satisfaction and comfort level on the part of the staff nurse, as well as growth in the nurse's ability to independently handle basic needs of the ostomy patient (i.e., emptying a pouch, changing a pouching system, and providing basic teaching). These outcomes can lead to better nurse retention and may also contribute to organizational performance outcomes.

Organizational Performance Outcomes

Organizational performance outcomes study Donabedian's structure and process categories within the health care system. Projects related to structure may focus on the WOC/ET nursing service itself. To accomplish goals of the health care system and the WOC/ET nursing service, appropriate staffing levels, WOC/ET nurse expertise, technology, secretarial support, and other position-related resources are required. WOC/ET nurse shortages are structure problems, as are the lack of technology resources that are key components in the tracking of outcomes data. Other structure-related examples include committee work within the health care system, such as collaborative practice committees, research committees, and product committees.

Process components in the WOC/ET nursing role center on the "how" of providing health care. Process examples include outpatient scheduling, notification of new inpatient referrals, and inpatient supply-ordering procedures. Each of these projects is a quality improvement effort that yields outcomes to be measured. A structure and process quality improvement initiative that is common to most WOC/ET nursing practices is the proper selection, use, and inventory of ostomy products within the health care system. These types of projects are frequently identified because of a complaint; a multidisciplinary team is then required to change organization processes. A process improvement project can also impact and change practice.

Examples of Outcomes Studies

Process Improvement. Several patients in 1 month (15%) responded on the ostomy outpatient satisfaction survey that there are long waiting periods before appointments and that they did not realize they should bring their own supplies to the examination. Inquiry into the process revealed that delays also resulted in schedule disruptions for the clinic staff and the WOC/ET nurse. Increased inventory was required in the clinic, and several emergency orders to Materials Management were made while patients waited. A process improvement project was developed that included the stakeholders involved in the process and a review of each step required to schedule patients. The desired outcome for the project was to achieve a 98% satisfaction rating in this area during the first month of change implementation. Added benefits of this study were increased clinic staff productivity and increased outpatient scheduling opportunity for the WOC/ET nurse.

Clinical: Preoperative Marking. Preoperative stoma site marking and education with a WOC/ET nurse was revealed to result in fewer ostomy complications when compared with those in patients who did not have the benefit of this intervention (Park et al, 1999; Bass et al, 1997). This type of outcomes information can lead to questions about whether an outpatient clinic is available for elective ostomy patients and reinforces the need for reimbursement for this service.

Clinical: Postoperative Patient Concerns. Pieper and Mikols identified the top-rated concerns before and after discharge, in a study published in 1996. Odor, participation in sports, leakage, changing the pouch, changes in body appearance, need for further treatment, and participation in sex were among the concerns identified by patients. This information provides an evidence base for teaching topics while the patient is in the hospital and areas of follow-up for return clinic visits (Pieper and Mikols, 1996).

Clinical: Posthospitalization Adjustment. Thomas presents a prospective study of 106 patients where the link is established between inadequate advice (teaching) and poor patient adjustment (Thomas, Madden, and Jehu, 1987).

Clinical: Posthospitalization. Another study with direct application to WOC/ET nursing was reported by Nordstrom's survey of 66 patients with urinary diversion; it pointed out that 58% of patients were using the same equipment as that which was first introduced to the patient 3 to 14 years earlier. This study also reviews body shape changes and the opportunity to correct potentially harmful techniques that could require continuing treatment or reoperation (Nordstrom, Borglund, and Nyman, 1990).

Clinical: Morbidity Related to Ostomy Equipment. Significant morbidity related to ostomy equipment has been reported. One retrospective study of persons with an ileostomy over long-term related to peristomal skin problems and leakage of pouching systems (Leong, Londono-Schemmer, and Phillips, 1994). This type of study is directly relevant to WOC/ET nursing practice, patient comfort, and expense. As most WOC/ET nurses know, patients with long-term problems may self treat. This frequently results in a significant increase in product use. Ostomy equipment is reimbursed by Medicare and other third-party insurers; untreated or unsuccessfully treated complications incur increased costs.

Clinical: Bowel Sounds. Folkedahl et al asked the question, "Why are bowel sounds assessed following surgery?" since the indicators of bowel function return are flatus, nondistended abdomen, and absence of nausea or vomiting. Their research identified that bowel sounds do not need to be assessed routinely for postoperative patients when those indicators of return of bowel function are present. Best practice is exemplified by the implementation of these results into practice (Folkedahl et al, 2002).

Quality of Life. Marquis, Marrel, and Jambon studied the quality of life for stoma patients with a validated quality of life index. A total of 618 stoma care (WOC/ET) nurses in 16 countries in Europe recruited 4739 patients following surgery. A longitudinal study was done that included the first year after surgery. Results from the study indicate that patients have significantly higher quality of life rating when they (1) were satisfied with the care provided, (2) had a good relationship with the stoma

care (WOC/ET) nurse, and (3) expressed a solid comfort with managing the pouching system. The study concludes by stating that the patient's quality of life index is higher when access to the stoma care nurse is provided for up to 6 months following surgery (Marquis, Marrel, and Jambon, 2003).

Cost Savings. A WOC/ET nurse noted, when initially establishing a WOC/ET department, that many boxes of different pouching systems were in the patients' rooms in the hospital. It was determined that this hospital routinely dispensed entire boxes of pouching systems from Central Supply for each patient. A cost analysis was performed that determined that a large cost savings would be realized by issuing pouching systems individually rather than in larger quantities. This cost savings was calculated and partially justified another WOC/ET nurse position. In addition, care was also influenced: no longer were boxes of inappropriate product used by the staff nurses, so that patients experienced fewer difficulties with appliance adherence, and incorrect supplies were sent home with the patient less frequently (Netsch, 1987).

Education. Outcomes of research have resulted in changes related to the prevention and treatment of colon and rectal cancer. Extensive education of patients and health care professionals, an emphasis on prevention and early detection, and clinical guidelines for treatment have become the norm (The National Comprehensive Cancer Network, 2002).

Application of the Research Process to Outcomes Management Programs

This chapter is not intended to provide a review of research design or the process to critique research. The advantage of one design over another, as well as the matching of design and methodology with the question posed, are beyond the scope of this chapter. The ability to see flaws in research design and the impact of subtle biases in methodology are important to consider when interpreting research results. The reader is encouraged to seek further reading on this topic. However, the reader should also be reassured that the value of an OM program is not in the complexity of the studies conducted.

Application of the Deming Wheel (*Plan, Do, Check, Act*) quite successfully allows investigation into system improvement projects. When a research methodology is anticipated, it is always wise to secure an additional team member, based on the type of question being asked, who is experienced in research design. This person could also serve as a resource when reviewing the literature in an attempt to identify levels of evidence.

Basic steps to designing a research project are outlined in Box 19-3. Key elements are easily reflected in the quality management program and include the fact that the topic should be one that is of interest and will make a difference. For example, a comparison study could be done on preoperative marking techniques to determine which method results in an adequately visible mark in the operating room (OR), least cost, and least amount of patient discomfort. Many times the topic can be a search for the answer to the classic queries: what if we did it this way, or why do we continue to do it that way? Only one question should be addressed at a time; additional questions present future research opportunities.

Data collection can be either quite laborious (i.e., manual chart reviews) or entail the use of readily available data (i.e., infection rates). Probably the most overlooked step in the OM program is the dissemination of the results, both good and bad. When this step is overlooked, the project will benefit only a very few and will not contribute to the pool of available literature that will ultimately guide changes in practice and quality of care. Finally, the long-term adoption of the practice innovation or change must be implemented to realize improvement in the process or care provided (Hickey, Ouimette, and Venegoni, 2000).

Implementing an OM Program for WOC Nursing

It is essential for the future of our profession that the WOC/ET nurse lead and champion an OM program for the ostomy patient population. However, it is not the sole responsibility of the WOC/ET nurse to create and conduct such a program. Rather the key to a successful OM program is the use of a strong and diverse interdisciplinary team (Gallagher, 2002).

It behooves the WOC/ET nurse to use the evidence-based practice available when creating a nursing care plan. It also behooves the WOC/ET nurse to question different approaches to old problems, and explore these further.

Although it may be distressing to realize that there is a paucity of published research studies and OM projects related to the care of the ostomy patient population, it also represents considerable opportunity (Gray, 1998). Furthermore, of the literature that is available concerning this specific patient population, many are case studies, consensus, or expert opinion. Although it is undeniable that the level of evidence represented by case studies and expert opinion is lower-level evidence, this literature has played an important role in the improvement of care for this patient population. However, WOC/ET nurses must seize the opportunity to build the evidence needed to substantiate the import and significance of the care provided. Nurses participate in our professional responsibility to build evidence by (1) publishing all outcome-related studies we conduct, and (2) designing appropriately sophisticated outcome-related studies to best answer the question posed.

Steps for Creating an OM Program

This chapter is based on the premise that OM projects will be used or implemented and not done only for the sake of performing research or in fulfillment of a work requirement. An OM program does not

BOX 19-3   Basic Steps of Research
....
1. Identify problem or research question.
2. Review literature related to the topic.
3. Define the research question or the problem to be studied.
4. Select the study design, data collection tools, plan for analysis, and personnel.
5. Conduct the study.
6. Analyze results.
7. Evaluate results (i.e., accept, reject, restudy).
8. Disseminate results.

need to be difficult. In fact, it should be logical and flow from one step directly into the next step.

The first step is to identify a problem, a potential innovation, or an area of interest to study. One method easy to understand and use involves the business technique of the identification of strengths, weaknesses, opportunities, and threats (SWOT). Looking at the department's SWOT may in fact identify a need for further OM projects, clinical pathways, or the implementation of best practice. It is certainly an excellent tool to evaluate the department from a different perspective (Wojner, 2001).

Perhaps the most important step is to assemble a team. The team should include change agents who contribute to the OM from different perspectives (e.g., a statistician, business office personnel, clinicians). It is extremely important that this team be interdisciplinary so the multiple facets of the project are identified and addressed. The project coordinator champions the project and keeps it moving forward (Gallagher, 2002). Once the team is assembled, the selection of an OM model is recommended. After a model has been identified, the team must implement and initiate the model with the designing of the identified OM project.

One member of this team may be a nurse specializing in nursing informatics. This is a nursing specialty newly recognized by the American Nurses Association. It integrates "nursing science, computer science, and information science to manage and communicate data, information, and knowledge in nursing practice." This specialized group of nurses is certified by the Nursing Informatics Association. However, the role is quite new. It encompasses the management of information technology and can be an important resource within research teams (Nursing Informatics, 2002).

Data Collection

The data collection portion of the OM project is perhaps the most labor intensive. The ANA recommends a simple yet effective approach to ensure thorough and complete data collection, using a who, what, when, where, and how system (Duffy and Korniewicz, n.d.).

Who? This identifies the actual data collectors. The data collectors can be clinicians, staff nurses, or the business office personnel; what is most important is they be precise and consistent. There must be interrater reliability to ensure the integrity of the data. It is essential that the data collectors have the same definitions, collection tools, and instructions and are trained for consistency.

What? This determines the question(s) being asked and the variables being measured. *What* also refers to operational definitions, research instruments used, protocols to be implemented, and identification of the sample and sample size. The data collectors must have access to all the aforementioned information. A statistician or a colleague in the research department is extremely helpful at this stage to determine the appropriate sample size and the best methods of the necessary data collection. It is helpful at this stage of the design process to identify the statistical test that will be used to compile the data. This can avoid pitfalls at the end of the study. Instruments are available for use based on the outcome being studied (Duffy and Korniewicz, 1999). Instruments may vary in type, including health status surveys, quality of life, laboratory values, functional status, and treatment protocols (Gallagher, 2002). In addition to these sources, the NOC provides appropriate tools that the WOC nurse can use to measure outcomes (Gallagher, 2003).

When? This refers to how often the data will be collected.

Where? This identifies the actual location where the data collection is to take place. Collection of the data can take place in a patient room, the medical records department, a nursing home, or on the phone.

How? This denotes the method or the instrument that will be administered. In addition to interviews, data collection methods include concurrent and retrospective chart review and observation; however, each must be used in an appropriate, accurate, and consistent manner. If the data are collected in a precise manner consistent with the above concerns, they are more likely to be accurate and reflect real life (Duffy and Korniewicz, 1999).

Statistical analysis tests are used to synthesize the data into the study findings. As previously discussed, the statistical method of analysis should be determined during the study design, before the data collection stage. The most common types of statistical tests performed for OM projects include descriptive statistics such as frequency distributions, as well as standard and means deviations. In addition, inferential statistics of regression analysis and variance analysis identify relationships or comparisons (Duffy and Korniewicz, 1999). Statistical packages such as MyStat and Statistical Package for Social Services (SPSS) help with data compiling and analysis.

Reporting the findings is essential. Report cards are a means of doing so (Figure 19-2). The term report card is used in OM to place the emphasis on the project summary and the accountability necessary to a complete and thorough project. Crucial aspects of the report card are brevity and prioritizing the information it carries. Busy colleagues, administration, and staff can glean the findings of the OM project quickly and identify its recommendations (Schriefer, Urden, and Rogers, 1997). The report card is an excellent tool to disseminate project findings efficiently.

Once the OM project has been completed, the project findings must be analyzed to determine if they should be implemented or rejected. Tools such as evidence-based practice and clinical pathways are valuable ways to use the results of the OM project. In fact, it is imperative that evidence-based practice and clinical pathways be based on research findings or OM projects.

WHAT DOES THE FUTURE HOLD?
Tradition-Based to Evidence-Based Practice

Moving away from tradition-based practice requires education of WOC/ET nurses and useful tools. In 1999, the WOCNS formed the Center for Clinical Investigation (CCI) in response to the member-driven movement to address evidence-based practice. The CCI's role is to promote and expand the evidence base for WOC/ET nursing by supporting clinical investigation programs of its members and by partnering with other agencies and professional organizations to expand efforts to increase the evidence base of practice. In short, the

CCI will support the membership to generate, synthesize, and disseminate evidence (Gray, 1999). Within this initiative, "Spotlight on Research," "Notes on Methodology," and "Report Cards" are now being published in the JWOCN.

The Society is currently establishing best practice-based ostomy fact sheets. Evidence-based practice involves reviewing all the pertinent research, determining the level of evidence, and incorporating the evidence into practice. The Society has identified the following five levels of evidence:

Level 1: More than one randomized, controlled trial supports safety and efficacy of intervention.

Level 2: Majority of randomized trials support safety and efficacy of intervention, but others are equivocal or fail to support efficacy.

Level 3: Quasi-experimental studies (nonrandomized trials) support safety and efficacy.

Level 4: Case series or case studies suggest potential for safety and efficacy.

Level 5: Consensus or expert opinion (best practice) (Gray et al, 2000).

Other Sources of Research

Some further research/OM projects are completed or underway, yet are not published in a manner conducive to wide dissemination. Master's theses provide an example. These are published, but frequently are not identified in electronic searches. Perhaps the CCI could call for all theses related to ostomy to be registered with the organization. Think of the studies that would be initiated if every WOC/ET nurse currently enrolled or soon to be enrolled in a graduate program would focus on an ostomy topic! There would be a surge in research studies or OM projects.

CONCLUSION

OM represents a philosophy and a culture, focused on the measurement of quality, that is based on results of care and care delivery. Within this framework, clinical, nursing support, and systems improvement outcomes may be identified and measured as they relate to the contributions of the

Pathway: write the name of the diagnosis here
ICD-9 or DRG or CPT4: ask your coders which codes to use   **Date:** update with each revision

This report is prepared pursuant to but not limited to (P. A. 368 of 1978). This report is a review function and as such is confidential and shall be used only for the purpose provided by law and shall not be a public record and shall not be available for court subpoena.

PATIENT CASE-MIX

Patient Descriptors This box is intended to describe the population which is targeted for use of the pathway. Data fields include: Avg cases per month, avg age, gender mix, payer mix, referral source. % with Comorbidities—smoking, HTN, diabetes, COPD, CHF, depression, etc.
Also included are:
Number of completed pathways _____
Number eligible for pathways _____
% with pathway used _____

CURRENT IMPROVEMENT ACTIVITIES

It is important to list all of the clinical, process and CQI/TQM activities related to the pathway diagnosis that are in progress. This will assist the team in tracking and documenting the multiple improvement initiatives. This box is used as a communication tool; and serves as a quick reference point with a summary of all improvement activities. It also serves to link QI and clinical process improvement activities which are required by regulatory agencies.

OUTCOMES

Patient Satisfaction
Indicators from the existing patient satisfaction tool deemed important to assess are evaluated; additional questions specific to the DRG may be added. Numerical scores (Likert in our case), and any high volume verbal complaints are tabulated and examined. In this box and all of the others be sure to include the data source, sample size and data range for data displayed in each box. This is critical!

Clinical Outcomes
This box contains the clinical outcome measures determined by the pathway team to be the most important to track. If you are unsure what they should be, review the clinical trials for the diagnosis and see what the researchers measure. We try to use the outcomes databases we have on site (such as NRMI for the MI path). If you don't have a clinical outcome database, you may have to review charts for these measures. It is important to develop a data definition and chart abstract form prior to chart abstraction in order to increase consistency.

Functional Health Status
This box includes information from standardized tools such as the Short Form 36 (SF-36) Health Status Tool from the Medical Outcomes Trust (617-426-4046). We display the scores by category before and 6 months after the pathway:
mental health   emotional role
social function   vitality
general health   pain
physical role   physical function

Other health status tools can be used for this box. Use the one that best measures the health status of your population.

Charges, Cost and Utilization
This box requires a strong partnership with the finance department. The automated claims data provides loss of this information. Again, try to compare one quarter to the next to show the trends. It is also helpful to break down total charge/cost into cost centers. This is the area to place length of stay, number of physician office visits, number of home visits, % going on to prevention programs, etc.

Figure 19-2   Report card. (From Schriefer J, Urden LD, Rogers S: Report cards: tools for managing pathways and outcomes, *Outcomes Management Nurs Pract* 1(1):14-19, 1997.)

WOC/ET nurse. Therein lies the evidence to justify the role of the WOC/ET nurse and maintain a continuous effort to improve care for patients with ostomy.

SELF-ASSESSMENT EXERCISES

Questions

1. Name two characteristics or indicators that encompass dimensions of quality.
2. Patient outcomes are the results of care.
   True _____ False _____
3. Name two reasons to measure outcomes in a WOC/ET nursing practice.
4. What are some of the obstacles to OM as related to a nursing practice?
5. Which of the following outcomes can the WOC/ET nurse target for assessment? (Select more than one.)
   a. Clinical
   b. Morbidity
   c. Nursing staff support
   d. Length of stay
   e. Organizational improvement
6. Name at least two clinical outcomes that can be measured in a WOC/ET nursing practice.
7. Discuss the benefit of examining nursing staff support outcomes.
8. The first step in creating an OM program is:
   a. Writing a proposal for funding.
   b. Discussing problems unique to WOC/ET nursing with colleagues.
   c. Identify a problem, innovation or area of interest to study.
   d. Create a template for action.
9. Describe the "who, what, when, where, and how system" for data collection recommended by the ANA.
10. One of the best methods to use the results of an OM project is via evidence-based practice and clinical pathways.
    True _____ False _____

Answers

1. Characteristics or indicators that encompass dimensions of quality include: safety, morbidity/mortality, accessibility, timeliness, patient satisfaction, prevention of disease, and the comprehensiveness and the effectiveness of care provided.
2. True; patient outcomes represent what happened to the patient as a result of care delivered.
3. Results are used by customers to make more informed decisions; provides evaluative feedback about care provided; can lead to evidence-based interventions; can assist in the development of standardized approaches to practice; can be used to demonstrate the contribution of the WOC/ET nurse.
4. The incidence and prevalence of the ostomy and CD patient population presents an obstacle to OM, as well as deficiencies in the supply of nurses, educational preparedness, technologic support, SCMs, and uniform nursing terminology.
5. a, c, and e; Morbidity and length of stay are typically influenced by medical practice patterns rather than WOC/ET nursing practice.
6. Clinical outcomes that can be measured in a WOC/ET nursing practice include: stoma site selection and marking, patient education, emotional support, family education and support, assessments (stoma, peristomal skin, mucocutaneous juncture, function/complications /treatment), technical skills acquisition (i.e., pouch emptying, assembly, change, basic peristomal skin care), discharge teaching (i.e., fluid and electrolytes, diet, complication recognition, emergency contacts), patient's sense of well-being, patient satisfaction with WOC/ET nursing care, patient satisfaction with staff nurses' ability to provide basic ostomy care, cause and effect relationship of preoperative activities to postoperative or long-term management, patient's sense of well-being, patient's return to school/ life work/social/sexual activities, patient satisfaction with WOC/ET nursing care, quality of life.
7. Decreases frustrations, providing the nursing staff with opportunities to provide ostomy patient teaching; increases nursing staff satisfaction and retention

8. c; identification of a problem, potential innovation, or area of interest to study

9. The *who* identifies the actual data collectors. The *what* determines the question and the variables being collected. The *when* refers to how often the data will be collected. The *where* identifies the actual location in which the data collection is to take place and the *how* is the method in which the instrument will be administered.

10. True; it is important that evidence-based practice and clinical pathways be based upon research findings or OM projects.

REFERENCES

Agency for Health Care Policy and Research (September 1999): *The outcome of outcomes research at AHCPR: final report. Summary.* Retrieved September 26, 2002, from website: www.ahrq.gov/cinic/outcosum.htm.

Agency for Healthcare Research and Quality (2000): *Outcomes research,* fact sheet, Publication No. 00-P011 ed. (brochure). Retrieved September 26, 2002, from Agency for Health Care Policy and Research website: www.ahrq.gov/clinic/outfact.htm.

Agency for Healthcare Research and Quality (1998): *The challenge and potential for assuring quality health care for the 21st century,* Publication No. OM 98-0009, prepared by the Department of Health and Human Services for the Domestic Policy Council, Washington, DC. Retrieved November 30, 2002, from website: www.ahrq.gov/qual/21stcenc.htm#references.

Alterescu V: Reflections upon the history and future of IAET, *J Enterostom Ther* 18:126-131, 1991.

American Academy of Family Physicians (1998): *Policy and advocacy, definition of quality care.* Retrieved December 27, 2002, from website: www.aafp.org/x6909.xml.

American Academy of Family Physicians (2002): *Quality Initiative.* Retrieved December 26, 2002, from website: www.aafp.org/x3843.xml.

Bass EM et al: Does preoperative stoma marking and education by the enterostomal therapist affect outcome? *Dis Colon Rectum* 40(4):440-442, 1997.

Brooks DC, editor: The Joint Commission on Accreditation of Healthcare Organizations. In Goldfield, N. and Nash, DB, editors: *Providing quality care: future challenges,* ed 2, Ann Arbor, Mich, 1995, Health Administration Press.

Brown-Etris M et al: ET goes home, *J Enterostom Ther* 14(1):4-11, 1987.

Centers for Medicare Services (December 2, 2002): *Nursing home quality measures.* Retrieved December 27, 2002, from website: www.medicare.gov/NHCompare/Search/Related/ImportantInformation.asp.

Centers for Medicare and Medicaid Services (October 10, 2002): *Glossary.* Retrieved November 30, 2002, from website://www.medicare.gov/Glossary/ShowTerm.asp?Language=English&term=quality.

Codman EA: The value of case records in hospitals, *Modern Hosp* 9:426-428, 1917.

Creech B., editor: *The five pillars of TQM,* New York, 1994, Truman Talley Books/Plume.

Cullen B: Outcomes management: an administrator's view, *JWOCN* 28(4):180-181, 2001.

Deming WE, editor: *Out of the crisis,* Knoxville, 1982, SPC Press.

Donabedian A: *The methods and findings of quality assessment and monitoring: an illustrated analysis,* Ann Arbor, Mich, 1985, Health Administration Press.

Donabedian A: The role of outcomes in quality assessment and assurance, *Qual Rev Bul* 18:356-360, 1992.

Duffy J R, Korniewicz DM: *ANA quality indicators: outcomes measurement using the ANA safety and quality indicators,* 1999. Retrieved November 11, 2002 from website:www.nursingworld.org/mods/working/QY/ceomfull.htm.

Ellwood PM: Outcomes management: a technology of patient experience (Shattuck lecture), *N Engl J Med* 318:1549-1556, 1988.

ET Quarterly (American Cancer Society) Fall:11-14, 1972.

Flarey DL: Patient care outcomes: a league of their own, *Outcomes Management Nurs Practice* 1(1):36-40, 1997.

Folkedahl B et al: Poster Presentation, WOCN Conference, Las Vegas, Nev, June, 2002.

Gallagher S: Outcome research and WOC nursing practice, *JWOCN* 29(6):278-282, 2002.

Gallagher S: Tools of outcome measurement in WOCN practice, *JWOCN* 30(1):7-10, 2003.

Gray M: Ostomy care? Show me the data! *JWOCN* 25(1):2-4, 1998.

Gray M (1999): *Initial finds for our first CCI member survey,* Center for Clinical Investigation. Retrieved October 26, 02, from website: www.wocn.org/clinical-inv/survey.htm.

Gray M (2000): *Selecting outcomes: the clinical value compass approach.* Retrieved October 26, 02, from website: www.wocn.org/pdf/WOCN_News_Iss_4_r4.pdf.

Guadagnoli E, McNeil BJ: Outcomes research: hope for the future or the latest rage, *Inquiry* 31:14-24, 1994, website: www.wocn.org/about/profile.htm

Hickey JV, Ouimette RM, Venegoni SL, editors: *Advanced practice nursing: changing roles and clinical applications,* Philadelphia, 2000, Lippincott, Williams & Wilkins.

Joint Commission on Accreditation of Healthcare Organizations (January, 2002). Retrieved November 25, 02 from website: www.jcaho.org/accredited+organizations/codman+award/codman_overview.htm.

Kynes TC et al: White paper on the cost-benefit analysis of ET nursing, *J Enterostom Ther* 1987.

Lang NM, Clinton JF: The classification of patient outcomes, *J Professional Nurs* 6:153-163, 1990.

Lange, NM, Marek KD, editors: *Patient outcomes research: examining the effectiveness of nursing practice.* Washington, D.C. 1992, Department of Health and Human Services, NIH Publication No. 93-3411.

Leong AP, Londono-Schimmer EE, Phillips, R, KS: Life-table analysis of stomal complications following ileostomy, *Br J Surg* 81:727-729, 1994.

Maas ML, Johnson M: Outcome Data Accountability, *Outcomes Management Nursing Pract* 2(1):3-5, 1988.

Marquis P, Marrel A, Jambon B: Quality of life in patients with stomas: the Montreaux study, *Ostomy/Wound Management* 49(2):48-55, 2003.

Motheral B: Outcomes management: they why, what and how of data collection, *J Managed Care Pharm* 3:00-00, 1997.

Nelson EC et al: Improving health care, Part 1: The clinical value compass, *Joint Commission Journal on Quality Improvement* 1996(22):243-58, 1996.

Netsch D: Cost savings report (unpublished internal document), Des Moines, Iowa, 1987, IMMC.

Newell, M: *Using nursing case management to improve health outcomes,* Gaithersburg, Md, 1996, Aspen.

Nordstrom GM, Borglund E, Nyman CR: Urostomy appliances and stoma care routines: the relation to peristomal skin complications, *Scand J Caring Sci* 4(1):35-42, 1990.

Nursing Informatics. (September 19, 2002): *Nursing informatics.* Retrieved December 29, 2002, from website: www.ania.org/ni/index.htm.

Oermann MH, Floyd JA: Outcomes research: an essential component of the advanced practice nurse role, *Clinical Nurse Specialty: J Advanced Nurs Pract* 16(3):140-144, 2002.

Pande PS, Neuman RP, Cavanagh R, editors: *The Sis sigma way,* New York, 2000, McGraw-Hill.

Park JJ et al: Stoma complications: the Cook County Hospital experience, *Dis Colon Rectum* 42(12):1575-80, 1999.

Pierce B (2002): Data collection and patient outcomes: strategies for success, Presentation at the WOCN Society Annual Conference.

President's Advisory Commission on Consumer Protection and Quality in the Health Care Industry. (March 12, 98). *Quality first: better health care for all Americans.* Agency for Healthcare Research and Quality, Publications Clearinghouse. Retrieved December 27, 2002, from website: http://www.hcqualitycommission.gov/final.

Pieper B, Mikols C: Predischarge and postdischarge concerns of persons with an ostomy, *JWOCN* 23(2):105-9, 1996.

Relman AS: Assessment and accountability: the third revolution in medical care, *N Engl J Med* 319:1220-22, 1988.

Rolstad BS, Scheel NR: Fiscal responsibility: prescription for survival, *J Enterostom Ther* 14(6):248-254, 1987.

Salive ME, Mayfield JA, Weissman NW: Patient outcomes research teams and the Agency for Health Care Policy and Research, *Health Serv Res* 25:697-708, 1990.

Schriefer J, Urden LD, Rogers S: Report cards: tools for managing pathways and outcomes, *Outcomes Management for Nursing Pract* 1(1):14-19, 1997.

The National Comprehensive Cancer Network (June 2002): *Colon and rectal cancer treatment guidelines for patients.* Retrieved September 27, 2002, from website: http://www.nccn.org/patient_gls/_english /_colon/index. htm.

Thomas C, Madden F, Jehu D: Psychological effects of stoma. II. Factors influencing outcome, *J Psychosom Res* 31(3):317-323, 1987.

Wojner AW: Outcomes management from theory to practice, *Crit Care Nurs Q* 19(4):115, 1997.

Wojner AW, editor: *Outcomes management: applications to clinical practice,* St Louis, 2001, Mosby.

Woodward CA (2000): Strategies for assisting health workers to modify and improve skills: developing quality health care—a process change. In editor: *Issues in health services delivery, improving provider skills* (pp 1-60), Geneva, World Health Organization. Retrieved December 0202, from website: www.who.int/health-services-delivery/disc_papers/Process_Change.pdf.

Wound, Ostomy and Continence Nurses Society (1999): *The patient information data system,* Laguna Beach, Calif, WOCN.

Wound, Ostomy, Continence Nurses Society (2002): *Profile of the WOCN membership.* Retrieved September 30, 02, from

RESOURCES

Agency for Quality and Research
www.ahcpr.gov/browse/evidmed.htm
http://www.ahcpr.gov/clinic/epc/
http://www.ahcpr.gov/clinic/epcquick.htm

American Society for Quality
http://www.asq.org/

Center for Evidence Based Medicine
http://cebm.jr2.ox.ac.uk/

Centre for Health Evidence
http://www.cche.net/che/home.asp
http://www.indigojazz.co.uk/cebm/levels_of_evidence.asp

Evidence-based Nursing
http://ebn.bmjjournals.com/

National Association for Health Care Quality
http://www.nahq.org/

Outcomes and Effectiveness
http://www.ahcpr.gov/clinic/outcomix.htm

Outcomes Management
http://www.nursingcenter.com/library/journalissue.asp?Journal_ID=54038&Issue_ID=240272

Resources for Practicing Evidence-based Medicine
http://pedsccm.wustl.edu/EBJ/EB_Resources.html

The ScHARR Guide
www.nettingtheevidence.org.uk
http://www.shef.ac.uk/~scharr/ir/netting/

The Cochrane Library
http://www.cochrane.de/cc/cochrane/cdsr.htm

Health Sciences Library Resources, Buffalo, New York
http://ublib.buffalo.edu/libraries/units/hsl/internet/ebn.html

The University of York
http://www.york.ac.uk/healthsciences/centres/evidence/updindex.htm

Core Library for Evidence-based Practice
http://www.shef.ac.uk/~scharr/ir/core.html

A listing of websites
http://www.med.ic.ac.uk/divisions/63/phcgp/ebmweb
sites.htm

Software/Internet
American Psychological Association website (1999)
Buros Institute of Mental Measurements website (1999)
HAPI (1999) (CD Rom with questionnaires, rating scales,
interview forms, checklists, tests)
MERLIN (1999) (online public access catalog of tests and
measures)
CONQUEST (2000)

Organizations/Institutes
Agency for Health Care Research and Quality, Clinical
Practice Guidelines, formerly the AHCPR, website:
www.ahcpr.gov.
Joint Commission of Health Care Organizations, Oakbrook
Illinois. Outcome indicators/measures with the ORYNX
initiative, which integrates performance measures into the
accreditation process, website: www.jcaho.org.

The Use of Telemedicine in Ostomy Management

....

ANNE SCHEURICH

OBJECTIVES

1. Identify three ways telemedicine can assist the nurse in caring for the ostomy patient in home care.
2. Discuss the process of video transmission.
3. Define criteria for patient selection of telemedicine services.
4. Relate how to perform an ostomy assessment using telemedicine equipment.
5. Discuss issues to consider when developing a telemedicine program.

INTRODUCTION

It has often been said that nursing is both an art and a science. For the wound, ostomy, and continence (WOC/ET) nurse, teaching, treating, and supporting the ostomy patient can be the perfect marriage of the art and the science. Nurses continue to be challenged to provide the best care for patients despite having less money, time, and personnel resources. As the scope of practice for the WOC/ET nurse continues to grow, so do the tools and technologies available to support that practice. One such technology is telemedicine. Telemedicine technology can assist the WOC/ET nurse in providing patient care. It's amazing to imagine being able to reach a patient who is 60 or 160 miles away just by means of a phone line and camera: no lengthy drive time, and no frustration trying to visualize an abdomen or an appliance based on only a description.

In June of 1999, the Congressional Telehealth Briefing Committee developed the following definition (American Telecare, Inc., n.d.):

Telemedicine uses information and telecommunications technology to transfer medical information for diagnosis, therapy, and education. The information may include medical images, live two-way audio and video, patient medical records, output data from medical devices, and sound files.

The telemedical interaction may involve two-way live audio and video visits between patients and medical professionals, sending patient monitoring data from the home to the clinic, or transmitting a patient medical file from a primary care provider to a specialist.

Simply put, *telemedicine* or *telehealth* is the exchange of medical information from one site to another using an electronic communication device. This exchange may be to improve patient care, for the health education of the patient, or the education of the health care provider. It allows providers to reach patients who may not be able to access services in any other manner. It allows the practitioner to actually see the problem rather than just hear a description. It permits direct access to the patient or caregiver in the patient's own environment or in the local clinic, both of which are generally more convenient. With technology evolving by the minute, it is unrealistic to try to address specific technology by name and parameters. This chapter addresses the general concepts and guidelines of telemedicine and its use for the WOC/ET nurse. How to select the type of services available is addressed first; patient selection comes next; and then, how to perform an assessment using telemedicine equipment is discussed. Finally, program development with the current available technology is addressed.

SELECTING SERVICES

In assessing the needs of the identified population, the types of services to be provided are evaluated. Historically, a variety of services have been provided to diverse populations via telemedicine, and the list continues to grow. In the short history of telemedicine, typical diagnostic groups served include respiratory, cardiac, psychiatric, and wound care patients. Serving the ostomy patient is a new frontier. Still, it is an exciting and valuable asset to offer the person with an ostomy. When evaluating services traditionally provided to the ostomy patient, the practitioner must assess which services might be provided from a distance and consider the essential tasks to be accomplished both before and after surgery (Box 20-1).

Many of these tasks can be carried out during the initial interview with the patient and a family member, a caregiver, or a significant other. Live video telemedicine equipment is a tool that can be effectively used in the preoperative patient interview. Many preoperative doctors' visits and laboratory evaluations are required of a patient. Meeting with the WOC nurse can add to an already overloaded schedule. If the preoperative interview can be performed at a convenient location or in the patient's home, the stress and the overwhelming feeling of surgery can be ameliorated slightly. The clinician can benefit from assessment of the patient's environment. This may help in decision making and decrease or actually prevent postoperative problems in the home. In addition, if postoperative teaching is to be done by way of telemedicine, it's good for everyone to get a chance to see and use the equipment in advance. Although cultural or social barriers may take time to overcome, early identification helps everyone involved.

Postoperative interventions such as education, counseling, and follow-up care can also be accomplished in this manner. Live video equipment acts as a "television camera" to allow both parties instant access to information. A question-and-answer session can be performed as it would be in person. The camera can be manipulated for viewing of the patient's care environment. The camera can also be manipulated for the clinician to assess the patient's abdomen and assess skin and stoma condition and function, as well as accurate pouching system placement. It can be extremely helpful to visualize the patient's abdomen as he or she is describing a problem on the phone. To have the ability to see the curves and contours of a patient's abdomen and be able to suggest a solution is extremely satisfying for both the patient and the clinician. Observing the patient on multiple occasions in the home or in a clinic space that is geographically convenient will accelerate patient learning and possibly prevent problems.

One area that does not appear to be conducive to telemedicine is preoperative stoma site selection and marking. The process of selecting and accurately marking a stoma site requires a hands-on approach. While many tasks can be achieved with telemedicine, some still require the personal touch.

SELECTING THE APPROPRIATE PATIENT

The first step in a telehealth program is identifying the appropriate patient. Not all patients should receive telemedicine services. Technology is a great

---

BOX 20-1   Items To Consider Before Providing Services From a Distance

- Physical, psychologic, mental, and emotional status
- Cultural, social, and philosophic attitudes
- Sensory perception
- Past experience
- Current meaning of the event
- Interest and motivation
- Actual knowledge
- Environment
- Presence and attitudes of others

From Hampton BG, Bryant RA, editors: *Ostomies and continent diversions: nursing management,* St Louis, 1992, Mosby.

tool, but it does not always apply to every situation and patient. Although no hard and fast rules currently exist from the governing bodies, Box 20-2 suggests guidelines.

PERFORMING THE VISIT

After selecting and enrolling the appropriate patient into the program, the visit process can begin. First and foremost, the clinician must obtain consent. The language of the current patient consent form must be checked. Does it contain a photography clause? If not, a separate consent for video and photography must be obtained.

Next, the clinician has to set a timetable and stick to it. Telemedicine patients need to be scheduled the same as inpatients or clinic patients. It can be easy to be distracted by patients, physicians, or projects that are in the clinician's plain view each day. It is advisable to set a day or time of day that is dedicated to telemedicine. The telemedicine patients can be thought of as patients that are come in to be seen in person. The success of a telemedicine program hinges on commitment. A dedicated room or office for the telemedicine program is necessary. This room should provide privacy for the caregiver and the patient. Sensitive images and information will be transmitted; the patient's privacy and confidentiality must be ensured as if the patient were being met in person. Good lighting at the base station is critical so that the practitioner can be viewed well by the receiving party. It is important to have all equipment in the room that might possibly be used in the teaching lesson. Now the visit can commence. The visits will get easier and more natural as the practitioner and the patient become familiar with the technology. See Box 20-3 for information on a successful telemedicine visit.

PATIENT RESPONSE

Patient response to this technology will be varied. The success of the program can be greatly influenced by how the program is explained to those

---

BOX 20-2   Guidelines To Consider in Selecting Patients for Telemedicine Services

- The patient and/or the caregiver should be alert and oriented to diminish the potential for confusion.
- The patient should have good cognition and hearing.
- A significant other or a caregiver should be present for all or most encounters.
- The patient or caregiver should demonstrate comfort with technology.
- Patients who do not have local access to a WOC practitioner or have developed a particular bond to the telemedicine practitioner would be good candidates.

Modified from Telemedicine Reimbursement Guidelines for Medicare Recipients. (n.d.), website: www.fcc.gov/e-file/ecfs.

BOX 20-3   Steps to a Successful Telemedicine Visit

1. Activate the equipment as directed by the manufacturer.
2. Greet patient as per routine. Encourage the operator of the equipment in the remote location to focus the camera on the patient's face at the beginning of the call. Acknowledge the patient and all parties present. Then ask whatever questions are pertinent. Now focus the camera on the patient's abdomen.
3. Discuss issues at hand and allow time for comments and discussion. Initial visits, until everyone is comfortable with the technology, may be lengthy.
4. Give clear, concise camera directions, such as "move to the middle of abdomen," or "toward the head." Avoid using words like "up" and "down." These can be misleading and end up frustrating everyone.
5. Take photo stills of each visit for records, research, and reference. Save these photos to the patient file.
6. Proceed with instructions, moving the camera back to the patient's face so the feeling of an in-person encounter is created.
7. Close the visit with a plan and a schedule for follow-up.

who participate. Patient responses range from excitement to fear and skepticism. Many patients have a concern about privacy. The patient must be assured that all routine privacy regulations will be maintained. No one can remotely access the camera without the patient's consent. No one can "spy" on the patient. A privacy statement complying with the Health Insurance Portability and Accountability Act of 1996 (HIPPA) guidelines can be provided on admission to the program. Often, patients can be quite excited by the technology. They feel they are getting something "extra," the latest and best technologic care. Patients may want to chat, share a joke, or comment on how the practitioner is looking or sounding that day.

DO'S AND DON'TS

With any new procedure and technology there are uncertainties the first time a clinician performs the task with a patient. Everyone is a bit nervous or anxious. It will take practice, but the more relaxed and confident the practitioner is on camera, the more at ease the patient will be. The practitioner should consider ways to relax encounters, for instance taking a few moments to discuss the way patients look, how they are dressed, or the weather. Time should be taken to train the camera operator at the remote site before the first visit. This may be the caregiver, the home health nurse, or a clinician in a virtual clinic. If the person operating the camera is comfortable with the equipment, the visit should go smoothly. Adequate time must always be allowed, especially in the early stages of the program. An initial visit generally lasts 30 to 45 minutes. Follow-up visits that do not involve major problem solving may only require 15 minutes. Everyone must give the technology a chance. Any new system will have bugs. It may be helpful to have a representative from the Informational Technology (IT) department at hand on the first day of calls to assist with any unexpected problems. The clinician must be confident and reassuring to those at the remote site. This is new to them as well.

The practitioner shouldn't try to replace human interaction with technology. While technology can allow geographic areas and patients to be reached who were previously inaccessible, it cannot and will not replace the human touch. There may be times when the hands-on approach will be the only solution. The practitioner must give the technology a chance, but should realize that a "live" visit may be required at times.

SELECTING THE TECHNOLOGY

Once the needs of patients and physicians have been assessed and the scope and goals of the program have been established, the next step should be identifying the type of equipment required. The field of technology is massive and will need to be narrowed to make the right selection.

Telemedicine systems vary greatly. There are three general categories of telemedicine equipment. The first consists of a device that provides access to emergency medical services. This mechanism transmits a coded message to a monitoring station when the user touches a button. It is battery-operated and worn around the neck or wrist. The system is only used to summon emergency assistance or personnel. The second type of device is a patient telemonitoring device, also known as *store and forward*. It collects and transfers patient data, inputted by the user, to the monitoring station. This device is used for monitoring respiratory patients. The patient performs routine spirometry, and the data are stored in the unit until a preprogrammed time, when it is transmitted to the monitoring station and/or the physician. Other common uses of store and forward devices are for hypertensive or diabetic patients (www.HomMed.com). The third type of device is the *televideo* patient monitoring system. This tool allows live, real time transmission of voice and video from the user to the monitoring station or clinician and allows visualization of the patient and the clinical situation. This type of technology has been used for monitoring and intervention of asthma and psychiatric patients, and most effectively with wound care patients (American Telecare, Inc., n.d.) Any of these systems can assist the WOC nurse to provide telephone reassurance and emergency intervention. However, the televideo system would be the most appropriate and effective system to use with the ostomy patient. Such support can increase patient independence and self-confidence. Being able to see the situation rather than just hearing about it can be a tremendous asset for both the patient and the health care provider.

Telemedicine can address many needs. Identifying these needs at the outset of developing a program is the important first step. Will the primary goal be patient instruction, ongoing monitoring, or strictly troubleshooting? Will the program be used to deliver educational programs to nurses or physicians? Will there be a "virtual clinic" or in-home assessments? Determining these needs will assist the practitioner in selecting the type of equipment and device that will be needed. For example, if home care is to be the primary setting for the program, a base station for the WOC/ET nurse and multiple field units to go in the patients' homes will be required. In contrast, a clinic-to-clinic, or clinic-to-physician's office setup will only require a base station and one or two field units.

ASSESSING NEEDS

Telemedicine has proven to be a great teaching tool. A telemedicine camera provided to the patient at discharge can make teaching in the home more effective. The cameras are sent home with the patient like any other piece of durable medical equipment. The patient and/or the home care nurse schedule a time for a joint visit, and the patient is seen in the home environment. This is a great advantage for the homebound patient or patients in rural areas with limited access to health care services. It is useful to imagine being able to watch the patient perform his or her ostomy care in the home environment. How much easier would it be to observe technique and identify problems? As the patient progresses or tries a new pouching system, the camera could be activated for follow-up and monitoring. Solutions to problems could be achieved so much faster.

If the patient population is not homebound, or if a large portion of the patient population travels a great distance to receive services, a virtual clinic may be the best use of telemedicine. A virtual clinic can exist anywhere. It may be in a physician's

office, or at a medical facility. By contrast, it may be a room at the local community center or in a senior citizens housing facility. In the virtual clinic mode, a room is set up as the receiving station where patients are seen. By setting the area aside, privacy is ensured. Regularly scheduled appointments are planned. The number of cameras required is generally limited to one (decreasing the financial investment) and the "clinic" can be staffed by a registered nurse or a licensed practical nurse and perhaps an office assistant or clerk. At regular times the system is activated and the patients seen, assessed, taught, or treated as necessary.

Telemedicine can also be a great teaching tool for the professional. Inservices can be provided without barriers such as distance and location. If a camera is placed in the physician's office, teaching and troubleshooting can be done with all pertinent staff present as needed. Teaching all the care providers at once in their environments saves time and money.

When beginning to plan to provide telemedicine services, the target population and end user are assessed. Current referral patterns (where and from whom) must be determined. If most referrals come from physician's offices, perhaps a virtual clinic between the physician's office and the WOC/ET nurse's office will fit the need. Will most visits be with patients in the long-term care setting or home care? Then more field cameras will be required and instruction to the staff on equipment planned. Who will benefit most from the technology, the patient, the caregivers, the practitioners, or physicians? Identifying this will give direction to marketing the program. Who are the stakeholders in the application, and how is support obtained? Planning ahead and getting the identified people involved from the start is best. The more people who understand and help build the program, the more successful it will be. Business management's support is vital to the financial success of the program. The clinicians' involvement in the program is key, otherwise they may see the program as a burden. If nursing staff understands the time savings and the patient advantages, their buy-in will come more easily. Overcoming patient fears is vital. The practitioner should develop a sheet of frequently asked questions and answers. As much information should be given up front as possible. This can become part of the preoperative teaching plan. If patients know what to expect, they will have an easier time in the postoperative period. It is useful to involve the IT department early in the assessment. It can be a valuable resource in evaluating equipment and software.

CHOICES OF TELEMEDICINE SYSTEMS

Once needs have been determined, the equipment can be selected. There are currently three basic scenarios of live video transmission. The first scenario uses a Plain Old Telephone System or POTS line.

One camera is in the patient's home, connected to a phone jack (Figure 20-1, *A*). This camera connects to the base station at the office using the standard phone connection. No other special lines are needed. The advantages of this system include easy implementation, relatively low cost, simple maintenance, and the fact that all hardware can be purchased "over the counter." The drawback to this system is that any software must reside in the office base station, which can limit software choices.

The second scenario is called the combination system (Figure 20-1, *B*). There is still a POTS connection between the patient's home and the office's base station, but there is an additional high-speed

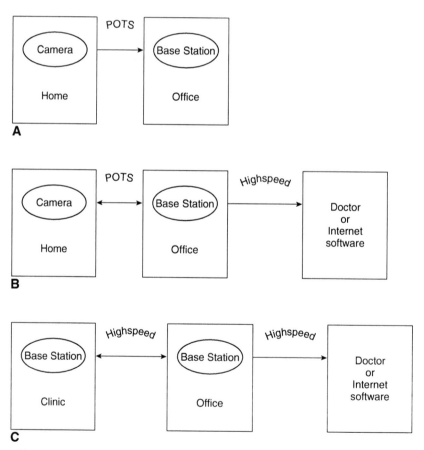

Figure 20-1   **A,** Plain Old Telephone System (POTS). **B,** Combination system. **C,** "Virtual Clinic" setup.

connection between the base station and the Internet. This system allows for most of the benefits discussed in Figure 20-1, *A,* but also allows the system to use Internet-based software, providing rapid uploading of documenting photos to offsite storage or to a doctor's files. There are few disadvantages to this type of system; one drawback is that the use of Internet software can leave an office dependent on the Internet connection to record the visit information. If the connection should go down, visits could still be made but not entered into the software. There is also the factor of the added expense of the software and high-speed connection. However, it should be noted that these costs appear to be decreasing with time and usage. The ability to send the physician or health care provider a photo of the patient's progress is a powerful tool.

The third system (Figure 20-1, *C*) shows a virtual clinic setup that uses a high-speed connection between two base stations. This setup gives the user a system that is always on and ready to make a visit, with no need to dial up. The equipment can be expensive but is no harder to use than the equipment in the previous two scenarios. Figure 20-1, *C,* also shows a high-speed connection to a doctor's office or to Internet software. This is not a necessary part of the system, but would be employed to use the Internet software discussed in Figure 20-1, *B.*

Telemedicine technology is rapidly evolving. Cell phones can capture and transmit pictures and will soon be telehealth-capable. The choice process should start with assessment of the current infrastructure available including questions about connectivity features. Each device has different requirements. The great advantage of POTS is that it is readily available in most areas. Video and voice transmission can be sent over the phone lines quite well. The only infrastructure that is required to turn any telemedicine system on is a phone line and an electrical outlet. Are the lines and cables needed available in the space planned, or will they have to be installed? Although high-speed Internet access can enhance the system, it is not an essential component. Most homes are not currently equipped with high-speed Internet service. This is important if dealing with a homebound or a senior population. If homebound patients are not part of the plan, then an Internet system may work. A high-speed Internet line may be required for photo downloads to off-site electronic files. A higher-speed transmission can also improve the quality of the image received. If plans include transmission of images and reports to physicians or health care providers in this manner, this is an important consideration. If transmission of images is desired, the quality of the in-field camera lens must be assessed. Its sensitivity to light and how light is transmitted will affect the quality of the image viewed and received. Also, the number of pixels captured per image must be known, since this will affect image quality. A minimum of 640 by 480 pixels is essential for quality photo documentation. Is the software located on the central system's hard drive or is it on the Internet? Where the software is to be located is important for security reasons and must be determined. It can be located either on the system's hard drive or on an Internet site. Most system-wide Internet servers have security walls or "fire walls" (i.e., protective programs that prevent outside or unauthorized users' access to patient information). IT services are helpful in evaluating these needs and how the current system will be able to adapt to them. Does the hardware and software comply with current HIPPA (1996) privacy standards?

Finally, costs must be looked at. Reimbursement of telemedicine is in the early stages. Congress continues to evaluate the need and the effectiveness of telehealth. Whether a practitioner can bill Medicare or Medicaid for a telemedicine visit currently depends on where the practitioner and the patient are located. Present Medicare standards cover telehealth only in rural areas. This is under constant review, and telehealth advocates continue to lobby for broad coverage (Telemedicine Reimbursement Guidelines for Medicare Recipients, n.d.). Private insurers have traditionally followed the trends of Medicare in coverage criteria. However, many practitioners are getting telemedicine visits covered on a case-by-case basis.

Other costs to consider include the cost of hardware, software, and potential Internet connections.

The use of off-the-shelf software can be considered, rather than custom designs, to keep costs low. The cost of training time for the staff and the IT department's time in implementing the program must be figured in.

CONCLUSION

The future of telemedicine is endless. Currently, trial programs are underway to record and evaluate surgical procedures. For the WOC nurse, this technology can be used to record and evaluate patient technique and provide follow-up care. Remote areas are using telemedicine during procedures in the operating room to provide clinical experts' advice and for troubleshooting. Telemedicine offers the practitioner and the patient increased access for teaching, providing and receiving support, and problem solving. Telemedicine gives new meaning to the phrase, "Reach out and touch someone!"

SELF-ASSESSMENT EXERCISES

Questions

1. When establishing telemedicine in a patient's home, the following basic equipment is required:
   a. Internet service and a separate telephone line.
   b. Digital camera.
   c. Television monitor.
   d. Telephone and camera.
2. A homecare agency would like to develop a telehealth service for their patients. Which of the following should be addressed first?
   a. Reimbursement
   b. Staff skill level
   c. Patient population needs
   d. Physician's acceptance
3. Which of the following patients would be a good candidate for a telehealth program in the home?
   a. An 80-year-old man with a new colostomy, living with his 82-year-old wife who is blind

   b. A 70-year-old man with a ileal conduit who was discharged from the hospital before being seen by the WOC nurse
   c. A 68-year-old woman with a new colostomy who only speaks Russian
   d. A 70-year-old woman with an ileostomy and end stage ovarian cancer
4. Virtual clinics can only be set up in a physicians' office.
   True _____ False _____
5. The most efficient method for a telemedicine system in the home relies on the availability of high-speed Internet service.
   True _____ False _____
6. Medicare will reimburse all telemedicine home care visits.
   True _____ False _____

Answers

1. d
2. c
3. b
4. False
5. True
6. False

REFERENCES

American Telecare, Inc. (n.d.), website: www.americantele care.com.
American Telemedicine Association (1999): *Report to Congress on Telemedicine,* website: www.atmeda.org/news/newres.htm.
Health Insurance Portability and Accountability Act of 1996 (HIPPA). Website: (www.fcc.gov/e-file/ecfs).
HomMed, Inc. (n.d.), website: www.HomMed.com
Joint Commission on Accreditation of Healthcare Organizations (JCAHO): *2001-2002 Comprehensive accreditation manual for home care.* Oakbrook Terrace, Ill, 2002, Author.
Retrieved from website: www.Motion-Media.com
Telemedicine Reimbursement Guidelines for Medicare Recipients (n.d.), website: www.fcc.gov/e-file/ecfs.

21 *Accelerated Surgical Stay*

·····································

HENRIK KEHLET and DORTHE HJORT JAKOBSEN

OBJECTIVES

1. Discuss the physiologic support for accelerated surgical programs.
2. Describe the most effective pain relief strategy following colorectal surgery, a major component of fast-track surgical programs.
3. Identify the type of surgical incision that has been suggested to reduce postoperative pain.
4. Relate the importance of staff and patient education to the success of an accelerated surgical program.
5. List several of the perioperative factors that may delay postoperative recovery.

INTRODUCTION

Despite major improvements in anesthesiology and surgery with newer effective and short-acting anesthetics, modern principles of multimodal perioperative analgesia, and development of minimally invasive surgery, major gastrointestinal operations are still beset with undesirable morbidity. Thus cardiopulmonary morbidity, ileus, thromboembolic and infectious complications, fatigue, and the need for a postoperative hospital stay and convalescence remain common features in these patients.

In recent years an increased understanding of perioperative pathophysiology and effective pain control, as well as a revision of perioperative surgical and nursing care programs, has led to a faster recovery and an assumed reduction in morbidity (Kehlet and Wilmore, 2002). With this increased knowledge, programs have been developed that advocate a faster convalescence, as well as a postoperative recovery with fewer complications; these care programs have various names such as "accelerated recovery programs," "fast-track surgery," or "clinical pathways."

This chapter reviews the physiologic background for accelerated postoperative recovery programs and presents results from interventions from various colorectal procedures. A detailed description follows of the nursing care involved, along with an outline of future strategies within the concept of "fast-track surgery."

PHYSIOLOGIC BACKGROUND FOR ACCELERATED RECOVERY PROGRAMS
Stress-Induced Organ Dysfunction

It is well established that existing comorbidities in the *preoperative* period (mostly cardiopulmonary and neurological diseases and disability) may contribute to postoperative morbidity, and every effort should be made to institute preoperative optimization of organ dysfunction (Kehlet and Wilmore, 2002). The *postoperative* period is characterized by multiple factors that may contribute to prolonged recovery and hospital stay, morbidity, and convalescence (Box 21-1).

The main contributory factor to postoperative morbidity and prolonged recovery is the surgical stress response, which is released by two main mechanisms. The first mechanism, afferent neural stimuli from the surgical area, induces various reflex responses to the endocrine glands. This results in secretion of catecholamines and cortisol with subsequent hypermetabolism and catabolism.

The second mechanism is a complicated humoral cascade response with complement activation and release of cytokines from the white blood cells. This contributes to the inflammatory response with leucocytosis, acute phase protein release, fever, loss of appetite, and fatigue (Kehlet and Wilmore, 2002). The purpose of the complicated surgical stress response has still not been fully elucidated, but there is no question that an amplified and continued response adds to morbidity and that techniques to reduce surgical stress improve outcomes. On the other hand a certain amount of surgical stress is important for wound healing and defense against infections and cancer cells. Future research will, it is hoped, define the optimal balance between undesirable and desirable effects of the surgical stress responses.

The most effective technique to reduce surgical stress is an afferent neural blockade with spinal or epidural local anesthetic, especially if continued postoperatively (Holte and Kehlet, 2002a; Kehlet and Wilmore, 2002). Thus the catabolic hormonal response is reduced with subsequent improved protein economy and reduced loss of muscle tissue. Also, this technique is the most effective for postlaparotomy pain relief (Jørgensen et al, 2002; Kehlet, 1999a) and ileus (Holte and Kehlet, 2002a; Kehlet and Holte, 2001). Importantly, to obtain the advantages of continuous epidural analgesia, appropriate insertion of the catheter at the level of surgical injury, (i.e., thoracic epidural analgesia for major colorectal procedures) is required. Also, epidural analgesia requires an optimal composition with local anesthetics and only a small amount of opioid. Epidural analgesia with opioids alone has no advantageous metabolic effects (Holte and Kehlet, 2002a).

The inflammatory cascade responses are most effectively reduced by minimally invasive surgery (Kehlet, 1999b), which, however, has only relatively minor effects on endocrine-metabolic responses. The inflammatory responses may also be reduced by preoperative glucocorticoid administration, which may reduce pain, nausea and vomiting, and pulmonary dysfunction (Holte and Kehlet, 2002b). The advantageous effects of preoperative glucocorticoids are well established in minor, laparoscopic procedures, whereas further studies are needed regarding its potential to improve outcomes in major colorectal procedures.

Postoperative Pain

Mobilization-induced pain is dominant after major colorectal procedures; it may inhibit mobilization and contribute to pulmonary dysfunction, reduced nutritional intake, sleep disturbances, and fatigue (Kehlet and Wilmore, 2002; Kehlet, 1999a). Every effort should be made to optimize pain relief, allowing early mobilization. The most effective technique is continuous epidural analgesia with local anesthetics and a small contributory dose of opioid (Jørgensen et al, 2002). Therefore such a regimen is one of the main components of most fast-track surgical programs after colorectal procedures (Box 21-2). In addition, multimodal analgesia with acetaminophen and nonsteroidal antiinflammatory drugs (NSAIDs) is recommended, especially after cessation of the epidural analgesia (Kehlet, 1999a). Patient-controlled opioid analgesia (PCA) may increase patient satisfaction but has no important effect on surgical stress, and it is debatable whether outcomes are improved by reducing morbidity (Kehlet, 1999a). Furthermore, PCA is not very effective on mobilization-induced pain (Jørgensen et al, 2002; Kehlet, 1999a). The optimal analgesic regimen for colorectal procedures is therefore a continuous

BOX 21-2 **An Example of a Perioperative Care Program for Fast-Track Recovery After Colonic Resection**

Premedication
None

Epidural Catheter (Intraoperative)
Right hemicolectomy: T_6-T_7
Sigmoid resection: T_9-T_{10}
Test: lidocaine 2% 3 ml with epinephrine
Bupivacaine 0.5% (6+6) ml
Bupivacaine 0.25% 5 ml 2 hourly intraoperative
Morphine 2 mg if <70 year
Morphine 1 mg if ≥70 year

General Anesthesia
Remifentanil 1 µg/kg/min
Propofol 2-4 mg/kg/h
Cisatracium 0.15 mg/kg
Hydroxyethyl starch (HAES) 500 ml
   Saline 1500 ml (max)
   Ondansetron 4 mg
   Ketorolac 30 mg
   Bupivacaine 0.25% 20 ml (incision)

Incision
Transverse or curved

Continuous Epidural Analgesia (postoperative/2 days):
Bupivacaine 0.25% 4 ml and morphine 0.2 mg/h

Breakthrough Pain
Ibuprofen 600 mg orally
Bupivacaine 0.125% 6 ml epidurally
Morphine 10 mg orally (last choice)

Medications: Starting Day of Surgery
Acetaminophen (slow-release) 2 g 12 hours
Magnesia 1 g q12h
Cisapride 20 mg q12h

Food
Protein drink ~60-80 g protein/day, start the night
   of surgery

Activity
Mobilization beginning the day/night of surgery as
   tolerated
Patient to be out of bed for minimum of 4 hours in
   morning, in afternoon, and in evening (total 12
   hours), include walking at least three times in 24
   hours.

First Postoperative Day
Remove bladder catheter in the morning

Second Postoperative Day
Remove the epidural catheter in the morning
Discharge after lunch

Modified from Basse L et al: Accelerated postoperative recovery programme after colonic resection improves physical performance, pulmonary function and body composition, *Br J Surg* 89:446-453, 2002a; and Basse L et al: A clinical pathway to accelerate recovery after colonic resection, *Ann Surg* 232:51-57, 2000.

thoracic epidural analgesia with local anesthetic and opioids for 2 to 3 days, followed by multimodal analgesia with acetaminophen, NSAIDs, or the newer COX-2 inhibitors and with systemic opioids only for break-through pain.

Nausea, Vomiting, and Ileus

Postoperative nausea and vomiting are common complaints after colorectal procedures and may limit recovery and hospital discharge. Modern antiemetic treatment includes use of multimodal opioid-reduced analgesia, droperidol, and ondansetron (or other, similar drugs) (Kehlet and Wilmore, 2002). Metoclopramide (e.g., Reglan), which often is used for antiemetic prophylaxis and treatment, has been found ineffective (Kehlet and Wilmore, 2002).

Postoperative ileus is an important factor contributing to delayed recovery. The pathogenesis is multifactorial and includes activation of inhibitory intestinal nerve reflexes (afferent neural stimuli from the surgical area), a local inflammatory response in the intestine, and postoperative opioid analgesia (Kehlet and Holte, 2001). As a result, several treatment regimens exist to reduce ileus, including continuous epidural analgesia with local anesthetics, which is very effective (Jørgensen et al, 2002), and minimally invasive surgery (laparoscopic surgery) (Kehlet and Holte, 2001; Kehlet, 1999b). The effect of early oral feeding on ileus development is probably relatively minor (Kehlet and Holte, 2001), but when combined with epidural analgesia, early normalization of gastrointestinal function is observed after colorectal surgery (Basse, Madsen, and Kehlet, 2001). The use of laxatives may seem rational, and has often been included in fast-track care programs, but so far there is no firm evidence from randomized trials to support their use. The common use of nasogastric tubes has no ileus-reducing effect and may add to atelectasis formation and thereby pulmonary morbidity. Efforts should be made to adjust postoperative care programs and avoid routine use of nasogastric tubes in elective colorectal procedures (Kehlet and Wilmore, 2002).

In summary, the well-known gastrointestinal side effects to major abdominal surgery—nausea, vomiting, and ileus—can be effectively managed with antiemetic prophylaxis and the use of continuous epidural local anesthetics, as well as minimally invasive surgeries (i.e., laparoscopic), which may have beneficial effects, thereby allowing early oral nutrition (Bisgaard and Kehlet, 2002) and decreased length of stay.

Hypoxemia

Postoperative hypoxemia may occur as a result of stress-induced pulmonary dysfunction, immobilization, and sleep disturbances (Kehlet and Wilmore, 2002). Every effort should be made to avoid postoperative hypoxemia, and effective techniques to do so include enforced postoperative mobilization (Basse et al, 2002a; Kehlet and Wilmore, 2002), opioid-induced analgesia, and/or oxygen administration in high-risk patients when supine. Early postoperative oxygen administration has been shown to reduce infectious complications after major colorectal procedures. The role of postoperative hypoxemia in postoperative cerebral dysfunction is controversial, although most data suggest that hypoxemia may increase risk of myocardial complications (i.e., arrhythmia and ischemia) (Kehlet and Wilmore, 2002).

In summary, efforts should be made to avoid postoperative hypoxemia by mobilization, opioid-reduced analgesia, and oxygen administration in supine position in high-risk patients.

Perioperative Fluid Excess

Perioperative care principles often include administration of large volumes of fluid, but recent data suggest that such fluid excess may have detrimental effects by prolonging recovery and maintaining or precipitating postoperative organ dysfunction (Holte, Sharrock, and Kehlet, 2002). Thus postoperative fluid excess may add to pulmonary and cardiac complications, as well as thromboembolic complications, and recent studies have also shown that perioperative fluid excess may prolong postoperative ileus (Holte, Sharrock, and Kehlet, 2002). Every effort should therefore be made to adjust perioperative fluid management to maintain preoperative weight and fluid balance and prevent fluid overloading.

Immobilization

Although every surgeon and surgical nurse knows that postoperative immobilization should be avoided, patients are often physiologically immobilized after major operations as a result of inadequate pain relief and fatigue. Furthermore, hospitals rarely offer a "daily living room" in the surgical units, which may hinder early recovery of normal activity. A daily living room provides patients a place to walk to and encourages them to stay out of their rooms (and beds) for longer periods of time. Postoperative immobilization is undesirable and may add to pulmonary and thromboembolic complications, as well as loss of muscle function (Harper and Lyles, 1988) and should therefore be avoided. Effective treatment includes optimal dynamic pain relief combined with enforced mobilization as part of the postoperative nursing care. Such efforts have led to a pronounced improvement in postoperative mobilization, which may contribute to the maintenance of normal organ functions in the postoperative period (Basse et al, 2002a).

Semistarvation

Inadequate postoperative nutrition may occur because of nausea, vomiting, and ileus, as well as loss of appetite, unnecessary use of nasogastric tubes, and "restrictions" usually not founded on scientific data. Recent studies from randomized trials have shown that early oral feeding after elective abdominal surgery is feasible, safe, and in addition reduces catabolism and infectious complications (Bisgaard and Kehlet, 2002). Every effort should therefore be made to include early oral feeding as an enforced care principle after major abdominal operations to improve outcome, and such principles have usually been included in fast-track care programs. Since postoperative appetite is reduced, adequate protein and energy intake may often be facilitated by supplementary protein drinks in addition to normal food.

Fatigue

Postoperative fatigue is a paradoxic event and may occur even after otherwise successful anesthesia and surgery (Christensen and Kehlet, 1993; Rubin and Hotopf, 2002). The most important pathogenic factors of postoperative fatigue are loss of muscle tissue and function, reduced cardiovascular adaptation to exercise, and preoperative fatigue (Christensen and Kehlet, 1993; Rubin and Hotopf, 2002). Every effort should be made to reduce catabolism by means of afferent neural blockade with epidural analgesia, minimally invasive surgery, enforced mobilization, and oral intake. Therefore these principles are included in fast-track programs with subsequent reduction of fatigue after discharge (Jakobsen et al, 2002).

Traditional Postoperative Care Principles

Guidelines for perioperative care should be based on scientific data. However, many postoperative practices have evolved from traditions without scientific documentation (Kehlet and Wilmore, 2002; Wexner, 1998). In recent years, several studies have demonstrated that various common postoperative care principles must be revised (Wexner, 1998). Thus, routine use of nasogastric tubes should be avoided (Kehlet and Wilmore, 2002), and the requirement for drains and urinary catheters should be reconsidered (Kehlet and Wilmore, 2002). Furthermore, a reconsideration of other principles (e.g., monitoring and restrictions) is required. The choice of surgical incision in elective colorectal procedures may influence postoperative recovery, since randomized trials suggest that horizontal or curved incisions may lead to less postoperative pain and improved pulmonary function and are therefore to be preferred whenever possible (Kehlet and Wilmore, 2002).

In summary, many factors may influence recovery after major colorectal procedures (see Box 21-1), and a revision of the perioperative care program is desirable and should be adjusted to existing scientific data (Kehlet and Wilmore, 2002). Outcomes data suggest that effective strategies to improve recovery and reduce morbidity must consist of a multimodal approach (Kehlet and Wilmore, 2002). Such strategies include optimized patient information, reduction of surgical stress, and optimal dynamic pain relief, combined with enforced mobilization and oral feeding within the context of a "fast-track surgery program" (Kehlet and Wilmore, 2002).

CARE PRINCIPLES: FAST-TRACK PROCEDURES

Several fast-track colorectal procedures publications have been reported, but only a minority provide detailed information about the perioperative care program (Basse et al, 2002a; Basse, Billesbølle, and Kehlet, 2002; Basse et al, 2000; Basse et al, 2001; Basse et al, 2002b). An example of a perioperative care program for standard segmental colonic resection (Basse et al, 2002a; Basse et al, 2000) is shown in Box 21-2. It is seen that the approach is multimodal and aims at stress reduction, with intraoperative and postoperative epidural analgesia with local anesthetics (and a small dose of opioid) and with a focus on optimized pain treatment allowing early mobilization. Also, early institution of food intake is included, as well as well-defined standards for fluid management, choice of surgical incision, and removal of epidural and bladder catheters. The care principles that should be present in a fast-track colorectal surgical program include preoperative patient and family education, development and use of a care map or a similar tool, adequate staff/patient ratios, and staff education.

Introduction of fast-track programs in surgical patients seems to be a major advantage resulting in improved postoperative organ function and reduction of hospital stay. These programs provide a nursing challenge in that the plan of care for this group of patients must be altered. A tool to assist in the care of patients using the fast-track program is the establishment of a care map. Care map use is a method to standardize surgical and nursing care by focusing on daily goals; it can result in more structured and focused care. The care map should include details on assessments, observations, and goals and outcomes, and specifics such as oral intake, hours out of bed, planned day of discharge, and nutrition. Furthermore, the map provides documentation of care and represents a working tool for the staff and a help to eliminate undesirable variations in postoperative care.

As noted above, fast-track programs can result in shorter hospital stays, which subsequently results in fewer days available to educate the patient. In addition, patients and their families must be educated about the benefits of the fast-track program to elicit their participation. Patients are more likely to participate in their care if they understand the rationale for each step. For many patients (and for that matter, staff), the normal expectation is that the hospital stay will be 5 to 7 days, and that they will not be ambulating or eating for several days. By providing them with preoperative information that includes the expectation that they will be eating the evening of surgery, that their hospital stay may last only 3 to 4 days, and that they will spend the majority of their postoperative hospital stay out of bed, they are helped to understand the rationale and become active participants in their postoperative care. For these reasons a detailed preoperative information session is required in the outpatient setting with the surgeon and the advanced practice nurse. In addition to preparing the patient and family, attention must be given to preparing and supporting the patient care staff. Several areas

must be addressed: the shift in the organizational staffing and the manner of delivering care and staff education.

The transition from conventional to accelerated care requires a shift in nursing interventions from more physical interventions to more teaching and learning interventions. The hours per patient day are nearly the same with a fast-track program but are divided into fewer days, which can mean an increased workload per day, and a decreased hospital stay. The number of nurses on duty at different time intervals within the department must be reconsidered. In some institutions, staffing patterns require readjustment to allow for increased acuity and shorter inpatient stays. It may be helpful to schedule fast-track surgery at the beginning of the work week to facilitate discharge before the weekend. This can allow for use of maximal staffing during the week, since on the weekends, available resources are generally lower. Establishment of expert patient care teams can facilitate a change of traditions and introduce new programs to provide patient care. Fast-track programs demand a well-educated staff with a profound knowledge of the background and principles of the program; otherwise, deviations will occur. Finally, the management of the surgical unit must support the decision to run fast track and to champion the overall program.

If fast-track programs are going to be successful, the staff must understand perioperative pathophysiology. The multidisciplinary team involved must be thoroughly educated and have discussions about the goals and plans for the patients. Presentation of study results and follow-up (e.g., by meeting with the patients after discharge in the outpatient clinic) may be necessary to convince and support the staff, especially in the introduction period. Such education is crucial to demonstrate that fast-track nursing care is the most appropriate principle of care.

Results from Fast-track Recovery Programs in Colorectal Procedures

The results from accelerated recovery programs in standard segmental open colonic resection have shown a median hospital stay of 2 to 3 days, even including high-risk patients (Basse et al, 2002a;

Basse et al, 2000; Basse et al, 2001). Medical morbidity has been very low, with no pulmonary morbidity in 100 consecutive patients despite an average age of 73 years, and only limited cardiac morbidity (Basse et al, 2001). So far the care programs have included a liberal policy for readmission, which has led to about a 15% to 20% readmission rate but mostly for short stays and benign conditions. In no reported case has a patient been readmitted in severe condition, including the few cases with anastomotic dehiscence (Basse et al 2000; Basse et al, 2001). Importantly, the fast-track care program has documented very efficient pain relief (Werner et al, 2002) and normalization of defecation within 48 hours in more than 95% of patients (Basse et al, 2000; Basse et al, 2001; Basse et al, 2001). The normalization of the entire gastrointestinal function has been documented by normal transit of a radioactive indium compound instilled into the stomach postoperatively and followed by repeated scans for the next 48 hours (Basse et al, 2001). A detailed analysis of various organ functions in patients undergoing open colonic resection with fast-track rehabilitation as compared with conventional care has demonstrated improved mobilization, pulmonary function, oxygen saturation, and physical performance, and lean body mass has been preserved in contrast to the usual reduction in organ functions with conventional care (Basse et al, 2002a). In addition, a more detailed study of patient functions during follow-up after discharge has shown increased activity and reduced fatigue and need for sleep with fast-track rehabilitation care as compared with conventional care, and without increased need for a home care nurse or visits to general practitioners (Jakobsen et al, 2002). Similar care programs have also documented improved energy, protein intake, and preservation of muscle force (Henriksen et al, 2002a; Henriksen et al, 2002b). Therefore, in summary, the literature reports that the institution of a multimodal fast-track rehabilitation program accomplishes the following:

1. Reduces the risk of postoperative organ dysfunction and the usual postoperative decrease of physical performance.

2. Reduces the period of convalescence fatigue and increased need for sleep, without the need for increased secondary support after early discharge.

Establishment of the fast-track program has also met with similar success with other procedures such as abdominal rectopexy for prolapse (Basse et al, 2002), external anal sphincter repair (Rosenberg and Kehlet, 1999), colostomy closure after Hartmann's procedure (Basse et al, 2002b), and ileocolic resections for Crohn's disease (Andersen and Kehlet, 2002). Other studies have shown similar fast-track recovery and reduced hospital stay in more complex colorectal procedures (Delaney et al, 2001) even without the use of epidural analgesia. However, patients in these series were 20 to 30 years younger than those in studies from open colonic resection (Basse et al, 2000; Basse et al, 2001). Nevertheless, these interesting observations (Delaney et al, 2001) call for future studies on the need for continuous epidural analgesia in subgroups of patients to elucidate the relative role of the different components of the fast-track care program.

The role of laparoscopic surgery to reduce hospital stay and facilitate recovery is controversial, since most studies have not included a revised, optimized, over-all perioperative care program, thereby hindering sufficient interpretation (Kehlet, 2002). However, from centers where traditional care principles have been revised with no use or only short-term use of nasogastric tubes and early institution of oral feeding, laparoscopic-assisted colonic resection has also been demonstrated to have a very short (i.e., 2- to 3-day) hospital stay with very low morbidity and readmission rate (Bardram, Funch, and Kehlet, 2000; Senagore et al, 2002; Senagore, 2001). Future studies are needed to evaluate the potential for laparoscopic-assisted colorectal surgery to further enhance recovery. In this context, it is important to combine the advantageous physiologic effects of laparoscopic surgery (i.e., reduced stress, pain, and ileus) with a revised care program focusing on early recovery. It may be assumed that such a combined effort will further improve outcomes and reduce risk of morbidity after colorectal surgery in high-risk patients in the future (Kehlet, 2002).

Most of the fast-track rehabilitation studies have so far considered patients without stomas, and there is an urgent need to include such patients in an integrated rehabilitation program, as well as patients undergoing acute abdominal procedures. Preliminary experience from the Cleveland Clinic suggests that even major complex colorectal procedures including a stoma may be included in such short-stay programs with success (Delaney et al, 2001). Future studies should evaluate the optimal overall care program for such patients.

CONCLUSION

Recent advances in the understanding of the pathophysiologic responses to surgery and their influence on postoperative organ functions have led to improvements in perioperative care principles with a focus on optimized patient information, stress reduction, dynamic pain relief, and enforced mobilization and oral nutrition. These data suggest that recovery after colorectal procedures may be enhanced with a pronounced reduction in the length of hospital stay needed, a potential major reduction in medical morbidity, and early recovery of normal daily functions, thereby limiting fatigue and convalescence. These advances may be further improved by defining the role of minimally invasive (i.e., laparoscopic) procedures. Future studies should focus on safety aspects and readmission rates, and should clarify whether medical and surgical morbidity is modified by such fast-track, accelerated recovery programs. The studies available so far have demonstrated that improved patient care can only be obtained by a close, multidisciplinary collaboration between the patient, the anesthesiologist, the surgeon, and the nursing staff, calling for increased attention to the field of "perioperative medicine" (Dahl and Kehlet, 2002).

SELF-ASSESSMENT EXERCISES

Questions

1. Part of the fast-track surgical plan of care to reduce surgical stress and control postoperative pain includes:
   a. Epidural local anesthesia used only in the operating room.
   b. Epidural local anesthesia used in the operating room, continued after surgery, followed by analgesia with acetaminophen, NSAIDs, or COX-2 inhibitors.
   c. Epidural local anesthesia used in the operating room and a patient-controlled anesthesia used for the entire hospital stay.
   d. Epidural local anesthesia used in the operating room and continued after surgery, and weaned as aggressively as the patient tolerates.

2. The use of nasogastric tubes had no ileus-reducing effects and may add to the development of atelectasis.
   True _____ False _____

3. Discuss the benefits of the institution of a multimodal fast-track surgical rehabilitation program.

4. When planning implementation of a fast-track surgical program, what issues should be considered?
   a. A potential increase in staffing needs to accommodate the increased acuity
   b. Preparation of the staff, the patients, and their families to accept a short postoperative stay
   c. Collection of data on satisfaction levels and complication rates
   d. All of the above

5. Reports in the literature regarding fast-track surgical procedure have noted that after hospital discharge, patients demonstrate increased activity, reduced fatigue, and less need for sleep when compared to conventional care.
   True _____ False _____

Answers

1. b
2. True
3. The fast-track program can provide adequate pain relief allowing the patient to ambulate, decreasing muscle loss, preventing atelectasis, preventing ileus formation, and allowing early feeding. Oral feeding (as reported in the literature) can reduce catabolism and infectious complications. Overall the institution of a

fast-track surgical program can decrease the surgical stress response, which in turn improves outcomes (i.e., faster return of bowel function, ability to ambulate, fewer complications, and early discharge with less fatigue).

4. d

5. True

REFERENCES

Andersen J, Kehlet H: Fast-track open ileo-colic resections for Crohn's disease, *Scand J Gastroenterol* 2002 (submitted).

Bardram L, Funch JP, Kehlet H: Rapid rehabilitation in elderly patients after laparoscopic colonic resection, *Br J Surg* 87:1540-1545, 2000.

Basse L et al: A clinical pathway to accelerate recovery after colonic resection, *Ann Surg* 232:51-57, 2000.

Basse L et al: Accelerated rehabilitation after colonic resection, *Ugeskr Laeger* 163:913-917, 2001.

Basse L, Madsen L, Kehlet H: Normal gastrointestinal transit after colonic resection using epidural analgesia, enforced oral nutrition and laxative, *Br J Surg* 88:1498-1500, 2001.

Basse L, Billesbølle P, Kehlet H: Early recovery after abdominal rectopexy with multimodal rehabilitation, *Dis Colon Rectum* 45:195-199, 2002.

Basse L et al: Accelerated postoperative recovery programme after colonic resection improves physical performance, pulmonary function and body composition, *Br J Surg* 89:446-453, 2002a.

Basse L et al: Colostomy closure after Hartmann's procedure with fast-track rehabilitation, *Dis Colon Rectum* vol 45, 2002b.

Bisgaard T, Kehlet H: Early oral feeding after elective abdominal surgery—what are the issues? *Nutrition* 18:944-948, 2002.

Christensen T, Kehlet H: Postoperative fatigue, *World J Surg* 17:220-225, 1993.

Dahl JB, Kehlet H: Perioperative medicine—a new subspecialty, or a multi-disciplinary strategy to improve perioperative management and outcome? *Acta Anaesthesiol Scand* 46:121-122, 2002.

Delaney CP et al: "Fast-track" postoperative management protocols for patients with high co-morbidity undergoing complex abdominal and pelvic colorectal surgery, *Br J Surg* 88:1533-1538, 2001.

Harper CM, Lyles UM: Physiology and complications after bed rest, *J Am Geriat Soc* 36:1047-1054, 1988.

Henriksen MG et al: Early oral nutrition after elective colorectal surgery: influence of balanced analgesia and enforced mobilisation, *Nutrition* 18:263-267, 2002a.

Henriksen MG et al: Enforced mobilization, early oral feeding and balanced analgesia improve convalescence after colorectal surgery, *Nutrition* 18:147-152, 2002b.

Holte K, Sharrock NE, Kehlet H: Pathophysiology and clinical implications of perioperative fluid excess, *Br J Anaesth* 89:622-632, 2002.

Holte K, Kehlet H: Epidural anaesthesia and analgesia—effects of surgical stress responses and implications for postoperative nutrition, *Clin Nutr* 21:199-206, 2002a.

Holte K, Kehlet H: Perioperative single-dose glucocorticoid administration: pathophysiologic effects and clinical implications, *J Am Coll Surg* 195:694-712, 2002b.

Jakobsen DH et al: Convalescence after colonic resection with a fast-track versus conventional care programme, *Br J Surg* 2002 (submitted).

Jørgensen H et al: Epidural local anaesthetic versus opioid-based analgesic regimens on postoperative gastrointestinal paralysis, PONV and pain after abdominal surgery (Cochrane Review). In The Cochrane Library, issue 1, 2002, Oxford, Update Software.

Kehlet H: Clinical trials and laparoscopic surgery. The second round will require a change in tactics, *Surg Laparosc Endosc Percut Tech* 12:137-138, 2002.

Kehlet H: Acute pain control and accelerated postoperative surgical recovery, *Surg Clin North Am* 79:431-443, 1999a.

Kehlet H: Surgical stress response: does endoscopic surgery confer an advantage? *World J Surg* 23:801-807, 1999b.

Kehlet H, Holte K: Review of postoperative ileus, *Am J Surg* 182:3S-10S, 2001.

Kehlet H, Wilmore DW: Multimodal strategies to improve surgical outcome, *Am J Surg* 183:630-641, 2002.

Rosenberg J, Kehlet H: Early discharge after external anal sphincter repair, *Dis Colon Rectum* 42:457-459, 1999.

Rubin GJ, Hotopf M: Systematic review and meta-analysis of interventions for postoperative fatigue, *Br J Surg* 89: 971-984, 2002.

Senagore AJ: Epidural anesthesia—analgesia shorten length of stay after laparoscopic segmental colectomy for benign pathology, *Surgery* 129:672-676, 2001.

Senagore AJ et al: Cost structure of laparoscopic and open sigmoid colectomy for diverticular disease, *Dis Colon Rectum* 45:485-490, 2002.

Werner MU et al: Does postoperative pain influence gastrointestinal recovery and length of stay after colonic resection with multimodal rehabilitation? *Anesth Analg* 2002 (submitted).

Wexner S: Standard perioperative care protocols and reduced length of stay after colon surgery, *J Am Coll Surg* 186:589-593, 1998.

22 *Intestinal Transplantation*

·······························

KATHLEEN SHORTRIDGE, ALAINE KAMM, and DAVID C. CRONIN, II

OBJECTIVES

1. Identify factors that have influenced improvement in the small bowel transplant procedure.
2. Describe primary indications for intestinal transplant.
3. Identify medical events that occur in the adult that may require a small bowel transplant.
4. Describe complications with long-term total parenteral nutrition.
5. Discuss contraindications for intestinal transplant.
6. Relate the preoperative assessment and workup for the transplant recipient.
7. Identify postoperative complications following intestinal transplant.
8. Describe the three grades of acute cellular rejection.
9. Identify immunosuppressant medications prescribed for the patient following intestinal transplant.
10. Discuss the graft-versus-host disease following an intestinal transplant.

INTRODUCTION

Small bowel transplantation has advanced as a treatment option for some patients with irreversible intestinal failure. Significant improvement in patient and graft survival has been obtained thanks to improvements in immunosuppression therapy, surgical techniques, and a better understanding of the immunologic and physiologic aspects of intestinal transplantation (Sudan et al,

2000). An increased number of intestinal transplants continue to be performed each year (Figure 22-1). As of May 31, 2001, the Intestinal Transplant Registry listed 55 centers performing intestinal transplants worldwide. Those 55 transplant centers performed 696 intestinal transplants in 651 patients. Of the 696 transplants performed, 41.8% were isolated small bowel transplants, 44.5% were combined liver and small bowel transplants, and 13.6% were cluster (multivisceral) transplants (i.e., stomach, pancreas, liver, and small intestine). At the time of reporting, 335 of the 651 patients were still alive. Intestinal transplantation is performed at 24 medical centers within the United States (Intestinal Transplant Registry, 2003).

INTESTINAL FAILURE: ANATOMIC AND PHYSIOLOGIC CAUSES

There are several reasons why the intestine fails to such an extent that intestinal transplant is required (Box 22-1). Failures of the small intestine can be categorized as one of the following:

- Anatomic (i.e., insufficient length for absorption)
- Physiologic (i.e., defective absorption or motility)
- A combination of both

Demographically nearly two thirds of patients waiting for an intestinal transplant are children. Unfortunately, many of the problems resulting in short-gut syndrome among adult patients are terminal events. Short-gut syndrome describes a condition in which the anatomic length of the small intestine is insufficient to sustain life with enteral

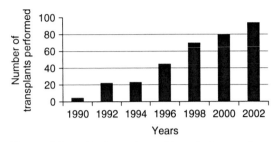

Figure 22-1 Total number of intestinal transplants performed in the United States as of August 1, 2002. (From Organ Procurement and Transplantation Network, Annual Report, OPTN/SRTR, website: www.optn.org/, 2003.)

BOX 22-1   Causes of Intestinal Failure
· ·

Anatomic (Short-Gut Syndrome)
Pediatric patients
Necrotizing enterocolitis
Gastroschisis
Volvulus
Trauma
Intestinal atresia
Tumor resection
Adult patients
Superior mesenteric artery occlusion (hypercoagulation state, embolism, thrombosis)
Mesenteric venous occlusion
Desmoid tumor resection
Trauma
Crohn's disease
Volvulus

Physiologic
Impaired enterocyte absorption
Defective intestinal motility (dysmotility syndrome)
Hirschsprung's disease (pediatric)
Pseudoobstruction (pediatric/adult)

---

nutrition. Loss of more than 70% of the small intestine results in inadequate nutrient and fluid absorption.

The most common cause of short-gut syndrome is surgical resection of the small intestine. The most common diseases that require surgical resection of the small intestine are necrosis and autoimmune disease.

Preterm, low birth-weight newborns infants are at high risk for necrotizing enterocolitis (Kamitsuka, Horton, and Williams, 2000). Surgical resection in this disease process can leave the child with an inadequate length of intestine, necessitating nutritional and fluid supplementation. Other causes of intestinal loss within the pediatric group include gastroschisis and volvulus. Intestinal atresia is a congenital defect of intestinal development resulting in variable length deficiencies in newborns (Reyes et al, 1998).

In adults, embolic or thrombotic occlusion of the superior mesenteric artery can result in infarction and necrosis of the small intestine. Although many of these patients do not survive surgery, those who do often have life-threatening complications in the perioperative period. These survivors depend totally on parenteral hyperalimentation for nutrition and hydration. In addition, mesenteric venous thrombosis is an unusual cause of chronic gastrointestinal bleeding, which may require intestinal transplantation as the only means of treatment. Other causes of short-gut syndrome secondary to intestinal resection include Crohn's disease (Krupnick and Morris, 2000), volvulus, tumor resection (Calne et al, 1993), and trauma.

Physiologic derainment of cellular function can also result in intestinal failure despite an adequate length of intestine. Impaired enterocyte absorption (IEA) occurs when the intestinal cells or enterocytes have a substantially reduced ability to absorb water and other vital nutrients. Causes of IEA range from microvillus inclusion disease (Reyes et al, 1998; Bunn et al, 2000) to selective autoimmune neuropathy, radiation enteritis, and massive intestinal polyps (Hogenauer and Hammer, 2002).

Another type of physiologic dysfunction results from defective integration of the neuromuscular network within the gut. Defective intestinal motility or dysmotility syndrome is one such example with many causes. Dysmotility can be caused by pseudoobstruction (Sigurdsson et al, 1999; De Goyet, 1999), hollow visceral myopathy, extensive visceral neuropathy, or total intestinal aganglionosis (Hirschsprung's disease), which is an absence of nerve cell groups resulting in intestinal dilation and dysmotility (De Goyet, 1999; Gambarara et al, 2002).

COMPLICATIONS ASSOCIATED WITH TOTAL PARENTERAL NUTRITION

Signs and symptoms of intestine insufficiency can include chronic diarrhea and dehydration, muscle wasting, malnutrition, failure to thrive, frequent infections, weight loss, and fatigue. To maintain adequate enteral nutrition, a minimum length of functional intestine is required. In situations of intestinal failure, basic nutrients can be provided through the intravenous route. Total parenteral nutrition (TPN), also referred to as hyperalimentation, is an intravenously administered formulation of electrolytes, essential amino acids, lipids, and glucose. Formula modifications are made to provide trace elements and medications required by the individual patient. Because of the high osmolality of this intravenous formula, central venous administration is required. Therefore, in addition to the side effects associated with intravenous nutrition, complications associated with the indwelling central venous catheter can occur (e.g., loss of vascular access, line sepsis, and thromboembolic episodes). Long-term TPN is associated with a variety of acute and chronic complications, the most severe of which is liver failure. TPN-induced liver failure secondary to diminished gut hormone secretion, reduced bile flow, and cholestasis can occur in as many as 40% to 60% of infants receiving long-term parenteral nutrition for intestinal failure (Kelly, 1998). Since intestinal transplantation may provide an alternative treatment option for patients with irreversible intestinal failure, management of TPN therapy and reduction of related complications is paramount (Kelly, 1998; Dionigi et al, 2001). Complications associated with TPN for intestinal failure can be life-threatening and frequent. The overall probability of 5-year survival was 60% in a 20-year retrospective study (Scolapio et al, 1999). Therefore, in appropriate selected patients, intestinal transplantation may provide a life-saving therapeutic alternative.

INTESTINAL TRANSPLANTATION: INDICATIONS AND CONTRAINDICATIONS

The primary indication for intestinal transplantation is irreversible intestinal failure compounded by life-threatening complications secondary to parenteral nutrition. The majority of patients with this diagnosis acquire the irreversible intestinal failure secondary to surgical resection, as previously outlined.

Fortunately, many children who undergo intestinal resection do not require intestinal transplantation and are supplemented with hyperalimentation for short periods of time. In the adult population, those patients who suffer intestinal resection for an intraabdominal vascular catastrophe usually do not survive the perioperative period. However, for those patients in whom hyperalimentation represents greater than 50% of total caloric support, long-term management and success depends on an experienced, multidisciplinary approach. Patients who have irreversible intestinal failure should be identified early and referred to a center that is experienced in long-term TPN management and intestinal transplantation (Gruessner and Sharp, 1997; Calne et al, 1993). Optimization of nutritional support, reduction in complications, close follow-up, and early listing for small bowel transplantation should improve overall survival (Kaufman et al, 2001). Efforts should be directed toward avoiding hyperalimentation-induced hepatic failure and cirrhosis (Kelly, 1998). Although combined liver–small bowel transplant can be performed, the surgical procedure is more difficult because the recipient is sicker at the time of transplant, and the patient and graft survival rate is generally inferior to isolated small bowel transplantation (Sudan et al, 2001).

Patients referred late for evaluation are primarily those with significant complications from prolonged hyperalimentation. Loss of vascular access sites and hepatic dysfunction with hepatitis and fibrosis are common causes for referral. Primary graft loss after intestinal transplant and poor quality of life secondary to intestinal failure are also qualifications for a small bowel transplant.

Absolute contraindications to intestinal transplant include current or recent malignancy, HIV infection, active bacterial or fungal infection, and inability to resolve psychosocial issues such as compliance or drug addiction. Relative contraindications include cardiopulmonary dysfunction and limited vascular access.

Cost

Just as a balance exists between the risks and the benefits associated with continued parenteral nutrition support and the risks and the benefits associated with intestinal transplantation, there is also a financial balance between the two therapies. Successful intestinal transplantation represents a cost savings when compared to continuation of parenteral nutrition therapy. The estimated average cost of an isolated intestinal transplant is $135,285. A combined liver-intestine transplant averages approximately $214,716, and a cluster (multivisceral) transplant is estimated at $219,098. In addition, the costs of immunosuppressive drugs and associated medical expenses average $20,000/year. This is contrasted to the costs associated with continued parenteral nutrition: the average annual cost of TPN therapy is about $150,000 per patient, exclusive of hospital visits, necessary medical equipment, and home nursing care (Silberman, 1999). Therefore it is reasonable to conclude that isolated small bowel transplantation represents an overall decreased health care expenditure at approximately 1.5 to 2 years after successful transplantation.

Preoperative Workup

The transplant evaluation serves to determine the patient's need for small bowel transplant, establish a time line for transplantation, examine the patient's current state of health, and to educate the patient and family about intestinal transplantation. The patient and family will meet with, and be reviewed by, the multidisciplinary transplant team. The transplant workup can be performed on an inpatient or outpatient basis and can be completed within days to several weeks depending on the patient's acuity, the facility, and the patient's availability (Andersen et al, 2000). Successful

intestinal transplantation requires a lifelong commitment to medications and medical follow-up. It is essential that the patient and family understand and be compliant with the many demands imposed by intestinal transplantation.

Consultation with a gastroenterologist who is experienced in nutrition, as well as a dietitian, should occur early in the evaluation process. Their evaluation may identify significant nutritional deficiencies (e.g., vitamin and trace elements) that must be corrected. In addition, an accurate assessment of the patient's nutritional reserve, metabolic expenditure, and functional status must be performed to ensure adequate nutritional supplementation. This team will also be actively involved in the management of parenteral nutrition after intestinal transplant (Dionigi, Alessiani, and Ferrazi, 2001).

Evaluation of the cardiac, pulmonary, renal, and especially hepatic subsystems are conducted to assess the risk of transplantation, identify other organs that might benefit from replacement, and identify contraindications to transplant. Determination of the patency of mesenteric, central, and peripheral venous system is important. This can be accomplished with a variety of modalities including duplex Doppler mapping of the peripheral veins, magnetic resonance angiography (MRA), or venography of the mesenteric and central venous system. Evaluation is especially important in those patients who have limited vascular access, have had extensive abdominal surgery, or have evidence of portal hypertension. A hematologic workup, including investigation of potential hypercoagulable states, should be done with all patients, especially in those with a history of embolic or thrombotic disease. A brief listing of some of the evaluation tests required in the evaluation of the small bowel transplant candidate is given in Box 22-2.

During evaluation of hepatic function a liver biopsy may be indicated. If liver function tests or radiologic imaging indicate that significant hepatic dysfunction is present, the possible presence of fibrosis or cirrhosis must be investigated. Demonstration of fibrosis or cirrhosis indicates the presence of significant liver damage. Although

BOX 22-2   Laboratory, Radiologic, and Diagnostic Tests for Intestinal Transplant Workup

....

Cardiac
Electrocardiogram, echocardiogram, stress thallium*
Right heart catheterization*

Pulmonary
Pulmonary function tests, chest x-ray

Hematologic
Blood typing, complete blood count, differential, platelets, hypercoagulation profile

Infectious Disease
Serology
Human immunodeficiency virus, hepatitis C and B, cytomegalovirus, Epstein-Barr virus, alpha-fetoprotein
Blood culture

Gastrointestinal
Duplex Doppler ultrasonography evaluation of mesenteric and hepatic vasculature
Mesenteric venogram/MRA
Contrast study

Hepatic Evaluation
Liver function studies
PT/ PTT
Hepatic ultrasound
Liver biopsy*
Abdominal CT scan
MRI

Kidney evaluation
Serum electrolytes
Creatinine clearance

Nutritional Assessment
Body mass index
Nutrient assessment (trace elements, vitamins)
Growth chart
Bone density assessment

CT, computed tomography; *MRA,* magnetic resonance angiography; *MRI,* magnetic resonance imaging; *PT/PTT,* prothrombin time/partial thromboplastin time.
*As needed if indicated by preliminary tests.

hepatic fibrosis can resolve after isolated small bowel transplantation (Sudan et al, 2000), cirrhosis requires a combined liver-small bowel transplant.

Assessment of kidney function is also an important element of the transplant workup. Many electrolyte and acid/base disturbances may be secondary to continued parenteral nutrition and losses from the remaining gut. However, functional assessment of the kidney is important because many of the required immunosuppressive medications have deleterious effects on the kidney (Cronin et al, 2000). If renal function is declining and cannot be improved, combined kidney-small bowel transplantation may be required.

The psychologist or social worker will evaluate the psychologic status of the patient and/or the caregiver. Potential recipients must demonstrate a strong support system and be free of alcohol and drug addiction, abuse, or dependency. The wound, continence, and ostomy nurse will also meet with the patient and family to provide information on the adjustment to living with a stoma, as well as to mark the stoma site.

Transplant Guidelines

Once identified as an acceptable small bowel transplant candidate by the transplant team, the patient is listed with the United Network for Organ Sharing (UNOS). UNOS is a nonprofit organization contracted by the federal government to administer the nation's Organ Procurement and Transplantation Network. UNOS facilitates organ allocation through regional subdivisions and local Organ Procurement Organizations. Patients may wait weeks to months until an appropriate donor becomes available. Approximately 27% of patients waiting for an intestinal transplant die while on the waiting list and 2.4% are removed because they are too sick to undergo the operation (Organ Procurement and Transplantation Network, 2003).

SURGICAL PROCEDURE
Donor Selection

The majority of grafts used in small bowel transplantation are provided by cross match-negative, ABO blood group–identical, deceased heart-beating donors. Live donors represent less than 4%

of transplants performed, and to date evidence to support an improved outcome is insufficient (Gruessner and Sharp, 1997; Calne et al, 1993; Pollard, 2002). Improvements in patient and graft survival and diminished posttransplant complications begin with donor selection.

Enterocytes lining the small intestine are exquisitely sensitive to the detrimental effects of hypotension. Consequently, ideal cadaveric donors are those who have not experienced prolonged or significant systemic hypotension or did not require pharmacologic support of perfusion pressure. Both of these clinical situations can result in significant enterocyte cellular damage and death. Transplantation of the small intestine requires the coincident transplantation of a large mass of donor lymphoid tissue contained in the mesentery. Currently it is hypothesized that this mass of donor lymphoid tissue may predispose the recipient to virally mediated infections secondary to cytomegalovirus (CMV) and Epstein-Barr virus (EBV), or EBV-induced malignancies such as posttransplant lymphoproliferative disorder. Consequently, selection of donors with CMV- and/or EBV-negative results of serology study is desirable.

In addition to standard criteria used in selection of solid organs for transplantation, other desirable selection criteria include a short hospitalization (<3 days), absence of infection, age greater than 40 years, good general health preceding the events associated with death, absence of malignancy, and no evidence of gastrointestinal disease. Many programs have their own donor selection protocols and treatments.

Donor procurement follows generally accepted surgical and storage procedures. Many programs have a special cocktail of antibiotics and antifungal medication that are instilled into the proximal small intestine before its removal. The isolated small intestine graft is procured with preservation of the superior mesenteric artery and the portal vein. Proximal intestine division usually occurs at the level of the ligament of Treitz, whereas distal division can be at the terminal ileum or across the right colon. The graft is flushed in situ with iced preservation solution and stored under hypothermic conditions. Cold storage time should be as short as possible to minimize cellular damage induced by ischemia reperfusion.

The time spent in the preoperative planning for small bowel transplantation is critical to a successful outcome. Many candidates for bowel transplantation, both pediatric and adult, have had significant intraabdominal surgeries and intestinal resections in the course of their illness. Consequently, the abdominal cavity is much smaller than would be anticipated in an age-matched, size-matched patient without the prior surgical history. Therefore, selection of the appropriately sized donor is of great importance to the technical aspect of the transplant. Usually a donor-to-recipient weight ratio of 2:1 is appropriate for most transplants. Additionally, this anatomic restriction of intraabdominal space may limit the size of the patient considered for transplantation. Restrictions on the minimal weight of a potential recipient vary among programs. Patients who undergo small bowel transplantation for pseudoobstruction, microvillus disease, and other dysmotility syndromes, and who have not had a prior resection, can receive a size-matched donor organ.

Recipient Surgery

Because most patients have been maintained on long-term parenteral nutrition with central venous access, they have a high incidence of venous thrombosis and sclerosis that may affect operative management. Preoperative venography, duplex Doppler mapping, or MRA is required in most recipients. A mesenteric venogram or duplex Doppler ultrasonogram should be performed to assess the patency of the portal vein. Lack of venous outflow is a contraindication for the transplant. If the inferior vena cava is occluded, a portal-to-portal anastomosis can be used as venous outflow. Defining the patency of other deep venous systems may be of value for the perioperative intravenous resuscitation and continued parenteral nutrition requirements in the postoperative period. Some programs consider fewer than three central venous access sites a contraindication for small bowel transplantation. Operative planning should seek to optimize use of previous incisions, prospectively map sites for ostomy placement, and obtain closure of the abdomen at the end of the transplant. In some situations, residual bowel must be resected before implantation. Arterial inflow to the graft can be obtained with direct anastomosis to the aorta or with use of an arterial conduit between the aorta and the superior mesenteric artery of the graft. Venous drainage of the graft can be obtained by direct connection to the vena cava. If the vena cava is diseased as a result of thrombosis or sclerosis, direct end-to-side anastomosis to the native portal vein can be performed.

Intestinal continuity can be provided in various ways and is dependent on the recipient's intestinal anatomy and the type of graft performed. Proximally, the end of the intestinal graft is connected to the distal end of the most proximal bowel. Size disparities between bowel segments can be accommodated by different operative techniques. An alternative is creation of a proximal stoma with an end-to-side intestinal anastomosis between the recipient and the graft. This proximal stoma allows for endoscopic evaluation of the proximal graft after transplant. The distal graft is usually fashioned as an end stoma with a more proximal end-to-side anastomosis between the recipient large bowel, if present. This anatomic configuration allows for postoperative graft surveillance with endoscopic access through the stoma and evaluation of the graft output and vascular perfusion. Once engraftment has been established and the risk of acute rejection diminished, the stoma sites can be resected and closed, reestablishing intestinal continuity without reentering the abdomen.

Immune Responses

Transplantation of allogeneic tissue stimulates various cellular mechanisms responsible for humoral and cellular immunity. The small bowel possesses such a high density of immune cellular components that it is a significant challenge to control the host's immune response against the foreign graft while controlling the graft's immune response against the host.

The occurrence of acute cellular rejection is the single most common cause for intestinal graft loss.

Its occurrence and severity has been diminished with the use of current immunosuppressive agents, but it has not been eliminated. It is hypothesized that ischemia-reperfusion injury is a significant, nonimmunologic stimulus for the development of acute cellular rejection. Therefore, limitation of the time spent in cold preservation storage is important. In addition, it appears that the occurrence of acute cellular rejection predisposes to development of chronic rejection, which manifests itself as fibrosis (Perez et al, 2002), scarring, and diminished absorption capacity of the intestine.

The transplanted intestine can potentially trigger immunologic consequences in the host. In addition to stimulating rejection, the high density of lymphocytes in the graft can exert immunologic effects against the host. The human gastrointestinal tract and associated mesentery contains as much lymphoid tissue as the spleen. Of the immunoglobulin-producing cells in the body, 80% are located in the intestinal mucosa (Sartor, 2002). This immunologic capacity of the intestine can manifest in the form of graft-versus-host disease (GVHD). This is a difficult and sometimes fatal disease seen in patients who have received a significant amount of immunocompetent cells (e.g., bone marrow transplant, small bowel transplant). The goal of immunosuppressive therapy is to prevent both host-versus-graft disease (i.e., rejection), by blocking the host's immune system, and GVHD, by allowing the host's immune system to react against the donor lymphoid cells.

Immunosuppressive Medications

Common immunosuppressive agents used in intestinal transplantation are listed in Box 22-3. The introduction of tacrolimus-based immunosuppression to small bowel transplant protocol in the early 1990s was associated with improved long-term intestinal graft survival (Reyes et al, 1993). Tacrolimus suppresses cytokine production by interfering with the transcription of many cytokines. Dosage is patient-specific and adjusted based on blood trough levels. Usual doses range from 0.05 mg/kg to 0.1mg/kg per day given in two divided doses at twelve-hour intervals, with early

BOX 22-3   Immunosuppressive Medications

Calcineurin Inhibitors
Tacrolimus (Prograf)
Cyclosporine (Neoral, Sandimmune)

Monoclonal Antibodies
Basiliximab (Simulect)
Daclizumab (Zenapax)
Muromonab-CD3 (Orthoclone OKT-3)

Polyclonal Antibodies
Antithymocyte globulin (rabbit) (Thymoglobulin)
Lymphocyte immune globulin (equine) (ATGAM)

Antiproliferative Agents
Sirolimus (Rapamune)
Mycophenolate mofetil (CellCept)

Glucocorticoids
Prednisone (Deltasone, generic)

---

target trough levels of 15 to 20 ng/ml. Blood trough levels are monitored daily, and adjustments in dosing are made to maintain therapeutic levels. Over time, trough blood levels are decreased based on individual patient care and the institution's protocol.

Steroid therapy is also used for immunosuppression. Steroids act at many sites in the immunologic cascade. Generally they depress hypersensitivity reactions and decrease cytotoxic T cell proliferation. Recipients usually receive a bolus of high-dose glucocorticoids during the transplant, and then the dose is tapered to a maintenance dose. Although there is much excitement in the transplant community surrounding immunosuppressive protocols that do not include steroids, the immunosuppressive protocol for the intestinal transplant recipient will continue to include steroids because of the high incidence of acute cellular rejection (Ghanekar and Grant, 2001).

Sirolimus is a relatively new immunosuppressive drug that is also commonly used in the intestinal transplant recipient. This agent is generally referred to as an antiproliferative drug, but it has many other effects on the immune system. Similar in structure to tacrolimus, it binds with the same

intracellular protein, FK-506 binding protein. However, its mechanism of action is different from that of tacrolimus. The site of action for sirolimus is mTOR, which blocks the lymphocytes' proliferative response to cytokines (IL-2). Unlike tacrolimus, sirolimus is not associated with nephrotoxic side effects. Although a potent immunosuppressive drug, sirolimus is also associated with diminished fibroblast activity and consequently delayed wound healing. This side effect has caused some centers to delay introduction of sirolimus into the immunosuppressive cocktail until later in the postoperative period.

Mycophenolate mofetil is another antiproliferative agent. It inhibits the proliferation of lymphocytes and can also be used to prevent rejection of the transplanted intestine. Mycophenolate has a unique mechanism of action, which is specific for lymphocytes. Basiliximab and daclizumab are two monoclonal antibodies specific for the IL-2 receptor on T cells. These anti–IL-2 FK-506 binding protein receptor monoclonal antibodies block the interaction of IL-2 (T cell growth factor) with its receptor on the T cell and thereby inhibit IL-2–induced proliferation of the T cell. These antibodies are given intraoperatively at the time of the transplant and again in the postoperative period. Their blocking effect lasts for at least 1 to 2 months after dosing, and they are relatively devoid of side effects. Either of these agents can be used and are referred to as induction agents (Cronin et al, 2000; Sudan et al, 2002).

Bone marrow infusions from the donor are given at some transplant centers to induce immunogenic tolerance between the recipient and the intestinal graft. Graft irradiation is also being investigated as a method of immunosuppression. Combined liver-intestine recipients may exhibit decreased incidences of rejection (Abu-Elmagd et al, 2001).

POSTOPERATIVE COMPLICATIONS
Fluid and Electrolyte Imbalance

Because of dependency on parenteral nutrition, along with intraoperative fluid administration and the difficult and lengthy surgery, patients may have a variety of fluid and electrolyte abnormalities in the immediate postoperative period. These derangements are compounded by the diminished absorptive capacity of the transplanted graft. In addition, edema and ischemia-reperfusion injury of the mucosa contribute to large secretory losses from the graft. The amount of graft output should be continuously monitored and quantified. Replacement fluids should be directed at correcting the electrolyte abnormalities identified on frequent serum assessment. Resuscitation with albumin-based solutions may limit the amount of edema and intestinal "leakiness."

Enteral feeding should be initiated with the return of gut motility. Despite institution of enteral feeding, total protein and calorie support should be continued with TPN. Weaning from TPN should begin after the absorptive capacity of the gut has been determined and the patient has recovered from the immediate postoperative phase. It can be expected that between 60% and 75% of intestinal transplant recipients will become free of the need for parenteral nutrition (Dionigi, Alessiani, and Ferrazi, 2001).

Administration of enteral pharmaceutical agents should also be avoided until the absorptive capacity of the gut has been demonstrated. Immunosuppressive drugs such as tacrolimus, mycophenolate mofetil, steroids, and monoclonal and polyclonal antibody preparations can and should be administered intravenously.

Technical

Technical complications associated with the transplantation of the intestine can be broadly categorized as vascular or graft-related. The most dreaded vascular complication would be arterial thrombosis. This complication results in infarction of the graft and requires its removal. Frequent examination of the stoma site is the most informative bedside evaluation of arterial patency (Table 22-1). Meticulous vascular technique during the arterial anastomosis aided by use of the operative microscope should minimize this complication.

Because of the lack of collateral outflow, venous thrombosis can be equally disastrous. Secondary to venous outflow obstruction, the bowel swells, edema worsens, and intravascular stasis occurs, eventually leading to arterial thrombosis and graft loss. Efforts to reduce the occurrence of venous thrombosis include avoidance of vascular conduits and prevention of graft torsion.

Reoperative abdominal surgery is always associated with the risk of enterotomy. Patients undergoing intestinal transplant are no exception. In fact, the occurrence of an unsuspected enterotomy in these immunosuppressed patients is life-threatening. Delayed enteric leaks also occur secondary to impaired healing at the anastomotic site, technical error, or regional vascular insufficiency. Before the institution of enteral nutrition, many programs evaluated the integrity of the intestinal graft by means of a contrast study.

Types of Rejection

Most intestinal transplant recipients experience some degree of rejection during the postoperative period (Misiakos et al, 1999). The Intestinal Transplant Registry reports that the removal of the intestinal graft required by 57% of patients was due to rejection. Ten percent of

TABLE 22-1 **Stoma Management Considerations in the Intestinal Transplant Patient**

INTERVENTION	RATIONALE
Use a two-piece pouching system with a floating flange	Nontraumatic removal of pouch for weekly scope and biopsy
Monitor stoma output for volume and consistency	Assessment of stoma functioning, potential for dehydration or abnormal function
Monitor stoma daily for color, mucosal appearance, or signs of bleeding	Assessment for signs of rejection

intestinal transplant deaths are caused by graft rejection (www.intestinaltransplant.org, 2003).

Intestinal transplantation can be very successful with prevention or early treatment of rejection. Unfortunately, there are no specific clinical markers or laboratory tests to diagnose rejection. D-xylose absorption studies and fecal fat analysis may be used as markers for intestinal absorption and reflect small bowel absorptive function; however, abnormal results are not specific for rejection. Clinical surveillance with endoscopy and biopsy appears to be the best method to assess intestinal health and the presence of acute cellular rejection. Clinically silent acute cellular rejection of the intestinal graft often occurs in multiple isolated areas throughout the graft. Consequently, multiple random and directed deep mucosal biopsies are taken throughout the entire intestine graft. Zoom videoendoscopy, which magnifies the mucosa up to 100 times, can be used to facilitate a more detailed and accurate evaluation (Kato et al, 2000).

The stoma facilitates access for frequent intestinal endoscopies, performed at least once a week in the early postoperative period. If no rejection is noted, the interval between endoscopic biopsies is slowly increased. Once the stoma is reversed, usually 6 to 12 months after transplantation, esophagogastroduodenoscopy and colonoscopy are used to obtain intestinal biopsies (Kato et al, 2000).

Clinical manifestations of acute cellular rejection within the intestinal graft include increased or bloody stoma output, a change in the consistency of the output, changes in the texture or color of the stoma, and increased friability or intolerance of enteral feedings. Sudden absence of bowel sounds, abdominal pain, nausea, vomiting, and diarrhea are important indicators of rejection or infection in the transplanted graft (Funovits et al, 1993). Prompt evaluation with endoscopic biopsy is required. If suspicion is high, institution of treatment, including pulse steroid therapy, should begin while awaiting pathologic findings.

Acute rejection is graded as mild, moderate, or severe based on morphologic examination and immunohistochemistry. Mild acute rejection can be difficult to diagnose and easily confused with infectious diseases (Damotte, 1999). Histologic changes include cryptic epithelial apoptosis and increased inflammatory cell infiltration. Typical treatment for mild and moderate rejection is steroid bolus administration and increased dosage of maintenance immunosuppression. Treatment for severe rejection may include more potent doses of immunosuppression such as OKT3 or thymoglobulin. Careful clinical follow-up and frequent endoscopic surveillance is imperative (Kato et al, 2000).

Chronic rejection is a progressive deterioration of intestinal function, the mechanism and causes of which are poorly understood. There is no known treatment with the exception of graft removal and retransplantation. Clinical presentation may be subtle, consisting of chronic diarrhea and nonhealing ulcerations in the mucosal lining of the intestinal graft. Histologic changes include villous atrophy and fibrosis. Episodes of acute cellular rejection and CMV infection are thought to be factors stimulating chronic rejection (Damotte, 1999).

Infections

Heavy colonization of microorganisms in the intestine, continued central line access for posttransplant TPN, and high doses of immunosuppression predispose intestinal transplant recipients to infectious complications including primary and nosocomial infections, community-acquired pathogens, and reactivation of latent viruses. Close clinical and histologic monitoring is necessary to diagnose and manage the delicate balance between infection and rejection (Green et al, 1999).

Patients are maintained postoperatively on prophylactic antiviral, antifungal, and antibacterial medications. These drugs lower the incidence of posttransplant infections caused by such pathogens as *Cytomegalovirus*, EBV, *Candida*, *Aspergillus*, and *Pneumocystis carinii*.

In particular, CMV and EBV have a high rate of occurrence along with a prolonged disease state and are associated with increased morbidity and mortality in the intestinal transplant recipient. Prevention of CMV and EBV may be achieved by matching donor and recipient serostatus before transplantation and through aggressive monitoring and institution of antiviral therapy when indicated (Green et al, 1999; Farmer et al, 2002).

Cytomegalovirus

CMV is a herpes virus occurring commonly in the general population. It usually causes no significant illness; however, in an immunocompromised patient it may have life-threatening complications. CMV infection is diagnosed through histologic staining of tissue or demonstration of CMV antigenemia. Clinical manifestations include fever, myalgias, headache, arthralgias, leukopenia, and thrombocytopenia. Treatment typically involves prolonged intravenous ganciclovir in combination with cytomegalovirus immune globulin (CMV-IVIG, Cytogam, Medimmune), and a reduction in baseline immunosuppression (Bowden, Ljungman, and Payan, 1998a). Despite improved patient survival with the introduction of ganciclovir therapy, infection with CMV is associated with a high incidence of acute cellular rejection. Therefore the frequency of surveillance graft biopsies should be increased during and immediately after CMV infection.

Epstein-Barr Virus

EBV is a herpes virus and the causative agent for mononucleosis in the general population. In the immunosuppressed recipient of a small bowel transplant, EBV can infect and transform B cells. Those transformed B cells can proliferate independently and produce an unusual malignancy referred to as posttransplant lymphoproliferative disorder (PTLD). Clinical manifestations include fever, malaise, flulike symptoms, headache, sore throat, and/or lymphadenopathy. Diagnosis is made though histologic analysis of graft biopsy or affected lymph node specimens. Recently, surveillance for the presence of EBV in serum with polymerase chain reaction has become an important prognostic device to detect impending PTLD. Treatment of EBV infection includes intravenous administration of ganciclovir and reduction of immunosuppression. Once EBV infection has evolved into PTLD, the management may require traditional chemotherapy (Kaufman, 2001; Bowden, Ljungman, and Paya, 1998b).

Graft-Versus-Host Disease

GVHD is an interesting and often fatal complication of transplantation. Although more commonly seen in recipients of bone marrow transplants, it does occur in recipients of solid organ transplants. The development of GVHD among recipients of solid organ and intestinal transplants appears related to the relatively large burden of passenger lymphatic cells that accompany the graft. In addition to initiating acute cellular rejection, these lymphocytic cells can recognize the donor as foreign and begin an attack against the recipient (a type of rejection response of the donor cells against the recipient). Once established, these donor cells attack the recipient lymphocytes, marrow elements, epithelial cells, and other members of the immune system, further depressing the host immunity and increasing susceptibility to infections. Clinical manifestations include skin rash, fever, diarrhea, and pancytopenia. Diagnosis is confirmed by histopathologic criteria, and treatment usually involves administration of high-dose steroids. Although the small intestine is rich in lymphoid tissue, GVHD does not have a higher incidence of occurrence in intestinal recipients than other solid organ transplants (Damotte, 1999).

QUALITY OF LIFE

Quality of life in small bowel transplant recipients has not been researched or defined thoroughly in the literature. One reason for this deficit is the relative newness of small bowel transplantation as a legitimate therapeutic option for irreversible intestinal failure. In addition, the relatively small number of patients who receive transplants at any one center further complicates the conducting of such studies. One study demonstrated an improved quality of life among the participants not on TPN, whether it was before their illness or after transplantation, as compared to being on TPN (DiMartini et al, 1998). Others state that although the quality of life immediately after an intestinal transplant is similar to that while being maintained on hyperalimentation, over time the quality of life continues to improve after the transplant (Rovera et al, 1998). In addition, the stress and burden placed on the family and the patient further serve to modify the quality of life after transplant or with continued parenteral nutrition (Brook, 1998).

As with any new medical procedure, the quality of life it brings to its recipients must be investigated. An awareness is needed of how these particular patients view their quality of life. Through educational efforts, support, and empathy, the staff, the care-providers, and the patients can have an improved quality of life before, during, or after small bowel transplantation.

CONCLUSION

For patients suffering from irreversible intestinal failure, intestinal transplantation has become a reasonable treatment option. Recent improvements in immunosuppression, surgical technique, and management of posttransplant infection have resulted in increased patient and graft survival. Recently, 1-year patient and graft survival rates have been reported as high as 93% and 71%, respectively (Sudan et al, 2000). However, many impediments to widespread application exist. First, the decision to proceed with intestinal transplantation must be weighed against the risks associated with such an intervention, and against the benefits and the risks associated with continued parenteral nutrition. Currently, patients who have experienced a complication, or who are at increased risk of experiencing a life-threatening complication associated with parenteral nutrition, should be considered for intestinal transplantation. Early identification of this patient cohort, as well as early referral to a transplant center and prompt evaluation, should avoid many of the problems associated with parenteral nutrition, nutritional deficiencies, and transplant candidacy. Unfortunately, many patients are referred late in their course of therapy with difficult problems such as total lack of venous access or hepatic failure with cirrhosis. Second, as with other solid organ transplants, there is an absolute lack of adequate donors to meet the demand. This disparity will only increase as intestinal transplantation becomes more successful and has wider applicability.

Postoperative management of the intestinal transplant patient is one of vigilance. In the early postoperative period, correction of fluid and electrolyte abnormalities, monitoring for infection and rejection, and continued parenteral nutritional support are essential. Stoma management considerations are found in Table 22-1. As the patient recovers, assessment of bowel absorption and surveillance for opportunistic infections and rejection is required. Once engraftment is stable, most patients are independent of parenteral nutrition and report greater satisfaction with their lives as compared to the pretransplant period.

Although many advances have occurred in small bowel transplantation, success is limited to a small number of centers treating a highly select group of patients. Clear comprehension of the physiology and immunology of the small intestine is essential to the continued success of this new therapy. Increasing patient survival, improving the recipient's quality of life, and maintaining a cost-effective alternative to continued parenteral nutrition will only increase the demand for and benefits of small bowel transplantation.

SELF-ASSESSMENT EXERCISES

Questions

1. List three factors that have influenced improvements in intestinal transplant procedures.
2. Which of the following diseases may result in intestinal failure requiring surgical resection?
   a. Ulcerative colitis
   b. Necrotizing enterocolitis
   c. Colorectal cancer
   d. Prune belly syndrome
3. Nearly two thirds of the patients waiting for an intestinal transplant are children.
   True _____ False _____
4. Long-term TPN in the person with short-gut syndrome can result in which of the following complications?
   a. Renal failure
   b. Cardiac arrhythmia
   c. Liver failure
   d. Dizziness and headaches

5. List three contraindications for intestinal transplant surgery.
6. Intestinal transplant recipients will no longer require parenteral nutrition.
   True _____ False _____
7. Sirolimus is one of the first immunosuppressive drugs used in the intestinal transplant recipient.
   True _____ False _____
8. Name two pathogens that can cause infection after intestinal transplant.
9. GVHD in intestinal transplantation is related to the large burden of lymphatic cells in the graft.
   True _____ False _____
10. Postoperative assessment for rejection of the intestinal transplant is performed by endoscopic examinations via the _____.

Answers

1. Three factors that have influenced improvements in intestinal transplant procedures: (a) improved immunosuppression therapy; (b) improved surgical technique; (c) better understanding of immunologic and physiologic aspects of intestinal transplantation
2. b
3. True
4. c
5. Three contraindications for intestinal transplant surgery: (a) HIV infection; (b) active bacterial or fungal infection; (c) recent or current malignancy
6. False; only 60% to 75% of transplant recipients will no longer require parenteral nutrition.
7. False
8. Two pathogens that can cause infection after intestinal transplant are cytomegalovirus and Epstein-Barr virus.
9. True
10. The endoscopic examinations is performed via the stoma.

REFERENCES

Abu-Elmagd K, Reyes J, Bond G, et al: Clinical intestinal transplantation: a decade of experience at a single center, *Ann Surg* 234:404-16; discussion 416-417, 2001.

Andersen D et al: Intestinal transplantation in pediatric patients: a nursing challenge: part one: evaluation for intestinal transplantation, *Gastroenterol Nurs* 23:3-9, 2000.

Brook G: Quality of life issues: parenteral nutrition to small bowel transplantation—a review, *Nutrition* 14:813-816, 1998.

Bunn SK et al: Treatment of microvillus inclusion disease by intestinal transplantation, *J Pediatr Gastroenterol Nutr* 31:176-180, 2000.

Calne RY et al: Intestinal transplant for recurring mesenteric desmoid tumour, *Lancet* 342:58-59, 1993.

Cronin DC et al: Modern immunosuppression, *Clin Liver Dis* 4(ix):619-655, 2000.

Damotte D: Pathology of intestinal transplantation, *Curr Op Organ Transpl* 4:355-367, 1999.

De Goyet JD: Pseudo-obstruction in children: transplant or wait? *Gut* 45:479-480, 1999.

DiMartini A et al: Quality of life after small intestinal transplantation and among home parenteral nutrition patients, *J Parenter Enteral Nutr* 22:357-362, 1998.

Dionigi P, Alessiani M, Ferrazi A: Irreversible intestinal failure, nutrition support, and small bowel transplantation, *Nutrition* 17:747-450, 2001.

Farmer DG et al: Effectiveness of aggressive prophylactic and preemptive therapies targeted against cytomegaloviral and Epstein-Barr viral disease after human intestinal transplantation, *Transplant Proc* 34:948-949, 2002.

Funovits M et al: Small intestine transplantation: a nursing perspective, *Crit Care Nurs Clin North Am* 5:203-213, 1993.

Gambarara M et al: Indication for small bowel transplant in patients affected by chronic intestinal pseudo-obstruction, *Transplant Proc* 34:866-867, 2002.

Ghanekar A, Grant D: Small bowel transplantation, *Curr Opin Crit Care* 7:133-137, 2001.

Green M et al: Unique aspects of the infectious complications of intestinal transplantation, *Curr Opin Organ Transpl* 4:361-371, 1999.

Gruessner RW, Sharp HL: Living-related intestinal transplantation: first report of a standardized surgical technique, *Transplantation* 64:1605-1607, 1997.

Hogenauer C, Hammer H: Maldigestion and malabsorption. In Feldman M et al, editors: *Sleisenger and Fordtran's gastrointestinal and liver disease*, Philadelphia, 2002, WB Saunders.

Intestinal Transplant Registry, Website: www.intestinaltransplant.org/ Vol. 2003.

Kamitsuka MD, Horton MK, Williams MA: The incidence of necrotizing enterocolitis after introducing standardized feeding schedules for infants between 1250 and 2500 grams and less than 35 weeks of gestation, *Pediatrics* 105:379-384, 2000.

Kato T et al: Improved rejection surveillance in intestinal transplant recipients with frequent use of zoom video endoscopy, *Transplant Proc* 32:1200, 2000.

Kaufman SS: Small bowel transplantation: selection criteria, operative techniques, advances in specific immunosuppression, prognosis, *Curr Opin Pediatr* 13:425-428, 2001.

Kaufman SS et al: Indications for pediatric intestinal transplantation: a position paper of the American Society of Transplantation, *Pediatr Transplant* 5:80-87, 2001.

Kelly DA: Liver complications of pediatric parenteral nutrition—epidemiology, *Nutrition* 14:153-157, 1998.

Krupnick AS, Morris JB: The long-term results of resection and multiple resections in Crohn's disease, *Semin Gastrointest Dis* 11:41-51, 2000.

Misiakos EP et al: Clinical outcome of intestinal transplantation at the University of Miami, *Transplant Proc* 31:569-571, 1999.

Organ Procurement and Transplantation Network: Transplant recipient characteristics, 1992 to 2001, intestine recipients, OPTN/SRTR, website: www.optn.org/, 2003.

Patel R, Paya C: Cytomegalovirus infection and disease in solid organ transplant recipients. In Bowden R, Ljungman P, Paya C: *Transplant infections*, Philadelphia, 1998a, Lippincott-Raven.

Perez MT et al: Temporal relationships between acute cellular rejection features and increased mucosal fibrosis in the early posttransplant period of human small intestinal allografts, *Transplantation* 73:555-559, 2002.

Pollard S: Living-related small bowel transplantation, *Curr Opin Organ Transpl* 7:214-217, 2002.

Preiksaitis JK, Cockfield SM: Epstein-Barr virus and lymphoproliferative disorders after transplantation. In Bowden R, Ljungman P, Paya C: *Transplant infections*, Philadelphia, 1998b, Lippincott-Raven.

Reyes J et al: Small bowel and liver/small bowel transplantation in children, *Semin Pediatr Surg* 2:289-300, 1993.

Reyes J et al: Current status of intestinal transplantation in children, *J Pediatr Surg* 33:243-254, 1998.

Rovera GM et al: Quality of life of patients after intestinal transplantation, *Transplantation* 66:1141-1145, 1998.

Sartor R: Mucosal immunology and mechanisms of gastrointestinal inflammation. In Feldman M et al, editors: *Sleisenger and Fordtran's gastrointestinal and liver disease*, Philadelphia, 2002, WB Saunders.

Scolapio JS et al: Survival of home parenteral nutrition-treated patients: 20 years of experience at the Mayo Clinic, *Mayo Clin Proc* 74:217-222, 1999.

Sigurdsson L et al: Intestinal transplantation in children with chronic intestinal pseudo-obstruction, *Gut* 45:570-574, 1999.

Silberman S: Pittsburgh team labels intestinal transplants life-saving and cost effective, website: www.ccfa.org, accessed 1999.

Sudan DL et al: Isolated intestinal transplantation for intestinal failure, *Am J Gastroenterol* 95:1506-1515, 2000.

Sudan DL et al: A new technique for combined liver/small intestinal transplantation, *Transplantation* 72:1846-1848, 2001.

Sudan DL et al: Basiliximab decreases the incidence of acute rejection after intestinal transplantation, *Transplant Proc* 34:940-941, 2002.

CHAPTER

23 Minimally Invasive Surgical Techniques

PETER W. MARCELLO

OBJECTIVES

1. Identify indications for laparoscopic stoma surgery.
2. List advantages of laparoscopic colorectal surgery as compared to open surgical techniques.
3. Discuss three different methods for stoma creation.
4. Describe complications related to laparoscopic procedure.
5. Explain the laparoscopic ileostomy procedure.
6. Compare outcomes for the laparoscopic colorectal surgery to the open surgical technique.

INTRODUCTION

Since the worldwide acceptance of laparoscopic cholecystectomy as the preferred approach for resection of the gallbladder, surgeons have gradually applied laparoscopic techniques to the treatment of various colorectal diseases. Naturally seeking the same advantages seen in laparoscopic cholecystectomy, surgeons have found laparoscopic colorectal surgery to present greater challenges, especially in resection for colorectal malignancies. The first laparoscopic colectomy was reported by Jacobs, Verdeja, and Goldstein in 1991 and began the surgeons' struggle to master laparoscopic colectomy. Successful laparoscopic surgical therapy of the large intestine is different from other procedures because it requires operating over multiple quadrants, and is associated with the need to retract the small intestine away

from the operative field and dissection of broad tissue planes.

However, the construction of a stoma, either an ileostomy or colostomy, may be one of the best indications for laparoscopy, since only minimal tissue dissection is required, the mesenteric vessels do not need to be divided, and the intestine does not require intracorporeal resection. For surgeons starting out in laparoscopic intestinal surgery, laparoscopic stoma formation is one of the easiest procedures to complete and can be utilized successfully early in their experience.

INDICATIONS AND CONTRAINDICATIONS

The indications for laparoscopic surgery for colorectal disease have expanded in accordance with advances in both operative technique and instrumentation. As surgeons and anesthesiologists become more experienced with laparoscopic surgery for colorectal disease, the contraindications for laparoscopic stoma creation have become more relative than absolute (Milsom and Bohm, 1996), with the exception of known extensive adhesion formation or sepsis (Box 23-1). However, with a higher morbidity rate reported after conversion from laparoscopic to open procedures (Slim et al, 1995), careful preoperative and intraoperative assessment of the patient's condition and disease extent is mandatory.

The primary benign indications for laparoscopic stomas are perineal sepsis or incontinence. It may also be used after complex anorectal surgery when a temporary diversion is required to protect the

BOX 23-1   **Indications and Contraindications of Laparoscopic Stoma Creation**

··

Major Indications

Colorectal tumors
  Familial adenomatous polyposis (proctocolectomy)
  Colorectal malignancies:
    Palliation
    Temporary diversion for near obstructing lesion
Inflammatory diseases of the intestine
  Diverticulitis
  Mucosal ulcerative colitis (proctocolectomy)
  Crohn's disease
    Temporary
    Permanent (with resection)
Functional disorders
  Constipation
  Incontinence

Contraindications

- Cardiovascular instability or failure
- Severe or unstable chronic obstructive pulmonary disease
- Coagulopathy not correctable preoperatively
- Extreme obesity (body mass index > $35 kg/m^2$)
- Pregnancy
- Carcinomatosis
- Diffuse peritoneal contamination with perforation
- Obstruction of the intestine with abdominal distention
- Extensive adhesion formation, especially at the stoma site

surgical site. In cases in which advanced colorectal carcinoma is diagnosed preoperatively or intraoperatively, laparoscopic surgery can permit a variety of palliative measures such as limited resection of the primary tumor, intestinal bypass, or stomal diversion without the need for a large incision. For patients with near-obstructing rectal cancer, who require preoperative chemoradiation therapy, a laparoscopic loop ileostomy is the preferred method of temporary fecal diversion. Without a midline incision, the subsequent rectal resection can be performed without the need for extensive adhesiolysis, and the loop ileostomy may remain for temporary fecal diversion following a low colorectal anastomosis.

The creation of the stoma may be the only procedure performed, or it may be combined with resection. For example, proctocolectomy with end ileostomy for ulcerative colitis or familial adenomatous polyposis may be performed laparoscopically. Also, laparoscopic restorative proctocolectomy with a temporary loop ileostomy is not only feasible, but for many is the preferred method of performing this procedure (Marcello et al, 2000). Laparoscopic total colectomy with end ileostomy for acute colitis can be performed by an experienced laparoscopist (Marcello et al, 2001).

BENEFITS AND DRAWBACKS OF LAPAROSCOPIC COLORECTAL SURGERY: AN OVERVIEW

The initial clinical reports of laparoscopic colorectal surgery suggested many advantages in comparison to conventional (open) techniques. These included reduced postoperative pain, earlier recovery of bowel function, shorter length of hospital stay, and earlier return to normal activities (Monson et al, 1992; Phillips et al, 1992). However, later studies have not been as favorable (Senagore et al, 1993; Ortega et al, 1995; Bergamaschi and Arnaud, 1997). To date, there appear to be no significant differences in perioperative complications or mortality between laparoscopic and open colorectal surgery, and short-term outcomes seem equivalent. Despite a trend toward a reduced length of stay, the overall cost of laparoscopic surgery has historically been higher. This has been related, in part, to longer operative time and higher equipment costs, both inflating the overall operative charges. Many of the expenses of laparoscopic surgery are expected to fall, since advances in both laparoscopic equipment design and surgical technique will reduce the surgeon's operative time and costs. More recent studies have confirmed this, demonstrating a cost savings for elective laparoscopic sigmoid and ileocolic resections.

Some of the specific complications related to laparoscopic techniques include port-site herniation, inadvertent organ injury, complications of pneumoperitoneum, and resection of the wrong segment of bowel (Ota, 1995). Alterations in tactile sensation and view magnification that are inherent to laparoscopic surgery may result in some of these complications early in a surgeon's experience. Conversely, laparoscopic techniques could potentially decrease adhesion formation and thereby lower the incidence of delayed small bowel obstruction. In the future, a faster recovery and potentially lower risks of both short- and long-term complications could offset some of the total health care cost of laparoscopic surgery.

LAPAROSCOPIC STOMA CREATION

There are basically three different methods of creating a stoma as a primary operation:

1. Conventional laparotomy
2. "Trephine" method (Senapati and Phillips, 1991; Anderson et al, 1992)
3. Laparoscopy (Fuhrman and Ota, 1996; Ludwig et al, 1996; Oliviera et al, 1997; Hollyoak, Lumley, and Stitz, 1998; Schwandner, Schiedeck, and Bruch, 1998; Young, Eyers, and Solomon, 1998)

A laparotomy permits exploration of the entire abdominal cavity, but this generally requires a fairly large incision. If the patient has had previous surgery, the laparotomy also permits lysis of adhesions and mobilization of the intestine so it will reach without tension to the abdominal wall.

With a trephine stoma, the surgeon uses the stoma opening as a "minilaparotomy" to explore the abdomen and retrieve the relevant bowel segment. This method averts the need for a large incision and is simple, but neither allows for a thorough exploration nor permits adhesiolysis over a wide area (which is needed in some cases). The trephine method may also require moderate dilation of the stoma aperture to effectively bring the bowel to the anterior abdominal wall, which could predispose to stomal herniation.

The laparoscopic method appears to have all the advantages of the other procedures with none of their disadvantages. This is the simplest of the laparoscopic colorectal procedures and can be one of the most satisfying to both the patient and the health care team. Either colostomy or ileostomy can be created, and the abdomen thoroughly explored at the same time. Adhesions can be lysed if necessary, and any intraabdominal abnormality can also be sampled for biopsy if this is indicated. Fecal diversion may also be combined with resection or strictureplasty if indicated. This has been done in cases of Crohn's disease involving the proximal small bowel and anus; the proximal obstruction is relieved and the fecal stream diverted to assist in the management of suppurative anal Crohn's disease.

TECHNIQUE
Laparoscopic Ileostomy

The patient should be marked preoperatively for the site of the stoma. The patient is placed supine on the operating table, and a urinary catheter is placed to decompress the bladder. A 10-mm trocar is placed over the site of the proposed ileostomy. This should be performed with a direct cutdown over the rectus fascia and muscle to avoid injury to the inferior epigastric vessels. If the patient has had prior abdominal surgery or the stoma site is questionable, a 10-mm trocar is placed at the umbilicus to allow an initial diagnostic laparoscopy. One or two smaller, 5-mm trocars are placed on the left side of the abdomen. A thorough exploration of the abdomen is easily performed and the terminal ileum located. The loop of bowel for the stoma is identified; if it will reach to the camera port at the stoma site, there is adequate reach. If not, the cecum and terminal ileum can be partially mobilized. This is often necessary in the obese patient. Once the loop has been verified to reach, a small clip applier is passed intracorporeally to mark the proximal and distal limbs of the ileostomy. Typically, four clips are placed on the proposed afferent limb of the ileostomy and two on the efferent limb. The clips are placed at the border of the bowel and mesentery. If the afferent and efferent limbs are not marked inside the abdomen, there is the potential to evert the wrong side of the stoma at the end of the procedure. With the clips in place, the camera is switched to one of the 5-mm ports, and the loop of bowel is brought through the 10-mm trocar in the stoma site. A rod is placed beneath the bowel and a pneumoperitoneum is reestablished to ensure that the mesentery to the loop ileostomy is not twisted. Once the orientation is confirmed, the pneumoperitoneum is released, the trocar sites are closed, the clips are removed, and the stoma is matured in the usual fashion.

Laparoscopic Colostomy

The procedure for a laparoscopic loop sigmoid colostomy is the mirror image of the ileostomy. However, the patient is placed in a modified lithotomy position to allow access to the perineum. In some cases, having the ability to perform rigid or flexible endoscopy can facilitate the later stages of the procedure. The trocar sites are nearly reversed. Suprapubic and right lower quadrant 5-mm trocars are placed after pneumoperitoneum is established. In nearly every case, it will be necessary to mobilize the sigmoid colon laterally to have the loop reach the abdominal wall without tension. The proximal and distal sides of the loop are marked intracorporeally with clips to maintain orientation. The loop is brought through the stoma site in a nonrotated

fashion, and a pneumoperitoneum is reestablished to confirm that the mesentery is not twisted. Once the loop is exteriorized it is possible to pass a flexible sigmoidoscope up to the distal limb to again confirm orientation. This will be done when planning to make an end loop colostomy, where the distal limb will be stapled and buried in the subcutaneous space. With this type of stoma, maturing the wrong side of the loop can lead to the afferent limb inadvertently being stapled off instead of the efferent limb, causing a bowel obstruction.

OUTCOMES

A number of studies over the past 10 years have demonstrated not only the feasibility of laparoscopic stoma creation, but superior results, in a few comparative studies, as measured against conventional surgery (Table 23-1) (Fuhrman and Ota, 1996; Ludwig et al, 1996; Oliviera et al, 1997; Hollyoak, Lumley and Stitz, 1998; Schwandner, Schiedeck, and Bruch, 1998; Young, Eyers, and Solomon, 1998). For diverting procedures alone, operative times varied from 40-75 minutes depending on the series. This compares favorably with conventional surgery. Since there is little dissection and mobilization, conversion to traditional surgery during laparoscopic stoma formation is rare (<5 %). This likely relates to the simplicity of the procedure,

TABLE 23-1   Outcomes of Laparoscopic Stoma Creation

AUTHOR	YEAR	NO. OF ILLEOSTOMIES/ NO. OF COLOSTOMIES	LOS (DAYS)	COMMENTS
Fuhrman	1996	2/15	NS	Feasible, some as part of an abdominoperineal excision
Ludwig	1996	16/8	6.0	4% conversion Median operation time: 60 minutes
Oliviera	1997	25/7	6.2	Temporary or permanent loop ileostomy
Hollyoak	1998	40	7.4	5 % conversion Favorable as compared to open procedure group
Schwandner	1998	7/35	13.0	One conversion Mean operative time: 74 minutes
Young	1998	1/18	8.0	Case control study, favorable results

LOS, Length of stay; *NS*, not stated.

but also to case selection. Laparoscopic attempts were not made in most series with patients with known dense adhesion formation or significant intraabdominal sepsis. Return of bowel function was faster in the laparoscopic group, as expected. Length of stay was shorter in the laparoscopic group, but in some cases the length of stay was dictated by the patients' concomitant procedures rather than the creation of a diverting stoma alone.

In the comparative case studies the patients were not randomized, but procedures were performed during the same operative period. In the series by Hollyoak from Australia, (1998) 40 patients undergoing laparoscopic stoma formation were compared to 15 open procedure patients. The mean operative time was slightly less in the laparoscopic group (54 minutes versus 72 minutes) as was return of bowel function (1.6 days versus 2.2 days). The mean hospital stay was also shorter in the laparoscopic group when compared to the open procedure patients (7.4 days versus 12.6 days). A length of stay of 7.4 days seems long by American standards, but represents a significant reduction from the longer hospital stays typically seen in the United Kingdom, Europe, and Australia.

In another comparative study by Young, (1998) similar results were reported, with a significant reduction in the time until diet was advanced in the 19 laparoscopic patients as compared to 23 open procedure patients (2.1 days vs 3.7 days). Intravenous narcotic usage, a measure of early postoperative pain, was lower in the laparoscopic group, as was the median hospital stay (8 days versus 11 days). Postoperative complications were also slightly fewer in the laparoscopic group (5% versus 23%). Other series have confirmed a low rate of conversion and postoperative complications when an experienced team performs laparoscopic fecal diversion.

Combining the results of all the published series, there is an overwhelming impression that a laparoscopic stoma procedure is safe and feasible and has significant advantages over conventional surgery.

CONCLUSION

As compared to conventional (open) surgery, the use of laparoscopic techniques offers several advantages to patients requiring stoma creation. Future studies will likely confirm the reduced postoperative pain, earlier return of gastrointestinal function, and shorter recovery time seen in previous reports. The procedure does not require extensive tissue dissection, vascular ligation, or colon resection, and therefore can be accomplished in the majority of cases. For patients who require temporary or permanent fecal diversion, a laparoscopic approach will likely replace conventional techniques in the vast majority of cases.

SELF-ASSESSMENT EXERCISES

Questions

1. Which of the following cases would offer the best candidate for laparoscopic stoma surgery?
   a. A 25-year-old female, 4 months pregnant, with perforated diverticulitis
   b. A 60-year-old male with COPD diagnosed with rectal cancer
   c. A 19-year-old male with familial adenomatosis polyposis (FAP) and colorectal tumor
   d. A 40-year-old obese female with obstructing rectal cancer
2. List three advantages of laparoscopic surgery compared to open surgery.
3. Laparoscopic stoma creation is one of the easiest procedures to complete.
   True _____ False _____
4. Laparoscopic surgery continues to be very expensive and will probably remain so in the future.
   True _____ False _____
5. Name the three different methods for creating a stoma as a primary operation.
6. Laparoscopic stoma procedure should only be done for permanent fecal diversion.
   True _____ False _____
7. A complication specific to colorectal laparoscopic procedure is:
   a. Port side herniation.
   b. Hemorrhage.
   c. Ileus.
   d. Infection.

8. The laparoscopic ileostomy procedure requires placement of 4 trocars.

True _____ False _____

Answers

1. c

2. Three advantages of laparoscopic surgery appear to be (a) shorter length of stay, (b) earlier return of bowel function, and (c) less postoperative pain.

3. True

4. False

5. Stomas can be created by (a) conventional laparotomy, (b) the trephine method, and (c) laparoscopically.

6. False

7. a

8. False

REFERENCES

Anderson ID et al: An improved means of faecal diversion: the trephine stoma, *Br J Surg* 79:1080, 1992.

Bergamaschi R, Arnaud JP: Immediately recognized benefits and drawbacks after laparoscopic colon resection for benign disease, *Surg Endosc* 11:802, 1997.

Fuhrman GM, Ota DM: Laparoscopic intestinal stomas, *Dis Colon Rectum* 37:444, 1996.

Hollyoak MA, Lumley J, Stitz RW: Laparoscopic stoma formation for faecal diversion, *Br J Surg* 85:226, 1998.

Jacobs M, Verdeja JC, Goldstein HS: Minimally invasive colon resection (laparoscopic colectomy), *Surg Laparosc Endosc* 1:144, 1991.

Ludwig KA et al: Laparoscopic techniques for fecal diversion, *Dis Colon Rectum* 39:285, 1996.

Marcello PW et al: Laparoscopic restorative proctocolectomy: a case-matched comparative study with open restorative proctocolectomy, *Dis Colon Rectum* 43:604, 2000.

Marcello PW et al: Laparoscopic total colectomy for acute colitis: a case control study, *Dis Colon Rectum* 44:1441, 2001.

Milsom JW, Bohm B: Indications and contraindications. In Milsom JW, Bartholomäus B: *Laparoscopic colorectal surgery*, New York, 1996, Springer-Verlag.

Monson JRT et al: Prospective evaluation of laparoscopic-assisted colectomy in an unselected group of patients, *Lancet* 340:831, 1992.

Oliviera L et al: Laparoscopic creation of stomas, *Surg Endosc* 11:19, 1997.

Ortega AE et al: Laparoscopic bowel surgery registry. Preliminary results, *Dis Colon Rectum* 38:681, 1995.

Ota DM: Laparoscopic colectomy for cancer: a favorable opinion, *Ann Surg Oncol* 2:3, 1995.

Phillips EH et al: Laparoscopic colectomy, *Ann Surg* 216:703, 1992.

Schwandner O, Schiedeck THK, Bruch HP: Stoma creation for fecal diversion: is the laparoscopic technique appropriate? *Int J Colorect Dis* 13:251, 1998.

Senagore AJ et al: Open colectomy vs. laparoscopic colectomy: are there differences? *Am Surg* 59:549, 1993.

Senapati A, Phillips RK: The trephine colostomy: a permanent left iliac fossa end colostomy without recourse to laparotomy, *Ann R Coll Surg Engl* 73:305, 1991.

Slim K et al: High morbidity rate after converted laparoscopic colorectal surgery, *Br J Surg* 82:1406, 1995.

Young CJ, Eyers AA, Solomon MJ: Defunctioning of the anorectum: historically controlled study of laparoscopic vs. open procedures, *Dis Colon Rectum* 41:190, 1998.

Innovative Approaches to Fecal Incontinence

AMY J. THORSEN and ROBERT MADOFF

OBJECTIVES

1. Discuss the population demographics of fecal incontinence.
2. List four medical therapies for treatment of fecal incontinence.
3. Describe the Malone (ACE) procedure.
4. Discuss the use of neosphincters in the treatment of fecal incontinence.
5. Describe the artificial anal sphincter and how it is used to manage fecal incontinence.
6. Explain the use of sacral nerve stimulation for treatment of fecal incontinence in patients with intact anal sphincters.
7. Define internal sphincter augmentation and how it can be used to treat patients with anal sphincter dysfunction.
8. Explain how the Procon incontinence device can be used as a noninvasive treatment for fecal incontinence.

INTRODUCTION

Although considered a benign medical condition, fecal incontinence has a significant effect on quality of life (Johanson and Lafferty, 1996). Incontinent patients are embarrassed by their condition, limit their activities, and experience pain and discomfort resulting from perianal skin irritation, all of which can lead to social isolation, low self-esteem, and sexual dysfunction (Sangwan and Coller, 1994). Because of embarrassment, only one third of those with fecal incontinence mention it to their physi-

cian. A population-based study revealed that less than one fourth of elderly persons with defecation disorders reported seeking medical treatment (Talley et al, 1992).

According to other population-based studies, the prevalence of fecal incontinence is 1.4% to 4.4% (Johanson and Lafferty, 1996; Nelson et al, 1995; Perry et al, 2002). Incontinence is more common in women (Nelson et al, 1995), the elderly, and people with diabetes mellitus (Bytzer et al, 2001) and multiple sclerosis (Hinds, Eidelman, and Wald, 1990), as well as other neurologic diseases. Symptoms of incontinence can occur with inflammatory bowel disease, after pelvic irradiation for malignancy, and after surgical reconstruction of the rectum for irritable bowel disorder or cancer.

MEDICAL THERAPY

Medical therapy for fecal incontinence includes dietary modification, use of antidiarrheals, bowel regimens, and biofeedback. All patients should initially undergo a trial of medical therapy; those with mild to moderate symptoms of incontinence respond best to medical therapy.

Dietary Modification

Fecal incontinence associated with diarrhea or loose stools may often respond to dietary modification. If infectious causes of diarrhea are not suspected, then food intolerances (including lactose intolerance, gluten sensitivity, and fat malabsorption) should be investigated. Other dietary causes of diarrhea include caffeine, alcohol, and certain fruits and vegetables. Patients may need to experiment with their diet by withholding the specified foods suspected of offending.

The addition of fiber, by dietary means or through the use of supplements, may enhance gastrointestinal absorption of water and improve stool consistency. Patients should gradually increase fiber intake to a goal of 25 to 30 g per day (Bliss et al, 2001). Side effects include abdominal bloating, cramping, and increased flatus. Fiber supplements are available in powder, pill, and granule forms. If patients become noncompliant with one form of supplement, another may be more suitable.

Antidiarrheals

Patients with a history of terminal ileal resection or postcholecystectomy diarrhea may respond to cholestyramine, a bile salt–binding resin. Opiates, which include diphenoxylate, loperamide, codeine phosphate, and tincture of opium, increase luminal water absorption and prolong gastrointestinal transit time. Since opiates are habit-forming, loperamide (e.g., Imodium) is most frequently used because of its inability to cross the blood-brain barrier. Loperamide may also improve continence by increasing anal sphincter pressures (Read et al, 1982).

Bowel Regimens

Bowel regimens are best suited for patients with overflow incontinence and poor rectal sensation, including people with spina bifida, spinal cord injuries, and neurologic diseases (such as diabetes and multiple sclerosis). A survey of patients with spinal cord injury found that a chemical rectal stimulant (e.g., bisacodyl, dioctyl sodium sulfosuccinate, or senna) was the most frequently used agent (Kirk et al, 1997). In patients who experience incomplete evacuation, routine use of enemas may prevent stool leakage after defecation. In patients with overflow incontinence associated with severe constipation, the addition of oral laxatives may be necessary.

Biofeedback

Biofeedback is a noninvasive behavioral therapy that has been successfully used to treat fecal incontinence. Motivated patients with intact rectal sensation and the ability to actively contract the external anal sphincter are appropriate candidates for biofeedback. The presence of an external sphincter defect does not appear to affect the clinical response of biofeedback (Leroi et al, 1999). Using sensory, electromyography, or manometric feedback, patients learn to contract the pelvic floor and the external sphincter muscles in response to rectal distention. A minimum of five weekly treatment sessions was recently found to be a positive predictor of success (Gilliland et al, 1997). In that and other studies, symptoms improved for 50% to 90% of biofeedback patients (Cerulli, Nikoomanesh, and Schuster, 1979; Gilliland et al, 1997; Haskell and Rovner, 1967; Jensen and Lowry, 1997; MacLeod, 1983; MacLeod, 1987; Sangwan et al, 1995). In a retrospective study analyzing the long-term effects of biofeedback, Pager et al (2002) reported improved continence in 75% of patients and improved quality of life in 83% of patients (mean follow-up, 42 months). Biofeedback has also been successful for patients who did not improve after sphincteroplasty (Jensen and Lowry, 1997).

Familiar Medications and New Uses

Amitriptyline (e.g., Elavil) is a tricyclic antidepressant commonly used to treat many psychiatric and neurologic conditions. Doses as low as 20 mg per day may increase anal sphincter pressure and improve continence scores (Santoro et al, 2000). Through its anticholinergic properties, amitriptyline may inhibit colonic motility, thereby decreasing frequency of bowel movements and symptoms of urgency (Farrar, 1982). Amitriptyline should be used with caution in patients with cardiovascular disease, liver dysfunction, and glaucoma. It is contraindicated in patients taking monoamine oxidase inhibitors.

Hormone replacement therapy may also have a role in treating fecal incontinence. In both men and women, the smooth muscle fibers of the anal canal have estrogen and progesterone receptors (Franz, Wendler, and Oettling, 1996). In a study by Donnelly, O'Connell, and O'Herlihy (1997), 20 postmenopausal women with fecal incontinence who underwent 6 months of hormone replacement therapy experienced improvements in resting pressure, squeeze pressure, and maximum tolerated volume. Their clinical symptoms of incontinence also improved; in fact, one fourth of the women became asymptomatic.

Topical phenylephrine, by stimulating the α-adrenergic receptors of the internal anal sphincter, may be effective in treating idiopathic fecal incontinence. Concentrations varying from 10% to 40% have been shown to increase resting sphincter pressure for about 2 hours (Cheetham, Kamm, and Phillips, 2001). A randomized controlled trial of patients with incontinence after ileoanal pouch construction showed that topical phenylephrine improved continence and eliminated nocturnal incontinent episodes in some patients (Carapeti et al, 2000). However, a randomized controlled trial of patients with fecal incontinence treated with 10% topical phenylephrine did not show any significant benefit (Carapeti, Kamm, and Phillips, 2000).

SURGICAL THERAPY

The first surgical techniques used to treat fecal incontinence were aimed at correcting the anatomic defects thought to contribute to incontinence. Newer reconstructive techniques include anal sphincter replacement with transposed skeletal muscle or artificial devices. For patients with intact anatomy, sacral nerve stimulation (see later section), a minimally invasive operation, may improve function.

Overlapping Sphincteroplasty

Karoui et al (1999) demonstrated sonographic sphincter defects in 65% of 335 incontinent patients; this rate increased to 88% inpatients with a history of childbirth or proctologic surgery. The technique of overlapping sphincteroplasty was first described by Parks and McPartlin in 1971. The two ends of the sphincter muscles are mobilized adequately to allow an overlapping repair. Scar tissue is preserved, to assist in suture fixation. The internal sphincters may occasionally be isolated and plicated separately (Wexner, Marchetti, and Jagelman, 1991), and an anterior levatoroplasty may be added to increase anal canal length. Routine fecal diversion (to divert stool from the surgical area) does not appear to improve functional outcome or prevent wound infection (Hasegawa, Yoshioka, and Keighley, 2000; Slade et al, 1977; Young et al, 1998).

After overlapping sphincteroplasty, continence generally improves in 70% to 90% of patients (Engel et al, 1994; Fleshman et al, 1991; Hasegawa, Yoshioka, and Keighley, 2000; Simmang et al, 1994; Young et al, 1998). A review of the University of Minnesota experience of 191 consecutive sphincteroplasties revealed that advanced age was a predictor of poor functional outcome (Nancy N. Baxter, unpublished data, 2002). However, other investigators have not found the patient's age to be a predictor of outcome (Simmang et al, 1994; Young et al, 1998). The presence of pudendal neuropathy in addition to a sphincter defect may lead to suboptimal continence after sphincteroplasty (Gilliland et al, 1998; Sangwan et al, 1996), yet significant improvements in function may still be observed (Buie et al, 2001; Chen et al, 1998). In patients with poor results after overlapping sphincteroplasty, repeat attempts at sphincter repair should be considered when a persistent sonographic defect is observed; continence may be improved in over 50% of such patients (Giordano et al, 2002; Pinedo et al, 1999).

The long-term results of overlapping sphincteroplasty have recently been evaluated. After 3 to 4 years of follow-up, success rates may deteriorate to 26% to 57% (Ctercteko et al, 1988; Engel, van Baal, and Brummelkamp, 1994; Yoshioka and Keighley, 1989). In a telephone survey of 49 patients who underwent sphincteroplasty at the Cleveland Clinic (mean follow-up, 69 months) 54% were incontinent to liquid or solid stool, and only 14% were fully continent (Halverson and Hull, 2002). The University of Minnesota experience through 2002 (mean follow-up, 10 years) is similar: 57% of patients were incontinent to solid stool; 16% were incontinent to flatus only; and only 6% were fully continent (Nancy N. Baxter, unpublished data, 2002). Despite this deterioration in results over time, overlapping sphincteroplasty is still considered the best initial treatment for incontinence in the presence of a sphincter defect.

Malone (ACE) Procedure

In a survey of 115 outpatients, Glickman and Kamm (1996) demonstrated the prevalence of bowel disorders following spinal cord injury. Constipation, diarrhea, and nausea were all significantly more common after injury. Over 60% of patients admitted to occasional fecal incontinence, and 11% of patients were incontinent of stool at least once a week; 54% of patients acknowledged that their bowel regimen was a source of emotional distress. The Malone procedure can be used for spinal cord injury (SCI) patients, and in adults it is probably used more for this group than any other adult patient group.

Malone, Ransley, and Kiely (1990) first described a technique to administer antegrade continence enemas (ACE) in children with neurogenic bowel complications secondary to myelomeningocele. The appendix or a segment of bowel is used to create a stoma, which empties into the ascending colon and can be easily catheterized. Antegrade tap water enemas can then be administered through the stoma, facilitating bowel care without the need for laxatives or traditional enemas. The ACE procedure is well accepted and has successfully been used to treat this pediatric population. The most frequent complication is stomal stenosis, which occurs in 12% to 30% of cases (Ellsworth et al, 1996; Koyle et al, 1995; Mor et al, 1997).

Teichman et al (1998) evaluated the ACE-Malone procedure in seven adults with quadriplegia or paraplegia: six of these patients underwent a synchronous urinary procedure, and six of the seven patients were compliant with the self-administered antegrade colonic enemas. All six of these patients reported regular anal and stomal continence, as well as decreased toileting time and improved quality of life. Complications occurred in four patients: stomal stenosis requiring dilation (1), superficial wound infection (1), small bowel obstruction requiring lysis of adhesions (1), and urinary incontinence in a patient who had a synchronous urinary diversion (1). Although the experience in the adult population is limited, the ACE procedure appears to be a safe and effective treatment for SCI patients who may otherwise choose a colostomy to facilitate bowel care.

Neosphincters

When surgical repair of the anal sphincters has failed or is not possible, sphincter replacement should be considered. A neosphincter can be constructed out of transposed skeletal tissue, or an artificial device may be implanted to restore continence. Sphincter replacement is indicated only in patients with severe refractory fecal incontinence, i.e., frequent incontinence to solid stool.

The passive gracilis wrap was described by Pickrell et al in 1952. This technique, initially devised for children with spina bifida, has been associated with variable clinical results. Sonnino et al (1991) reported good long-term results in a series of 7 pediatric patients (mean follow-up, 4.4 years). Corman (1985) reported late results (median follow-up, 77 months) in 14 patients: 7 had excellent results, 4 fair, and 3 poor. Faucheron et al (1994) reviewed the results of graciloplasty in 22 patients: 18 improved, but results frequently deteriorated with time, and only 1 patient was fully continent. Kumar, Hutchinson, and Grant (1995) performed bilateral gracilis transposition in 10 patients and reported restoration of continence in 9.

Several authors have used transposition of the gluteus maximus to treat refractory incontinence. Published results have been generally positive: Pearl et al (1991) reported improvement in 6 of 7 patients, Devesa et al (1992) in 9 of 10, Christiansen, Hansen, and Rasmussen (1995) in 3 of 7, and Guelinckx, Sinsel, and Gruwez (1996) in 9 of 11. However, the quality of continence varied within each of those series, with many patients enjoying only partial restoration of function.

Results after muscle transposition procedures are suboptimal because patients cannot maintain constant voluntary contraction of the transposed muscle and because the transposed muscle is composed of predominately type II muscle fibers. These muscle fibers, of the "fast twitch" variety, are well suited to rapid intermittent contraction, but poorly suited to long-term tonic contraction because of the rapid onset of fatigue.

Laboratory work has demonstrated that type II muscle can be converted to type I muscle by graded electrical stimulation (Salmons and Vrbova, 1969).

By increasing the intensity of stimulation over several weeks, type II muscle fibers can be converted to slow twitch, fatigue-resistant type I fibers. This finding led Baeten et al (1991) in Maastricht, Netherlands, and Williams et al (1991) in London to devise the electrically stimulated skeletal muscle neosphincter. The first case was reported by Baeten, Spaans, and Fluks in 1988. With this technique, a standard gracilis wrap is performed around the native sphincter using two circumanal incisions. Electrodes are placed either within the muscle or on its nerve; they are then attached to an implantable pulse generator, usually located in the subcutaneous tissue of the lower abdominal wall. The transposed gracilis is trained over an 8-week period using a protocol of increasing stimulation. Once the muscle is fully trained, it is maintained in tonic contraction. When patients wish to defecate, the stimulator is deactivated using a hand-held transmitter or magnet, at which time the neosphincter relaxes. After defecation is complete, the neosphincter is reactivated.

In Baeten's own series of 52 patients treated with dynamic graciloplasty for fecal incontinence, 38 (73%) became continent (median follow-up, 2.1 years) (Baeten et al, 1995). Their frequency of defecation decreased, and their ability to defer defecation and retain a phosphate enema improved. Success rates (categorized by cause of incontinence) were 92% for trauma, 64% for pudendal neuropathy, and 50% for anal atresia. Successfully treated patients enjoyed improved quality of life, as documented by Part 2 of the Nottingham Health Profile, as well as decreased anxiety and decreased social isolation.

Two large multicenter trials have evaluated the safety and efficacy of dynamic graciloplasty in treating fecal incontinence. The first included 128 patients treated at 12 centers (Madoff et al, 1999). Success was defined as a greater than 70% decrease in solid stool incontinence for patients without preexisting stomas, and as no solid stool incontinence for patients with stomas. Some graciloplasty patients start off with stomas because of their incontinence, and these cannot be evaluated in relation to their baseline because they do not have accidents per anum. Success rates were 66% for all patients, 71%

for patients with acquired incontinence, and 50% for those with congenital incontinence. There were 138 complications, including major wound infections (32%), minor wound problems (29%), pain (22%), and device-related problems (11%); 48% of the complications required at least one reoperation. The most consequential problem was a major wound infection, which led to failure of dynamic graciloplasty in 41% of patients. Two centers in this trial had previous experience with dynamic graciloplasty; their complication rates were lower and their results better than those of inexperienced centers.

The second multicenter study included 123 patients treated at 20 centers (Baeten et al, 2000). This study differed from the first in two important respects. First, a daily continence diary (rather than patient recall) was used to assess continence (these lead to a more rigorous accounting of incontinent events). Second, offsetting the effect of the diary, success in the second study was defined less stringently than in the first. For patients without stomas, success was defined as a 50% decrease in the number of incontinent events. For patients with stomas, for whom no baseline measurement was possible, success was defined as 50% of stools being continent.

In the second multicenter study, overall success rates for patients without stomas were 63% at 12 months and 57% at 18 months. Quality of life studies demonstrated a decrease in both bowel amounts and bowel accidents during 10 activities of daily living, as well as a decrease in the limitation of participation in the same 10 activities due to a fear of incontinent events. Good to excellent bowel control, as rated by the patients, increased from 7% before graciloplasty to 49% at 12 months ($p < 0.001$). Functional and quality of life improvements were generally sustained in this cohort of patients at 2 years (Wexner et al, 2002).

Of the 123 patients in the second multicenter study, 91 experienced a total of 189 complications; 1 of them died from pulmonary embolism. Other complications included 18 major infections, 31 minor infections, 17 noninfectious wound problems, 9 muscle complications, 34 instances of pain, and 20 device-related complications. As in the first multicenter study, major wound infections were associated with a markedly decreased success rate of 15%.

Dynamic graciloplasty has been described as a technique for anorectal reconstruction after abdominoperineal resection for rectal cancer (Cavina et al, 1998; Rongen et al, 1999; Rouanet et al, 1999; Rullier et al, 2000). It has also been used successfully in pediatric patients (Ruckauer, 2001). It is available in specialty centers in Europe and Canada, but Food and Drug Administration (FDA) approval has not been sought in the United States because of its high complication rate and the availability of alternative therapies.

The artificial anal sphincter (Acticon Neosphincter) is the treatment of choice for sphincter replacement in the United States. It is an implantable device, composed of a silicone elastomer that maintains continence by means of a fluid-filled cuff surrounding and compressing the anal canal (Figure 24-1). To deflate the cuff and allow the passage of stool, patients squeeze a pump (placed in the labia or scrotum) 9 to 12 times. Squeezing forces fluid from the cuff into the reservoir, which is implanted in the space of Retzius. The cuff then automatically inflates, usually within 5 minutes, to restore continence. Advantages of the artificial sphincter (as opposed to dynamic graciloplasty) include the need for only one surgical procedure, less postoperative pain, and activation 6 weeks postoperatively without any need for muscle conditioning.

Since Christiansen and Lorentzen (1987) first described the artificial anal sphincter in 1987, many authors have reported their experience with this device. As with dynamic graciloplasty, local complications substantially affect success rates, and both complications and results appear related to experience. Published results must be interpreted with some caution, because reported successes are often based on the number of patients with functional sphincters in place, rather than on the total number who underwent implantation.

Device explantation may be required because of early or late complications. O'Brien and Skinner (2000) explanted 10 of 13 devices. Lehur, Roig, and Duinslaeger, (2000) explanted devices in 7 of 24

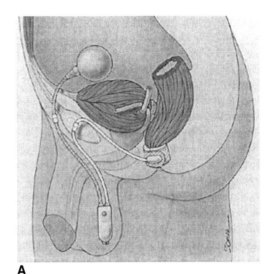

A

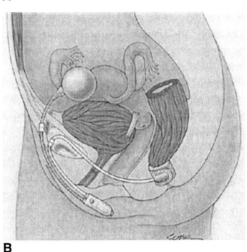

B

Figure 24-1 Acticon Neosphincter. **A,** Male placement. **B,** Female placement. (Courtesy American Medical Systems, Minnetonka, MN.)

patients but were able to reimplant 3. Michot et al (2003) explanted devices from 6 of their first 12 patients but only from 5 of their next 25. Ortiz et al (2002) noted early complications in 10 and late complications in 10 of 22 patients (mean follow-up, 28 months). In those four studies the cumulative probability of device explantation was 44% at 48 months. Late complications included infection, erosion, pump migration, unbuttoning of the cuff, anal pain, and impaired rectal emptying. Obstructed defecation after artificial sphincter implantation is often related to a short duration of cuff opening (Savoye et al, 2000).

Functional results in patients who have retained a functioning artificial sphincter tend to be good, with most patients regaining control of solid and liquid stool (Michot et al, 2003; O'Brien and Skinner, 2000); standardized continence scores improve markedly (Altomare et al, 2001; Devesa et al, 2002; Lehur, Roig, and Duinslaeger, 2000). Devesa et al (2002) reported significant improvement in all four scales of the Fecal Incontinence Quality of Life (FIQL) Scale (Rockwood et al, 2000), although the assessment was retrospective and involved only half of the patients in his series.

Wong et al (2002) reported the results of a prospective multicenter clinical trial that evaluated the artificial anal sphincter in 112 patients. Patients were evaluated by a quality of life questionnaire, physiologic testing, and a fecal incontinence score (ranging from 1 to 120) devised specifically to validate the study. To qualify for the study, patients were required to have a stoma or a minimum fecal incontinence score of 88 (incontinent of stool more than once per week). At 1 year of follow-up, 67% of patients had functioning devices. Infections occurred in 25% of patients, and nearly half (46%) of all patients required revisional surgery. At 1 year the mean fecal incontinence score dropped from 105 (daily incontinence of liquid and solid stool) to 48 (incontinent to seepage). Quality of life and anal canal resting pressures improved significantly in patients with functioning devices.

The chapter authors' long-term experience with the artificial anal sphincter at the University of Minnesota involves two groups of patients: (1) 10 patients who underwent device implantation from 1989 through 1992, and (2) 35 patients from 1997 through 2001. In group 2, 49% still have a functional artificial anal sphincter (mean follow-up, 39 months). Patients with a functioning device decreased their fecal incontinence score by a mean of 90 points (minimum follow-up, 24 months). Of the 6 patients in group 1 with a functioning device,

this improvement in continence was maintained at over 10 years of follow-up (Congilosi et al, 2002).

Unlike dynamic graciloplasty, the artificial anal sphincter may be contraindicated, or less successful, in patients who lack sufficient perineal soft tissue. However, in such patients, preliminary reconstruction with gluteal rotation flaps and implantation at levels higher in the anal canal are possible. Both dynamic graciloplasty and artificial anal sphincter implantation have high complication rates, but patients with successful procedures can likely expect long-term improvement in continence and quality of life.

Sacral Nerve Stimulation (SNS)

For patients with intact anal sphincters and severe fecal incontinence, sacral nerve stimulation (SNS) is a minimally invasive surgical option. It was first used to treat urinary incontinence. Matzel et al (1995) first described the use of sacral nerve stimulation for fecal incontinence in 1995. An electrode is placed in the S2, S3, or S4 sacral foramen to stimulate the nerve roots that enhance pelvic floor contraction, with minimal stimulation to the lower extremity. After optimal placement (usually S3), the lead is attached to a temporary external pulse generator for a test period of stimulation. A diary monitoring continence is kept over the 3-week test period; if sufficient improvement in continence is observed, the pulse generator is implanted during a second small procedure under light sedation.

Most published series have described the success of SNS in small numbers of patients (Ganio et al, 2001; Kenefick et al, 2002a; Malouf et al, 2000; Matzel et al, 2001; Rosen et al, 2001). Rosen et al (2001) attempted SNS in 20 patients, 16 of whom had a satisfactory acute response and went on to permanent stimulator implantation. The mean number of incontinent episodes per 21 days decreased from 6 to 2; the mean enema retention time increased from 2 to 7.5 minutes. Quality of life, as determined by the FIQL score, improved significantly. Similar results were reported by Kenefick et al (2002a) in a group of 15 patients from St. Mark's Hospital: all 15 patients improved (mean follow-up, 24 months), with a decrease in accidents from a median of 11 to 0 per week, and an improvement in the ability to defer defecation from less than 1 to 8 minutes. In the largest series to date, Ulludag and Baeten (2002) reported an 80% success rate in 44 patients, with an average decrease in weekly incontinent episodes from 8.66 to 0.67. Patients were also able to postpone defecation for 10 to 15 minutes.

In contrast to dynamic graciloplasty and artificial anal sphincter implantation, complications after SNS have been few and relatively minor. Rosen et al (2001) reported three infections and two lead dislodgements (both in one patient, leading to abandonment of therapy). Kenefick et al (2002a) reported no infections and no device explantations; two patients with lead dislodgements underwent successful reimplantation, and three patients had transient pain from the temporary subcutaneous lead used during the test stimulation period.

The mechanism of improvement after sacral nerve stimulation remains unknown. Physiologic studies after SNS demonstrate an increase in resting and squeezing anal pressures, as well as improved rectal sensitivity (Ganio et al, 2001; Kenefick et al, 2002a; Rosen et al, 2001). Ambulatory manometry shows a qualitative decrease in rectal motor complexes and in episodes of spontaneous anal relaxation (Vaizey et al, 1999), suggesting autonomic nerve effects from SNS. However, possible alternative mechanisms include slowing of gastrointestinal transit, dampening of rectal contractility, and improved coordination of anorectal sensorimotor function. SNS impulses can proceed in both afferent and efferent directions, and the exact nerves effecting changes in incontinence are unknown. Which nerves are stimulated depends both on electrode placement and on the diameter of the nerve in the electrode's vicinity. Because the largest nerves have the lowest stimulation thresholds, it is most likely that somatic motor efferents and sensory afferents are involved. However, the physiologic findings also suggest that smaller autonomic nerve fibers are also being stimulated.

Internal Sphincter Augmentation

Anal canal bulking agents, originally used to treat urinary sphincter dysfunction, aim to increase the resting tone of the anal canal. Injectable materials include autologous fat, collagen, silicone, and carbon-coated beads (Bernardi, Favetta, and Pescatori, 1998; Davis and Kumar, 2002; Feretis et al, 2001; Kenefick et al, 2002b; Kumar, Benson, and Bland, 1998; Shafik, 1995). Kenefick et al (2002b) treated six patients, all with fecal incontinence attributed to internal anal sphincter dysfunction, with an injectable silicone biomaterial. This technique involves three circumferential, transsphincteric injections, at or above the dentate line, performed under local anesthesia. At a median follow-up of 18 months, five of six patients had significantly improved continence and quality of life. Improved continence was also associated with increased resting and squeeze pressures. Glutaraldehyde crossed-link collagen injections into the anal canal significantly improved anal continence in 11 of 17 patients (Kumar, Benson, and Bland, 1998).

Durasphere carbon-coated beads appear to be as effective as collagen in treating urinary sphincter dysfunction, with more durable results (Lightner et al, 2001). Preliminary results suggest this material may also successfully treat fecal incontinence (Davis and Kumar, 2002). ACYST carbon-coated beads were evaluated in 10 patients at the Cleveland Clinic in Florida (Weiss et al, 2002). All injections were performed under local anesthesia in an outpatient setting. An increase in mean resting and squeeze pressure was seen in 80% of patients. A 23% improvement in continence scores was seen at 3 months, and this increased to 30% at 6 months. One patient had extravasation of beads into the skin, which required removal of the material in the office.

Expandable microballoons, placed in the submucosa of the anal canal, have led to improved continence without morbidity in a small series of patients (Feretis et al, 2001). Although the long-term results of anal canal bulking agents are unclear, they appear to be a relatively safe method of treating incontinence in these small series of patients.

Radiofrequency energy has also been evaluated as a technique to augment resting sphincter tone. Under local anesthesia with intravenous sedation, temperature-controlled radiofrequency energy is delivered to the sphincter muscles via multiple needle electrodes. The resulting thermal injury appears to increase collagen contractility and tighten the anal canal while preserving the overlying mucosa. In a series of 10 patients, Takahashi et al (2002) demonstrated improved continence at 12 months after radiofrequency ablation. However, 4 of these 10 patients experienced postprocedure bleeding. A multicenter study trial is now underway to further evaluate the technique (Fleshman and Efron, 2002).

At this time, augmentation procedures are not widely available to most patients. However, they appear to be a promising mode of treatment for patients who are poor candidates for sphincter reconstruction or SNS, and for patients whose primary symptom is seepage.

Noninvasive Devices

For patients with severe incontinence for whom surgery has been unsuccessful or who have chosen less invasive treatments, the Procon incontinence device may be a simple option for preventing episodes of fecal incontinence. The device consists of a flexible, disposable catheter with an infrared sensor and flatus vent holes, which is inserted into the rectum. A silent, vibrating signal is received by the paging device worn at the waistline when stool is sensed by the electrode. A 20-cc cuff is inflated in the rectum, preventing inadvertent stool leakage. To allow the passage of feces, the balloon is deflated and the catheter removed.

Giamundo et al (2002) evaluated the effect of the Procon device in seven patients over a 2-week period. All patients were evaluated by manometry, endoanal ultrasound, and pudendal nerve terminal motor latency assessment before the study. Of these seven patients, two had a known sphincter injury, four had idiopathic incontinence, and one had a known neurologic disorder. Patients kept a diary of bowel activity and quality of life. The Procon device was shown to significantly reduce incontinence scores and improve quality of life. The device has since been modified and further clinical trials are presently underway.

CONCLUSION

In the past, the treatment of fecal incontinence consisted mainly of medical management, biofeedback, sphincteroplasty, and even colostomy. For patients with minor incontinence, newer pharmacologic options and anal canal bulking agents may be promising. Patients with extensive perineal damage and patients with an unsuccessful or deteriorating sphincteroplasty are candidates for sphincter replacement with dynamic graciloplasty or artificial anal sphincter implantation. SNS, which has had excellent results in treating urinary incontinence, appears to be an effective treatment for fecal incontinence that could benefit a large range of patients, with minimal morbidity. For patients with severe incontinence for whom surgery has been unsuccessful or who have chosen less invasive treatments, the Procon incontinence device may be an option that leads to improved continence and quality of life.

SELF-ASSESSMENT EXERCISES

Questions

1. Dietary assessment of the person with fecal incontinence includes all of the following *except*:
   a. The time of day that meals are ingested.
   b. Food intolerances (e.g., lactose intolerance, gluten sensitivity, fat malabsorption).
   c. Caffeine and alcohol intake.
   d. Certain fruits and vegetables.
2. What is the recommended daily goal of fiber intake that may enhance gastrointestinal absorption of water and improve stool consistency?
   a. 40 to 50 g per day
   b. 25 to 30 g per day
   c. 10 to 15 g per day
   d. 20 to 25 g per day
3. What is the mechanism of action of opiates?
4. Hormone replacement therapy may have a role in treating fecal incontinence.
   True _____ False _____
5. The best initial treatment for incontinence in the presence of sphincter defect is believed to be:
   a. Diverting loop colostomy.

b. Biofeedback.
c. Malone procedure.
d. Overlapping sphincteroplasty.

6. Describe the Malone ACE procedure.
7. What is the treatment of choice for sphincter replacement in the United States?
   a. Dynamic graciloplasty
   b. Collagen implants
   c. Artificial anal sphincter
   d. Gluteal muscularis flap
8. Describe how the implantable artificial anal sphincter works.
9. Sacral nerve stimulation applies an electrode in the S2, S3, or S4 sacral foramen to stimulate the nerve roots that enhance pelvic floor contraction.
   True _____ False _____
10. Internal sphincter augmentation is:
    a. Achieved by ingesting over 40 mg of fiber daily and providing bulk into the anal canal.
    b. A surgical procedure that tightens the sphincter muscles preventing involuntary passage of stools.
    c. Injectable materials that aim to increase the resting tone of the anal canal.
    d. Placement of a gracillis flap to augment the sphincter tone.
11. Describe how a noninvasive device like the Procon incontinence device can prevent episodes of fecal incontinence.

Answers

1. a
2. b
3. Opiates increase luminal water absorption and prolong gastrointestinal transit time.
4. True; The smooth muscle fibers of the anal canal have estrogen and progesterone receptors.
5. d
6. A stoma is created from the appendix or a segment of the bowel; antegrade tap water enemas are administered through the stoma, allowing for bowel cleansing without the need for laxatives or traditional enemas.
7. c
8. A fluid-filled cuff surrounds and compresses the anal canal. To deflate the cuff (and allow stool to pass), a pump that is implanted in the labia or scrotum is squeezed. The squeezing forces fluid from the cuff into a reservoir, deflating the cuff; the cuff automatically inflates in approximately 5 minutes, restoring continence.
9. True
10. c
11. This device uses a catheter with a 20-ml balloon catheter and an infrared sensor with flatus vent holes. The catheter is placed in the rectum and the cuff is inflated. When stool enters the rectum a signal is received by a paging device worn by the user. The balloon is deflated and the catheter removed to allow stool to be drained from the rectum.

REFERENCES

Altomare DF et al: Multicentre retrospective analysis of the outcome of artificial anal sphincter implantation for severe faecal incontinence, *Br J Surg* 88(11):1481-1486, 2001.

Baeten CG, et al: Dynamic graciloplasty for treatment of faecal incontinence, *Lancet* 338(8776):1163-1165, 1991.

Baeten CG, et al: Anal dynamic graciloplasty in the treatment of intractable fecal incontinence, *N Engl J Med* 332(24):1600-1605, 1995.

Baeten CG, et al: Safety and efficacy of dynamic graciloplasty for fecal incontinence: report of a prospective, multicenter trial. Dynamic graciloplasty therapy study group, *Dis Colon Rectum* 43(6):743-751, 2000.

Baeten CG, Spaans F, Fluks A: An implanted neuromuscular stimulator for fecal continence following previously implanted gracilis muscle. Report of a case, *Dis Colon Rectum* 31(2):134-137, 1988.

Bernardi C, Favetta U, Pescatori M: Autologous fat injection for treatment of fecal incontinence: manometric and echographic assessment, *Plast Reconstr Surg* 102(5):1626-1628, 1998.

Bliss DZ, et al: Supplementation with dietary fiber improves fecal incontinence, *Nurs Res* 50(4):203-213, 2001.

Buie WD, et al: Clinical rather than laboratory assessment predicts continence after anterior sphincteroplasty, *Dis Colon Rectum* 44(9):1255-1260, 2001.

Bytzer P, et al: Prevalence of gastrointestinal symptoms associated with diabetes mellitus: a population-based survey of 15,000 adults, *Arch Intern Med* 161(16):1989-1996, 2001.

Carapeti EA, et al: Randomized, controlled trial of topical phenylephrine for fecal incontinence in patients after ileoanal pouch construction, *Dis Colon Rectum* 43(8): 1059-1063, 2000.

Carapeti EA, Kamm MA, Phillips RK: Randomized controlled trial of topical phenylephrine in the treatment of faecal incontinence, *Br J Surg* 87(1):38-42, 2000.

Cavina E, et al: Anorectal reconstruction after abdominoperineal resection. Experience with double-wrap graciloplasty supported by low-frequency electrostimulation, *Dis Colon Rectum* 41(8):1010-1016, 1998.

Cerulli MA, Nikoomanesh P, Schuster MM: Progress in biofeedback conditioning for fecal incontinence, *Gastroenterology* 76(4):742-746, 1979.

Cheetham MJ, Kamm MA, Phillips RK: Topical phenylephrine increases anal canal resting pressure in patients with faecal incontinence, *Gut* 48(3):356-359, 2001.

Chen AS, et al: Pudendal nerve latency. Does it predict outcome of anal sphincter repair? *Dis Colon Rectum* 41(8):1005-1009, 1998.

Christiansen J, Hansen CR, Rasmussen O: Bilateral gluteus maximus transposition for anal incontinence, *Br J Surg* 82(7):903-905, 1995.

Christiansen J, Lorentzen M: Implantation of artificial sphincter for anal incontinence, *Lancet* 2(8553):244-245, 1987.

Congilosi S, et al: The artificial bowel sphincter: long-term experience at a single institution, *Dis Colon Rectum* 45(4):A26, 2002 (abstract).

Corman ML: Gracilis muscle transposition for anal incontinence: late results, *Br J Surg* 72 Suppl:S21-22, 1985.

Ctercteko GC et al: Anal sphincter repair: a report of 60 cases and review of the literature, *Aust N Z J Surg* 58(9):703-710, 1988.

Davis K, Kumar D: Clinical evaluation of an injectable anal sphincter bulking agent (Durasphere) in the management of patients with persistent faecal incontinence secondary to an internal anal sphincter defect. Paper presented at: Tripartite 2002 Colorectal Meeting; October 27-30, 2002; Melbourne, Australia.

Devesa JM et al: Total fecal incontinence—a new method of gluteus maximus transposition: Preliminary results and report of previous experience with similar procedures, *Dis Colon Rectum* 35(4):339-349, 1992.

Devesa JM et al: Artificial anal sphincter: Complications and functional results of a large personal series, *Dis Colon Rectum* 45(9):1154-1163, 2002.

Donnelly V, O'Connell PR, O'Herlihy C: The influence of oestrogen replacement on faecal incontinence in postmenopausal women, *Br J Obstet Gynaecol* 104(3):311-315, 1997.

Ellsworth PI et al: The Malone antegrade colonic enema enhances the quality of life in children undergoing urological incontinence procedures, *J Urol* 155(4):1416-1418, 1996.

Engel AF et al: Anterior anal sphincter repair in patients with obstetric trauma, *Br J Surg* 81(8):1231-1234, 1994.

Engel AF, van Baal SJ, Brummelkamp WH: Late results of anterior sphincter plication for traumatic faecal incontinence, *Eur J Surg* 160(11):633-636, 1994.

Farrar JT: The effects of drugs on intestinal motility, *Clin Gastroenterol* 11(3):673-681, 1982.

Faucheron JL et al: Is fecal continence improved by non-stimulated gracilis muscle transposition? *Dis Colon Rectum* 37(10):979-983, 1994.

Feretis C et al: Implantation of microballoons in the management of fecal incontinence, *Dis Colon Rectum* 44(11):1605-1609, 2001.

Fleshman JW, Efron J: Multicenter open label prospective trial evaluating the safety and effectiveness of temperature controlled radio-frequency energy delivery to the anal canal (secca procedure) for treatment of fecal incontinence. Paper presented at: Tripartite 2002 Colorectal Meeting; October 27-30, 2002; Melbourne, Australia.

Fleshman JW et al: Anal sphincter reconstruction: anterior overlapping muscle repair, *Dis Colon Rectum* 34(9): 739-743, 1991.

Franz HB, Wendler D, Oettling G: Immunohistochemical assessment of steroid hormone receptors in tissues of the anal canal. Implications for anal incontinence? *Acta Obstet Gynecol Scand* 75(10):892-895, 1996.

Ganio E et al: Short-term sacral nerve stimulation for functional anorectal and urinary disturbances: results in 40 patients: evaluation of a new option for anorectal functional disorders, *Dis Colon Rectum* 44(9):1261-1267, 2001.

Giamundo P et al: The Procon incontinence device: a new nonsurgical approach to preventing episodes of fecal incontinence, *Am J Gastroenterol* 97(9):2328-2332, 2002.

Gilliland R et al: Outcome and predictors of success of biofeedback for constipation, *Br J Surg* 84(8):1123-1126, 1997.

Gilliland R et al: Pudendal neuropathy is predictive of failure following anterior overlapping sphincteroplasty, *Dis Colon Rectum* 41(12):1516-1522, 1998.

Giordano P et al: Previous sphincter repair does not affect the outcome of repeat repair, *Dis Colon Rectum* 45(5): 635-640, 2002.

Glickman S, Kamm MA: Bowel dysfunction in spinal-cord-injury patients, *Lancet* 347(9016):1651-1653, 1996.

Guelinckx PJ, Sinsel NK, Gruwez JA: Anal sphincter reconstruction with the gluteus maximus muscle: anatomic and physiologic considerations concerning conventional and dynamic gluteoplasty, *Plast Reconstr Surg* 98(2):293-302, 1996.

Halverson AL, Hull TL: Long-term outcome of overlapping anal sphincter repair, *Dis Colon Rectum* 45(3):345-348, 2002.

Hasegawa H, Yoshioka K, Keighley MR: Randomized trial of fecal diversion for sphincter repair, *Dis Colon Rectum* 43(7):961-964; discussion 964-965, 2000.

Haskell B, Rovner H: Electromyography in the management of the incompetent anal sphincter, *Dis Colon Rectum* 10(2):81-84, 1967.

Hinds JP, Eidelman BH, Wald A: Prevalence of bowel dysfunction in multiple sclerosis. A population survey, *Gastroenterology* 98(6):1538-1542, 1990.

Jensen LL, Lowry AC: Biofeedback improves functional outcome after sphincteroplasty, *Dis Colon Rectum* 40(2):197-200, 1997.

Johanson JF, Lafferty J: Epidemiology of fecal incontinence: the silent affliction, *Am J Gastroenterol* 91(1):33-36, 1996.

Karoui S et al: Prevalence of anal sphincter defects revealed by sonography in 335 incontinent patients and 115 continent patients, *AJR Am J Roentgenol* 173(2):389-392, 1999.

Kenefick NJ et al: Medium-term results of permanent sacral nerve stimulation for faecal incontinence, *Br J Surg* 89(7):896-901, 2002a.

Kenefick NJ et al: Injectable silicone biomaterial for faecal incontinence due to internal anal sphincter dysfunction, *Gut* 51(2):225-228, 2002b.

Kirk PM et al: Long-term follow-up of bowel management after spinal cord injury, *SCI Nurs* 14(2):56-63, 1997.

Koyle MA et al: The Malone antegrade continence enema for neurogenic and structural fecal incontinence and constipation, *J Urol* 154(2 Pt 2):759-761, 1995.

Kumar D, Benson MJ, Bland JE: Glutaraldehyde cross-linked collagen in the treatment of faecal incontinence, *Br J Surg* 85(7):978-979, 1998.

Kumar D, Hutchinson R, Grant E: Bilateral gracilis neosphincter construction for treatment of faecal incontinence, *Br J Surg* 82(12):1645-1647, 1995.

Lehur PA, Roig JV, Duinslaeger M: Artificial anal sphincter: prospective clinical and manometric evaluation, *Dis Colon Rectum* 43(8):1100-1106, 2000.

Leroi AM et al: Pudendal neuropathy and severity of incontinence but not presence of an anal sphincter defect may determine the response to biofeedback therapy in fecal incontinence, *Dis Colon Rectum* 42(6):762-769, 1999.

Lightner D et al: A new injectable bulking agent for treatment of stress urinary incontinence: results of a multicenter, randomized, controlled, double-blind study of durasphere, *Urology* 58(1):12-15, 2001.

MacLeod JH: Biofeedback in the management of partial anal incontinence, *Dis Colon Rectum* 26(4):244-246, 1983.

MacLeod JH: Management of anal incontinence by biofeedback, *Gastroenterology* 93(2):291-294, 1987.

Madoff RD et al: Safety and efficacy of dynamic muscle plasty for anal incontinence: lessons from a prospective, multicenter trial, *Gastroenterology* 116(3):549-556, 1999.

Malone PS, Ransley PG, Kiely EM: Preliminary report: the antegrade colonic enema., *Lancet* 336:1217-1218, 1990.

Malouf AJ et al: Permanent sacral nerve stimulation for fecal incontinence, *Ann Surg* 232(1):143-148, 2000.

Matzel KE et al: Electrical stimulation of sacral spinal nerves for treatment of faecal incontinence, *Lancet* 346(8983):1124-1127, 1995.

Matzel KE et al: Chronic sacral spinal nerve stimulation for fecal incontinence: long-term results with foramen and cuff electrodes, *Dis Colon Rectum* 44(1):59-66, 2001.

Michot F et al: Artificial anal sphincter in severe fecal incontinence: outcome of prospective experience with 37 patients in one institution, *Ann Surg* 237(1):52-56, 2003.

Mor Y et al: Combined Mitrofanoff and antegrade continence enema procedures for urinary and fecal incontinence, *J Urol* 158(1):192-195, 1997.

Nelson R et al: Community-based prevalence of anal incontinence, *JAMA* 274(7):559-561, 1995.

O'Brien PE, Skinner S: Restoring control: the Acticon Neosphincter artificial bowel sphincter in the treatment of anal incontinence, *Dis Colon Rectum* 43(9):1213-1216, 2000.

Ortiz H et al: Complications and functional outcome following artificial anal sphincter implantation, *Br J Surg* 89(7):877-881, 2002.

Pager CK et al: Long-term outcomes of pelvic floor exercise and biofeedback treatment for patients with fecal incontinence, *Dis Colon Rectum* 45(8):997-1003, 2002.

Parks AG, McPartlin JF: Late repair of injuries of the anal sphincter, *Proc R Soc Med* 64(12):1187-1189, 1971.

Pearl RK et al: Bilateral gluteus maximus transposition for anal incontinence, *Dis Colon Rectum* 34:478-481, 1991.

Perry S et al: Prevalence of faecal incontinence in adults aged 40 years or more living in the community, *Gut* 50(4):480-484, 2002.

Pickrell KL et al: Construction of a rectal sphincter and restoration of anal continence by transplanting the gracilis muscle; a report of four cases in children, *Ann Surg* 135(6):853-862, 1952.

Pinedo G et al: Results of repeat anal sphincter repair, *Br J Surg* 86(1):66-69, 1999.

Read M et al: Effects of loperamide on anal sphincter function in patients complaining of chronic diarrhea with fecal incontinence and urgency, *Dig Dis Sci* 27(9):807-814, 1982.

Rockwood TH et al: Fecal Incontinence Quality of Life Scale: Quality of life instrument for patients with fecal incontinence, *Dis Colon Rectum* 43(1):9-16; discussion 16-17, 2000.

Rongen MJ et al: Secondary coloperineal pull-through and double dynamic graciloplasty after miles resection—feasible, but with a high morbidity, *Dis Colon Rectum* 42(6):776-780; discussion 781, 1999.

Rosen HR et al: Sacral nerve stimulation as a treatment for fecal incontinence, *Gastroenterology* 121(3):536-541, 2001.

Rouanet P et al: Anal sphincter reconstruction by dynamic graciloplasty after abdominoperineal resection for cancer, *Dis Colon Rectum* 42(4):451-456, 1999.

Ruckauer KD: Dynamic graciloplasty in children with fecal incontinence: a preliminary report, *J Pediatr Surg* 36(7):1036-1039, 2001.

Rullier E et al: Morbidity and functional outcome after double dynamic graciloplasty for anorectal reconstruction, *Br J Surg* 87(7):909-913, 2000.

Salmons S, Vrbova G: The influence of activity on some contractile characteristics of mammalian fast and slow muscles, *J Physiol* 201:535-549, 1969.

Sangwan YP, Coller JA: Fecal incontinence, *Surg Clin North Am* 74(6):1377-1397, 1994.

Sangwan YP et al: Can manometric parameters predict response to biofeedback therapy in fecal incontinence? *Dis Colon Rectum* 38(10):1021-1025, 1995.

Sangwan YP et al: Unilateral pudendal neuropathy. Impact on outcome of anal sphincter repair, *Dis Colon Rectum* 39(6):686-689, 1996.

Santoro GA et al: Open study of low-dose amitriptyline in the treatment of patients with idiopathic fecal incontinence, *Dis Colon Rectum* 43(12):1676-1681; discussion 1681-1682, 2000.

Savoye G et al: Manometric assessment of an artificial bowel sphincter, *Br J Surg* 87(5):586-589, 2000.

Shafik A: Perianal injection of autologous fat for treatment of sphincteric incontinence, *Dis Colon Rectum* 38(6):583-587, 1995.

Simmang C et al: Anal sphincter reconstruction in the elderly: does advancing age affect outcome? *Dis Colon Rectum* 37(11):1065-1069, 1994.

Slade MS et al: Sphincteroplasty for acquired anal incontinence, *Dis Colon Rectum* 20(1):33-35, 1977.

Sonnino RE et al: Gracilis muscle transposition for anal incontinence in children: long-term follow-up, *J Pediatr Surg* 26(10):1219-1223, 1991.

Takahashi T et al: Radio-frequency energy delivery to the anal canal for the treatment of fecal incontinence, *Dis Colon Rectum* 45(7):915-922, 2002.

Talley NJ et al: Prevalence of gastrointestinal symptoms in the elderly: a population-based study, *Gastroenterology* 102(3):895-901, 1992.

Teichman JM et al: Malone antegrade continence enema for adults with neurogenic bowel disease, *J Urol* 160(4):1278-1281, 1998.

Ulludag O, Baeten C: Sacral neuromodulation for faecal incontinence: Paper presented at: Tripartite 2002 Colorectal Meeting; October 27-30, 2002; Melbourne, Australia.

Vaizey CJ et al: Prospective comparison of faecal incontinence grading systems, *Gut* 44(1):77-80, 1999.

Weiss E et al: Submucosal injection of carbon-coated beads is a successful and safe office-based treatment of fecal incontinence, *Dis Colon Rectum* 45(4):A46-47, 2002 (abstract).

Wexner SD et al: Long-term efficacy of dynamic graciloplasty for fecal incontinence, *Dis Colon Rectum* 45(6):809-818, 2002.

Wexner SD, Marchetti F, Jagelman DG: The role of sphincteroplasty for fecal incontinence reevaluated: a prospective physiologic and functional review, *Dis Colon Rectum* 34(1):22-30, 1991.

Williams NS et al: Development of an electrically stimulated neoanal sphincter, *Lancet* 338:1166-1169, 1991.

Wong WD et al: The safety and efficacy of the artificial bowel sphincter for fecal incontinence: results from a multicenter cohort study, *Dis Colon Rectum* 45(9):1139-1153, 2002.

Yoshioka K, Keighley MR: Sphincter repair for fecal incontinence, *Dis Colon Rectum* 32(1):39-42, 1989.

Young CJ et al: Successful overlapping anal sphincter repair: relationship to patient age, neuropathy, and colostomy formation, *Dis Colon Rectum* 41(3):344-349, 1998.

APPENDIX

A   DISCHARGE RESOURCES

························

CONNIE KELLY

This appendix contains examples of discharge resources. The following examples are included: patient instruction sheet, the use of digital photography for patient instruction, contact information, support group information, and supply information.

The number of days patients are hospitalized following ostomy surgery has progressively decreased over the last several years. It is true that the patient and the patient's significant other are given instruction in ostomy care during the hospital stay; however, they also need to be given detailed reference material upon discharge. There are many sources of instructional material available to the person with an ostomy. The wound, ostomy and continence/enterostomal therapy (WOC/ET) nurse can develop individualized instruction sheets. Many manufacturers of ostomy equipment provide materials that cover pouch changes, as well as problem solving, that are available in written format and on videotape. Companies such as Pritchett & Hull Associates also have discharge instruction sheets. The United Ostomy Association provides supportive information regarding adjustment issues and general overview of living with a stoma. This information can offer the patient additional education and support while at home.

Discharge information/equipment should include:

- Supply list with step-by-step instructions for the pouch change procedure and simple problem solving (e.g., skin irritation interventions)

- Nutritional guidelines (see Appendix C)

- Contact information, including whom to call and when (telephone and e-mail addresses, Box A-1)

- Support group information (Box A-2)

- List of ostomy retail options, including local dealers and mail order companies (Box A-3)

- Supplies for at least three pouching system changes

BOX A-1 Template for Contact Information

Your WOC (ostomy) nurse's name: _____

Telephone/voice mail number: _____

To page, call telephone number: _____

Mailing address: _____

_____

E-mail address: _____

Location and phone number of the outpatient clinic: _____

After your discharge from the hospital, please call to set up an outpatient appointment. It is important to routinely see **the WOC/ET nurse** to help you adapt to living with an ostomy, as well as to address any problems with your skin or pouching system.

Call **the WOC/ET nurse** should the following occur:

- Skin irritation lasting for more than a few days (redness, itching, or burning)
- No bowel movement for more than 2 days (colostomy) or 6 hours (ileostomy)
- If you have any questions or problems with pouching or leakage
- To receive additional information or if you have questions about activities of daily living

Call your doctor if any of the following occur:

- Stoma changes color from pink/red to purple/black
- Excessive bleeding from the stoma
- Continuous bleeding between stoma and skin
- Unusual bulging around your stoma
- Any unusual problems with abdominal pain, continuous nausea, vomiting and/or severe diarrhea

BOX A-2 Template for Support Group Information

The United Ostomy Association (UOA) is a volunteer-based organization dedicated to assisting people who have had or will have intestinal or urinary diversions. Its purpose is to offer mutual aid and moral support from people who have learned to live with their ostomies. At monthly meetings, open to any one who is interested, members exchange practical experiences about their ostomies, see ostomy equipment displayed, and listen to knowledgeable speakers. Call the national office to receive the contact person for the chapter in your area.

Join the national association and receive the magazine, *Ostomy Quarterly*. Write to:

United Ostomy Association
36 Executive Park, Suite 120
Irvine, CA 92714-6744
1-800-826-0826
Website: www.uoa.org

United Ostomy Association Chapter Directory (example of local listings to be tailored to individual practice area)

Aurora Chapter
Second Tuesday, 7:00 PM
Mercy Center
1325 N. Highland Ave., Blue Room
Aurora
Contact person and phone number:

Chicago, Illiana Chapter
Second Monday, 7:30 PM
Alternates: Olympia Fields, Ingalls, South Suburban, and St James Hospitals
Contact person and phone number:

BOX A-3   Retailer Information[*]

• •

Ostomy Retailers

This is a partial list of retailers who sell ostomy supplies. Check with the individual retailer to learn if Medicare or private insurance assignment is accepted. Contact your insurer to check on reimbursement issues before your first purchase of ostomy supplies. Many of these retailers will take phone orders and deliver to your home.

Becker Prof. Pharmacy   Phone: _____
4744 N. Western Ave.
Chicago, IL 60625

Doubek Pharmacy   Phone: _____
11350 S. Cicero
Alsip, IL 60803

Mail-Order Companies

American Ostomy Supply   Phone: _____
1-800-xxx-xxxx

AARP Pharmacy Service   Phone: _____
1-800-xxx-xxxx

Edgepark Surgical Inc.   Phone: _____
1-800-xxx-xxxx

---

[*]Example to be tailored to individual needs and practice area.

OSTOMY CARE USING A ONE-PIECE POUCHING SYSTEM

The following material provides an example of an instruction sheet for a patient with a fecal diversion who is using a one-piece pouching system.

Supplies

Pouch number: _____
Manufacturer: _____
Stoma pattern, pen, and scissors
Skin barrier paste: _____
Manufacturer: _____
Washcloth or paper towels
Plastic garbage bag

Directions

1. Gather supplies.
2. Trace stoma pattern onto the back of the pouch and cut out. Be careful not to cut through the front of the pouch. Place aside.
3. Empty, then remove the soiled pouch; save the clamp and place the soiled pouch in the plastic garbage bag.
4. Wipe any stool from your skin with a washcloth or paper towel. Wash the skin around the stoma with warm water. Pat dry.
5. Remove the paper backing from the tan-colored adhesive on the pouch. Put a small bead of skin barrier paste around the cut edge. Center the pouch over the stoma, and press down. Remove the outside paper backing from the adhesive tape on the pouch.
6. Smooth adhesive down on all sides.
7. Place clamp on the bottom of pouch.

Important

1. As your stoma heals it may change in size, and you will need to change your pattern as this occurs. The skin barrier on the pouch must fit up to the stoma, protecting the skin around the stoma.
2. You may shower or bathe with the ostomy pouch on. The tape around the edges is waterproof and should be dried off after showering or bathing.
3. To treat red, irritated skin, sprinkle skin barrier powder onto the red skin. Brush off excess. There should only be a light dusting left on the skin. The powder will absorb moisture and allow the pouch to adhere to the irritated skin.
4. Do not use products on the skin around the stoma that may contain creams or oils, such as soap. They may leave a greasy build-up and interfere with the pouch seal.

PICTORIAL GUIDE DEMONSTRATING POUCH CHANGE

It may be very helpful for the patient with a new ostomy to be given a personalized step-by-step picture guide of the pouch change procedure. While the patient is changing the pouch, pictures can be taken of each of the critical steps. The benefit of the digital picture guide is that the pictures will be demonstrating the patient's own equipment and may assist the patient to remember critical steps. Digital photography has the advantage of providing an immediate print-out and thus contributes to a personalized instruction sheet that can be quickly assembled.

Example of Pouching System Directions Using Digital Photography.

1. Apply strip paste into skin fold below the stoma. Look at picture to remember the amount of strip paste that is appropriate.

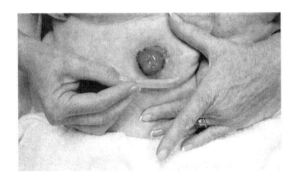

2. Center the stoma in the opening of the skin barrier. Press the skin barrier down, around the stoma.

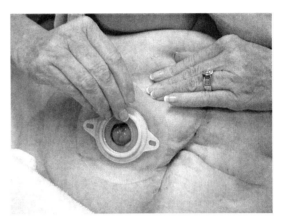

B OSTOMY-RELATED RESOURCES: CLINICIAN AND PATIENT RELATED

BEVERLY FOLKEDAHL

Professional Education and Support

The following are professional organizations and agencies whose members specialize in the care of the person with an ostomy and/or provide information and support necessary for professionals caring for a person with an ostomy:

American Pseudo-Obstruction and
    Hirschsprung's Disease Society, Inc.
P.O. Box 772
Medford, MA 02155
617-395-4255
www.tiac.net/users/aphs/

This society was formed to answer the needs of families, patients and health care professionals facing a myriad of challenges posed by gastrointestinal motility disorders in infants and children. As an international, not-for-profit organization, APHS promotes public awareness of conditions such as chronic intestinal pseudo-obstruction syndrome, Hirschsprung's disease, gastroesophageal reflux, gastroesophageal reflux disease, and intestinal neuronal dysplasia, as well as other serious disorders that significantly affect gastrointestinal motility.

American Society of Colon and
    Rectal Surgeons
85 W. Algonquin Rd., Suite 550
Arlington Heights, IL 60005
847-290-9184
www.fascrs.org

The American Society of Colon and Rectal Surgeons is a professional society representing more than 1000 board-certified colon and rectal and other surgeons dedicated to advancing and promoting the science and practice of the treatment of patients with diseases and disorders affecting the colon, rectum, and anus.

Canadian Association of Enterostomal
    Therapists
P.O. Box 48069
60 Dundas St. E.
Mississauga, ON L5A 1W4
Canada
caet@on.aibn.com

The Canadian Association for Enterostomal Therapy (C.A.E.T.) is a professional organization founded to represent Enterostomal Therapy Nursing. The C.A.E.T. endorses the Canadian Nurses Association Vision of Nursing and believes that all persons with the following conditions are entitled to the comprehensive services of an Enterostomal Therapy Nurse: abdominal stomata, fistulas, draining wounds, and selected disorders of the integumentary, gastrointestinal, and genitourinary systems.

Centers for Medicare and
    Medicaid Services
www.cms.hhs.gov/coverage/

Centers for Medicare and Medicaid Services is the governmental agency responsible for tracking emerging technologies and patterns of care to determine applicability of existing national coverage policy and to assess the need for policy change.

International Foundation for
    Functional Gastrointestinal
    Disorders
P.O. Box 17864
Milwaukee, WI 53217
414-964-1799
888-964-2001
www.iffgd.org

The International Foundation for Functional Gastrointestinal Disorders is a nonprofit education and research organization that addresses the issues surrounding life with gastrointestinal functional and motility disorders and increases the awareness about these disorders among the general public, researchers, and the clinical care community.

Medicare
Region A:
Ostomy policy: www.umd.nycpic.com/ostomy.html
Region B:
Ostomy policy: www.astar-federal.com/anthem/affiliates/adminastar/dmerc/suppmanualbychapters.html
Region C:
Ostomy policy: www.pgba.com/palmetto/main.nsf/allframesets/pro_dmer.html
Region D:
Ostomy Policy: www.cignamedicare.com/dmerc/supman/C09/sm0928.html

Medicare Part B, a governmental agency, provides subscribers with partial coverage for ostomy products. For Medicare administrative purposes the United States is divided into regions, and each region has a local administrator who handles Medicare policy. The reimbursement policies are found at the respective region's website.

National Digestive Disease Information
  Clearinghouse
2 Information Way
Bethesda, MD 20892-3570
301-654-3810
www.niddk.nih.gov/

The NDDIC website provides information about many different health topics, current research and clinical trials, advances and initiatives, grant application procedures, and useful links. Descriptions of the major research projects being conducted by NIDDK laboratories are listed.

Society of Urologic Nurses
East Holly Ave., Box 56
Pitman, NJ 08071-0056
888-TAP-SUNA
856-256-2335
www.suna.inurse.com

The Society of Urologic Nurses and Associates is a professional organization committed to excellence in patient care standards and a continuum of quality care, clinical practice, and research through education of its members, patients, families, and community.

World Council for Enterostomal Therapy
P.O. Box 48099
60 Dundas St. East
Mississauga, ON L5A 4G8
Canada
905-848-9400
info@wcetn.org

The World Council for Enterostomal Therapy is an international association of enterostomal therapy nurses and is dedicated to ongoing professional education through publication of a journal, as well as education for people who have ostomies and people who suffer from incontinence, wounds, or other problems in tissue integrity.

Continued

Wound Ostomy Continence
Nurses Society
4700 W. Lake Ave.
Glenview, IL 60025-1485
888-224-WOCN
www.wocn.org

The Wound, Ostomy and Continence Nursing Society (WOCN) is a professional organization that provides support for WOC/ET nurses and other professionals caring for people with ostomies. The WOCN offers fact sheets for both the professional and the layperson; opportunities to network through discussion forums; educational offerings; a professional journal; and guidelines of care for the person with an ostomy.

Wound Ostomy Continence Nursing
Certification Board
611 East Wells St.
Milwaukee, WI 53202
888-496-2622
www.wocncb.org

Wound Ostomy Continence Nursing Certification Board is the certification entity for registered nurses who are eligible to become certified in the care of persons with ostomies (as well as wound and continence care).

Consumer Education and Support

The following organizations provide support and information for the person with an ostomy and the professional:

American Cancer Society
2200 Century Pkwy, Ste 950
Atlanta, GA 30345
800-ACS-2345
www.cancer.org

The American Cancer Society provides cancer information to professionals and lay people about various types of cancer, sponsors support groups, and funds cancer related research.

American College of Gastroenterology
4900 B South 31st St.
Arlington, VA 22206-1656
703-820-7400
www.acg.gi.org/

This professional society provides information or pamphlets on request. Tap into the "Digest This!" section of their site for "Understanding Your GI Tract" and "Digestive Health Tips."

American Gastroenterological Association
7910 Woodmont Ave., 7th Floor
Bethesda, MD 20814
301-654-2055
www.gastro.org/

The website of this professional association of gastroenterologists features a digestive health section for patients.

Association for the Bladder Exstrophy
Community
P.O. Box 87954
Fayetteville, NC 28304
www.bladderexstrophy.com/

The Association for the Bladder Exstrophy Community is an international support group network comprising individuals with bladder exstrophy, local parent exstrophy support groups, and health care providers who work with patients and families living with bladder exstrophy. Resources, talent, and information are available to assist patients and families living with bladder exstrophy to help them master the medical and psychosocial issues relating to exstrophy.

Continent Diversion Network (Division of UOA) P.O. Box 23401 Shawnee Mission, KS 66283 800-456-7494	A national support group for people who have or plan to have an internal intestinal pouch replace the bladder, any part of the colon, or the rectum.
Crohn's and Colitis Foundation of America 396 Park Ave. South, 17th floor New York, NY 10016-8804 212-685-3440 800-343-3637 www.ccfa.org	Crohn's and Colitis Foundations of America's mission is to cure and prevent Crohn's disease and ulcerative colitis through research, and to improve the quality of life of children and adults affected by these digestive diseases through education and support. Informational pamphlets are available for both the professional and the layperson. Several areas also have local chapters that sponsor educational meetings, support groups, and newsletters for lay people affected by inflammatory bowel disease.
Centers for Medicare and Medicaid Services www.cms.hhs.gov/coverage/	Centers for Medicare and Medicaid Services is responsible for tracking emerging technologies and patterns of care to determine applicability of existing national coverage policy and to assess the need for policy change.
Crohn's and Colitis Foundation of Canada 60 St. Clair Ave. East, Suite 600 Toronto, ON M4T 1N5 Canada 416-920-5035 800-387-1479 www.ccfc.ca.	The Crohn's and Colitis Foundation of Canada is a national not-for-profit, voluntary medical research foundation. Its mission is to find the cure for inflammatory bowel disease. To achieve its mission, the Foundation is committed to raising increasing funds for medical research.
European Ostomy Association Smidkova 5a CZ 61600 Brno Czech Republic 42-045-43-248517 europeanregion@ostomyinternational.org	This is a region of International Ostomy Association and contains a directory of the European Ostomy Association.
International Foundation for Functional Gastrointestinal Disorders P.O. Box 17864 Milwaukee, WI 53217 414-964-1799 888-964-2001 www.iffgd.org	This foundation provides support and educational information for people affected by functional bowel disorders, including irritable bowel syndrome.

Continued

International Ostomy Association
Kakatahi RD 15
Wanganui 5021
New Zealand
64-634-28-808
www.ostomyinternational.org

The purpose of the International Ostomy Association is to provide a world council for the benefit of ostomates, run by ostomates to represent the viewpoint of ostomates at the international level.

Friends of Ostomates Worldwide USA
400 North June St.
Los Angeles, CA 90004-1002.
www.fowusa.org

Friends of Ostomates Worldwide USA is a not-for-profit, volunteer-run organization that provides ostomy supplies and educational materials to help ostomates in need throughout the world.

Interstitial Cystitis Association
110 N. Washington St, Suite 340
Rockville, MD 20850
800-helpica
301-610-5300
www.ichelp.org

The Interstitial Cystitis Association (ICA) is a not-for-profit, health dedicated to providing patient and physician educational information and programs, patient support, public awareness, and research funding. The ICA works nationwide on behalf of all IC patients.

J-Pouch Group
www.j-pouch.org

The J-pouch group is an online website that provides information, support and discussion about ileoanal anastomosis, or the "J-Pouch" operation.

Medicare
Region A: Ostomy policy:
www.umd.nycpic.com/ostomy.html
Region B: Ostomy Policy:
www.astar-federal.com/anthem/
affiliates/adminastar/dmerc/
suppmanualbychapters.html
Region C: Ostomy policy:
www.pgba.com/palmetto/main.nsf/
allframesets/pro_dmer.html
Region D: Ostomy Policy:
www.cignamedicare.com/dmerc/
supman/C09/sm0928.html

Medicare Part B, a governmental agency, provides subscribers with partial coverage for ostomy products. For Medicare administrative purposes the United States is divided into regions, and each region has a local administrator who handles Medicare policy. The reimbursement policies are found at the respective region's website.

Pediatric Crohn's & Colitis
Association, Inc.
P.O. Box 188
Newton, MA 02168
617-489-5854
pcca.hypermart.net

PCCA is committed to helping children with inflammatory bowel disease and their families better understand Crohn's disease and ulcerative colitis. As parents coping with inflammatory bowel disease, its members are there to share concerns and offer emotional support.

Quality Life Association, Inc.
124 Gray St.
Millen, GA 30442
912-982-2340
www.qla-ostomy.org

The Quality Life Association is a not-for-profit nationwide association aimed at meeting the special needs of the person with a continent diversion and educating others of the latest advances in ostomy options.

The Pull-Thru Network
2312 Savoy St.
Hoover, AL 35226-1528
205-978-2930
www.pullthrough.org

The Pull-Thru Network, part of the United Ostomy Association, is one of the largest organizations in the world dedicated to the support and information needs of the families of children born with imperforate anus, cloaca, cloaca exstrophy, bladder exstrophy, VATER Syndrome, Hirschprung's disease, and other, related birth anomalies.

Spina Bifida Association of America
4590 MacArthur Blvd., NW, Suite 250
Washington, DC 20007-4226
202-944-3295
sbaa@sbaa.org

The association was founded to address the specific needs of the spina bifida community and serves as the national representative of almost 60 chapters.

United Ostomy Association
19772 MacArthur Blvd, Suite 200
Irvine, CA 92612-2405
www.uoa.org

The United Ostomy Association is a volunteer-based health organization dedicated to providing education, information, support, and advocacy for the person with an ostomy. The organization offers educational booklets and educational offerings and sponsors a youth camp for children ages 12-17 with ostomies. Local chapters also sponsor monthly or quarterly meetings and provide newsletters to members with helpful information for the person with an ostomy. Links to websites of local and international groups can be founds on the UOA site.

United Ostomy Association of Canada
P.O. Box 825-50 Charles St. East,
Toronto ON M4Y 2N7
Canada
416-595-5452
888-969-9698
www.ostomycanada.ca

This is a volunteer-based health organization offering mutual aid and moral support for people in Canada who have had ostomy surgery.

World Ostomy Resource
www.powerup.com.au/~takkenb/
OstomySites.htm

The primary function of this site is to list links to all ostomy sites in the world, making it easier for everyone to locate available information.

Continued

Product Manufacturers, Education, and Support

Many of the following manufacturers of ostomy-related products provide ostomy education and support for both the professional and the layperson. Printed information may be available in different languages and/or in video format. Company representatives provide updated lists of support products.

Coloplast Corporation
1955 West Oak Circle
Marietta, GA 30062
800-533-0464
www.us.coloplast.com

Coloplast manufactures ostomy pouches and related products. The company provides educational information, reimbursement information, and samples for the professional and the layperson.

ConvaTec
P.O. Box 5254
Princeton, NJ 08543-5254
800-422-8811
www.convatec.com

ConvaTec manufactures ostomy pouches and related products. The company also provides educational and reimbursement information and samples for the professional and layperson. ConvaTec sponsors the Better Together Club, a support and information group for people with ostomies.

Cook Wound Ostomy Continence
1100 West Morgan St.
P.O. Box 266
Spencer, IN 47460
812 829-4891
800 843-4851
www.cookwoc.com

Cook Wound Ostomy Continence manufactures nonadhesive ostomy pouch systems for people with urinary and fecal diversions.

Cymed Ostomy Company
1440C Fourth St.
Berkeley, CA 94710
800-582-0707 or 510-558-1926
www.cymed-ostomy.com

Cymed manufactures ostomy pouches and related products and provides samples for the professional and the layperson.

Dansac-Incutech
Incutech Inc., P.O. Box 1608
Kernersville, NC 27285-1608
800-699-4232
www.colostomy.com

Dansac-Incutech manufactures ostomy pouches, including pouches for premature infants, and related products.

Hollister Incorporated
2000 Hollister Drive
Libertyville, IL 60048
800-323-4060
www.hollister.com

Hollister manufactures ostomy pouches and related products. The company also provides educational and reimbursement information and samples for the professional and the layperson.

Marlen Manufacturing Co.
5150 Richmond Rd.
Bedford, OH 44146
216-292-7060
www.marlenmfg.com

Marlen manufactures both reusable and disposable ostomy pouches and accessories.

Nu-Hope Laboratories, Inc.
P.O. Box 331150
Pacoima, CA 91333-1150
800-899-5017 1-818-899
www.nu-hope.com

Nu-Hope manufactures general and custom-made ostomy pouches and related products.

Torbot Group, Inc.
1367 Elmwood Ave.
P.O. Box 3564
Cranston, RI 02910
800-545-4254
www.torbot.com

Torbot manufactures reusable ostomy pouches and related equipment. The company also makes custom pouches for difficult ostomy problems.

C NUTRITIONAL RESOURCES

CRINA V. FLORUTA

GENERAL CONSIDERATIONS

- If the person with a new ostomy is in a facility, consultation with nutritional therapist is appropriate.
- A well-balanced diet will provide adequate amounts of all nutrients.
- Dietary needs are individualized and related to the type of surgery.

Basic Food Groups and Daily Recommendations

Food Group	Daily Recommendations
Dairy: Milk, yogurt, and cheese	2-3 servings
Meat, poultry, and fish	2-3 servings
Breads and cereal	6-11 servings
Fruits	2-4 servings
Vegetables	3-5 servings

Essential Vitamins and Minerals Necessary to Improve Healing

Vitamins	Food Source
A	Egg yolk, milk fat, liver, kidney; yellow, orange, and dark green leafy vegetables such as spinach, broccoli, carrots, winter squash, sweet potatoes; fruits such as cantaloupe, apricots, pink grapefruit
B complex	Milk and dairy foods, pork, organ meats, egg, fish, poultry, enriched cereals and breads, green leafy vegetables, legumes
C	Citrus fruits, tomatoes, melons, peppers, raw green cabbage, potatoes, strawberries, pineapple
K	Vegetable oils, green leafy vegetables, tomatoes, cauliflower

Minerals	Food Source
Sodium	Table salt, seafood, milk, eggs; abundant in most foods except fruit
Potassium	Fruits and fruit juices, milk, meat, cereal, vegetables, and legumes
Iron	Liver, meat, egg yolk, dark green vegetables, whole or enriched grains
Zinc	Lean meats, liver, egg, milk, whole wheat breads

Dietary Guidelines: First 6 Weeks Following Bowel Surgery

General Considerations

Postoperative stoma edema may be present up to 6 weeks following surgery. The intestine's diameter is narrowed as a result of edema, and high fiber foods may have difficulty passing through the stomal lumen.

- Eat a well-balanced diet, choosing from all food groups.
- Include the necessary vitamins, minerals, and calories needed for good health and healing.
- Eat a low-fiber diet for 6 weeks after surgery.
- Eat at least the minimum servings from each group.
- Eat small, frequent meals, up to 5-6 times per day.
- Consider past tolerance before eating any food in large amounts. Introduce one new food at a time daily to determine tolerance.
- Eat slowly and chew food well.
- Eat foods that are tender, well-cooked, and thoroughly chewed.
- A fruit or vegetable is tender if it can be cut with the side of the fork and the food falls apart easily.
- Drink 8 glasses of liquids (8 ounces each) per day.

- Choose nutritious beverages such as milk, fruit juices, and sports drinks, as well as water.
- Avoid drinking liquids through a straw and chewing gum, to decrease intestinal air.
- Beverages that contain caffeine (such as regular coffee, tea, colas) can lead to dehydration if taken in excess.

Foods That May Cause Bowel Blockage

- Corn
- Dried fruit
- Bean sprouts
- Celery
- Raw vegetables eaten in excess
- Bamboo shoots
- Mushrooms
- Raw fruits eaten in excess
- Fruits with seeds and skin
- Citrus fruit membrane
- Nuts, peanuts
- Popcorn

Foods That May Loosen Stool

- Fruit juices (apple and prune in particular)
- Baked beans
- Highly spiced foods
- Cabbage
- Broccoli

- Milk
- Prunes
- Fried foods
- Fresh fruit
- Raw vegetables

Foods That May Thicken Stool

- Applesauce
- Bananas
- Potatoes (no skin)
- Cheese
- Boiled rice and pasta
- Creamy peanut butter
- Whole wheat bread
- Tapioca pudding
- Marshmallows

Foods That May Cause Gas and Odor

- Asparagus
- Cabbage family
- Eggs (especially hard-boiled)
- Fish
- Strong-flavored cheeses
- Spiced foods
- Onions
- Dried beans and peas
- Carbonated beverages
- Beer

D WOCN SOCIETY PUBLICATIONS

BASIC OSTOMY SKIN CARE: A GUIDE FOR PATIENTS AND HEALTHCARE PROVIDERS

People who have a stoma often share many of the same questions and concerns. This Best Practice document provides answers to some of the common questions that people ask about the day-to-day care of the stoma and the surrounding skin. The answers are directed to a person who has a stoma but may also be helpful for healthcare providers as a teaching tool.

People with a stoma often worry that their skin may become irritated from the stool, urine, or pouching system. It is important to treat the skin gently, protect it from stool, urine, and chemicals, and use products correctly to decrease the chance for skin problems.

The Basic Rule Is To Keep It Simple

Understand the reasons for doing what you do. Follow your Wound, Ostomy, Continence (WOC/ET) Nurse or healthcare provider's recommendations and the directions from product manufacturers. When fewer products are used on the skin, there is less chance for developing skin problems.

If you have questions about the information in this document, problems with leakage, or skin problems around your stoma, contact your WOC/ET Nurse or your healthcare provider.

From the Wound, Ostomy Continence Nurses Society, 2003. Used with permission.

Caring for Yourself

How often should I change my pouching system?

- How often you will need to change your pouching system depends on the type of stoma, the location of the stoma, and the kind of drainage from the stoma. There are three basic types of ostomies. Urostomies are for urine; colostomies are for drainage of the large bowel; and ileostomies are for drainage of the small bowel. Using the right type of pouching system and putting it on the right way will also affect how long you can wear it. Wear time may be affected by other factors such as activity level, body shape, and perspiration.

- Many pouching systems are made to be worn for 3 to 7 days. However, there are some pouching systems that are made to be changed every day. The type of pouching system you think is best for you is a personal decision. However, issues of reimbursement from Medicare or your private insurance company may influence this decision.

- Contact your WOC/ET Nurse or healthcare provider if you are changing your pouching system more often than expected, or suddenly more frequently than your normal wear time.

When is a good time to change my pouching system?

- Choose a day and time that is best for you. Try to pick a time when you won't be disturbed and when your stoma is not putting out a lot of drainage.

- The best time to change the pouching system is different for everyone. For most people, the stoma is less active before eating or drinking in the morning. Some people will do their care while they take their bath or shower. Other people may choose to do their care at the end of the day or at least 2 hours after a meal.

How do I remove my old pouching system?

- Take your time when you remove your pouching system. You do not want to rip it off because this may hurt your skin. Try to remove it in the direction your hair grows.
- Loosen and lift the edge of the pouching system with one hand and push down on the skin near the skin barrier with the other hand. You may find it helpful to start at the top and work down to the bottom so you can see what you are doing, which would also allow the pouch to catch any drainage.
- Some people use warm water to remove the pouching system and other people may use adhesive remover. If you use adhesive remover it is very important to wash off all the adhesive remover from your skin with soap and water and dry the skin completely before you put on your new pouching system.
- Sometimes your skin may look pinker, redder, or darker right after you take off your pouching system. This should fade away in a few minutes.

How do I clean around my stoma?

- To clean the skin around your stoma, all you really need to use is warm water and a washcloth, or good quality, soft paper towels. The use of gauze or gloves is not necessary and can be expensive.
- It is not necessary to use soap to clean around your stoma. But if you prefer to use soap, use a very mild soap. Avoid using soaps and cleansers with oils, perfumes, or deodorants since these can sometimes cause skin problems or keep your skin barrier from sticking.
- Rinse the soap off the skin around your stoma very well because the residue may keep your skin barrier from sticking and may also cause skin irritation.
- If you are using paste, it may be easier to remove the paste before you wet the area. Some people

may use adhesive remover. Do not worry if a little bit of paste is left on your skin.
- Always dry your skin well before putting on your new pouching system.
- Sometimes you may see a small amount of blood on your cloth. The stoma tissue contains small blood vessels and may bleed a small amount when cleaned. Any bleeding that does not stop should be reported to your health care provider. The stoma has no nerve endings, so you are not able to feel, if you are rubbing too hard. Therefore, use a gentle touch when cleaning around the stoma, **do not** scrub.
- **Do not** use alcohol or any other harsh chemicals to clean your skin or stoma. They may be irritating to your skin and stoma.
- **Do not** use moistened wipes, baby wipes, or towelettes that contain lanolin or other oils, these can interfere with the skin barrier sticking and may irritate your skin.
- Unless recommended, **do not** apply powders or creams to the skin around your stoma because they can keep your skin barrier from sticking.

What should I do with my soiled supplies after I change my pouching system?

- Put your soiled pouching system into a plastic bag and throw it away in your household garbage. It is recommended to empty your pouch into the toilet first.
- For odor control with disposal when away from home, carry one to two plastic storage bags in a pocket or purse.
- If you used soft paper towels to wash your skin, you can throw them away with your pouching system in your household garbage.
- If you used washable items such as a washcloth to wash your skin, they may be washed with your household laundry.
- Some people who wear a two-piece pouching system choose to remove the pouch to empty it and then attach a clean one. They may decide to rinse out the soiled pouch and reuse it later.
- Some people use reusable pouching systems, which can be used again and again. If you use this type of pouching system, follow the cleaning instructions from the manufacturer.

- If you use a clamp to close your pouch, remember to save it.
- Carry an extra clamp with you in case it breaks.
- If you wear a urostomy pouch, the connector for use at bedtime should be saved and used again.
- The clamp and connector should be washed with soap and water.
- **Do** wash your hands after taking care of your ostomy. You do not need to wear gloves.

Can I get my pouching system wet?

- Yes. You can shower, bathe, swim, or even get in a hot tub with your pouching system on.
- It is a good habit to empty the pouch before showering, bathing, or other water activities.
- You can bathe or shower every day. On the day you plan to change your pouching system you can either leave it on or you can take the whole thing off to take your bath or shower.
- Some people may choose to shower or bathe without their pouching system. Because the stoma has no muscle, urine or stool may drain from your stoma while showering or bathing.
- Water won't hurt your stoma or go inside you. If the water pressure is strong, do not let it hit your stoma directly. Only use a gentle spray of water on your stoma.
- Check your pouching system before and after water activities. If you are in the water for a long time the pouching system may start to loosen up from your skin. Some people may find it helpful to wait an hour or so after changing their pouching system before swimming.
- Pouching systems are waterproof. However, you may feel more secure if you wear an ostomy belt or put tape around the edges of your skin barrier when you are in the water.
- Some people will secure the edges of the skin barrier with waterproof tape. Other people prefer to use paper tape and then wipe the paper tape with a skin sealant to make it more waterproof.
- If you have sensitive or fragile skin, the use of paper tape may be gentler on your skin than a waterproof tape. If you do put tape around the skin barrier edges, do not remove the tape after water activities. Removing the tape may cause the skin barrier to loosen.

- Some people wear tight biking style shorts when swimming to keep their pouch close to the body and help keep it from "floating."
- Gas filters do not work after they get wet. Therefore, it is best to protect the filter with waterproof tape before water activities.
- After bathing or swimming you may use a towel or a hairdryer on the coolest setting to dry the tape and cloth backing of the pouching system to prevent skin irritation from wetness.

What are some ways to keep my skin from getting irritated?

- The best skin protection is a well-fitted and comfortable pouching system. Your WOC/ET Nurse or healthcare provider will help you choose the system that works best for you.
- The opening of your skin barrier should be no more than 1/8 inch away from the edge of your stoma unless otherwise instructed by your WOC/ET Nurse or healthcare provider.
- Measure your stoma once a week for the first 6 to 8 weeks after your ostomy surgery. Your stoma shrinks while it is healing and you need to keep measuring so you can make sure that the opening in the skin barrier is the right size for your stoma. Remeasure your stoma if any irritation develops between the stoma and skin barrier wafer.
- It is helpful to hold your skin smooth as you put your pouching system on to avoid wrinkles that may lead to leakage.
- Check your skin and the back of your skin barrier each time you change your pouching system. You can use a mirror to check your skin under the stoma. Look for any places where stool or urine may have leaked under the skin barrier and on to your skin. When you apply your next pouching system these areas may need some extra reinforcement with skin barrier strips, rings, or paste. There are a variety of "paste" products available. Your WOC/ET Nurse or healthcare provider will advise you when this is recommended.
- When you have a stoma that drains urine or loose stool you may want to consider using an extended wear skin barrier because it will give your skin added protection. Ask your WOC/ET

Nurse or healthcare provider for help with selecting an extended wear skin barrier.

I have sensitive skin. Will the skin barrier irritate my skin?

- If your skin is sensitive, it is helpful to tell your WOC/ET Nurse or healthcare provider. A skin patch test may be necessary to see if you have any reaction to the different skin barriers and tapes. For the most part, the ingredients in the skin barriers do not cause skin irritation.
- If you are having a "reaction" to the skin barrier or tape, most of the time you will see skin changes that match the shape of the product. Inform your WOC/ET Nurse or healthcare provider so he or she can determine the cause of the irritation and recommend another product, if needed.
- Itching or burning under the skin barrier may indicate that you have leakage, a skin rash, or a skin infection. You need to remove your pouching system as soon as possible to check your skin for any irritation.

How can I prevent infection?

- The stoma is your bowel. It is protected by mucus so stool or urine won't hurt it. A stoma rarely becomes infected.
- The most important thing is to protect the skin around your stoma. A correctly fitted pouching system is the best way to prevent an infection of your skin.

If there is a small leak under my skin barrier, is it okay to patch it with tape or paste?

- Always change your pouching system at the first signs of leakage.
- **Do not** try to patch the pouching system with tape or paste. A leak under the skin barrier should not be fixed. Leaving a leaking pouch on can cause skin irritation.

How can I prevent leakage?

- Always empty your pouch before it is half full.
- Release gas before the pouch gets too full. If you have a lot of gas, you may want to consider using a pouch with a vent or filter.
- There are some medications that may be used to reduce gas. Check with your WOC/ET Nurse,

healthcare provider, or pharmacist to learn more about these medications.

I perspire a lot. How can I get the Pouching system to stick better?

- You can dust the skin with an ostomy skin barrier powder to help absorb perspiration. Then dab skin sealant on top of the powder so the pouching system will stick to the skin.
- There are additional ostomy adhesives available in sprays, wipes, skin cements, and tapes.

What can I do to remove hair from around my stoma?

- Some people shave with an electric razor while some dry shave with an ostomy skin barrier powder using a safety razor. Other people may use a safety razor and shave with mild soap and water. If a person decides to use shaving foam it is important to avoid a foam that has moisturizers or perfumes that may irritate the skin or keep the pouching system from sticking to the skin. Always wash the skin well with water after shaving.
- Shaving or clipping excess hair around the stoma in the direction of hair growth may limit skin irritation.

Ostomy Care Products

Should I use a skin sealant?

- A skin sealant, sometimes called barrier film, **does not** have to be used. The sealant puts a plastic-like coating on the skin. It comes in the form of sprays, wipes, and gels.
- A skin sealant may help if you have skin that tears easily, have problems with leakage, or are using an ostomy skin barrier powder. Some people who have dry or oily skin find that their pouching system sticks better when they use a skin sealant.
- Most skin sealants contain alcohol and if the skin has an open area the sealant will cause a burning feeling when applied. Alcohol-free (nonsting) skin sealants are available.

 A tip for use: Make sure the skin sealant dries completely before putting the pouching system on your skin.

Should I use adhesive remover?

- Remember the basic rule that you do not want to use too many products on your skin. So if the pouching system can be gently removed with water, then you do not need to use adhesive remover.

- Do use adhesive remover if you have skin that tears very easily. Sometimes people will use adhesive remover to prevent a build up of sticky residue on their skin.

- Adhesive remover often contains alcohol and feels oily.

A tip for use: After using adhesive remover always wash well with water and a mild soap to remove the oily coating on the skin. Then rinse the skin well with water and dry completely.

Convex Pouching Systems: a Fact Sheet for Patients

What is a convex pouching system?

There are flat and convex pouching systems. A flat pouching system lies flat on the skin around a stoma. A convex pouching system is different because a skin barrier, faceplate, or ring curves outward against the skin. The outward curve presses down on the skin and causes a person's stoma to stick out more and better empty into the pouching system.

Why use a convex product?

Convex products may:

- Stop urine or stool leakage.
- Make you feel more comfortable and secure.
- Prevent or stop skin irritation.
- Improve wear time of pouching system.
- Save you time and money.

When may a convex product be used?

Convex products may be used to:

- Prevent frequent pouch leakage caused by:
  A stoma that empties at or below skin surface.
  Wrinkles, scars, or creases in the skin near the stoma.
  Very soft abdomen around the stoma.
- Improve wear time for patients who have 3 days or less wear time with a flat pouching system.

What else should I know about convex products?

- A convex pouching system should be fitted by a WOC/ET nurse.
- A follow-up visit may be needed to make sure the convex pouching system is working for you.
- Convex products may leave a mark on your skin.
- If you use a belt, it should be snug but not too tight.
- Some convex products may be less flexible and less comfortable than nonconvex products.
- Depending on the appearance of your stoma and abdomen, a convex pouching system with a shallow, medium, or deep outward curve may be needed.
- Some convex products may be more expensive than flat products but may save money if longer wear time is possible.
- A convex pouching system is not the solution for all leakage problems. It is important to see a WOC/ET nurse so he or she can recommend a pouching system that is right for you.

What are the different types of convex Products?

Cut-to-fit convex: This is a one- or two-piece pouching system that allows you to cut the opening in the skin barrier to fit your stoma. This is especially recommended if your stoma is not round.

Precut convex: This is a one- or two-piece pouching system that has various-sized openings in the skin barrier.

Convex insert: These presized plastic rings are for use in the flange of a flat two-piece pouching system.

Barrier strips/rings: These products can be molded to different shapes or sizes.

Custom-made convex product: A product with built-in convexity that is made for you by a special company.

Faceplate: This is a reusable product with built-in convexity.

Ostomy belts and binders: These products may be used to give you extra support.

Where can I buy convex products?

Look in a telephone directory or on the Internet for:

- Local medical supply companies.
- Mail-order medical supply companies.
- Ostomy manufacturers (some may supply samples).

When should I call a WOC/ET nurse?

Call a WOC/ET nurse if you have:

- Problems with your stoma, such as bumps, cuts, bruises, bleeding
- Problems with the skin around your stoma, such as irritation or rash, bleeding, pain, burning, itching, open sores, skin color changes that do not return to normal after you remove the pouching system
- Continued frequent leakage of pouching system
- Weight gain or loss.

Where can I get more information?

For more information, contact

- Wound, Ostomy and Continence Nurses Society (WOCN), 888/224-9626, www.wocn.org
- United Ostomy Association (UOA), 800/826-0826, www.uoa.org

This fact sheet is provided by
Name
Contact

Convex Pouching Systems: A Fact Sheet for Clinicians

Convex pouching systems

A convex pouching system has a skin barrier, faceplate, or ring designed with an outward curve. The rigid convex surface presses down on the skin around the stoma and causes the stoma to protrude more into the opening of the pouching system, creating an improved seal with the skin. There are varying convexity levels—shallow, medium, and deep.

Indications for use

Convex pouching systems should be considered if the following indications are present:

- Flush stoma
- Peristomal creases, wrinkles, scars
- Retracted stoma
- Protruding or flabby abdomen
- Stomal opening at or below skin level
- Wear time of less than 3 days with a flat pouching system.

Precautions

Factors	Rationale
Ulcerations (e.g., pressure, pyoderma gangrenosum, Crohn's, malignancy)	May cause increased pain, further breakdown, and impaired healing
Caput medusa (peristomal varices)	May damage distended blood vessels at stoma/skin junction, causing bleeding
Mucocutaneous separations	May cause deeper tissue destruction and impaired healing at the stoma/skin junction
Parastomal hernia	May cause pressure ulcers, stoma laceration, and loosening of the pouching system as the abdominal contour fluctuates when the hernia moves

Factors to consider

- Convex pouching systems should be fitted by a WOC/ET nurse.

Evaluate the need for convexity postoperatively and again within 8 weeks to assess if initial pouching system remains appropriate after stoma and surgical abdominal swelling have resolved.

Reevaluate within 4 weeks following any initial fitting to assess for any potential complications.

- Weight gain or loss requires reevaluation of pouching system.
- Convex products may leave an imprint on the skin.

Caution: Monitor for signs of excessive tissue pressure.

- Convex products may be less flexible than nonconvex pouching systems.
- Some convex products (e.g., rings and inserts) require increased dexterity or hand strength.
- Some convex products may have a higher initial cost but may be a more cost-effective long-term solution because of less frequent changes.
- Belt or binder use may be necessary to hold the pouching system in place.

Patient education*

Patients should be encouraged to contact a WOC/ET nurse if any of the following occurs:

- Stomal changes—bumps, cuts, bruises, or worrisome bleeding
- Peristomal skin changes—irritation, rash, color change, bleeding, pain, itching, or lesions
- Continued frequent leakage of pouching system
- Weight gain or loss.

Expected outcomes

The patient will attain or maintain:

- Intact peristomal skin.
- Comfort and satisfaction with pouching system.
- Increased wear time compared to previous pouching system.
- Cost-effective stomal management.

From the Wound, Ostomy Continence Nurses Society, 2002. Used with permission.

*More information for patients is available in "Convex Pouching Systems: A Fact Sheet for Patients." For more information or to order call WOCN at 888/224-9626 or visit www.wocn.org.

Convexity Products and Devices[†]

Precut convex barrier: A skin barrier manufactured in specific sizes with built-in convexity; available in one- or two-piece pouching systems.

Cut-to-fit convex barrier: A skin barrier manufactured with built-in convexity that can be cut to a specific stoma size; available in one- or two-piece pouching systems.

Custom-made convex product: A product with built-in convexity, manufactured for a specific patient.

Faceplate: A reusable product with built-in convexity.

Convex insert: Presized plastic rings for use in the flange of a two-piece pouching system.

Barrier strips/rings: Products that can be molded to different shapes and sizes.

Belts and binders: These products may be used to provide extra support.

Research recommendations

A literature search revealed that the evidence base for convexity consists of expert opinion and data from two retrospective studies. More research is needed in this area. Suggestions for descriptive or exploratory studies include:

- Identify the percentage of people with ostomies who use convexity.
- Describe the frequency of the use of belts or binders with convex pouching systems.
- Identify patient characteristics and risk factors associated with complications related to the use of convex products.
- Describe the change in wear time that occurs when a patient changes from a flat to a convex pouching system.
- Describe the effect that weight gain or loss may have on the need for a convex pouching system.
- Identify criteria for establishing a standard for convexity levels.

Glossary

Convex: A surface that is curved or rounded outward.

Flange: The rigid ring on a two-piece skin barrier (wafer) that the pouch snaps on to.

Pouching system: A device, worn over your stoma, that acts as a reservoir for the urine or stool that empties out of the stoma. There are many different pouching system choices.

Skin barrier (wafer): A solid square or round piece of adhesive material that is used to protect the skin from urine and stool.

Stoma: A surgically created opening in the intestine or urinary system that is brought out onto the skin of your abdomen.

WOC(ET) Nurse: A nurse with specialized training in caring for people who have wounds, stomas, and/or bladder and bowel problems.

[†]For more details, refer to Table d-1, Convex Pouching Systems: Products and Devices.

Resources

Black P: *Holistic stoma care*, London 2000, Harcourt.

Blakley, P. (1998). *Practical stoma, wound and continence management*, Vermont, Victoria, Australia: Research Publications.

Colwell J, Goldberg M, Carmel J: The state of the standard diversion, *J Wound, Ostomy, Continence Nurs* 28: 6–17, 2001.

Davis S: *A retrospective study of the use of convexity and associated stomal characteristics.* Paper presented at the 31st annual meeting of the Wound, Ostomy, Continence Nurses Society, Minneapolis, Minn, 1999.

Erwin Toth P: Prevention and management of peristomal skin complications, *Adv skin wound care* 13(4): 175–179, 2000.

Hampton B, Bryant R, editors: *Ostomies and continent diversions: nursing management*, St Louis, 1992, Mosby.

O'Connor, E. (1988). Challenges in creating convexity: a management method, *J Enterostomal Ther* 15(4), 171–173, 1988.

Rolstad B, Boarini J: Principles and techniques in the use of convexity, *Ostomy Wound Management* 42(1) 24–32, 1996.

Wells, J, Doughty D: Pouching principles and products. *Ostomy/Wound Management*, 40(6): 50–63, 1994.

Wound, Ostomy, and Continence Nurses Society: *Guidelines for management: caring for a patient with an ostomy*, Laguna Beach, Calif, 1998, Author.

TABLE D-I Convex Pouching Systems: Products and Devices

Convex Equipment and Description	Companies*
Skin barrier with flange, standard wear with built-in convexity (wafer for a two-piece system)	
Cut-to-fit	CP, H, M
Precut	CP, C, H, M
Varying degrees of convexity	M
Skin barrier with flange, extended wear with built-in convexity (wafer for a two-piece system)	
Cut-to-fit	CP, H
Precut	CP, C, H
Pouch, drainable, standard wear barrier attached, with built-in convexity (one-piece system)	
Cut-to-fit	CP, M, N
Precut	CP, H, M, N
Varying degrees of convexity	M, N
Pouch, drainable, extended wear barrier attached, with built-in convexity (one-piece system)	
Cut-to-fit	CP, H
Precut	CP, C, H, N
Varying degrees of convexity	N
Pouch, urinary, standard wear barrier attached, with built-in convexity (one-piece system)	
Cut-to-fit	CP, H, M, N
Precut	CP, H, M, N
Varying degrees of convexity	M, N
Pouch, urinary, extended wear barrier attached, with built-in convexity (one-piece system)	
Cut-to-fit	CP, H, N
Precut	CP, C, H, N
Varying degrees of convexity	N
Custom-made convex pouch (one-piece system)	
Drainable, standard wear	N
Drainable, extended wear	N
Urinary, standard wear	N
Urinary, extended wear	N
Ostomy accessory, convex insert	C, H, K
Ostomy faceplate (reusable)	
Standard	M, N, P
Custom-made	P
Varying degrees of convexity	M, N, P, T
Ostomy faceplate equivalent, silicone ring (reusable)	V, T
Varying degrees of convexity	T
Skin barrier rings, strips, solid wafers (standard wear)	CP, C, H, N
Skin barrier rings, strips, solid wafers (extended wear)	C, H, N
Ostomy belt	CP, C, H, M, N
Ostomy hernia support belt	N

Manufacturer Legend and Contact Number (Contact manufacturers for more information about available products and sizes.)
CP = Coloplast, 800/533-0464   C = ConvaTec, 800/422-8811   H = Hollister, 800/323-4060
K = King Medical, 800/207-8322   M = Marlen, 216/292-7060   N = NuHope, 800/899-5017
P = Perma-type, 800/243-4234   T = Torbot, 800/545-4254   V = VPI, 800/843-4851
WOCN Society does not expressly promote or endorse the products or companies mentioned here. Efforts were made to include known convexity products and manufacturers. However, it is possible that inadvertent omissions were made.

GLOSSARY

· ·

Abdominoperineal resection A procedure using an abdominal and perineal approach for the resection of rectal cancer. The procedure involves the removal of the rectum, anus, and perirectal lymphatics and construction of a permanent colostomy.

Anal transitional zone Area in the anal canal, in which tissue transitions from columnar to squamous epithelium, 6 to 12 mm proximal to the dentate line.

Antegrade continence enema (ACE) The instillation of liquid into the intestine through a cecostomy. This enema is used for those persons (generally children) who have failed to respond to traditional bowel management and allows the patient to evacuate the entire colon (from the stoma to the anus) on a regular basis.

Atresia Absence or closure of a normal body opening.

Coloanal anastomosis A surgical procedure in which the entire rectum above the sphincter is removed and the colon is sewn or stapled at or above the sphincter muscle.

Crohn's disease An idiopathic transmural inflammatory bowel disease that can affect the entire gastrointestinal tract and presents with varied disease patterns according to the location and pattern of gastrointestinal tract inflammation.

Cystostomy An opening into the urinary bladder.

Detubularization A technique in which a piece of bowel is surgically opened length-wise to disrupt normal peristaltic contractions of the bowel. When the involved bowel is used to create a continent pouch, this procedure prevents contractions from raising the pressure within the pouch.

Diastasis An abnormal separation of parts normally joined together.

Diverticulitis Occurs when diverticula become inflamed and/or infected.

Diverticulosis A condition in which pouches of intestinal lining balloon out through weakened areas of intestinal wall. The pouches are called *diverticula*.

Double-barrel stoma An opening into the gastrointestinal tract that entails the resection of the involved bowel segment, anastomosis of the two limbs of the bowel to the abdominal wall as side-by-side skin flush end stomas, and the use of a crushing clamp to create a fistula between the proximal and the distal stomas, performed to reestablish intestinal continuity.

End stoma An opening into the bowel, created by division of the intestine in which the proximal end of the intestine is brought through the abdominal wall, everted, and attached to the skin.

Epispadias A congenital anomaly in the male in which the urethral opening in the penis is located anywhere on the top surface of the penis between the glans and the base, or behind the penis in the perineum (between the anus and testicles); occurs rarely in females, in whom the opening is above the clitoris.

Enterocutaneous fistula An abnormal connection between the small intestine and the skin.

Evidence-based practice The integration into practice of outcomes research to improve patient outcomes and care delivery.

Familial adenomatous polyposis (FAP) An autosomal dominant condition that presents with over 100 adenomatous polyps in the large bowel. If left untreated, colorectal cancer will develop by the mean age of 39 years.

Fistula An abnormal opening between two organs.

Folliculitis Inflammation of hair follicle commonly due to *Staphylococcus aureus*.

Gastroschisis An extrusion of nonrotated midgut through an opening in the abdominal wall to the right of the umbilicus.

Granuloma Granulation tissue that occurs at the junction of the skin and stoma in areas of retained or reactive suture material.

Haustra Ringlike "pockets" (sacculations) characteristic of the colon, created by longitudinal bands and circular bands along the colon wall.

Hartmann procedure Resection of involved bowel, closure of distal stump, and creation of a proximal stoma. The distal stump is referred to as the Hartmann's pouch.

Ileocecal valve One-way valve located at the junction between the ileum and the large intestine, which prevents the backflow of fecal contents from the colon to the small intestine and prevents the contents of the ileum from passing into the cecum prematurely.

Ileal pouch anal anastomosis A surgical procedure that involves a colectomy and construction of an ileal reservoir with ileoanal anastomosis.

Ileus The temporary absence of the normal contractile movements of the intestinal wall.

Indiana pouch Continent urinary diversion, created from the cecum, part of the transverse colon, and 10-12 cm of terminal ileum. The ureters are brought through the back of the cecum; the catheterizable limb is fashioned from the ileum. The ileocecal valve is plicated, and this acts as a continence mechanism.

Intussusception Invagination of a length of the intestine into the lumen of an adjoining part, usually causing an obstruction.

Ischemic colitis An unusual condition of the bowel that results from hypoperfusion. The condition occurs when inadequate mesenteric blood flow causes an imbalance between metabolic demands of the colon and available oxygen, resulting in cellular injury.

Kock pouch A continent urinary or fecal reservoir created from ileum with an intussuscepted nipple valve. The reservoir or pouch is emptied by periodic intubation.

Loop stoma A loop of bowel is brought through the abdominal wall and supported by a rod. A transverse opening is made in the bowel to allow the passage of stool.

Low anterior resection A surgical procedure that involves mobilization of the rectum and an anastomosis that is performed below the peritoneal reflection. It is generally accepted that low anterior resection is the treatment of choice for carcinomas located in the upper and middle thirds of the rectum.

Malone procedure The appendix or a segment of bowel is used to create a stoma, which empties into the ascending colon and can be easily catheterized. This procedure is generally performed to allow the administration of an antegrade continence enema to attempt to achieve fecal continence.

Meckel's diverticulum A rare condition in which a blind, pouchlike sac arises from the free border of the ileum.

Mucocutaneous junction Connection of stoma and skin.

Mucous fistula The defunctionalized portion of the intestine.

Mucosal transplantation Seeding of viable intestinal mucosa along the suture line onto the peristomal skin.

Neobladder An internal urinary reservoir constructed from a portion of the ileum or colon in which the urethra is anastomosed to the reservoir, also referred to as orthotopic bladder.

Neosphincter A device constructed out of transposed skeletal tissue, or an artificial device that is implanted to restore continence.

Omphalocele Protrusion of abdominal contents through an opening at the navel, usually occurring as a congenital defect.

Orthotopic diversion A urinary pouch that is connected to the native urethra.

Osteotomy Surgical division, cutting, or repositioning of bones in treatment of deformed joints or bones.

Peristomal plane Three to four inches of skin surface surrounding an abdominal stoma.

Peristomal pyoderma gangrenosum A rare ulcerative skin condition of unknown etiology that occurs in the area surrounding the stoma. Peristomal pyoderma gangrenosum is thought to start as one or more pustules, which break open and form full-thickness ulcers with irregular, ragged, overhanging margins. A necrotizing inflammatory process extends peripherally from the primary lesion, resulting in a necrotic ulcer with undermined edges. The surrounding skin becomes red and purple, and the entire area is very painful.

Pouchitis Inflammation of an internal pouch.

Prolapse The telescoping of the bowel through the stoma.

Pseudoverrucous lesion Wartlike lesion in the peristomal area.

Pyocystis Collection of infected fluid in a defunctionized bladder.

Radiation enteritis A malfunction of the large and/or small bowel that occurs due to iatrogenic damage occurring during radiation treatment for another disease or disorder.

Stenosis A narrowing.

Stricture A tight band of scar tissue that constricts the intestine or anal opening, interfering with the ability to pass stool.

Strictureplasty A surgical procedure that widens narrow segments of intestine (strictures) that can cause obstruction or obstructive symptoms. The intestine is incised, opened lengthwise, and closed in the opposite direction.

Taeniae coli Muscle bands that create sacculations in the colon wall known as haustrations.

Tenesmus Ineffectual urge to evacuate the rectum or urinary bladder.

Total proctocolectomy Removal of the entire colon, the rectum, and the sphincters. The terminal ileum is exteriorized as an end ileostomy.

Toxic megacolon Acute nonobstructive dilation and inflammation of the colon.

Ulcerative colitis Disease of unknown etiology that causes continuous, superficial inflammation of the colonic mucosa.

Valves of Houston Rectal mucosa formed from three folds in rectum.

Vesicostomy An opening directly into the urinary bladder.

Index

· ·

CPSIA information can be obtained at www.ICGtesting.com
Printed in the USA
LVOW121935140212

268702LV00002B/8/P